W0231908

Cellular and Humoral Immunological Components of Cerebrospinal Fluid in Multiple Sclerosis

NATO ASI Series

Advanced Science Institutes Series

A series presenting the results of activities sponsored by the NATO Science Committee, which aims at the dissemination of advanced scientific and technological knowledge, with a view to strengthening links between scientific communities.

The series is published by an international board of publishers in conjunction with the NATO Scientific Affairs Division

A	**Life Sciences**	Plenum Publishing Corporation
B	**Physics**	New York and London
C	**Mathematical and Physical Sciences**	D. Reidel Publishing Company Dordrecht, Boston, and Lancaster
D	**Behavioral and Social Sciences**	Martinus Nijhoff Publishers
E	**Engineering and Materials Sciences**	The Hague, Boston, Dordrecht, and Lancaster
F	**Computer and Systems Sciences**	Springer-Verlag
G	**Ecological Sciences**	Berlin, Heidelberg, New York, London,
H	**Cell Biology**	Paris, and Tokyo

Recent Volumes in this Series

Volume 126—Crystallography in Molecular Biology
edited by Dino Moras, Jan Drenth, Bror Strandberg, Dietrich Suck, and Keith Wilson

Volume 127—The Organization of Cell Metabolism
edited by G. Rickey Welch and James S. Clegg

Volume 128—Perspectives in Biotechnology
edited by J. M. Cardoso Duarte, L. J. Archer, A. T. Bull, and G. Holt

Volume 129—Cellular and Humoral Immunological Components of Cerebrospinal Fluid in Multiple Sclerosis
edited by A. Lowenthal and J. Raus

Volume 130—Individual Differences in Hemispheric Specialization
edited by A. Glass

Volume 131—Fat Production and Consumption: Technologies and Nutritional Implications
edited by C. Galli and E. Fedeli

Volume 132—Biomechanics of Cell Division
edited by Nuri Akkas

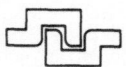

Series A: Life Sciences

Cellular and Humoral Immunological Components of Cerebrospinal Fluid in Multiple Sclerosis

Edited by

A. Lowenthal

Born-Bunge Foundation
Universitaire Instelling Antwerpen
Wilrijk, Belgium

and

J. Raus

Dr. L. Willems Instituut
Diepenbeek, Belgium

Springer Science+Business Media, LLC

Proceedings of a NATO Advanced Research Workshop on
Cellular and Humoral Immunological Components of Cerebrospinal Fluid
in Multiple Sclerosis,
held April 20–24, 1986,
at the Congress Complex, Hengelhoef, Limburg, Belgium

ISBN 978-1-4899-5350-6 ISBN 978-1-4899-5348-3 (eBook)
DOI 10.1007/978-1-4899-5348-3

© 1987 Springer Science+Business Media New York
Originally published by Plenum Press, New York in 1987
Softcover reprint of the hardcover 1st edition 1987

All rights reserved. No part of this book may be reproduced, stored in a retrieval system, or transmitted in any form or by any means, electronic, mechanical, photocopying, microfilming, recording, or otherwise, without written permission from the Publisher

FOREWORD

Multiple Sclerosis (MS) is a disease almost exclusively defined by clinical neurology, neurophysiology, neuroimaging and the analysis of cerebrospinal fluid (CSF). Even though disciplines such as virology, biochemistry, genetics and epidemiology have added a great deal to our knowledge, they hardly improved our knowledge on the pathological mechanisms of the disease.

The study of the cellular and humoral components in the CSF of patients with MS could furnish some important key elements. As these components most likely are correlated with the activity of the immune system, the workshop devoted to the study of these anomalies in the CSF could provide us with a better definition of the immunological anomalies in MS and by the same token open new perspectives in MS research.

Nearly 25 years ago an immunological anomaly, later called oligoclonal reaction or restricted heterogeneity of the immunoglobulins, was discovered in the CSF of MS patients. Based on this observation numerous immunological studies were performed on postmortem brain tissue or on blood or CSF from MS patients. These studies gave rise to the hypothesis that MS is characterized by an overactivation of the immune system possibly due to the persistence of an antigen. Neither the antigen, nor the antibodies produced, nor the type of immune dysregulation which favours the persistence of the antibodies have been defined.

The purpose of the workshop was not only to compare recent data obtained by neurologists, neuroimmunologists, immunologists and biochemists, but most importantly to stimulate interdisciplinary new ideas and new guidelines for research. This meant that by starting from the observed anomalies in the CSF or the blood of MS patients we hoped to get out of the present stagnation and to open new prospects for future research.

Several other diseases such as experimental allergic encephalomyelitis in its chronic relapsing form, corona virus meningoencephalomyelitis, subacute sclerosing panencephalitis etc. were confronted and compared with the MS disease process.

Several fundamental questions were raised. Against which antigens are the oligoclonal antibodies directed? Is the oligoclonal reaction a nonsense reaction? Which antigens are triggering the immune system to raise the oligoclonal reaction? Is this oligoclonal reaction essential in the disease process? Does myelin basic protein play a role in the disease process? Do other central nervous system proteins play a role? Is the immunological reaction an autoimmune reaction? Can one consider the immunological reaction seen in MS as a localized intrathecal reaction or can it be considered as a generalized phenomenon? Can MS be characterized by specific T cells and how can one identify the different specific T cell types? What is the relation between the oligoclonal reaction and the anomalies observed in the T cells? Is it possible that a critical regulatory mechanism is affected which gives rise to humoral and cellular immune abnormalities?

Almost 100 scientists from 22 different countries were invited to contribute to the workshop.

To organize this workshop we obtained important financial help from different organisations: The International Federation of Multiple Sclerosis Societies, The National Multiple Sclerosis Society (US), The National Institute of Neurological and Communicative Disorders, Wetenschappelijk Onderzoek Multiple Sclerose (WOMS), Belgische Studiegroep voor Multiple Sclerose, Nationaal Fonds voor Wetenschappelijk Onderzoek, The National Multiple Sclerosis Society (Switzerland), The National Multiple Sclerosis Society (Germany), The National Multiple Sclerosis Society (Great Britain), Belgische Vereniging voor Neurologie, The Towbes Foundation, NATO, Ministerie voor Nederlandse Kultuur, Provinciebestuur Limburg, Acade Diagnostic Systems, Beun de Ronde, Boehringer Ingelheim, Eurogenetics, Hoechst, Janssen Pharmaceutica, Merck Sharp & Dohme, Roche, Sandoz, Byk Belga, UCB.

Aside from this financial support, we would like to mention the moral and scientific support of the World Federation of Neurology and in particular the enthousiastic help received from the members of the scientific committee: B. Arnason, D. McFarlin, B. Waksman, H. Weiner and H. Wekerle.

We greatly appreciate the technical and adminstrative assistance of: Agnes Delsaer, Edith de Meyer, Lucrèce Marescau and Toni Marx.

We hope that the proceedings of this workshop will stimulate research in multiple sclerosis all over the world.

Dr. A. Lowenthal
Dr. J. Raus

CONTENTS

CEREBROSPINAL FLUID IMMUNOGLOBULIN ABNORMALITIES IN MULTIPLE SCLEROSIS

Dale E. McFarlin, Michael L. Pierce, Andrew Goodman,
Elizabeth S. Mingioli and Henry F. McFarland

Neuroimmunology Branch, IRP, NINCDS, NIH, Building 10
Room 5B-16, 9000 Rockville Pike, Bethesda, MD 20892

INTRODUCTION

Although the pathogenesis and etiology of multiple sclerosis (MS) are unknown, some of the most widely studied aspects of the disorder are immunoglobulin abnormalities in the cerebrospinal fluid (CSF). Immunoglobulins (Igs) are increased in quantity, as initially described by Kabat et al. (1,2), and are relatively homogeneous in charge; because of the latter fact IgG in concentrated CSF migrates in a few discrete bands which have been designated as "oligoclonal bands" (OCB) by Lowenthal et al. (3). OCB have been demonstrated by electrophoresis (2-8), isoelectric focusing (IEF) (5,6,9-13) and isotachophoresis (14). It is widely accepted that elevated CSF Igs are due to increased synthesis within the CNS, and techniques such as Tourtellotte's empirical formula for measuring CSF IgG synthesis (15) and an IgG index (16) have been developed. The measurements of IgM and IgA in the CSF require sensitive immunoassays (17-21). These have shown that approximately 50% of MS patients have elevated CSF IgM, and a smaller but significant number have increased IgA (17-21).

Although to date the specificity of most CSF Igs in (MS) has not been identified, it is currently common practice to follow abnormalities of CSF Igs as part of the assessment of experimental therapeutic agents in the disease. Since concentration of CSF can, at least theoretically, induce artifacts, our group previously developed a highly sensitive IEF for detecting OCB in uncentrated CSF (13). This procedure was standardized so that a constant amount (150μg) of IgG is studied in each IEF lane. It is our practice to assay several specimens of unconcentrated CSF from a given patient at the same Ig concentration to detect changes in OCB during the course of the disease, including treatment with experimental therapeutic agents. In addition, our group recently has been using enzyme linked immunosorbent assay (ELISA) to measure CSF Ig. The report describes the development and standardization of ELISA procedures for quantitating CSF Ig, as well as modification in the IEF technique (13) for the detection of OCB currently used in our laboratories. The findings in a group of MS patients with clinically definite (MS) are described.

MATERIALS AND METHODS

Clinical Samples

CSF specimens were collected and stored frozen at -70°C in 1-3cc aliquots as described previously (18) until studied. These were obtained from: (1) 29 normal volunteers; (2) noninflammatory neurologic disease controls (NINDC) including patients with motor neuron disease, Parkinsons disease, multiple system atrophy, Tourettes syndrome, benign intracranial hypotension, and peripheral neuropathy; (3) inflammatory neuropathies including meningovascular syphilis and SSPE; and (4) sporadic cases of MS. The findings in 14 of the normal volunteers and the patient with syphilis were reported previously (13) but the findings in the other specimens have not been described.

Radioimmunoassay (RIA)

CSF IgG, IgA and IgM were quantitated by competitive double antibody RIA using the procedures and reagents previously described by Mingioli, et al. (18). Total protein was measured by the Lowry procedure using human serum albumin as the standard.

ELISA

Preparation of antisera: Antisera against each of the human immunoglobulins to be assayed, were produced in sheep. Antisera specific for each class were purified by affinity chromatography using previously isolated immunoglobulins covalently-linked to CNBr-activated sepharose 4B (Pharmacia Inc., Piscataway, NJ, USA). Each sheep anti-human antiserum was tested by Ouchterlony and immunoelectrophoresis to assure that all non-specific binding had been removed. These antisera were placed in borate buffered saline (pH 8.0) containing .02% sodium azide, sterile filtered through a .45 μm filter and stored in the dark at 4°C. Enzyme-labelled anti-human immunoglobulin conjugates were prepared by the method described by Avrameas, et al. (22). The alkaline phosphatase used for labeling had a specific activity of 1000 units/mg protein (Type VII-S, Sigma Chemical Company, St. Louis, Mo. USA). Conjugates were diluted to 4.0 ml with Tris buffer (pH 8.0) containing 1.0% BSA and .02% sodium azide, sterile filtered through a .45 μm filter, and stored in the dark at 4°C.

The IgG, IgA and IgM in a normal human serum were quantitated by radial immunodiffusion and found to have values of 11.0 mg/ml, 0.97 mg/ml and 1.60 mg/ml respectively. Appropriate dilutions of that serum were used as standards for IgG and IgM ELISAs, but, as will be discussed below, preliminary experiments indicated that the use of a monomeric IgA standard would be preferable. This was isolated from the serum of a patient with an IgA myeloma by ion-exchange chromatography and gel filtration. The resulting IgA monomer was quantitated by absorption using $E^{280}_{1\%}$ of 12.0. Secretory IgA was purchased from Cappel.

ELISA was conducted using the double antibody sandwich method described by Voller et al. (23) Immulon-1 microelisa plates (Dynatech Laboratories, Alexandria, VA, USA), were coated with specific anti-human immunoglobulin overnight at 4°C using a carbonate buffer, pH 9.6. Plates were coated with 150 μl/well at 3μg, 2μg, and .75 μg/well for anti-IgG, anti-IgA, and anti-IgM respectively. For each well coated with specific antiserum an adjacent well was coated with normal sheep serum (NSS) 1 μg/150μl and used to assess background binding. After overnight incubation, plates were washed with PBS containing .05% Tween 20. Standard solutions and CSF samples were diluted into the 1.5 - 50 ng/100 μl range with PBS containing .05% Tween 20 and 1% NSS and added to the washed plate at 100 μl/well.

The plate was incubated two hours at room temperature and washed; the appropriate alkaline phosphatase anti Ig conjugate diluted in PBS containing .05% Tween 20 and 1% NSS was added at 100 μl/well and incubated for two hours at room temperature. Following incubation, plates were washed, and 100 μl of 1 mg/ml p-nitrophenylphosphate (Sigma Chemical Co., St. Louis, MO, USA) in diethanolamine buffer, PH 9.8, was added to each well. Plates were read at 405 nm on a Titertek Multiscan interfaced to a Wang 2200 computer. Data points were fitted to reference curves drawn from the formulas described by Davis et al. (24) and the concentration of Ig calculated.

Detection of OCB

The method previously described (13) was used with the following modifications: (1) Each sample consisted of 15 μl applied to the 5x10 mm piece of filter paper which was placed on the IEF gel. (2) IEF was performed for 1.5 hours at 4°C with 25 watts for an entire 24 cm-long Ampholine PAG plate (LKB, Stockholm, Sweden). Wattage was considered proportional to the length of the PAG plate being used, i.e., the wattage for a 12 cm length gel would be 12.5 watts. Transblotting to nitrocellulose was performed as described (13) with two modifications: the transblot buffer used was 0.7% acetic acid with 20% methanol (v/v) and the procedure was performed for 3 hours at 125 constant volts. The blot was cooled with a refrigerated circulator at 4°C. Visualization of OCB was performed by direct immunoperoxidase staining, following the minor modifications of Mattson's (5) technique outlined previously, with the exception that nitrocellulose paper was incubated with the rabbit anti-Human IgG peroxidase conjugate (Dako, Copenhagen, Denmark) at a dilution range of 1:200 to 1:400.

RESULTS

Development of ELISA to quantitate CSF immunoglobulins

RIA previously was used by our laboratory to measure CSF immunoglobulins (18). Initial efforts involved developing optimal conditions, described above, to quantitate IgG by ELISA. Subsequently, the values obtained in 30 specimens by this procedure were compared with those obtained using RIA (Fig.1). There was good agreement in the findings obtained by the two methods. The upper limit of normal (M + 2 SD) was 4.9 mg/dl. IgM concentrations measured by both methods were compared in the same patients. Again, there was good agreement, although the values obtained by ELISA tended to be higher (Fig.2). The upper limits of normal (M + 2 SD) by RIA was 36 μg/dl and ELISA 54 μg/dl.

When IgA was measured by ELISA the values were significantly higher than those obtained by RIA. The discrepancy between the two assays was greatest at highest values. In both assays dilutions of a normal serum were used as standards. The molecular form(s) of IgA in this serum were not known, and, in order to determine if this was an important variable, a number of experiments were conducted. First, a specimen containing a known amount of secretory IgA was assayed by ELISA using the normal serum as a standard; a low value was obtained. Secondly, the IgA in eight CSF specimens was assayed using two different standard curves: one generated with the normal serum and the second with the (11S) secretory protein. The values of all specimens were higher by approximately 50 percent when the secretory specimen was used as a standard. Thirdly, monomeric IgA was prepared from the serum of a patient with an IgA paraprotein and used as a standard. The same eight specimens were reassayed; the highest values were obtained using secretory IgA as the standard; the lowest values were obtained using the monomeric IgA as a standard; values using serum for the standard were intermediate. Subsequently, 25 CSF specimens were assayed

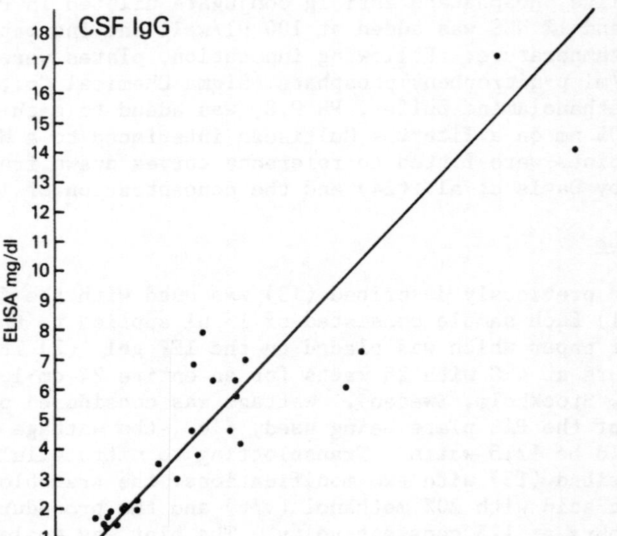

Fig.1. Quantitation of IgG in CSF by RIA and ELISA.

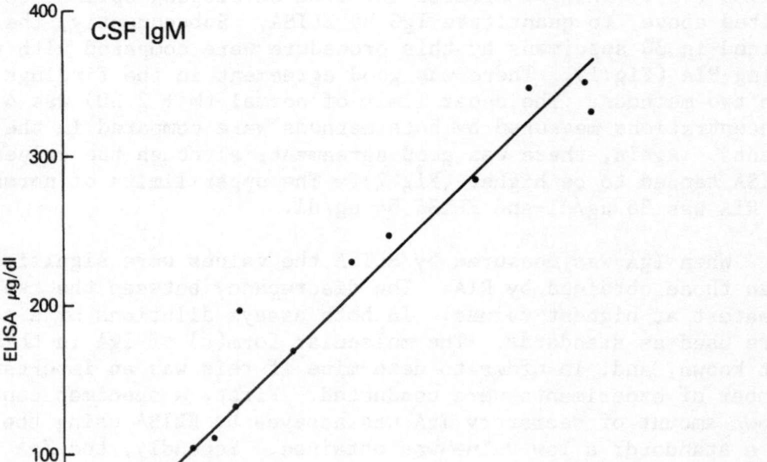

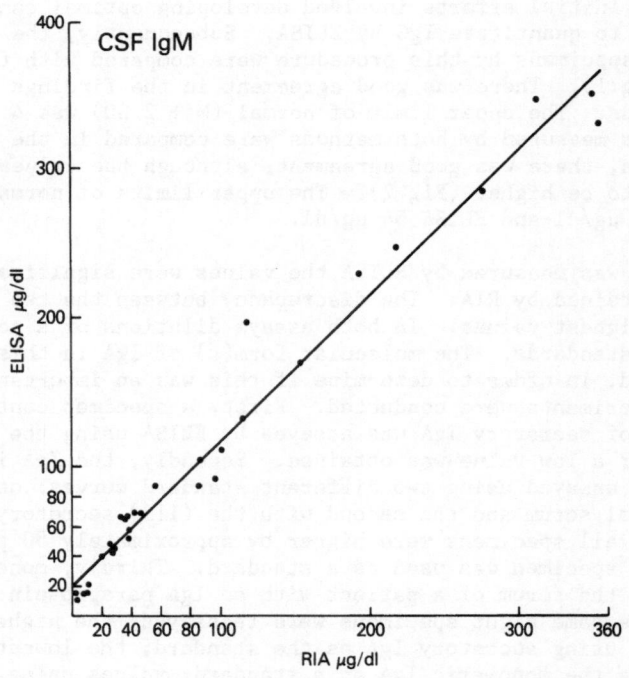

Fig.2. Quantitation of IgM in CSF by RIA and ELISA.

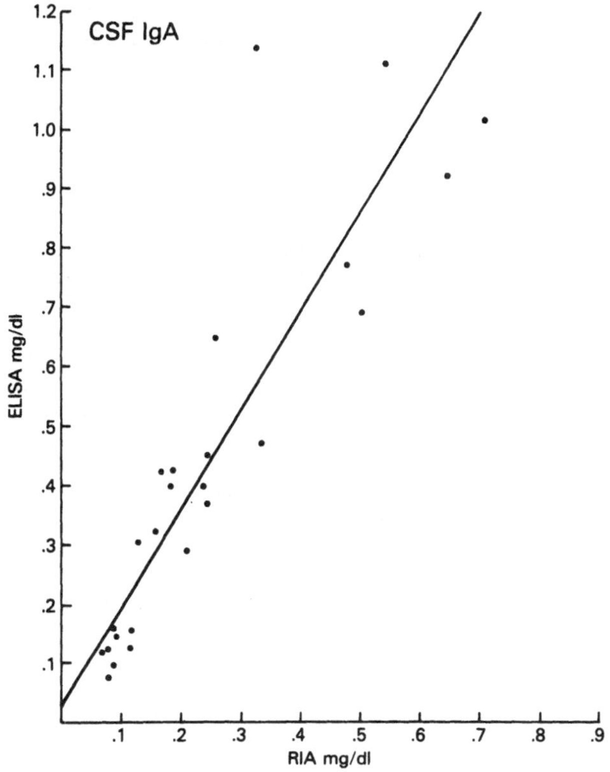

Fig.3. Quantitation of IgA in CSF by RIA using a diluted serum standard and by ELISA using monomeric IgA standard.

using the monomeric IgA standard. The values by ELISA were 1.7 times higher than those obtained by RIA (Fig.3). Because of these observations, it was concluded that the molecular form of IgA in the standard is an important variable in the ELISA. Because no evidence of secretory IgA in the CSF has been reported, it was decided to use monomeric IgA as a standard. Based on this approach, the upper limit of CSF IgA was established at 0.67 mg/dl.

Detection of OCB

The procedure previously described by us for the detection of OCB consists of IEF, transblotting of the Igs to nitrocellulose and immunostaining (13). Because this is highly sensitive, it is essential that a standard amount (15 µl containing 150 ng) of CSF be applied. The most recent technical modification in our procedure, using acetic acid as the buffer and changing the transblotting conditions, rendered the technique even more sensitive. To date, approximately 200 specimens have been analysed by the modified procedure, and frequently 2-3 bands were observed at pI 7.0 to 8.0. Because these were observed in CSF from a variety of neurological conditions and even some normal CSF, it was initially suspected that these represented artifacts or that nonimmunoglobulins such as serum catalases were being detected. These possibilities were studied in subsequent experiments. Omitting the anti Ig reagent did not show bands even at high concentrations of CSF, which excluded the possibility that CSF catalase was responsible. The bands were identified in some sera diluted to the same IgG concentration (10 µg/ml) as CSF; IgG purified from one serum also showed the same bands. Consequently, it was concluded that these probably represent serum IgG molecules which have diffused into the CSF. Bands with pI between 7.0 and 8.0 have been designated as "common bands" in our laboratory and are ignored in the interpretation of CSF OCB.

After developing the modified method for detecting OCB, specimens of CSF from 58 patients were analyzed. "Common bands" were seen in most specimens and disregarded. No additional bands were observed in 29/30 CSF specimens from normals. It was of interest that the remaining "normal" CSF showed eight bands. This specimen had been given to us by another investigator and the "normal" donor was not available for clinical or laboratory evaluation. The four INDC including three with SSPE and one with syphilis showed 10 or more bands. Specimens from 46 NINCD were evaluated: no bands were observed in 36, 1 band was seen in 4 and 2 were observed in 2. Four of the 46 specimens had greater than two bands. These included two specimens from patients with multiple system atrophy which had 8 bands and one specimen from a patient with Tourettes syndrome which had three bands. Specimens from the 27 patients with definite MS were studied. Four or more bands were seen in 23 of these patients; two bands were seen in three specimens and 3 bands in one specimen. Because of these observations, it is our current practice to consider the presence of four or more bands as definitely abnormal.

CSF findings in a group of clinically definite MS patients

Specimens from fifty patients who met McAlpine's criteria for a clinical diagnosis of definite MS were studied. All but one of these had white matter lesions consistent with MS by MRI. Many of these patients subsequently participated in a therapeutic trial. CSF from 49 of these individuals had at least one Ig abnormality, i.e. elevation of an Ig or more than 3 bands. The most frequent abnormality was OCB which was observed in 42 (84%); IgG was elevated in 29 (58%), IgA in 7 (14%) and IgM in 36 (72%). Isolated increase in IgG was seen in 6 specimens, isolated IgM in 13. Isolated elevations of CSF IgM have been observed previously (18,19). Specimens from 43 of these patients have also been studied by the Clinical Pathology Department at our institution. Although different techniques were used, similar conclusions were reached. OCB were observed in 42/43 and the IgG index was elevated in 36/43.

DISCUSSION

A broad objective of the Neuroimmunology Branch at the National Institute of Neurological and Communicative Disorders and Stroke has been to investigate clinical and laboratory abnormalities in MS. These efforts in recent years have been extended to include experimental therapeutic trials in the disorder. Our research has been facilitated by the participation of many patients and other research subjects such as family members including identical and nonidentical twins (13) of affected individuals. An important aspect of this research has been the investigation of CSF Ig abnormalities in the disorder. It has been our view that such efforts would be most meaningful if CSF from our well-characterized patients could be used for a variety of immunological, virological, and clinical studies which might provide useful information. Accordingly, a goal of our studies has been to develop highly sensitive techniques to investigate CSF abnormalities which would provide reproducible results and, if possible, to conserve CSF for other investigations.

Over the past decade RIA (18) has been useful for quantitating CSF Ig and although this procedure is sensitive and specific, the use of radioactivity requires special equipment and the adherence to certain procedures to insure safety to laboratory workers and the environment. Also, radiolabeled reagents in our experience are only reliable for 1-2 weeks and then new preparations are required. Consequently, it has been our practice to defer RIA until a large number of specimens (usually 100-150) were accumulated. This practice, however, limits the clinical use of our CSF studies for diagnosis and management. Use of ELISA to measure Ig avoids the above problems and is more expedient. Enzyme-linked reagents are relatively inexpensive, and once prepared, are stable for years.

Other investigators (20,21) have reached similar conclusions. Kobatake et al. (20) developed an ELISA to measure CSF IgG, IgA, and IgM; Forsberg et al. (21) studied CSF IgM using this technique. Our values, particularly for IgM, compare favourably with these two groups of investigators. This is also true of IgG; in the present study, the upper normal level (M + 2 SD) was 4.9 μg/dl which is higher, but in agreement with 4.2 μg/dl reported by Kobatake, et al. (20). Thus, it is likely that ELISA will be useful for assaying CSF IgG, and IgM.

In evaluating CSF IgA, there are additional variables which will require standardization. This is reflected in a discrepancy between our findings and those of others (20). In the current study, the upper limits of normal was 67 μg/dl when an IgA monomer was used as a standard. Higher values would have been obtained if dilutions of a normal serum had been used, which probably would have been closer to the upper normal limit of 377 μg/dl reported by Kobatake et al. (20). These results indicate that IgA values vary when different standards are used and point out that it will obviously be important for various laboratories investigating CSF IgA to use the same standards in order to compare findings.

Because CSF Ig are present in minute concentrations, it is essential to express the findings in terms of a reference to some other protein(s). In our initial study using RIA (18), each Ig was expressed as a ratio to total protein. The ELISA findings of Kobatake et al. (20) are also expressed in this manner; however, Forsberg et al. (21) have determined CSF/serum IgM ratios and calculated an IgM index which corrects for changes in blood-brain-barrier permeability. It is of interest that when these various parameters were used to assess CSF from patients with MS, it was concluded that "the diagnostic sensitivities for the three IgM variables were not significant" (21). Further, in the study by Forsberg et al., 66% of MS CSF had elevated IgM which is similar to 72% observed in the present study.

CSF IgD and IgE have also been evaluated in two studies (17,16), but not by us. Sindic et al. (26) have detected IgE in MS CSF but concluded that in most patients this was not due to local synthesis.

The procedures which our laboratory uses for the detection of OCB conserves CSF, is highly sensitive, and has been standardized to analyse a consistent amount of IgG. This facilitates determinations during longitudinal studies, minimizes the quantity of CSF utilized and avoids potential artifacts associated with CSF concentration. The results with this procedure compare favourably with those used by others including the clinical pathology laboratory at our institution (25).

REFERENCES

1. E.A. Kabat, H. Landow and D.H. More. Electrophoretic patterns of concentrated cerebrospinal fluid. Proc. Soc. Exp. Biol. Med. 49:260-9 (1942).

2. E.A. Kabat, M. Glusman and V. Knaub. Quantitative estimation of the albumin and gamma globulin in normal and pathologic cerebrospinal fluid by immunochemical methods. Am. J. Med. 4:653-62 (1948).
3. A. Lowenthal, M. van Sande and D. Karcher. The differential diagnosis of neurological diseases by fractionating electrophoretically the CSF gamma-globulins. J. Neurochem. 6:51-6 (1960).
4. H. Link. Oligoclonal immunoglobulin G in multiple sclerosis brain. J. Neurol. Sci. 16:103-14 (1972).
5. D.H. Mattson, R.P. Roos and B.G.W. Arnason. Comparison of agar gel electrophoresis and iso-electric focusing in multiple sclerosis and subacute sclerosing panencephalitis. Ann. Neurol. 19:34-41 (1981).
6. J.E. Olsson and K. Nilsson. Gamma globulins of CSF and serum in multiple sclerosis: isoelectric focusing on polyacrylamide gel and agar gel electrophoresis. Neurology (NY) 29:1383-91 (1979).
7. K.G. Kjellin and A. Siden. Aberrant CSF protein fractions found by electrofocusing in multiple sclerosis: a study of 26 cases with clinically verified or probable multiple sclerosis and 2 cases with optic neuritis. Eur. Neurol. 15:40-50 (1977).
8. J.E. Olsson and B. Petterson. A comparison between agar gel electrophoresis and CSF serum quotients of IgG and albumin in neurological diseases. Acta Neurol. Scand. 53:308-22 (1976).
9. K.G. Kjellin and O. Vesterberg. Isoelectric focusing of CSF proteins in neurological diseases. J. Neurol. Sci. 23:199-213 (1974).
10. M.A.Laurenzi, M. Mavra, S. Kam-Hansen and H. Link. Oligoclonal IgG and free light chains in multiple sclerosis demonstrated by thinlayer polyacrylamide gel iso-electric focusing and immunofixation. Ann. Neurol. 8:241-7 (1980).
11. D.H. Mattson, R.P. Roos and B.G.W. Arnason. Immunoperoxidase staining of cerebrospinal fluid IgG in isoelectric focusing gels: a sensitive new technique. J. Neurosci. Methods. 3:67-75 (1980).
12. A. Siden and K.G. Kjellin. CSF protein examination with thin-layer iso-electric focusing in multiple sclerosis. J.Neurol. Sci. 39:131-46 (1978).
13. X. Xu and D.E. McFarlin. Oligoclonal bands in CSF, twins with MS. Neurology (NY) Vol 34, No 6, pp 769-774 (1984).
14. P. Delmotte. Evaluation of the blood/CSF permeability coefficients and of the intrathecal synthesis of IgG by capillary isotachophoresis. In: "Progress in multiple sclerosis research". H.J. Baner, S. Poser and G. Ritter, eds. New York: Springer-Verlag, Berlin, Heidelberg. 117-22 (1980).
15. W.W. Tourtellotte, S.M. Staugaitis, M.J. Walsh, P. Shapshak, R.W. Baumhefner, A.R. Potvin and K. Synduvko. The basis of intrablood-brain-barrier IgG synthesis. Ann. Neurol. 17:21-27 (1985).
16. A.K. Lefuert and H. Link. IgG production in the central nervous system: a critical review of proposed formulae. Ann. Neurol. 17:13-20 (1985).
17. S.T. Nerenberg and R. Prasad. Radioimmunoassay for IgG, A, M, D and in spinal fluids. Normal values of different age groups. J. Lab. Clin. Med. 86:887-898 (1985).
18. E.S. Mingioli, W. Stober, W.W. Tourtellotte, J.N. Whitaker and D.E. McFarlin. Quantitation of IgG, IgA and IgM in the CSF by radio-immunoassay. Neurology (NY). 28:991-995 (1978).
19. C.J.M. Sindic, C.L. Cambiaso, A. Depre, E.C. Laterre and P.L. Masson. The concentrations of IgM in the cerebrospinal fluid of neurological patients. J. Neurol. Sci. 55:339-350 (1982).
20. K. Kobatake, Y. Shinohara and S. Yoshimura. Immunoglobulins in cerebrospinal fluid enzyme-immunoassay. J. Neurol. Sci. 47:273-283 (1980).

21. P. Forsberg, A. Henriksson, H. Link and S. Ohman. Reference values for CSF-IgM, CSF-IgM/S-IgM ratio and IgM index, and its application to patients with multiple sclerosis and aseptic meningoencephalitis. Scand. J. Clin. Lab. Inves. 44:7-12 (1984).
22. S. Avrameas, T. Ternynck and J.L. Guesdon. Coupling of enzymes to antibodies and antigens. Scan. J. Immunol. 8 (Suppl 7):7-23 (1978).
23. A. Voller, D. Bidwell and A. Bartlett. Enzyme immunoassays in diagnostic medicine. Bull. WHO. 53:55-65 (1976).
24. S. Davis, P.J. Munson, M.L. Jaffe and D. Rodbard. Radioimmunoassay data processing with a small programmable calendar. J. Immunoassay. 1:15-25 (1980).
25. N.N. Papadopoulos, R. Costello, A.D. Kay, N.R. Culter and S.I. Rapoport. Immunochemical and electrophoretic determinations of proteins in paired and cerebrospinal fluid samples. Clin. Chem. 30-1814-1816 (1984).
26. C.J.M. Sindic, C.G.M. Magnusson, E.C. Laterre and P.L. Masson. IgE in the cerebrospinal fluid. J. Neuroimmunol. 6(5):319-324 (1984).

MAGNETIC RESONANCE IMAGING IN MULTIPLE SCLEROSIS: THE EXPERIENCE AT UBC

Joel Oger

Work done by the MS Research Group of the University of British Columbia at the Health Sciences Centre Hospital Vancouver, B.C., Canada, 2211, Wesbrook Mall

INTRODUCTION

Since the description of "Sclerose en Plaques" by Charcot (1), the final diagnosis of multiple sclerosis has always been given by the pathologist. Efforts to clinically delineate the scope of the disease have led to the adoption of a range of diagnostic criteria (2). These take into account multifocality of the disease as well as the existence of attacks and remissions. More recently, the notion of laboratory support to the clinical diagnosis has been introduced (3). It takes into account the existence of oligoclonal bands in the CSF, together with proof of multifocality as substantiated by visual and sensory evoked potentials. These tests, however, remain short of assessing the presence of the demyelinating and/or gliotic lesions that the pathologist recognizes. In the past few years, the advent of Magnetic Resonance Imaging has opened new perspectives in the diagnosis of multiple sclerosis. The large population of patients (1400) attending the MS clinic at the University of British Columbia, has prompted our group to study the capacity of MRI to help to diagnose and follow up patients suspected of having multiple sclerosis. We will summarize the preliminary results obtained by our group in four sections: 1. Abnormalities recognized by MRI in 130 clinically definite M.S.; 2. Clinical pathological correlates between MRI findings and autopsy results; 3. Use of MRI in 200 probable and possible MS patients; 4. MRI findings in 7 MS patients with relapsing remitting disease followed serially.

Clinically definite MS

130 MS patients with clinically definite MS by the criteria of Rose (4) had MRI of the brain done using a Picker 2000 with a .15 Tesla Cryogenic Magnet (5). In 93% of them, abnormalities of the MRI were recognized. They appeared as circumscribed area of increased signal on T2 weighted spin-echo and were found in the white matter of the hemispheres, cerebellum, brain stem, pons or medulla. These lesions had a sharp margin, were round when isolated, but often confluent in the deep white matter. Lesions with an increased signal were often found to outline the ventricules. The presence of more than 2 such lesions, one of them being periventricular, was found in 87% of this group. This is equal to the frequency of 87% oligoclonal bands (OGB) that we found in the CSF using agar gel electrophoresis. As expected, clinical signs and MRI abnormalities

did not correlate well: (1) Often no lesions were seen to explain brainstem findings. (2) MRI abnormalities were also noted as being far more extensive than clinically suspected (6). In a subgroup of 27 clinically definite patients with typical MRI abnormalities but with chronic progressive course, we have assessed the frequency of immune abnormalities - their results were compared to that of a group of 21 healthy controls (7). IgG secretion in vitro in response to Pokeweed mitogen was increased from 1306 ± 310 ng in controls to 25508 ± 278 ng in MS. Con A induced suppression was reduced from 27.2 ± 3.8% in controls to 8.8 ± 6.1% in MS. NK cell function measuring chromium release on K562 cells was also reduced at each of the target/effector cell ratio tested. It is noteworthy that among the lymphocyte markers studied (Leu 1, Leu 2, Leu 3, OKT 8, Leu 7 and Leu 11) only Leu 2 was significantly reduced.

MRI/Pathological correlation

This was studied in clinically definite long standing multiple sclerosis, using both immediate post mortem and fixed brains (8). All clinical diagnoses were confirmed at autopsy. We found that fixation reduced the grey-white contrast on inversion recovery as well as spin echo. A remarkable correlation was found between the size of the lesions, as recognized on MRI, and the extent of the pathological process recognized on gross sections. Demyelinated lesions were recognized down to a size of 3 mm. Heavily gliotic lesions had a greater signal intensity on spin echo and longer T1 than demyelinated lesions. Formalin fixation reduced this difference (9).

Prospective use of MRI in suspect MS

Overall, we found that 75% of 42 probable MS had MRI abnormalities, compatible with multiple sclerosis, as defined by the presence of at least two areas of increased signal intensity, one of them being in a periventricular topography. Only 69% showed OCB on electrophoresis. Of the 158 possible MS, 58% had abnormalities typical of multiple sclerosis, but only 42% showed OCB.

Nine patients had isolated optic neuritis without abnormal sensory evoked potentials (SEP), 5 of them (55%) had distinct MRI abnormalities outside the optic nerve confirming the presence of a multifocal disease (only 3 of these five had OCB). Among 21 patients with progressive myelopathy without abnormal visualized evoked potentials (VEP), 11 had distinct areas of increased signal intensity. The same 11 had OCB on CSF studies. These results indicate that in monosymptomatic MS, proof of multifocality can be obtained in more than half of the patients when MRI is used (10).

In this group of 130 possible and probable MS, 34 patients had normal CT, normal CSF, normal VEP and normal SEP, thus being non "laboratory supported". Seven of these (20%) had MRI abnormalities, suggestive of multiple sclerosis.

Serial study of relapsing remitting MS

7 patients with clinically definite MS of the relapsing remitting type were followed by monthly clinical examination, MRI of the head and immune function studies (11). Three patients had 5 clinical attacks. Two occurred clinically at the level of the spinal cord and would not be seen on MRI of the head. Three were made of a short episode (1-2 weeks) of double vision; no new lesion was seen. This can be attributed to the presence of lesions too small to be seen (even though we can visualize lesions down to 3 mm in diameter), alternatively diplopia may not represent the presence of a new lesion. Most strikingly, 2 patients showed the ap-

pearance, enlargement and disappearance of lesions measuring 2 to 3 cm in diameter (1 temporal, 1 frontal) without any clinical correlation. The nature of these lesions is not known. When compared to the results obtained in the MRI/pathological correlation study, the intensity of their signal was different from that found in gliotic lesions. Their waxing and waning over a 3 month period, suggests that they may more likely represent a mixture of oedema and inflammation, than demyelinated lesions. It is noteworthy that Con A induced suppression and NK cell functions were both reduced at the time the lesions reached their maximum volume but were both in the normal range at the time the new lesions appeared. Both functions had normalized before MRI abnormalities disappeared; this could suggest that the immune abnormalities could be secondary to the volume of the lesions.

CONCLUSION

There is no doubt through the experience of our group that MRI has added a new insight into the diagnosis of multiple sclerosis. MRI, however, should be integrated in the total clinical presentation of the patient. MRI may not be necessary to confirm the diagnosis of clinically definite MS. In our experience, we feel that MRI is a major adjunct to the clinical examination in the evaluation of suspected MS. It is also of a major value for the following up of MS patients, in as much as this is useful to judge the outcome of therapeutical trials or the correlation with immune abnormalities.

REFERENCES

1. J.M. Charcot. Gaz. Hop. Paris. 41:554-566 (1868).
2. J.R. Brown, G.W. Beebe, J.F. Kurtzke, R.B. Lowenson, D.H. Silberberg and W.W. Tourtellotte. Neurology. part 2, p.1-23 (1979).
3. C.R. Poser, D.W. Paty, L. Scheinberg, W.I. McDonald, F.A. Davis, G.C. Ebers, K.P. Johnson, W.A. Sibley, D.H. Silberberg and W.W. Tourtellotte. Ann. Neurol. 13:227 (1983).
4. A.S. Rose, G.W. Ellison and L.W. Myers. Criteria for clinical diagnosis of MS. Neurology. 26:20-22 (1976).
5. D.W. Paty, M. Bergstrom, M. Palmer, J. MacFadyen and D. Li. A quantitative magnetic resonance image of the multiple sclerosis brain. Neurology. 35 (Suppl.1), p.137 (Abstract), (1985).
6. D. Li, J. Mayo, S. Fache, W.D. Robertson, L. Kastrukoff, J. Oger and D.W. Paty. Lack of correlation between clinical manifestations and lesions of MS as seen by NMR. Neurology. 34 (Suppl.1), p.227 (Abstract), (1984).
7. J. Oger, L. Kastrukoff, M. O'Gorman and D.W. Paty. Progressive multiple sclerosis: abnormal immune functions in vitro and aberrant correlation with enumeration of lymphocyte subpopulations. J. Neuroimm. (in press).
8. W.A. Stewart, L.D. Hall, K. Berry and D.W. Paty. Correlation between NMR scan and brain slice data in MS. Lancet. ii, p.412 (1984).
9. W.A. Stewart, L.D. Hall, K. Berry, A. Churg, J. Oger, S.A. Hashimoto and D.W. Paty. Magnetic resonance imaging (MRI) in multiple sclerosis (MS): pathological correlation studies in eight cases. Neurology. 36 (Suppl.1), p.320 (Abstract), (1986).
10. D.W. Paty, S.A. Hashimoto, J. Hooge, A. Eisen, K. Eisen, S. Purves, V. Brandejs, W.S. Robertson and D.K. Li. Magnetic resonance imaging (MRI) in multiple sclerosis (MS): a prospective evaluation of usefulness in diagnosis. Neurology. 36 (Suppl.1), p. 186 (Abstract), (1986).

11. J. Oger, L. Kastrukoff and D.W. Paty. Multiple sclerosis: relationship between suppressor cell function, IgG secretion in vitro and the attacks of MS as studied by serial clinical and MRI examinations. Ann. Neurol. (in press) (Abstract), (1986).

A STUDY IN TWINS, AND THE CONTRIBUTION OF NUCLEAR MAGNETIC RESONANCE TO THE DIAGNOSIS OF MULTIPLE SCLEROSIS IN 288 PATIENTS

E. Moens[1], B. Appel[2], Ch. Mahler[3] and A. Lowenthal[1]

Departments of Neurology[1], Neuroradiology[2] and Endocrinology[3], Algemeen Ziekenhuis Middelheim, Antwerp, Belgium

Two male discordant twins, 21 years old, one of them suffering from multiple sclerosis, were studied. The first symptoms appeared in the affected brother at the age of 17, with episodes of vertigo and gait disturbances. The disease evoluated in a typical pattern of exacerbations and remissions. When last examined, there was a spastic paraparesis, nystagmus and intentional tremor. In his past history, we noted a severe bout of measles complicated by an encephalitis and an meningitis after mumps. Serologic examinations showed elevated measles and herpes zoster virus antibodies in peripheral blood as well as in cerebrospinal fluid (CSF). The unaffected twin brother had neither complaints, nor clinical signs.

Somatosensory evoked potentials (SEP) of upper and lower limbs revealed delayed thalamo-cortical responses to stimulation of the right and left median nerves, and no detectable responses to stimulation of the right and left peroneal nerves. The brainstem auditory responses (BAEP1) were within normal limits. The visual evoked potentials (VEP) demonstrated a marked loss of amplitude on stimulation of the right eye with P100 at ca. 150ms. There was also a significant reduction of amplitude to stimulation of the left eye with P100 at ca. 100ms. Electrophoresis of CSF proteins showed an oligoclonal reaction of the gammaglobulins, whereas the unaffected brother only proved to have slight similar changes in his CSF. HLA-A (A1,A2) and HLA-C (Cw3) antigens were identical. The HLA-B (B8,Bw60 and Bw61) differed. A nuclear magnetic resonance examination was not performed.

A series of 288 patients, all presented clinically as suffering from MS, were examined by magnetic resonance imaging (MRI), with a 0.15 Tesla resistive system. All underwent a single echo multislice technique, with a repetition time (TR) of 1500 msec and an echo time (TE) of 120 msec. In the majority of cases the most pathological image was controlled in a multiecho single slice technique (TR 1500, TE/30,60,...,240 msec). Lesions were found to be as well focal as diffuse, predominantly periventricular, but also present in the posterior fossa, brainstem or the spinal cord.

For a comparative study only those patients were kept who underwent, both, EP and an electrophoresis of the CSF proteins. These 120 remaining patients were subdivided as follows: a "definite" group where EP and CSF were positive for MS, a "probable " group where EP or CSF were compatible with MS and a "possible" group where neither CSF, nor EP were contributive. Sex and age distribution were as expected. In our "definite" group 83,3% of the patients had a positive MRI signal, figure comparable with the 85% mentioned in the litterature. The "possible" group still showed a positive MRI signal in 57,8% of the cases, despite EP and CSF were not contributive.

In the differential diagnosis of MRI signals, we have to reckon with different white matter diseases, such as multistroke, dementia, leucodystrophia, vasculitis and more recently AIDS. In particularly, the so called Binswanger disease proved to be the most challenging problem, however, age and clinical history are different.

In conclusion, MRI seems to be very sensitive for MS, with even a pathoglogical signal in 57,8% of our "possible" cases. But it still remains negative in 15% of those MS patients we considered as "definite".

We thank Mr. L. Toussaint, Ms. L. Van der Eycken and Technicare Belgium for their collaboration in this study.

COMPARISON BETWEEN LYMPHOCYTE ABNORMALITIES IN BLOOD AND CEREBROSPINAL FLUID AND THE IMMUNOPATHOLOGY OF LESIONS IN MULTIPLE SCLEROSIS AND EXPERIMENTAL AUTOIMMUNE ENCEPHALOMYELITIS

Ute Traugott and Labe C. Scheinberg

Departments of Pathology (Neuropathology), Neurology, Rehabilitation Medicine and the Rose F. Kennedy Center for Research in Mental Retardation and Human Development
Albert Einstein College of Medicine, Bronx, N.Y. 10461

Even though abundant detailed information has become available since the original clinical and pathologic description of multiple sclerosis (MS) more than a century ago (1), etiology and pathogenesis of this primary demyelinating disease are still largely unknown (2-4). The present concept, that a viral infection early during life preceeds the clinical manifestations of MS by years to decades, is based upon the results of epidemiologic and virologic studies (3,4). Furthermore, a wide spectrum of immunologic abnormalities are detectable in MS patients. These include increased antibody titers to a number of viruses; elevated levels of immunoglobulin (Ig)G in the cerebrospinal fluid (CSF) and oligoclonal bands which show a constant pattern for individual patients. At the cellular level, a decrease in the number and function of suppressor T cells and natural killer (NK) cells has been reported. The postulated close association between low numbers of circulating suppressor T cells and exacerbations in MS, however, remains an open issue (5-7). The presence of activation antigens on lymphocytes in both blood and CSF (8) together with other immunologic abnormalities, strongly suggests a basic dysregulation of the immune system in MS (3,4). Whether the latter is of significance for the pathogenesis of this disease or represents an epiphenomenon, is unknown. A detailed investigation of immunopathologic changes occurring within the central nervous system (CNS) during lesion development and their comparison to systemic abnormalities could help to evaluate the significance of the latter. Preliminary information on the immunopathology of MS lesions in situ indicated an important role of T4+ cells for the growth of lesions while active myelin breakdown seemed to depend upon the presence of Ia+ macrophages (9-11). More detailed studies on the time sequence of immunologic events and the exact correlation between the clinical, pathologic and immunopathologic picture require the introduction of an animal model such as experimental autoimmune encephalomyelitis (EAE) in the SJL/J mouse (12,13). The results of pilot studies on the immunopathology of lesions in the mouse model (14,15) correlated well to the MS findings.

To investigate a possible correlation between the immunopathology of CNS lesions and systemic immunologic abnormalities, the results on the localization of various components of the immune system in MS lesions and a CNS tissue from mice with EAE will be presented and will be correlated to quantitative changes in lymphocyte subsets in the blood and CSF of MS subjects.

IMMUNOPATHOLOGY OF LESIONS IN MULTIPLE SCLEROSIS AND EXPERIMENTAL ALLERGIC ENCEPHALOMYELITIS

Multiple Sclerosis

Material. For Immunocytochemical investigations, 302 blocks of CNS tissue were available from 18 MS patients: 2 with acute and 16 with chronic disease (12F, 6M; Age: 32-69y; disease duration: 4 mo-22y). Active chronic lesions were found in 36 out of 254 blocks from chronic MS cases. Control CNS tissue was obtained from patients with leukemia, carcinoma of the lung and systemic lupus erythematosus.

Pathology. In H + E stained sections, active chronic MS lesions show a sharply-demarcated lesion edge with hypertrophic astrocytes, a zone of inflammation (consisting of lymphocytes, macrophages and plasma cells) and a lesion center with large numbers of macrophages, containing myelin degradation products, as demonstrated by Oil-Red-O staining (2). Silent chronic MS lesions lack hypercellularity and the few foamy cells seen, indicate previously active disease (2,13).

Immunopathology. For the localization of components of the immune system in situ, frozen sections of brain and spinal cord tissue were stained by the avidin-biotin-peroxidase complex (ABC) or the peroxidase-antiperoxidase (PAP) technique and direct fluorescence using monoclonal antibodies (mAb) and conventional antisera (11,14). The markers used in this study are shown in Table 1.

Table 1. Markers used for immunocytochemical analysis.

Human System	Cell Type Function	Mouse system
T11	Pan T Cells	Lyt-1.2
T4	Helper/Inducer T Cells	L3T4
T8	Suppressor/cytotoxic T Cells	Lyt-2
TQ_1	Cytotoxic T4+ Cells	n.t.
Leu-7	NK and K Cells	n.t.
Ia	Class II MHC: B cells, macrophages, activated T cells; endothelial cells, astrocytes	Ia^{sf}
HLA-ABC	Class I MHC: nucleated cells	n.t.
Ig	B cells, Ig-containing macrophages	Ig
Mac-1	Monocytes	Mac-1
Interleukin-2 receptor	Activation Antigen	n.t.
Ig	Deposits	Ig
n.t.	Deposits	Albumin
MBP	Myelin antigen	MBP
GC	Myelin antigen	GC
$Interferon^{beta}$	Lymphokine	n.t.

MBP: myelin basic protein
GC: galactocerebroside

Active Chronic MS. In the center of active chronic MS lesions, large numbers of activated macrophages were found, most of which stained positively for Class I (HLA-ABC) and Class II (HLA-Dr, Ia) major histocompatibility (MHC) antigens. Towards the edge of the lesion and the adjacent normal white matter, the density of macrophage infiltrates decreased somewhat (Table 2). While most Ia+ cells displayed a vacuolated cytoplasm in the center of the lesion, at the lesion periphery, homogeneously staining macrophages were not uncommon in the parenchyma and perivascular cuffs, suggesting that they had not yet participated in myelin destruction. This pattern could suggest that Ia+ macrophages can be of hematogenous origin and do not all arise from local microglial cells. Class I and Class II-positive macrophages were not only found in the lesion, but were also present, though in small numbers, within the normal white and grey matter parenchyma. The close association occasionally observed between lymphocytes and Ia+ macrophages could suggest functional interaction, such as local antigen presentation. While a high density of Ia on macrophages indicates activation, Mac-1 antigen is found on monocytes only. In agreement with this, Mac-1 bearing cells were absent from lesions and were detectable throughout the CNS in small numbers in the Virchow-Robin spaces only.

The density of T cell infiltrates was inverse to that of macrophages (Table 2), in that the numbers of pan T cells and T cell subsets, which were least frequently found in the center of active chronic MS lesions, increased steadily towards the edge of the lesion and the adjacent normal-appearing white matter. More detailed analysis of T cell infiltrates revealed a tendency of T4+ (helper/inducer) T cells to infiltrate deeply into the normal-appearing white matter adjacent to an highly active lesion, while T8+ (suppressor/cytotoxic) T cells seemed to be more confined to the lesion edge. When the distribution of activated T cells was investigated, interleukin-2 (IL-2) receptor positive cells were found to be uncommon and when detectable, were mainly seen in close association with highly active lesions. In the latter, IL-2 receptor positive cells displayed a distribution pattern reminiscent to that of T4+ cells, indicating previous activation and an important role of this cell type for lesion pathogenesis. Thus, lymphokines released by activated T4+ cells might attract Ia+ macrophages from the circulation, which in turn cause myelin damage possibly via receptor-mediated phagocytosis. Further dissection of T4+ cells into cytotoxic and non-cytotoxic subsets by a monoclonal antibody against TQ_1(16) demonstrated only a few labelled cells and thus ruled out a major role of this cell type for lesion pathogenesis (Table 2). NK and K cells, labelled by anti-Leu-7 mAb, were also rare (Table 2).

The distribution of Ig+ cells (B cells, Ig-containing macrophages) was comparable to that of Ia+ cells (B cells, macrophages, activated T cells), in that they displayed dense infiltrates within the lesion, and a slight decrease towards the lesion edge. Ig deposits were predominantly found at the lesion edge and the adjacent normal white matter. There was also staining for Ig on some endothelial cells and hypertrophic astrocytes, a pattern which could be related to the presence of Fc receptors on these cells. In all chronic MS cases studied, a few hematogenous cells of all subtypes could consistantly be found throughout the white and grey matter parenchyma. While insignificant in regard to numbers, this observation is in contrast to normal CNS tissue, which contained virtually no hematogenous cells.

It is known that presentation of antigen to T cells requires Ia-expressing accessory cells of the immune system. When Ia expression was investigated within the CNS, no Ia+ cells could be demonstrated in normal brain tissue.

Table 2. Quantitative data on inflammatory cells in active and silent chronic multiple sclerosis lesions*

Active Chronic MS						
Center	178.7 ± 21.2	81.2 ± 48.7	60.0 ± 35.0	1.3 ± 0.2	3.4 ± 1.8	1241.2 ± 91.2
Edge	578.7 ± 208.7	421.2 ± 170.0	316.2 ± 243.7	2.6 ± 3.0	8.7 ± 3.7	783.7 ± 71.2
Normal WM	243.7 ± 126.2	491.2 ± 187.5	241.2 ± 68.7	0.5 ± 0.6	3.0 ± 2.4	321.2 ± 116.2
Silent Chronic MS						
Center	12.5 ± 15.7	6.2 ± 10.0	3.1 ± 6.2	0.6 ± 0.4	0.9 ± 0.2	31.2 ± 28.2
Edge	50.0 ± 61.2	22.5 ± 27.5	16.2 ± 18.7	0.8 ± 0.5	3.3 ± 9.0	178.7 ± 36.2
Normal WM	6.3 ± 4.5	4.5 ± 2.4	2.1 ± 3.7	2.3 ± 1.3	5.2 ± 1.4	18.7 ± 6.2

* given as numbers of labelled cells per mm2

However, in MS material, Ia+ endothelial cells and astrocytes could be detected. Ia+ endothelial cells showed a spotty, discontinuous distribution pattern and were demonstrable with comparable frequency in the lesion, the lesion edge and the normal white and grey matter parenchyma (Table 3). This random distribution of Ia+ endothelial cells was unexpected in a disease which primarily effects the white matter and might be related to the induction of Ia antigen by activated circulating T cells or products thereof, as has been suggested previously by studies in vitro (17,18). In the event that Ia+ endothelial cells participate in local antigen presentation in MS, this might effect the blood-brain-barrier (BBB) and, thus, might be related to the formation of new lesions. In addition to endothelial cells, Ia could also be demonstrated on some astrocytes in MS tissue (Table 3). In contrast to the ubiquitous presence of Ia+ endothelial cells, Ia+ astrocytes were mainly found in close association with active lesions and were absent from normal white and grey matter parenchyma. In the lesion area, Ia+ astrocytes were quite common, displaying a slightly higher frequency at the lesion edge and the adjacent normal white matter than in the center of the lesion. The observed localization of Ia+ astrocytes corresponded well to the distribution pattern of presumably activated (IL-2 receptor positive) T4+ cells, suggesting that activated infiltrating T cells can induce the expression of Class II MHC antigens on astrocytes. Thus, it was demonstrated in vivo that astrocytes also qualify as potential antigen presenting cells within the CNS (21), as has been suggested previously by studies in vitro (20). This notion might also be supported by the occasionally observed close association between Ia+ astrocytes and lymphocytes. Antigen presentation on astrocytes at the edge of active lesions, could result in a local reactivation of the immune response which then could lead to continuous growth of the lesion from its periphery. Additional support for a possible role of Ia+ endothelial cells and astrocytes was provided by the demonstration of myelin basic protein and galactocerebroside on both cell types.

Since the actual immunologic function of T4+ and T8+ cells, both of which have been demonstrated in active chronic MS lesions, depends on the Class of MHC antigen they are interacting with (16), the presence of HLA-ABC was also investigated. HLA-ABC was present on most CNS endothelial cells from normal and MS cases. It was also common on inflammatory cells, showing a distribution pattern similar to that of Ia+ cells. That Class I MHC antigens are normally present on endothelial cells, while Class II MHC antigens need to be induced by activated T cells suggests a close relationship between Ia antigen and lesion pathogenesis in MS. In this setting, T4+ cells demonstrated in active MS lesions, might, indeed, function as helper/ inducer T cells.

When an attempt is made to establish the typical picture of the immunopathology of active chronic MS lesions, the wide spectrum of changes seen by routine pathology in various active chronic MS lesions as well as between different areas of the same lesion have to be taken into consideration. Interestingly, lesion growth, associated with lymphocytic infiltrates, seems to occur more readily along nerve fibers than when myelinated fibers are encountered tangentially.

Table 3. Multiple sclerosis: Frequency of endothelial cells and astrocytes expressing Ia antigen or galactocerebroside

	Endothelial Cells		Astrocytes	
	Ia	GC	Ia	GC
<u>Active Chronic MS</u>				
Center	0.3 ± 0.18	0.25 ± 0.46	2.78 ± 2.1	2.3 ± 0.92
Edge	0.68 ± 0.26	0.4 ± 0.69	3.74 ± 2.6	3.5 ± 0.87
Normal WM close to lesion	0.70 ± 0.16	1.3 ± 0.7	2.94 ± 2.6	1.9 ± 0.61
remote from lesion	0.74 ± 0.40	0.6 ± 0.4	0.30 ± 0.14	0.28 ± 0.20
Normal grey matter	0.62 ± 0.28	0.3 ± 0.09	0.0	0.07 ± 0.14
<u>Silent Chronic MS</u>				
Center	0.36 ± 0.24	0.25 ± 0.26	0.1 ± 0.07	0.11 ± 0.16
Edge	0.50 ± 0.25	0.93 ± 0.65	0.04 ± 0.14	0.64 ± 0.26
Normal WM close to lesion	0.62 ± 0.34	0.71 ± 0.48	0.02 ± 0.1	0.48 ± 0.3
remote from lesion	0.72 ± 0.54	0.34 ± 0.12	0.0	0.01 ± 0.03
Normal grey matter	0.54 ± 0.32	0.0	0.0	0.0

* given as numbers of labelled cells per mm^2

Silent Chronic MS. In silent chronic MS, the lesion edge lacks hypercellularity and a few foamy cells are present, indicating previous disease. By immunocytochemistry, most of the macrophages were Ig-positive, while only a few stained for Ia. Within the lesion, and the normal CNS parenchyma, hematogenous cells were occasionally found and, in accord with the immunologic inactivity of this type of lesion, IL-2 receptor-bearing cells were absent. Leu-7+ cells could sometimes be seen in a focus-like accumulation in normal white matter close to a silent lesion, but the significance of this observation is not known. Surprisingly, the frequency of Ia-expressing endothelial cells was comparable to that of active chronic MS lesions, while Ia+ astrocytes were rare. Myelin antigens on endothelial cells or astrocytes were infrequently found.

Experimental Autoimmune Encephalomyelitis (EAE)

Material. Acute and chronic relapsing EAE was actively induced with isogeneic spinal cord in complete Freund's adjuvant in 6-8 week old female SJL/J mice according to methods described previously (12,13). Mice, inoculated for acute EAE were sacrificed between 24h and 22 days post inoculation (PI), and animals sensitized for chronic relapsing EAE were sampled at day 7 PI (pre-clinical); during the first episode of signs; during a relapse; and during chronic progressive and chronic silent disease.

Acute EAE. Mice sensitized for acute EAE, developed clinical signs (floppy tail, incontinence, paraparesis) between 12 and 20 days PI. As early as 24h PI, Ia was demonstrable on some endothelial cells in the brain. At this time, a few T cells were also present and perivascular deposits of Ig and albumin suggested a damage of the blood-brain-barrier (BBB). The extent of these changes increased slightly up to day 4 PI, when there was a transient decline, which was followed by even more extensive abnormalities at day 7 PI. At 7 days PI (which corresponds to about 5 days before onset of signs), Ia was expressed more frequently on some endothelial cells and also on a few astrocytes. In the moderately dense infiltrates, T cells, T cell subsets, Ia+ and Ig+ cells were randomly distributed. Myelin antigens could be demonstrated on some endothelial cells early during the disease and it as well as Ia antigen and some damage to the BBB remained detectable for the duration of the disease. With onset of signs, the numbers of infiltrating cells, all of which were evenly distributed, increased significantly. A similar random pattern of inflammatory cells has been described previously for lesions in acute MS, SSPE and lepromatous leprosy (11,21,22). While in the latter, the uniform distribution of infiltrating cells has been considered to be associated with the continuous presence of the eliciting antigen, the distinct distribution pattern of infiltrating cells seen in lesions of tuberculoid leprosy and in active chronic MS might reflect the successful elimination of the antigen, rather than a difference in basic pathogenetic mechanisms.

Chronic Relapsing EAE. After the first (acute) episode of signs (12-18 days PI), mice inoculated for chronic relapsing EAE, developed spontaneous relapses with good recovery, chronic progressive worsening of signs, or no further manifestations of the disease. Immunopathologic changes observed in the CNS during the acute stage of the chronic disease were reminiscent of those seen in acute EAE. However, as the disease entered the chronic phase, the distribution pattern of hematogenous cells in the lesions changed (15). In active lesions from mice with chronic progressive disease, displaying severe paraparesis, L3T4+ cells (helper/inducer T cells) predominated, while Lyt-2+ cells (suppressor/cytotoxic T cells) were virtually absent. Moderate numbers of Ig+ and Ia+ infiltrating cells were found within the lesion, and in the spinal cord, Ia-expressing astrocytes were detectable at the edge of the lesion. During relapses or chronic progressive disease with only mild clinical signs, the density of

L3T4+ and Lyt-2+ infiltrating cells appeared to be more balanced and Lyt-2+ cells sometimes predominated during the recovery phase. Overall, damage to the BBB was less extensive during chronic than during acute stages of the disease. Ia and myelin antigens were consistently present on a few endothelial cells and small numbers of all types of infiltrating cells were detectable throughout the normal CNS. The latter findings are similar to those described in CNS tissue from chronic MS cases. This low-grade infiltration of the CNS parenchyma in autoimmune demyelination, which is in contrast to the findings on normal CNS tissue, might either reflect an increased pool of recirculating lymphocytes or might be related to the presence of Ia+ endothelial cells which could facilitate the passage of hematogenous cells. Indicating a continuous disease activity, this low-grade infiltration might provide an essential prerequirement for reactivation of the disease process by various, yet unknown factors. The present results on chronic EAE in the SJL/J mouse showed a decline in the extent of edema during chronic stages of the disease, at which time cellular infiltrates became more organized. Should a similar change occur in MS, this could explain the well known benefit of Prednisone during early stages of the disease and its decrease in efficacy later on.

These studies on the immunopathology of autoimmune demyelinating lesions have shown that possibly activated T4+ (L3T4+ helper/inducer) T cells are present in very active chronic lesions, the presence of which proceeds the infiltration by hematogenous macrophages, which, serving as effector cells, cause demyelination, possibly via receptor-mediated phagocytosis and/or the release of enzymes. The presence of T8+ (Lyt-2+; suppressor/cytotoxic) T cells is more common in less active lesions and during repair (15). Low-grade infiltration of the normal CNS parenchyma is associated with chronic disease and might facilitate its reactivation. In both MS and EAE, antigen might be presented locally within the CNS on endothelial cells and astrocytes, a phenomenon which is possibly related to the development of new lesions or to the growth of the lesion from its periphery.

STUDIES ON LYMPHOCYTE SUBSETS IN THE BLOOD AND CEREBROSPINAL FLUID (CSF) IN MULTIPLE SCLEROSIS

To investigate a possible correlation between quantitative changes in lymphocyte subsets in the periphery and the immunopathology of lesions, percentages of T cells, T cell subsets, Ia+ cells and activation antigen-bearing cells were determined in the blood and CSF of 39 MS patients with chronic progressive disease (22F, 17M; age: 31.4y ± 10.7y). The disease duration ranged from 3 to 7 years; the Kurtzke EDSS from 3.5 - 8.0. In 12 patients, blood samples were studied longitudinally for up to 14 mo. In agreement with previous reports (5,8,23), a decrease in numbers of T8+ cells in blood and CSF was not uncommon. However, the results of our longitudinal studies on changes in the blood, suggested that individual patients display a certain "pattern" (Fig.3), which can be maintained over a prolonged time period. This can include constantly decreased or increased levels of T8+ cells or considerable fluctuations in numbers of most lymphocyte subsets without clear evidence for a coinciding change in clinical disease activity. Interestingly, when levels of T8+ cells were also compared to the mental status of MS patients, low numbers of T8+ cells seemed to show a better correlation with a depressive mood alteration (as expressed by a "depression score") than with worsening of neurologic signs (24). If this observation can be reconfirmed on a larger number of patients and on longitudinal studies, it might yet be another indication for an important interrelationship between the neuro-endocrine and the immune system. In addition to the observed low levels of T8+ cells, there was also a trend to elevated levels of T4+ cells in both compartments, which, however, was not statistically significant. In blood and CSF, the mean of the T4/T8 ratio was elevated and the high SD suggested a high variability (Figs.1 and 2). In both compartments, levels of Ia+ cells and Leu-11b+ cells were decreased. Activation antigens (Ia, transferrin-receptor, interleukin-2 receptor) were detectable in the majority of blood and CSF samples (60%-70%). While the mean values of the whole group showed no significant differences between blood and CSF, in individual patients, discordant changes were not uncommon and were also not restricted to a particular lymphocyte subset (Table 2).

A comparison of these findings from the periphery to the immunopathology of lesions, described here, suggested that the mildly increased levels of T4+ cells in the CSF and the high frequency of activation antigens on lymphocytes in both blood and CSF seem to be most relevant for lesion activity. The increased numbers of T4+ cells in the CSF, which represents a continuation of the extracellular space of the brain, could reflect the infiltrates of T4+ cells, present in highly-active lesions and activation-antigen-bearing lymphocytes could be directly related to the expression of Ia antigen on endothelial cells and astrocytes. An importance of helper T cells for lesion pathogenesis has further been supported by the observation that EAE can be transferred by specifically-sensitized Lyt-1+ (helper/inducer T cells) but not by Lyt-2+ cells (25). The significance of decreased levels of T8+ cells in the circulation of some MS patients is not clear and our data provide no evidence for a selective accumulation of this cell type in the CNS.

The rather complex situation in MS, a disease in which the development of lesions is based upon a dynamic immunologic process, which is active long before neurologic signs become apparent and in which more than one active lesion whether clinically evident or not, can be present at a given time, could account for the conflicting results on lymphocyte changes in the periphery (blood and CSF) and might make it difficult to establish a reliable correlation between the latter findings and the immunopathology of MS lesions.

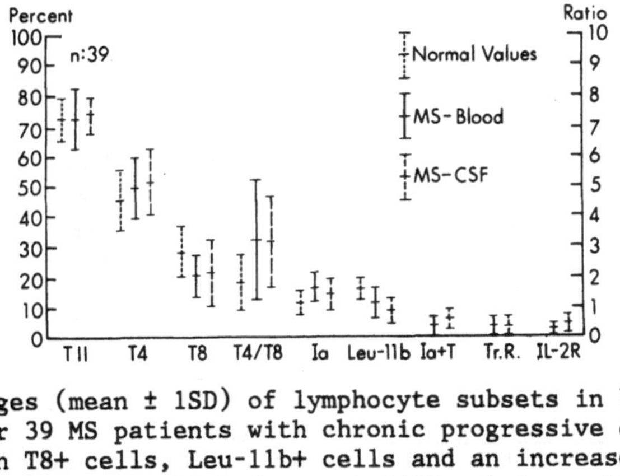

Fig.1. Percentages (mean ± 1SD) of lymphocyte subsets in blood and CSF are given for 39 MS patients with chronic progressive disease. A decrease in T8+ cells, Leu-11b+ cells and an increase in the T4/T8 ratio can be seen, which does not differ between blood and CSF. Activated T cells are present.

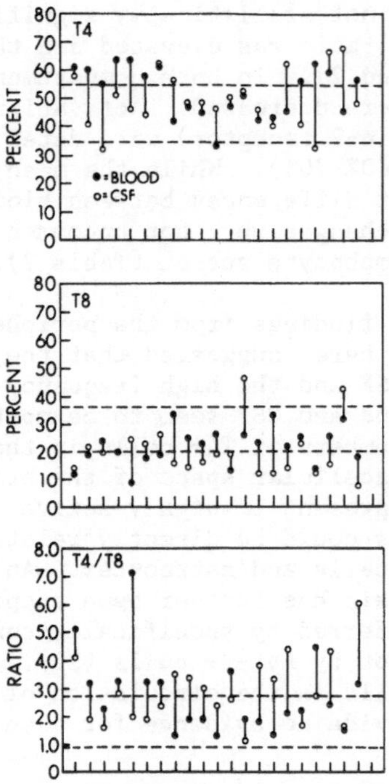

Fig.2. Blood and CSF values of T4+ cells, T8+ cells and the T4/T8 ratio are compared in individual patients. Note that discordant changes are not uncommon in all three panels. The normal range is indicated by the horizontal broken lines.

ACKNOWLEDGEMENTS

The authors thank Drs. J. Prineas, B. Bornstein and J. Powers for supplying some of the brain tissue; Patricia Lazzaro and Robyn Baff for expert technical help and Michele Griebel for typing the manuscript.

This work was supported in part by Grant RG-1664-B-1 and RG-1001-E-5 from the National Multiple Sclerosis Society, and by the National Institute of Health Grants, NS 11920, and RTC Grant G 008300040.

REFERENCES

1. J.M. Charcot. Histologie de la sclérose en plaques. Gaz. Hop. 41:554 (1968).
2. J.G. Greenfield and R.M. Norman. Demyelinating Diseases. In: "Greenfield's Neuropathology", W. Blackwood, W.H. McMenemey, A. Meyer, R.M. Norman and D.S. Russell, eds. Arnold, London p. 475 (1971).
3. D.E. McFarlin and H.F. McFarland. Multiple Sclerosis. N. Eng. J. Med. 307:1183 and 1246 (1982).
4. B.H. Waksman. Current trends in multiple sclerosis research. Immunol. Today 2:87 (1981).
5. E.L. Reinherz, H.L. Weiner, S.L. Hauser, J.A. Cohen, J.A. Distaso and S.F. Schlossman. Loss of suppressor T cells in active multiple sclerosis. N. Eng. J. Med. 303:125 (1980).
6. L.F. Kastrukoff and D.W. Paty. A serial study of peripheral blood T lymphocyte subsets in relapsing-remitting multiple sclerosis. Ann. Neurol. 15:250 (1984).

7. E.S. Mingioli and D.E. McFarlin. Leucocyte surface antigens in patients with multiple sclerosis. J. Neuroimm. 6:131 (1984).
8. D.A. Hafler, D.A. Fox, M.E. Manning, S.F. Schlossman, E.L. Reinherz and H.L. Weiner. In vivo activated T lymphocytes in the peripheral blood and cerebrospinal fluid of patients with multiple sclerosis. N. Eng. J. Med. 312:1405 (1985).
9. U. Traugott, E.L. Reinherz and C.S. Raine. Multiple sclerosis: Distribution of T cell subsets within active chronic lesions. Sci. 219:308 (1983).
10. J. Boose, M.M. Esiri, W.W. Tourtellotte and D.Y. Mason. Immunohistological analysis of T lymphocyte subsets in the central nervous system in chronic progressive multiple sclerosis. J. Neurol. Sci. 62: 219 (1983).
11. U. Traugott and C.S. Raine. Further lymphocyte characterization in the central nervous system in multiple sclerosis. Ann. N.Y. Acad. Sci. 436:163 (1984).
12. C.S. Raine, L.B. Barnett, A. Brown, T. Behar and D.E. McFarlin. Neuropathology of experimental allergic encephalomyelitis in inbred strains of mice. Lab. Invest. 43:150 (1980).
13. A. Brown, D.E. McFarlin and C.S. Raine. Chronologic neuropathology of relapsing experimental allergic encephalomyelitis in the mouse. Lab. Invest. 46:171 (1982).
14. U. Traugott, C.S. Raine and D.E. McFarlin. Acute experimental allergic encephalomyelitis in the mouse. Cell. Immunol. 91:240 (1985).
15. U. Traugott, D.E. McFarlin and C.S. Raine. Immunopathology of the lesion in chronic relapsing experimental autoimmune encephalomyelitis in the mouse. Cell. Immunol. (in press).
16. S.C. Meuer, S.F. Schlossman and E.L. Reinherz. Clonal analysis of human cytotoxic T lymphocytes: T4+ and T8+ effector T cells recognize products of different major histocompatibility complex regions. Proc. Nat. Acad. Sci. 79:4395 (1982).
17. D.R. Burger and R.M. Vetto. Vascular endothelium a major participant in T-lymphocyte immunity. Cell. Immunol. 70:357 (1982).
18. J.S. Pober, A. Gimbrone, R. Cotran, C. Reiss, S.J. Burakoff, W. Fierz and K.A. Ault. Ia expression by vascular endothelium is induced by activated T cells and by human gamma interferon. J. Exp. Med. 158: 1339 (1983).
19. U. Traugott, L.C. Scheinberg and C.S. Raine. On the presence of Ia-positive endothelial cells and astrocytes in multiple sclerosis lesions and its relevance to antigen presentation. J. Neuroimmunol. 8:1 (1985).
20. A. Fontana, W. Fierz and H. Wekerle. Astrocytes present myelin basic protein to encephalitogenic T cell lines. Nature 307:273 (1984).
21. U. Traugott. Characterization of inflammatory cells in situ in multiple sclerosis and subacute sclerosing panencephalitis. Ann. Neurol. 14:108 (1983).
22. R.L. Modlin, F. Hofman, P.R. Meyer, O.P. Sharma, C.R. Tayor and T.H. Rea. In situ demonstration of T lymphocyte subsets in granulomatous inflammation: leprosy, rhinoscleroma and sarcoidosis. Clin. Exp. Immunol. 51:430 (1983).
23. S.L. Hauser, E.L. Reinherz, C.J. Hoban, S.F. Schlossman and H.L. Weiner. CSF cells in multiple sclerosis: monoclonal antibody analysis and relationship to peripheral T cell subsets. Neurology. 33: 575 (1983).
24. F.W. Foley, A.H. Miller, U. Traugott, N.G. LaRocca and L.C. Scheinberg. Psychoimmunological factors in multiple sclerosis. Am. J. Psychiatry (submitted).
25. C.B. Pettinelli and D.E. McFarlin. Adoptive transfer of experimental allergic encephalomyelitis in SJL/J mice after in vitro activation of lymph node cells by myelin basic protein: requirement for Lyt 1+2- T lymphocytes. J. Immunol. 127:1420 (1981).

CORRELATION BETWEEN LEUCOCYTE SUBSETS IN CEREBROSPINAL FLUID (CSF), BLOOD AND SPINAL CORD LESIONS IN ACUTE ALLERGIC ENCEPHALOMYELITIS

H. Lassmann, K. Vass and Ch. Brunner

Institute for Brain Research, Austrian Academy of Sciences
Neurological Institute, Vienna University
Schwarzspanierstrasse 17, 1090 Vienna, Austria

SUMMARY

The dynamics of inflammatory reaction in the cerebrospinal fluid (CSF) and spinal cord tissue of rats with acute experimental allergic encephalomyelitis (EAE) was investigated by immunocytochemistry using monoclonal antibodies against T-cell subsets and Ia-antigen. Increased leucocyte numbers in the CSF were found as early as 5 days after sensitization, reaching maximal values during active CNS disease. We found a significant correlation between the total numbers of leucocytes in the CSF and disease severity or inflammatory reaction in the spinal cord. Furthermore, the absolute as well as relative numbers of Ia positive cells in the CSF proved to be an accurate marker for disease activity and inflammation in the CNS tissue. There were, however, no major fluctuations of T-cell subsets in the CSF during evolution of the disease and thus no correlation between T-cell subsets and their ratios between CSF and CNS lesions was observed. We found no significant correlation between T-cell subset ratios in blood and CSF samples respectively.

INTRODUCTION

Analysis of cerebrospinal fluid (CSF) is widely used in diagnostic neurology as an approach to screen for biochemical and immunological abnormalities in the central nervous system (CNS) tissue. Especially in inflammatory conditions of the brain and spinal cord the composition of CSF leucocytes as well as protein alterations allow diagnostically significant conclusions regarding the nature and activity of the disease process (Laterre 1974, Tourtellotte 1970, Link and Tibbling 1977). More recently, cloning of CSF leucocytes has been used in the search for antigen specificity of the inflammatory response and in the determination of functional properties of lymphocytes in human CNS diseases like multiple sclerosis (MS) (Hafler et al., 1984, Santoli et al., 1984). As a major problem of these studies, however, it is at present unresolved to what respect CNS inflammatory reaction is reflected by CSF leucocytes.

In the present study we have used the model of acute experimental allergic encephalomyelitis (EAE) to directly compare alterations of leucocyte subsets in the CSF with the composition of inflammatory infiltrates in meninges and CNS tissue.

MATERIAL AND METHODS

Induction of EAE

Acute EAE was induced in 35 young adult Sprague Dawley rats (200-250g body weight). The sensitization protocol, handling of animals and screening of neurological disease has been described in detail earlier (Lassmann et al., 1981; Lassmann 1983). Animals were sampled at 5, 8, 10, 11, 12, 15, 18, 24, 28 and 32 days after immunization. Unsensitized animals of the same age served as controls.

Preparation of Blood, CSF and CNS samples

Animals were sacrificed with an overdose of Thiopental and exsanguinated by cardiac puncture. Blood leucocyte numbers were counted in a Fuchs Rosenthal chamber and blood smears were prepared. After exsanguination CSF samples were obtained by suboccipital puncture. Small volumes of CSF (10-30 µl) were sedimented on precleaned glass slides. Blood smears and CSF samples were fixed with 4% paraformaldehyde (10 min) followed by acetone (10 min). They were then immunostained with monoclonal antibodies for T-cells, T-cell subsets and Ia-antigens (see below). Following CSF puncture the animals were perfused with 4% paraformaldehyde, the CNS tissue dissected and further immersed in the same fixative for additional 3 hours. Immunostaining was performed on paraffin sections and isolated leptomeninges (Kitz et al., 1981).

Immunostaining Procedure

The following monoclonal antibodies, purchased from Sera Lab (UK) were used for differentiation of leucocyte subsets: W3/13 (T-lymphocytes and granulocytes), W3/25 ("helper/inducer" T-cell subset), Ox 8 ("suppressor/cytotoxic" T-cells and NK cells) and Ox 6 and Ox 4 (common determinant of the Ia-antigen). Immunostaining was performed with a modified biotin/avidin technique (Lassmann et al., 1986; Vass et al., 1986).

Quantitative Evaluation of Immunostained Cells in Blood, CSF and CNS Tissue

At least 400 cells per immunocytochemical marker and animal were evaluated in blood smears and EAE CSF samples. In CSF preparations from control animals, the number of cells evaluated was lower (50-70 cells/animal and marker), because of the small number of total leucocytes in normal CSF. The % values of immunostained cells (Table 1) were calculated on the basis of total mononuclear cells (total leucocytes minus granulocytes).

In the CNS tissue, numbers of positively stained cells were evaluated in 15-20 standardized spinal cord cross sections in a total area of 40 mm^2 spinal cord tissue per animal and marker. Values are expressed in cells /mm^2. Perivascular cells were defined as immunostained cells located between the vessel wall and the perivascular glia limitans. Parenchymal cells represent inflammatory cells dispersed within the CNS tissue. Occasional intravascular cells and granulocytes stained by W3/13 antibody were not included in the counts. In isolated leptomeninges positive cells were counted in a total area of 4 mm^2 per animal and marker.

Statistical Analysis

Mean values of inflammatory cells at various stages of the disease were compared with each other by Student's T-test. Linear regression analysis was performed by the procedure of Pearson Corr of the statistical software package SSPS using a two tailed test of significance.

RESULTS

CSF Leucocyte Alterations in Acute EAE

Blood contamination of CSF samples. The average blood contamination in CSF samples of control and EAE animals was 50,0 erythrocytes/mm^3. No CSF samples contained more than 500 erythrocytes/mm^3.

CSF Leucocytes. CSF samples from normal unsensitized rats contained a small number of leucocytes (Table 1). The majority of these cells were positive with T-cell markers, $W3/25^+$ T-cells outnumbered Ox 8^+. During EAE an increase of total CSF leucocytes was present already during the incubation period (Table 1), the peak of CSF pleocytosis was reached 11 to 15 days after sensitization. During active disease a significant increase of granulocytes was noted. The relative number of T-lymphocytes and their subsets remained fairly constant during the evolution of the disease. This was also reflected by the lack of significant changes in the W3/25: Ox 8 ratio.

In contrast the number of Ia^+ cells in the CSF increased during active disease, reaching maximal values at the peak of acute EAE (Table 1).

Table 1. CSF leucocytes in acute EAE

	N	C	Leuco	% Gr	W3/13	W3/25	Ox 8	Ox 6
Controls	9	0	1.7±0.8	0.9±1.7	60±13	44±10	26±8	29±12
EAE								
5-10	8	0	8.7	5.7	47	33	29	36
11-15	13	0.8	203	<u>18</u>	50	42	28	34
18-24	4	3.0	146	<u>16</u>	48	32	18	55
25-40	10	1.5	36	4	51	34	22	43

N: number of animals.
C: clinical score.
Leuco: total CSF leucocytes (cells/mm^3).
% Gr: percentage of granulocytes in relation to total CSF cells.
W3/13, W3/25, Ox 8, Ox 6: percentage of mononuclear cells stained with these markers.
EAE 5-10: 5-10 days after sensitization; incubation period.
11-15: early clinical disease.
18-24: peak of clinical disease.
25-40: recovery phase.
Underlined values are significantly different from controls ($p<0.001$).

Composition of Inflammatory Infiltrates in Spinal Cord Lesions of Acute EAE Animals

A small number of T-lymphocytes and Ia-positive cells were found in the CNS tissue of normal control animals. In these animals the vast majority of leucocytes was located in the meninges. Within the tissue itself few T-lymphocytes were found scattered within the parenchyma, whereas Ia^+

cells were mainly found in perivascular position (Lassmann et al., 1986; Vas et al., 1986) (Table 2). During the incubation period of the disease some increase of T-lymphocytes was found mainly in the meninges, accompanied by increased numbers of Ia^+ cells in the nervous parenchyma. The peak of inflammatory reaction in the CNS tissue coincided with the peak of clinical disease (18-24 days after sensitization). Concerning T-lymphocyte subsets in the early phases, $W3/13^+$, Ox 8^- T-cells dominated, whereas during recovery most of the T-cells within the lesions carried the Ox 8 antigen. This shift in T-cell subpopulations was first noted in the meninges (as early as 11-15 days after sensitization) and then appeared with several days delay in the perivascular compartment and the parenchyma itself (Table 2). T-lymphocyte infiltration in acute EAE lesions was accompanied by massive expression of Ia-antigens on inflammatory cells in the lesions (Table 2).

No major fluctuations of leucocyte subsets were noted in the peripheral blood of acute EAE animals.

Table 2. Quantitative evaluation of leucocytes in the CNS of control and EAE animals (values given in cells/mm^2 of tissue).

	MENINGES			PERIVASCULAR			SPINAL CORD		
	W3/13	Ox 8	Ox 6	W3/13	Ox 8	Ox 6	W3/13	Ox 8	Ox 6
Controls	73	52	259	0.07	0.03	0.22	0.22	0.18	0.02
EAE									
5-10	107	29	205	0.08	0.02	0.20	0.13	0.04	0.20
11-15	264	182	440	6.5	2.9	14.2	14.7	2.8	27.3
18-24	<u>1106</u>	<u>656</u>	<u>1792</u>	<u>25.0</u>	<u>8.7</u>	<u>45.8</u>	<u>52.1</u>	<u>16.7</u>	<u>51.7</u>
25-40	<u>285</u>	<u>229</u>	435	<u>5.6</u>	<u>4.4</u>	<u>10.8</u>	<u>58.8</u>	<u>29.6</u>	<u>33.2</u>

The same animals were evaluated as listed in Table 1. The values represent means of counts (Cells/mm^2) obtained in individual animals of the representative groups. Underlined values are significantly elevated compared to controls ($p<0.001$).

Correlation between CSF Leucocytes and Inflammatory Reaction in the Spinal Cord Lesions

Evidently there was a significant correlation between the total number of CSF leucocytes and the number of T-lymphocytes and Ia^+ cells in the spinal cord tissue, reflecting the overall severity of the inflammatory process. (Table 3). There was, however, no correlation at all between the relative composition of T-cell subsets in the CSF and the spinal cord lesions. Accordingly, determination of W3/25 : Ox 8 ratio in the CSF did not allow conclusions on the composition of T-cell subsets in the lesions. We found, however, a weak negative correlation between the percentage of Ox 8^+ cells in the CSF and the overall severity of the inflammatory process in the CNS tissue.

The most clearcut correlation between CSF and spinal cord lesions was found regarding Ia^+ mononuclear cells. In general terms, the higher the percentage of Ia^+ cells in the CSF was found, the more intense and severe was the inflammatory process in the nervous tissue (Table 3).

Table 3. Correlation between CSF leucocytes and inflammatory reaction in meninges and spinal cord tissue in rat acute EAE

		MENINGES				SPINAL CORD		
		Clin	W3/13	Ox 8	Ox 6	W3/13	Ox 8	Ox 6
	Leuco	+*	n.s.	n.s.	+*	+**	+*	+***
C	% Gr	n.s.	n.s.	n.s.	n.s.	n.s.	n.s.	n.s.
	%W3/13	n.s.	n.s.	n.s.	n.s.	n.s.	n.s.	n.s.
S	%W3/25	n.s.	n.s.	n.s.	n.s.	n.s.	n.s.	n.s.
	%Ox 8	-*	-*	-*	-*	-**	-*	-*
F	H/S	n.s.	n.s.	n.s.	n.s.	n.s.	n.s.	n.s.
	%Ox 6	+***	+***	+***	+***	+***	+***	+***

Linear regression analysis.
+: positive correlation.
-: negative correlation.
*: $P < 0.05$.
**: $P < 0.01$.
***: $P < 0.001$.
n.s.: no significant correlation.
H/S: W3/25:Ox 8 ratio.

DISCUSSION

Although many studies have focused on the inflammatory reaction in EAE (Sriram et al., 1982; Hauser et al., 1984; Traugott et al., 1985; Sobel et al., 1984; Hickey et al., 1983; Wekerle 1984, Lassmann et al., 1986), relatively little information is available on the cellular composition of the CSF during evolution of the disease. There is good agreement, that in acute as well as chronic EAE the majority of CSF cells, regardless the stage of the disease, are T-lymphocytes (Wilkerson et al., 1978; Suckling et al., 1986). In addition, a variable number of monocytes has been described in EAE CSF, their percentage apparently increasing during active disease (Suckling et al., 1983, 1986). In contrast to our present study, the percentage of Ia^+ cells in the CSF was found to be high in all stages of acute and chronic EAE, without apparent relation to disease activity. This may be due to interspecies differences, since in guinea pigs a proportion of T-lymphocytes carries Ia-antigens even under normal conditions (Burger et al., 1984).

The increase in the percentage of Ia^+ cells in the CSF was found in our present study to be the best marker for disease activity, either when correlated with clinical disease or with the degree of inflammation in the CNS tissue. When adding the number of Ia^+ cells with total T-lymphocytes it was apparent that in addition to monocytes/macrophages also some T-lymphocytes carry Class II histocompatibility antigens. This finding is not surprising, since T-cells may become Ia^+ under stimulation conditions (Hammerling and Eichman 1976, Yamashita and Shevach 1977). A similar phenomenon was also found in the CNS lesions. In severely affected animals all inflammatory cells in perivascular cuffs were found to carry Ia antigens, in spite of the presence of numerous T-lymphocytes in this location (Lassmann et al., 1986). A similar, however less pronounced increase of Ia^+ mononuclear cells has been described in human CSF samples of patients with active multiple sclerosis (Kuroda and Shibasaki 1985), whereas others did not find a correlation between Ia-expression on CSF cells and disease activity (Hauser et al., 1985). This is surprising, since numerous Ia^+ cells are present in active multiple sclerosis lesions (Traugott et al., 1983). However, events occuring within the CNS tissue distant from the site of CSF puncture not necessarily have to be reflected by alterations in the spinal fluid (Kitz et al., 1984).

To our knowledge no studies are available on T-lymphocyte subsets in the CSF of EAE animals. In our present study we did not find correlations between T-cell subsets in the CSF and clinical disease activity or the inflammatory reaction in the spinal cord tissue respectively. Even more important was, that the relative composition of T-lymphocyte subsets in the CSF was entirely different compared to that in the CNS lesions and even to that in the meninges. Thus studies on antigen specificity and functional properties of T-lymphocytes obtained from CSF samples, may give little information about the actual events occuring in the CNS lesions of inflammatory diseases.

ACKNOWLEDGEMENTS

We are indebted to Mrs. H. Breitschopf, Ms. S. Katzensteiner and Ms. A. Cervenka for skillful technical assistance.

REFERENCES

1. R. Burger, I. Scher, S.O. Sharrow and E.M. Shevach. Non-activated guinea pig T cells and thymocytes express Ia antigens: FACS-analysis with alloantibodies and monoclonal antibodies. Immunology. 51:93-102 (1984).
2. D.A. Hafler, M. Buchsbaum, D. Johnson and H.L. Weiner. Phenotypic and functional analysis of T cells cloned directly from the blood and cerebrospinal fluid of patients with multiple sclerosis. Ann. Neurol. 18:451-458 (1984).
3. G.J. Hammerling and K. Eichmann. Expression of Ia determinants on immunocompetent cells. Eur. J. Immunol. 6:565-569 (1976).
4. S.L. Hauser, A.K. Bhan, M. Che, F. Gilles and H.L. Weiner. Redistribution of Lyt-bearing cells in acute murine experimental allergic encephalomyelitis: selective migration of Lyt-1 cells to the central nervous system is associated with a transient depletion of Lyt-1 cells in peripheral blood. J. Immunol. 133:3037-3042 (1984).
5. S.L. Hauser, E.L. Reinherz, C.L. Hoban, S.F. Schlossman and H.L. Weiner. CSF cells in multiple sclerosis: monoclonal antibody analysis and relationship to peripheral blood T-cell subsets. Neurology. 33:575-579 (1983).
6. W.F. Hickey, N.K. Gonatas, H. Kimura and D.B. Wilson. Identification and quantitation of T lymphocyte subsets in the spinal cord of the Lewis rat during acute experimental allergic encephalomyelitis. J. Immunol. 131: 2805-2809 (1983).
7. K. Kitz, H. Lassmann and H.M. Wisniewski. Isolated leptomeninges of the spinal cord: an ideal tool to study inflammatory reaction in EAE. Acta Neuropathol. Suppl. VII:179-181 (1981).

8. K. Kitz, H. Lassmann, D. Karcher and A. Lowenthal. Blood-brain-barrier in chronic relapsing experimental allergic encephalomyelitis: a correlative study between cerebrospinal fluid protein concentrations and tracer leakage in the central nervous system. Acta Neuropathol. 63:41-50 (1984).
9. Y. Kuroda and H. Shibasaki. Peripheral blood and CSF T-cell subsets in Japanese MS patients. Neurology. 35:270-273 (1985).
10. H. Lassmann. "Comparative neuropathology of chronic relapsing experimental allergic encephalomyelitis and multiple sclerosis." Springer Verlag, Berlin-Heidelberg. (1983).
11. H. Lassmann, K. Kitz and H.M. Wisniewski. Structural variability of demyelinating lesions in different models of subacute and chronic experimental allergic encephalomyelitis. Acta Neuropathol. 51:191-201 (1980).
12. H. Lassmann, K. Vass, Ch. Brunner and F. Seitelberger. Characterization of inflammatory infiltrates in experimental allergic encephalomyelitis. Progr. Neuropathol. Vol. 6, in press.(1986).
13. E.C. Laterre. Cerebrospinal fluid in pathology. La Ricerca Clin. Lab. 4:540-566 (1974).
14. H. Link and G. Tibbling. Principles of albumin and IgG analysis in neurological disorders. III. Evaluation of IgG synthesis within the central nervous system in multiple sclerosis. Scand. J. clin. Lab. Invest. 37:397-401 (1977).
15. D. Santoli, E.C. Defreitas, M. Sandberg-Wollheim, M.K. Francis and H. Koprowski. Phenotypic and functional characterization of T-cell clones derived from the cerebrospinal fluid of multiple sclerosis patients. J. Immunol. 132:2386-2392 (1984).
16. R.A. Sobel, B.W. Blanchette, A.K. Bhan and R.B. Colvin. The immunopathology of experimental allergic encephalomyelitis. I. Quantitative analysis of inflammatory cells in situ. J. Immunol. 132:2393-2401 (1984).
17. S. Sriram; D. Solomon, R.V. Rouse and L. Steinman. Identification of T-cell subsets and B lymphocytes in mouse brain experimental allergic encephalitis lesions. J. Immunol. 129:1649-1651 (1982).
18. A.J. Suckling, N.R. Wilson, J.A. Kirby and M.G. Rumsby. CR-EAE: CSF cytology and a comparison with meningeal and spinal cord pathology. Neuropathol. appl. Neurobiol. 9:237-249 (1983).
19. A.J. Suckling, P.W. Baron, U. Mauer, R. Burger and M.G. Rumsby. Quantitative analysis of the cellular constituents of the cerebrospinal fluid in chronic relapsing experimental allergic encephalomyelitis. J. Neuroimmunol. 11:57-66 (1986).
20. W.W. Tourtellotte. Multiple sclerosis cerebrospinal fluid. In: P.J. Vinken and G.W. Bruyn, eds. "Handbook of Clinical Neurology". North-Holland Publ. Comp. Amsterdam. (1970).
21. U. Traugott, E.L. Reinherz and C.S. Raine. Multiple sclerosis: distribution of T-cells, T-cell subsets and Ia positive macrophages in lesions of different ages. J. Neuroimmunol. 4:201-221 (1983).
22. U. Traugott, C.S. Raine and D.E. McFarlin. Acute experimental allergic encephalomyelitis in the mouse: Immunopathology of the developing lesion. Cell. Immunol. 91:240-254 (1985).
23. K. Vass, H. Lassmann, H. Wekerle and H.M. Wisniewski. The distribution of Ia antigen in the lesions of acute experimental allergic encephalomyelitis. Acta Neuropathol. In press (1986).
24. H. Wekerle. The lesion of acute experimental autoimmune encephalomyelitis: isolation and membrane phenotypes of perivascular infiltrates from encephalitic rat brain white matter. Lab. Invest. 51:199-205 (1984).
25. L.D. Wilkerson, R.P. Lisak and B. Zweiman. CSF lymphocytes in EAE. Clin. Exp. Immunol. 34:87-91 (1978).

ANALYSIS OF THE INTRATHECAL HUMORAL IMMUNE RESPONSE IN CORONA VIRUS INDUCED ENCEPHALOMYELITIS OF RATS

Rüdiger Dörries, Rihito Watanabe, Helmut Wege and Volker ter Meulen

Institute of Virology and Immunobiology, University of Würzburg, Versbacher Str. 7, D-8700 Würzburg
Fed. Rep. of Germany

INTRODUCTION

In recent years animal models of virus-induced primary demyelination in the central nervous system (CNS) have offered a promising approach to the understanding of pathological mechanisms leading to Multiple Sclerosis (MS), the most important demyelinating disease of man with an unknown etiology (1,2,3,4). Amongst these animal models, the induction of demyelination in rats by Coronavirus JHM, a mouse hepatitis virus, exhibits many interesting features with respect to possible immune-mediated mechanisms of myelin damage.

Intracerebral infection of rats with JHM virus result in different diseases, including acute lethal encephalitis (AE) and subacute demyelinating encephalomyelitis (SDE) (5). The outcome of the disease is influenced by the type of virus and the age and strain of animal. With respect to MS, the most interesting type of disease, SDE, is seen upon intracerebral infection of weanling Lewis rats with JHM wild type virus (JHM-WT) or suckling rats with TS 43, a temperature sensitive mutant of JHM (JHM-TS43) (6). Clinically, these animals suffer from hindleg paralysis, ataxic gait and severe impairment of growth. Histologically SDE animals exhibit plaques of primary demyelination in the brain and spinal cord, in the context of perivascular cuffs of mononuclear cells. Virus seems to persist for long times but viral antigens are demonstrable only in phases of clinically apparent disease (7,8,9,10). Some animals exhibit disease courses with remissions and relapses, even months after infection (11). The involvement of the immune system in the pathology of the disease is indicated by the findings of Watanabe et al. (12), who demonstrated, that lymphocytes from SDE animals upon transfer to healthy syngeneic recipients produce perivascular cuffs characteristic for experimental allergic encephalitis (EAE).

The Brown Norway (BN) rat, which is known not to be susceptible to the induction of EAE behaves differently upon intracerebral infection with JHM-WT virus. Although the AE type of the disease is induced sometimes, clinical signs of a delayed type of disease are extremely rare. However, histological examination of clinically healthy BN rats reveals marked demyelination in periventricular areas of the brain, often accompanied by signs of remyelination. Viral antigen is demonstrable several weeks after infection and cell infiltrates in demyelinated areas consist predominantly of plasma cells and not of macrophages, as in the case of the Lewis rat (13).

The significant plasma cell infiltration and absence of clinically noticable disease in BN rats is in contrast to the perivascular cuffs and macrophage infiltration in paralysed Lewis rats. Therefore, it seemed likely that a comparison of the humoral immune response in these two rat strains might give some insight into the role of antibodies in SDE. Therefore, paired serum- and cerebrospinal fluid specimens from Lewis rats suffering from clinically visible SDE and apparently healthy JHM virus inoculated BN rats were used to examine the state of the blood brain barrier (BBB) and the JHM-specific antibody response with respect to titers, site of synthesis and clonal distribution.

MATERIAL AND METHODS

Animals

Lewis rats. In order to get the highest possible rate of SDE, Lewis rats were infected intracerebrally with 10^4-10^5 plaque forming units (PFU) of the TS 43 variant of JHM virus. Rats showing clinical signs of SDE within the 4th to 18th week after virus inoculation were killed. Serum was collected by heart puncture and CSF was taken from the cisterna magna (14,15). Blood contamination of CSF samples was controlled by counting red blood cells (RBC) after staining an aliquot with crystal violet to discriminate nucleated cells from RBC. Samples containing more than 5×10^3 RBC per µl were not included in this study.

BN rats. BN rats were inoculated intracerebrally with 10^4-10^5 PFU of JHM-WT virus. Clinically healthy animals were killed between the 5th and 8th week after infection and examined for histopathological changes in the CNS. Only specimens from animals with noticable demyelination were analysed. Blood and CSF samples were taken as described for Lewis rats.

Virus

Virus (TS 43 and WT) was propagated in murine Sac(-) cells as described earlier (6). For the purposes of ELISA and immunoblots, viral antigens were extracted from the supernatant of tissue culture infected cells as described by Wege et al. (16). Virus antigen free control preparations were purified according to the same procedure as viral antigens.

Analysis of the Blood Brain Barrier (BBB)

The CSF/serum ratio of albumin was used to control the leakiness of the BBB for small proteins. The Ig-index, calculated according to Christensen et al. (17), was used to determine intrathecal Ig synthesis. Albumin concentrations in serum and CSF were determined by rocket immune electrophoresis and Ig concentrations by an ELISA (18). Normal reference values for CSF/serum ratios of immunoglobulins and albumin were calculated from healthy, noninoculated animals.

The virus specific antibody index determined from CSF/serum ratios of virus specific titers and albumin (19) was taken to evaluate intrathecal synthesis of JHM specific antibody. The reference index for specific antibodies was calculated from serum and CSF samples from animals hyperimmunized intraperitoneally with JHM virus, measles virus and a non-viral protein (keyhole limpet hemocyanine) by priming with 400 /µg protein precipitated in alaun and 10^{10} particles of pertussis bordetella. A booster injection was given 14-21 days later with 400 /μg of soluble protein.

Titration of JHM specific antibodies

Antibodies specific for JHM virus were titrated in serum and CSF specimens by an enzyme-immuno-assay (EIA) as described (16). Samples were considered to be positive for virus specific antibodies if the control antigen corrected absorbance at 496 nm was equal or higher than 0.2. The titer of a sample was defined as the last dilution exhibiting this cut-off value.

Isoelectric distribution of Ig and JHM-specific antibodies

Analysis of the electrophoretic distribution of total Ig and JHM-specific antibodies was done by a modified affinity-mediated immunoblot (AMI) (18,20). Serum samples were diluted to the same Ig concentration as determined in the corresponding CSF sample. Aliquots of 20 /μl were isoelectrically focused in a 0.5 mm thick agarose gel in the pH range 3.0 - 10.5. Immediately after electrophoretic separation of the proteins, the gel was overlayed by a nitrocellulose filter, passively loaded with either rabbit-anti-rat Ig (Rab-a-Rat Ig) or with JHM virus (EIA grade). After 60 min at room temperature filters were removed and passed through a cycle of 3 washings. To detect the pattern of total Ig on the Rab-a-Rat Ig coated filter and the pattern of JHM-specific antibody bound to the viral antigen coated filter, both filters were incubated for 60 min in Rab-a-Rat Ig labelled with horseradish peroxidase (Rab-a-Rat Ig^{POD}). After a further washing cycle filters were developed in 4-chloro-naphthol, a colourless substrate for peroxidase which is converted to a waterinsoluble blue-violet precipitate in the presence of H_2O_2. Stained bands on the filter indicate either the isoelectric pattern of total Ig (Rab-a-Rat Ig coated filter) or the isoelectric pattern of JHM virus-specific Ig (JHM antigen coated filter).

RESULTS

JHM-virus specific antibodies in serum and CSF

Virus-specific antibodies in serum and CSF were titered in both rat populations by enzyme-immuno-assay (EIA). Due to a shortage of CSF from SDE diseased Lewis rats, CSF titers could only be determined for 7 from 10 animals. The results are summarized in Fig.1. In Lewis rats JHM-specific antibody titers (> 1:100) were detected in 7 from 10 serum specimens and 4 animals from 7 displayed virus-specific antibodies in the CSF. In comparison, BN rats revealed virus-specific antibodies in serum more frequently, 10 from 10 animals, and 8 of these animals revealed JHM-specific antibodies in the paired CSF samples. Moreover, compared to the Lewis rats, the titers in BN rats were higher (approx. 5-fold in serum and 4-fold in CSF), thus supporting the idea, that the generation of high levels of virus-specific antibodies in the CNS compartment can protect the animal from severe clinical disease.

The titration of CSF specimens revealed the presence of JHM virus specific antibodies, but no conclusion could be drawn with respect to the site of synthesis of these antibodies. To answer this question, virus-specific antibody indices (SAB-index) were calculated in analogy to the Ig-indices. In this calculation, the CSF/serum ratio of JHM virus specific titers was divided by the CSF/serum ratio of albumin concentrations. As a reference SAB-indices were calculated in serum- and CSF specimens from healthy rats which had been hyperimmunized with JHM virus, measles virus and non-viral antigens intraperitoneally. The results are shown in figure 2. Taken together, these data show that a high proportion of the virus-specific antibodies of Lewis- as well as of BN rats are synthesized within the CNS, suggesting the intrathecal presence of antibody producing B-cells in these animals.

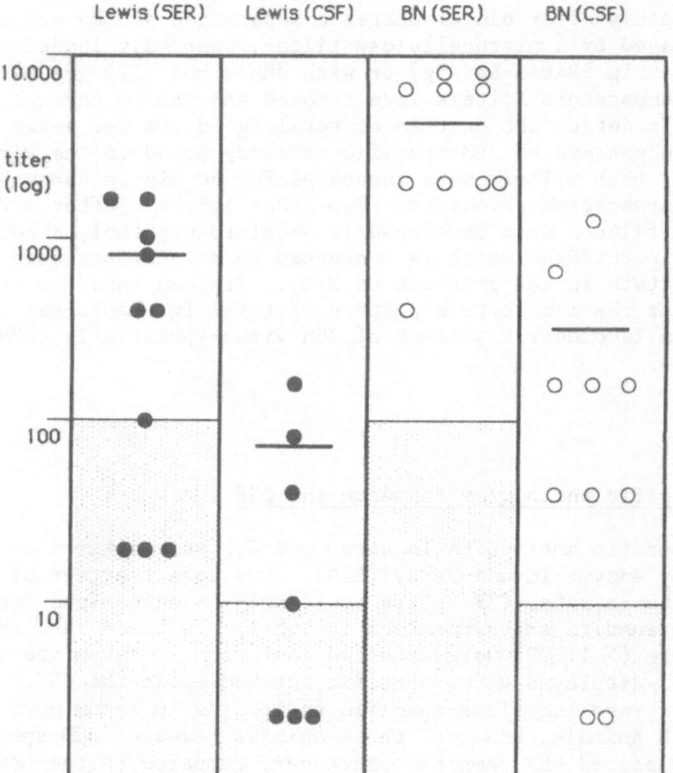

Fig.1. Virus-specific antibody titers in SDE diseased Lewis rats and clinically inapparent BN rats, after intra-cerebral infection with Coronavirus.

Each dot represents one animal. Dots in the shaded areas were scored as antibody negative. The solid horizontal bar in each box indicates the mean titer of that group.

● = Lewis rats ○ = BN rats

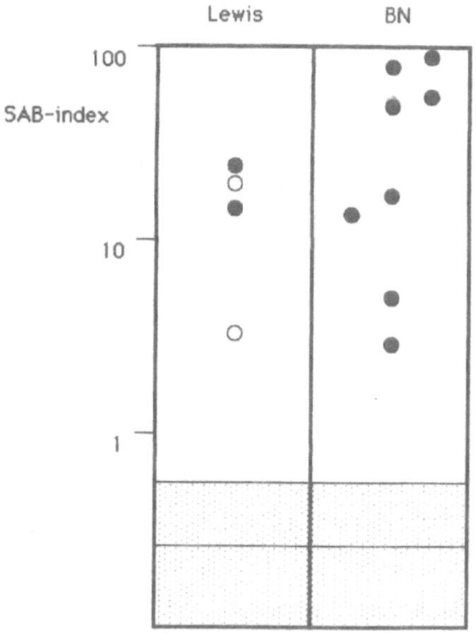

Fig.2. Virus-specific antibody indices in SDE diseased Lewis rats and clinically inapparent BN rats after intracerebral infection with Coronavirus.

Each dot represents one animal. The shaded area indicates the mean specific antibody index (2x the standard deviation added) of animals hyperimmunized with different viral antigens (JHM virus, measles virus) and a non-viral antigen (Keyhole Limpet Hemo cyanine). Animals falling outside this area do show intrathecal synthesis of JHM-specific antibodies.

● = CSF/serum ratio for albumin undisturbed
○ = CSF/serum ratio for albumin increased

State of the blood brain barrier

To evaluate the state of the BBB in the infected animals, Ig indices were calculated according to Christensen et al. (17). As a reference, normal Ig indices were calculated from non-inoculated Lewis- and BN rats (10 and 15 animals respectively) at the age of 5 to 10 weeks. The established mean Ig-index was 0.53 ± 0.28. Ig-indices higher than the cut-off value (mean value + 2x the standard deviation) were taken as an indication of intrathecal Ig synthesis. The calculated Ig-indices from infected Lewis and BN rats are shown in Fig.3.

The differences between the SDE diseased Lewis group and the clinically inapparent BN group were marginal. However, Lewis rats did show an increased permeability for small proteins, probably due to the severe disease process taking place in the CNS. The level of intrathecal Ig-synthesis was almost identical in both groups. However, by comparing the result of this analysis with the data on the intrathecal synthesis of JHM specific antibodies, an interesting observation can be made. Whereas BN rats synthesize JHM-specific antibodies intrathecally in 8 from 10 animals only 4 from 10 animals displayed increased Ig-indices. Obviously, intrathecal antibody responses to the virus infection did not necessarily cause an overall increase of CSF/serum ratio for total immunoglobulin. On the other hand, 3 from 10 Lewis rats were shown to have an increased Ig-index,

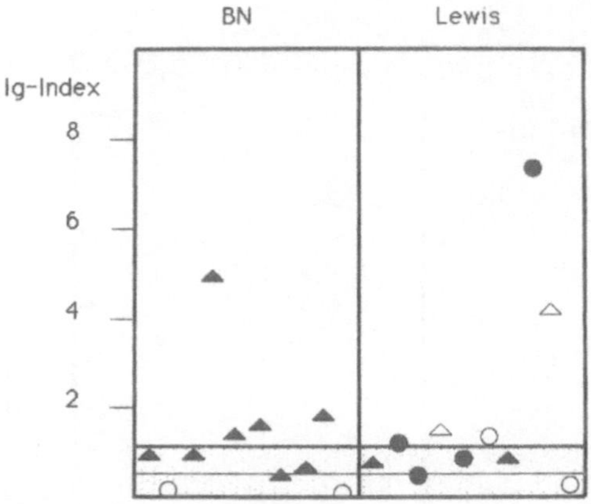

Fig.3. Immunoglobulin (Ig) indices in SDE diseased Lewis rats and clinically inapparent BN rats, after intracerebral infection with Coronavirus.

Dots and triangles represent individual animals. The shaded area indicates the mean Ig index (2x the standard deviation added) of healthy BN- and Lewis rats.

▲ = CSF/serum ratio for albumin undisturbed, intrathecal JHM virus-specific antibody synthesis

● = CSF/serum ratio for albumin undisturbed

△ = CSF/serum ratio for albumin increased, intrathecal, JHM virus-specific antibody synthesis

○ = CSF/serum ratio for albumin increased

but no detectable virus-specific antibody production in the CSF. This could probably indicate, that during the course of the SDE disease antibody reactions of an autoreactive nature were induced.

Isoelectric patterns of CSF derived immunoglobulins and JHM-specific antibodies

The intrathecal synthesis of antibodies in rats with a specificity for viral antigens as well as for unknown antigens raised the question of the clonal nature of these immunoglobulins. Therefore, attempts were made to characterize the CSF derived Ig, with respect to their isoelectric distribution and antigen-specificity using an affinity-mediated immunoblot. Due to a high sensitivity and specificity, this technique is able to detect the isoelectric distribution of total- as well as antigen specific immunoglobulins in small aliquots (20 /µl) of native CSF. Typical examples for this type of analysis are shown in Fig.4 to 6.

Two interesting observations have to be mentioned. Firstly, the virus-specific antibody response in Lewis- as well as in BN rats could be characterized as oligoclonal and intrathecal, since identical bands were not detectable in corresponding serum specimens, adjusted to the same Ig concentration as the paired CSF specimen. However, there were noticable differences in the quantity of bands detectable. Healthy BN rats (Fig.4) responded more vigorously to the virus than SDE diseased Lewis rats did (Fig.5). Secondly, those Lewis rats showing no intrathecal synthesis of

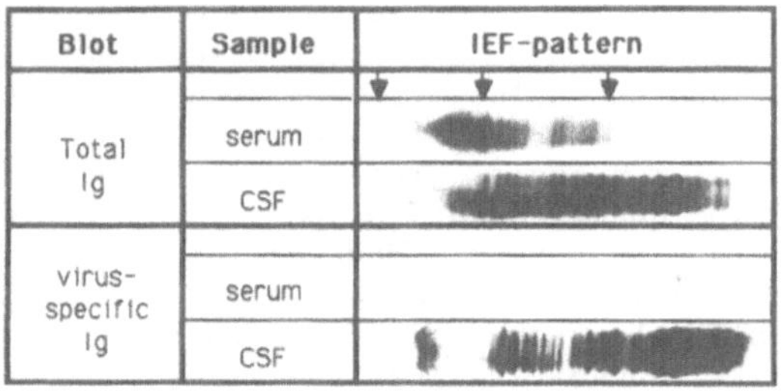

Fig.4. Isoelectric distribution of immunoglobulins in serum and CSF of a BN rat, clinically inapparent after intracerebral infection with Coronavirus.

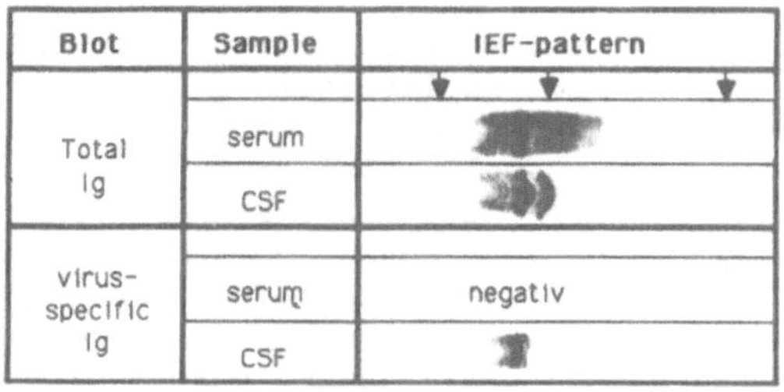

Blot
Sample
IEF-pattern
Total Ig
serum
CSF
virus-specific Ig
serum
negativ
CSF

Fig.5. Isoelectric distribution of immunoglobulins in serum and CSF of a Lewis rat, clinically diseased by SDE after intracerebral infection with Coronavirus.

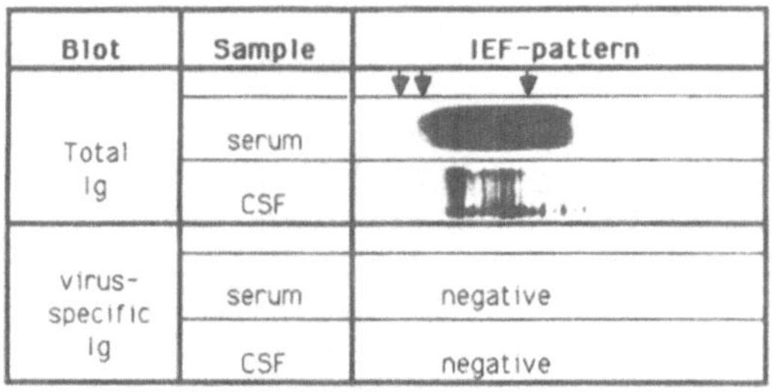

Blot
Sample
IEF-pattern
Total Ig
serum
CSF
virus-specific Ig
serum
negative
CSF
negative

Fig.6. Isoelectric distribution of immunoglobulins in serum and CSF of a Lewis rat, clinically diseased by SDE after intracerebral infection with Coronavirus.

JHM-specific antibodies sometimes revealed patterns of restricted heterogeneity of total immunoglobulins (Fig.6), even in cases where no elevated Ig-indices were detected. This finding strengthened the idea, that in animals which could not control the intracerebral infection, autoreactive immune reactions might have occurred as a consequence of severe tissue destruction.

DISCUSSION

In this study we have investigated the intrathecal humoral response in Lewis and BN rats following intracerebral infection with the murine coronavirus MHV JHM. In the first series of experiments, Coronavirus specific antibodies were titered in serum- and CSF specimens by micro-enzyme-immuno assay. Both groups raised JHM-specific antibody titers in serum- as well as in the CSF and the calculation of specific antibody indices revealed that the presence of JHM-specific antibodies in the CSF could be explained by intrathecal synthesis. The same observation was made by Sorensen et al. (21) who quantitated JHM specific antibodies in serum and CSF of inoculated Lewis Wistar rats. However, differences between the two types of rat were striking. The diseased Lewis rats responded less frequently and with considerably lower titers in the CSF compared to the clinically healthy BN rats, suggesting that the virus specific antibody response carries protective- rather than pathological character. This finding is supported by observations from another animal model of primary demyelination. In Canine distemper virus-induced demyelination in dogs, the presence of high titers of virus-specific antibodies is seen in clinically healthy animals, whereas animals suffering from the demyelinating late disease exhibit only moderate or low titers (22).

Interestingly, in both groups of animals intrathecal, JHM-specific antibody responses were not necessarily reflected by an increase of the Ig-index. In the BN rats twice as many animals were found to synthesize JHM-specific antibodies intrathecally than animals displaying increased Ig-indices. This leads to the conclusion that the absence of an increased Ig-index and clinically noticable disease, does not exclude an ongoing virus-induced demyelination process accompanied by a significant agent-specific antibody response. Similar observations have been made in Mumps-virus-induced meningitis of man (23), where in some cases the intra-blood-brain barrier synthesis of virus-specific antibodies did not result in an increased Ig-index.

On the other hand, in some Lewis rats there was a significant increase of the Ig-index but no detectable JHM virus specific intrathecal antibody synthesis. This suggests that the stimulation of intrathecal Ig-synthesis in JHM virus-induced demyelination is not only caused by the etiological agent itself, but may be triggered by non-viral, possibly autoantigens.

In the second series of experiments we studied the clonal distribution of CSF and serum derived JHM antibodies. In analogy to virus-induced demyelination in man, the analysis of the clonal distribution of CSF- and serum derived Ig revealed, in both BN and Lewis rats, the presence of oligoclonal Ig, carrying virus-specific nature. This points to the chronic persistent character of the intracerebral JHM virus infection in these animals. However, differences in the number and staining intensity of virus-specific antibody bands between the diseased Lewis- and the clinically healthy BN group, gave the impression that the severe disease in the Lewis rats is the consequence of the significantly lower intensity of the oligoclonal reaction in these animals. Either those antibodies, which are necessary to prevent the spread of the virus, were not produced at all or in an amount which is not sufficient to control the infection.

In the coronavirus animal model, the important role of individual virus-specific antibody clones for the outcome of the infection is suggested by the findings of Massa et al. (24) who were able to show that UV-inactivated JHM virus can induce immunoregulatory molecules (Ia) in embryonic astrocytes from Lewis rats. This induction event can be prevented by the presence of a monoclonal antibody specific for a virus-specific glycoprotein (E2). The full consequences of the virus-dependent induction of Ia on astrocytes are not yet known, but it is not unlikely that autoimmunological events may follow which are characterized by the generation of autoreactive lymphocytes (12) and the stimulation of a restricted number of B-cells producing immunoglobulins, as seen in the oligoclonal Ig-pattern displayed in some of the Lewis rats described in this study.

To examine differences in the nature of JHM-specific antibodies, as well as immunoglobulins of unknown specificity, synthesized intrathecally in SDE diseased and non-diseased but virus-inoculated rats, we are presently characterizing CSF and serum specimens for their specificity for individual viral proteins and/or self antigens of neural nature.

ACKNOWLEDGEMENT

This work was supported by the Deutsche Forschungsgemeinschaft and Hertie-Stiftung. We thank Andrea Deutscher for her expert technical assistance and Helga Kriesinger for preparing the manuscript.

REFERENCES

1. W.P.Weiner, R.T. Johnson and R.M. Herndon. Viral infections and demyelinating diseases. New. Eng. J. Med. 288:1103-1110 (1973).
2. P.W. Lampert. Autoimmune and virus-induced demyelinating diseases. Am. J. Pathol. 91:176-208 (1978).
3. M.C. Dal Canto and S.G. Rabinowitz. Experimental models of virus-induced demyelination of the central nervous system. Ann. Neurol. 11:109-127 (1982).
4. A. Friedman and Y. Lorch. Theiler's virus infection: A model for multiple sclerosis. Prog. med. Virol. 31:43-83 (1985).
5. H. Wege, S.G. Siddell and V. ter Meulen. The biology and pathogenesis of Coronaviruses. Curr. Top. Microbiol. Immunol. 99:165-200 (1982).
6. H. Wege, M. Koga, R. Watanabe, K. Nagashima and V. ter Meulen. Neurovirulence of murine Coronavirus JHM temperature sensitive mutants in rats. Infect. Immun. 39:1316-1324 (1983).
7. K. Nagashima, H. Wege, R. Meyermann and V. ter Meulen. Coronavirus induced subacute demyelinating encephalomyelitis in rats: a morpho logical analysis. Acta Neuropathol. (Berl.) 44:63-70 (1978).
8. K. Nagashima, H. Wege, R. Meyermann and V. ter Meulen. Demyelinating encephalomyelitis induced by a long-term Corona Virus Infection in rats. Acta Neuropathol. (Berl.) 45:205-213 (1979).
9. O. Sorensen, D. Percy and S. Dales. In vivo and in vitro models of demyelinating diseases. III. JHM Virus Infection of rats. Arch Neurol. 37:478-484 (1980).
10. M. Koga, H. Wege and V. ter Meulen. Sequence of Murine Coronavirus JHM induced neuropathological changes in rats. Neuropath. Appl. Neurobiol. 10:173-184 (1984).
11. H. Wege, R. Watanabe and V. ter Meulen. Relapsing subacute demyelinating encephalomyelitis in rats during the course of Coronavirus JHM Infection. J. Neuroimmunol. 6:325-336 (1984a).
12. R. Watanabe, H. Wege and V. ter Meulen. Adoptive transfer of EAE-like lesions from rats with Coronavirus-induced demyelinating encephalomyelitis. Nature. 305:150-153 (1983).
13. R. Watanabe. In preparation.
14. H. Reiber and O. Schunck. Suboccipital puncture of Guinea Pigs. Lab. Animals. 17:25-27 (1983).
15. J.O. Fleming, J.Y.P. Ting, S.A. Stohlman and L.P. Weiner. Improve ments in obtaining and characterizing mouse cerebrospinal fluid. J. Neuroimmunol. 4:129-140 (1983).
16. H. Wege and R. Dörries. Hybridoma antibodies to the murine Corona virus JHM: Characterization of epitopes on the Peplomer Protein (E2). J. Gen. Virol. 65:1931-1942 (1984b).

17. O. Christensen, J. Clausen and T. Fog. Relationships between abnormal IgG index, oligoclonal bands, acute phase reactants and some clinical data in multiple sclerosis. J. Neurol. 218:237-244 (1978).
18. R. Dörries, R. Watanabe, H. Wege and V. ter Meulen. Murine Coronavirus-induced encephalomyelitis in rats: analysis of immunoglobulins and virus-specific antibodies in serum and cerebrospinal fluid. J. Neuroimmunol. in press.
19. T. Arnadottir, M. Reunanen and A. Salmi. Intrathecal synthesis of virus antibodies in multiple sclerosis patients. Infect. Immun. 38:399-407 (1982).
20. R. Dörries and V. ter Meulen. Detection and identification of virus-specific oligoclonal IgG in unconcentrated cerebrospinal fluid by immunoblot technique. J. Neuroimmunol. 7:77-89 (1984).
21. O. Sorensen, M.B. Coulter-Mackie, S. Puchalski and S. Dales. In vivo and in vitro models of demeyelinating disease. IX. Progression of JHM virus infection in the central nervous system of the rat during overt and asymptomatic phases. Virology. 137:347-357 (1984).
22. S. Krakowa, R. Olsen, A. Confer, A. Koestner and B. McCullough. Serologic response to Canine distemper viral antigens in gnotobiotic dogs infected with Canine distemper virus. J. Infect. Dis. 132:384-392 (1975).
23. P. Ukkonen, M.L. Granström, J. Räsänen, E.M. Salonen and K. Pettinen. Local production of mumps IgG and IgM antibodies in the cerebrospinal fluid of meningitis patients. J. Med. Virol. 8:257-265 (1981).
24. P. Massa, R. Dörries and V. ter Meulen. Viral particles induce Ia antigen expression on astrocytes. Nature. 320: 543-546 (1986).

INTRATHECAL SYNTHESIS OF IMMUNOGLOBULINS IN MS PATIENTS

C.J.M. Sindic, L. Boon, M.P. Chalon and E.C. Laterre

Laboratory of Neurochemistry, University of Louvain Medical School, 53-59, Avenue E. Mounier, 1200 Brussels, Belgium

INTRODUCTION

In Multiple Sclerosis, the local intra-thecal production of IgG is a well-known feature, which is also observed in many persistent infections of the nervous tissue. However, all attempts at defining a MS-specific antigen have been unsuccessful and it is still not clear whether we are dealing with a response to a virus, an autoimmune reaction or some other manifestation of hypersensitivity unrelated to a putative MS-specific antigen.

The discrete bands observed in the cathodic region of agar gel electrophoresis represent the most frequent qualitative abnormality detectable in CSF from MS patients (Lowenthal et al., 1960). These bands have been demonstrated to represent mainly IgG produced by a limited number of B-cell clones, and the term "oligoclonal", as proposed by Laterre (1965) is now widely accepted to define these bands present in CSF but not or more faintly in blood. A high resolution technique such as isoelectric focusing may reveal up to 30 oligoclonal IgG bands; even in this case, some discrete IgG bands contain both kappa and lambda chains by immunofixation (Laurenzi et al., 1980, which indicates that they derive from more than one clone of cells. It should be also noted that some bands have been identified as kappa or lambda free light chains (Vandvik, 1977; Thompson and Vakaet, 1985). The presence of these free light chains is of uncertain significance. One explanation is the occurrence of a regulatory defect such as desynchronization between heavy and light chains assembly in antibody producing cells under intense immunogeic stimulation. Their presence was indeed strongly associated with pleocytosis and with recent exacerbation of the disease and thus perhaps, with a recent antigenic stimulation within the central nervous system (CNS) (Thompson and Vakaert, 1985).

The oligoclonal pattern is unique for each MS patient and seems very constant even when patients are studied over a long period or are in relapse (Olsson and Link, 1973; Vandvik,1977; Hershey and Trotter, 1980; Livrea et al., 1981; Walsh and Tourtellotte, 1986). However, Thompson et al. (1983) found sequential changes in oligoclonal pattern in 12 out of 25 patients who had a relapsing and remitting disease. By means of agar gel electrophoresis, we have also observed such changes in few patients. In any case, it should be noted that a relatively static electrophoretic pattern of IgG is not characteristic of repetitive antigenic stimulation (Montgomery and Pincus, 1973) and is different from what occurs in SSPE (Vandvik, 1977).

MEASUREMENT OF THE INTRA-THECAL SYNTHESIS OF IMMUNOGLOBULINS (Ig)

Several ratios or formulae have been proposed for the discrimination between the locally produced and the passively transudated IgG and for the quantitative assessment of this local production. The two most frequently used methods of calculation are the IgG index (Tibbling et al., 1977) and the Tourtellotte's formula (Tourtellotte et al., 1980).

Serum concentrations of Ig have a direct influence on their concentration in the CSF. In non-neurological patients, we found significant correlations between the serum and CSF concentrations of IgG ($N=52$; $r=0.35$; $p=0.01$), of IgM ($N=20$; $r=0.43$; $p=0.05$) and of IgA ($N=39$; $r=0.61$; $p<0.001$).

The index takes into account the influence of the serum concentration and the permeability of the blood-brain barrier (BBB), this latter factor being assessed by the gradient of albumin between the two compartments:

$$\frac{\text{CSF - Ig}}{\text{serum - Ig}} : \frac{\text{CSF albumin}}{\text{serum albumin}}$$

In presence of a BBB damage, each ratio should increase. The quotient between these two ratios, however, is expected to remain constant and of the same magnitude as in normal subjects (Tibbling et al., 1977). The Ig index is expected to increase only in cases where Ig are synthesized within the CNS. Our mean IgG index, 0.48, and the upper reference limit, 0.69, agree with the published values.

To test the validity of this method of calculation in case of BBB impairment, we have calculated an index for alpha$_2$-macroglobulin. If one admits that alpha$_2$-macroglobulin is never locally produced within the CNS and that the high molecular weight protein permeates the disturbed barrier in the same way as normal barrier, the index for alpha$_2$-macroglobulin must remain practically constant and independent of the BBB impairment, as assessed by the CSF/serum albumin ratio (Fig.1). This is true with only few exceptions, as in the acute phase of herpetic encephalitis; in this latter disease, one may expect a loss of the filtering function of the BBB due to the hemorhagic process (Sindic, 1985).

The formula of Tourtellotte et al. (1980) is also based on the use of albumin as a quantitative marker of the BBB permeability and on the proportional passage of IgG and albumin through an impaired BBB:

Local IgG synthesis in may per day :

$$\left\{\left(\text{CSF IgG}-\frac{\text{serum IgG}}{369}\right)-\left(\text{CSF albumin}-\frac{\text{serum albumin}}{230}\right)\left(\frac{\text{serum IgG}}{\text{serum albumin}}\right)0{,}43\right\} \times 5$$

where all concentrations actually found in patient's samples are expressed in mg/100 ml.

We used also this formula, slightly modified because our reference values for the serum/CSF ratio for albumin and IgG were 246 and 490 and not 230 and 369. However, it was not possible to use such a formula for

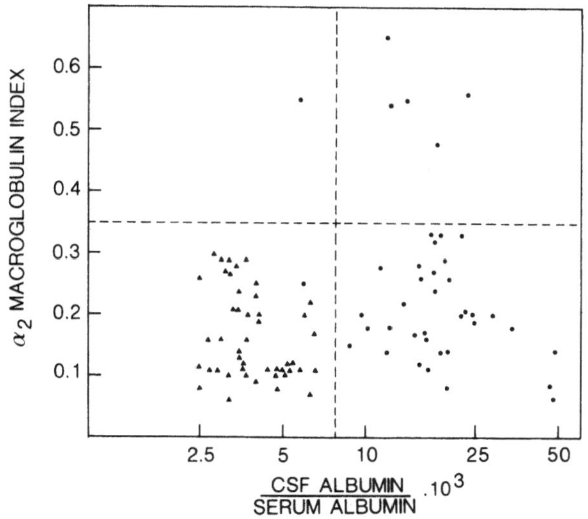

Fig.1. Relationship between the alpha$_2$-macroglobulin index and the BBB permeability assessed by the CSF/serum albumin ratio X 10^3, in 46 non-neurological patients (▲) and in 41 patients with various neurological disorders (●). Patients with post-traumatic hemorrhagic contusions, subarachnoid bleeding and brain hematoma were excluded. The index which remains practically constant and independent of the BBB impairment was however high in 4 patients with herpetic encephalitis (early sampling), 1 with pyogenic meningitis and 1 with MS.

the quantitative assessment of the local synthesis of IgM, IgA and IgE within the CNS, and we decided to choose the indices as method of calculation for the quantitative assessment of the local synthesis of these Ig isotypes.

THE IgM ASSAY IN CSF

IgM is present only in trace amounts in the normal CSF and was assayed by particle counting immunoassay (Sindic et al., 1982). In this automated technique, latex particles coated with antibodies are agglutinated by the antigen to be determined (Cambiaso et al., 1977; Masson et al., 1981). The use of F(ab')$_2$ fragments rather than whole antibody molecules prevents non-specific agglutination or inhibition of agglutination by proteins interacting with the Fc region of IgG. Agglutination is measured by counting residual unagglutinated particles in an optical cell counter whose electronics have been modified to ignore aggregates.

In a group of 50 non-neurological patients, the mean CSF IgM level, calculated on log values, was 130 µg/l with an upper reference limit of 400 µg/l (mean + 2 SD). In the serum of the control patients the mean, again calculated on log values, was 1,10 g/l and the mean serum/CSF ratio was therefore found to be 10,718. The IgM index had also a logarithmic normal distribution; the upper reference limit, which was set at 2 SD of log values above the mean (0.026) was found to be 0.079. Results of the determination of the IgM index in various neurological disorders are shown in Fig.2.

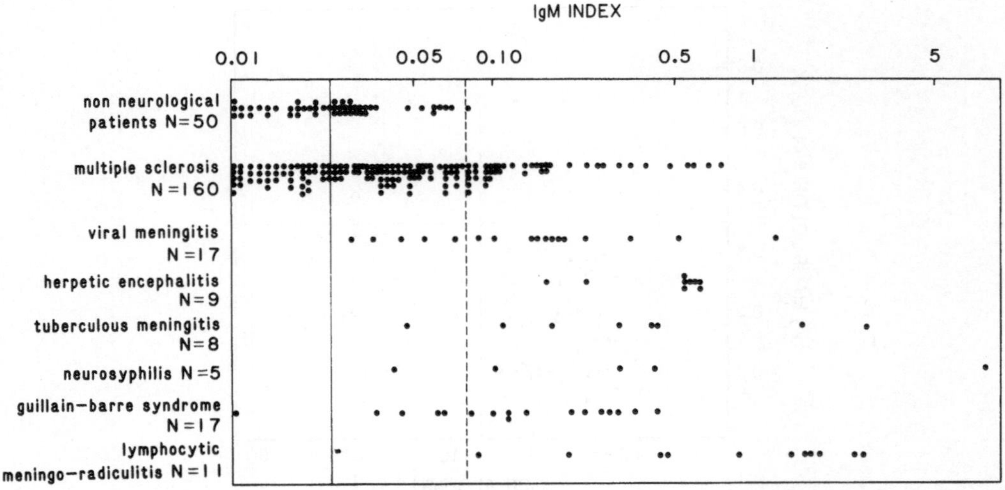

Fig.2. The IgM index in various neurological disorders. The continuous line represents the mean reference value (0.024), and the broken line, the upper reference limit (0.079). In this series of 160 MS patients, 42 (26%) had a high IgM index. Note the logarithmic scale.

It should be noted that a low molecular weight IgM (7 S-IgM/ is sometimes present in the serum of patients suffering from a variety of systemic disorders, including lupus erythematosus, rheumatoid arthritis, ataxia-telangiectasia, antibody deficiency syndrome and malignancy of the lymphoïd system. The presence of low molecular weight IgM in the serum could lead to the calculation of a falsely high IgM index since 7 S-IgM certainly penetrates the BBB more easily than pentameric IgM. However, to the best of our knowledge, the occurrence of 7 S-IgM in sera from MS patients had not been described.

THE IgA ASSAY IN CSF

IgA has different molecular forms, the monomeric one predominating in serum, and the polymeric one in secretions (Tomasi et al., 1985). In normal sera, the proportion of polymeric IgA varies between 5 and 22% with a mean of 13% (Delacroix et al., 1983). However, in vitro experiments have shown that blood lymphocytes in culture spontaneously secrete equal proportions of monomeric and polymeric IgA (Kutteh et al., 1982). After stimulation by various mitogens, the proportion of secreted polymeric IgA is even higher (Kutteh et al., 1980).

When immune reactions occur in the CNS, the lymphocytes invading the subarachnoid space have a blood origin (Oehmichen et al., 1982). Therefore, one may expect that CSF IgA when locally produced will have the characteristics of the IgA secreted by blood lymphocytes rather than those of serum IgA.

To estimate the local production of IgA, we calculated an IgA index, but, in this particular case, the index should ideally be calculated for both monomeric and polymeric IgA as their transudation rate is obviously different. A further problem is that most IgA immunoassays, except immunonephelometry, are dependent of the molecular size of IgA and underestimate the actual concentration of polymeric IgA (Delacroix et al., 1982b,

1982c). We tested therefore the effect of the IgA-size on its determination by particle counting immunoassay (Sindic et al., 1984a). Monomeric and dimeric polyclonal serum IgA were purified by preparative ultracentrifugation. On a same weight basis, the agglutinating activity of dimeric IgA was lower than that of monomeric IgA; the concentration of dimeric IgA was underestimated by a factor 2, which was approximately constant along the standard curve.

Keeping in mind that the calculation of an IgA index on total IgA levels in serum and CSF takes into account neither the relative proportions of monomeric and polymeric IgA in both fluids, nor the underestimation of dimeric CSF IgA by our immunoassay, for a matter of simplicity, however, we first calculated an IgA index based on these total IgA levels. The IgA index had also a logarithmic normal distribution ; the upper reference limit which was set at 2 SD of log values above the mean (0.23) was found to be 0.42. Only 16 out of 117 MS patients, as shown in Fig.3, had an IgA index higher than 0.42; however, there was a tendency towards higher values for the IgA index with the reference range, with a bimodal distribution not observed in non-neurological patients.

To assess the relative proportions of monomeric and dimeric IgA in CSF and in corresponding sera and to calculate the monomeric and dimeric IgA indices, 17 paired samples were studied by ultracentrifugation in isokinetic sucrose gradients: 3 samples from non-neurological patients, 3 samples with only an increased permeability of the BBB, 7 samples from MS patients, 3 samples from patients with herpetic encephalitis and 1 sample from a patient with tuberculous meningitis.

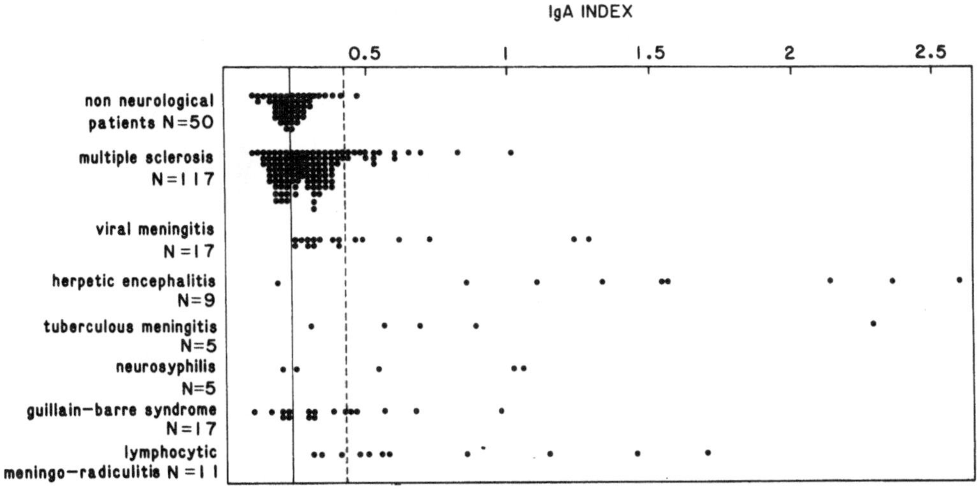

Fig.3. The IgA index calculated on total IgA levels in CSF and serum, in various neurological disorders. The continuous line represents the mean reference value (0.23), and the broken line, the upper reference limit (0.42). In this series of 117 MS patients, 16 (14%) had a high IgA index; note the bimodal distribution of the IgA index in this group.

In controls or in patients with an increased permeability of the BBB, CSF dimeric IgA was not detectable in one case while its proportion varied between 2.2 and 4.4% of total IgA in the other 5 cases (Fig.4). In contrast, in MS, the proportion of CSF dimeric IgA varied between 5 to 27.4% of total IgA; this proportion was sometimes higher in CSF than in serum. In the samples from patients with herpetic encephalitis or with tuberculous meningitis, the proportion of CSF dimeric IgA was even higher, from 16.1 to 53.9% (Fig.4). Consequently, the index calculated for the dimeric IgA increased much more (up to 199 times the mean) than the index for monomeric IgA (up to 6.5 times the mean) in case of local synthesis of IgA (Fig.5).

In conclusion, the local production of IgA is associated with a marked increase of the relative proportion of CSF dimeric IgA and consequently of the dimeric IgA index. These results are consistent with those of the analysis of IgA secreted by blood lymphocytes which release monomeric and polymeric IgA in equal amounts. the IgA index based on total values in both CSF and serum leads to an underestimation of the occurrence of local IgA synthesis as exemplified by the MS sample n° 7 (Fig.5): the total IgA index was in the normal range, while the index for dimeric IgA was abnormally high. These observations may explain the discrepancy between the presence of IgA producing cells in a great percentage of MS CSF samples and the low frequency of increased IgA index, as observed by Henriksson et al. (1985).

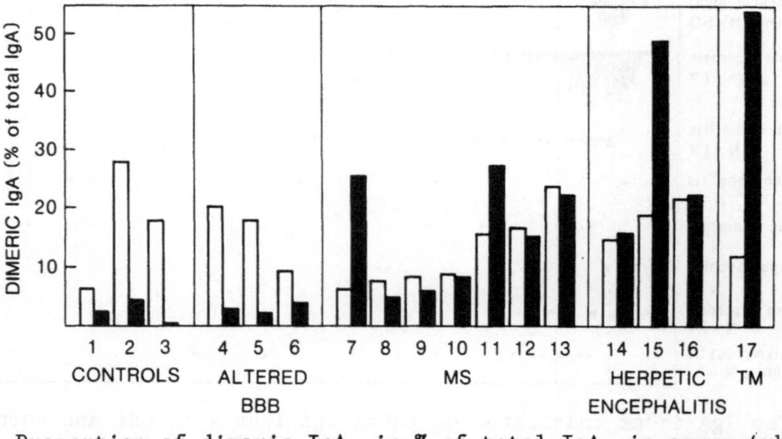

Fig.4. Proportion of dimeric IgA, in % of total IgA, in serum (white columns) and in CSF (black columns) from controls, patients with an increase of the BBB permeability (cervical disc prolapse, lumbar stenosis and metastatic compression of the spinal cord), and patients with MS, herpetic encephalitis and tuberculous meningitis (TM).

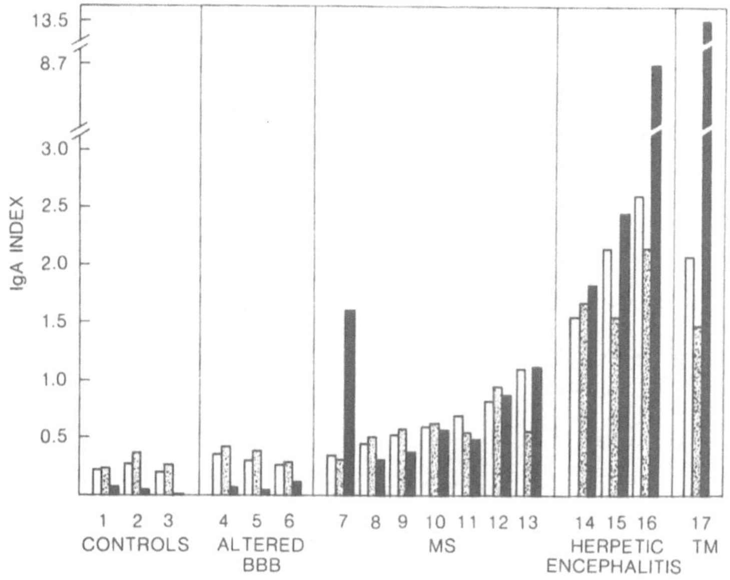

Fig.5. Indices for total IgA (white columns), monomeric IgA (dotted columns) and dimeric IgA (black columns) in controls and in patients with various neurological disorders (TM: tuberculous meningitis). MS patient No 7 had normal indices for total and monomeric IgA, but a very high index for dimeric IgA. The reference value for monomeric IgA index was 0.33 (SD: 0.08), and for dimeric IgA, 0.068 (SD: 0.028).

THE IgE ASSAY IN CSF

By particle counting immunoassay, IgE was detected neither in CSF of non-neurological patients (N=27) nor of patients with sciatica (N=13). IgE was present in the CSF of some patients with MS (13 out of 71) and in various infections of the CNS. We calculated the IgE index in each case where this immunoglobulin was detectable in CSF. Only patients with tuberculous meningitis had an increased IgE index. The mean IgE index calculated on the values of the samples from patients with MS or infectious meningitis, was 0.29 (SD: 0.12). As the mean IgG and monomeric IgA indices are 0.48 and 0.33 respectively, a value of 0.29 for IgE, which has a slightly higher molecular weight (180,000) could be expected. We concluded that the presence of IgE in most of these CSF samples was not related to local production (Sindic et al., 1984b).

THE LOCAL Ig PRODUCTION IN MS: CLINICAL CORRELATIONS

Results of CSF analyses from 299 patients with either probable or clinically definite MS were reviewed (Table 1). Presence of oligoclonal bands was the more frequent abnormality and was observed in 85% of patients. The IgG index was increased in 62% and the IgG synthesis calculated by Tourtellotte's formula, in 75%, these figures being similar to those reported by Verjans et al. (1983), i.e. 68 and 76% respectively in a group of 200 MS patients. The IgG index appeared therefore to be a rather insensitive method for the quantitative assessment of the local IgG synthesis. The Tourtellotte's formula was about 11% more sensitive than the calculation of the IgG index: the IgG synthesis calculated by this formula exceeded the reference value (2.7 mg/day) in 32 patients (out of 299) who had oligoclonal bands but a normal IgG index.

Table 1. Humoral immune abnormalities in MS CSF

		%
Oligoclonal bands	255/299	85
High IgG index (> 0.69)	187/299	62,5
High IgG synthesis* (> 2.7 mg/day)	223/299	75
High IgM index (> 0.079)	76/254	30
High IgA index (> 0.42)	54/211	26

* Calculated according to Tourtellotte's formula, modified by the use of our own reference values.

We analysed the relationship between the presence or absence of oligoclonal bands and the cell count, the Ig indices and the local IgG synthesis in 196 samples for which all these parameters were available (Table 2). The presence of these bands was significantly associated, as expected, with a high IgG index and a high IgG synthesis as calculated by Tourtellotte's formula ($p < 0.001$), but also with a high cell count ($p < 0.02$) and a high IgM index ($p < 0.05$). Among these 196 patients, only 16 (8.2%) had no signs of a local immune response (absence of oligoclonal bands, of high Ig indices and of abnormally high values with Tourtellotte's formula).

Table 2. X^2 analysis of the association of oligoclonal bands with cell count, Ig indices and IgG synthesis, in 196 CSF samples from MS patients

	Oligoclonal bands Absent N = 24	Oligoclonal bands Present N = 172
High cell count^xx^ (> 5/mm^3)	2	60
High cell inde^xxx^ (> 0.69)	1	117
High IgG synthesis^xxx^ (> 2.7 mg/day)	4	142
High IgM index^x^ (> 0.079)	2	53
High IgA index (> 0.42)	2	49

x Significant ($p < 0.05$)
xx Significant ($p < 0.02$)
xxx Significant ($p < 0.001$)

Table 3. Cell count, oligoclonal bands and Ig indices (abnormal values/total number of samples) in CSF from MS patients as function of the disease duration

	Interval between clinical onset and sampling					
	< 6 months	6 months to 2 years	2 to 5 years	5 to 10 years	10 to 20 years	≥ 20 years
High cell count (>5/mm^3)	11/30(37%)	25/48(52%)	12/39(31%)	4/32(13%)	7/28(25%)	5/14(36%)
Oligoclonal bands	27/31(87%)	43/51(84%)	32/39(82%)	29/35(83%)	25/28(89%)	12/14(86%)
High IgG index (> 0.69)	18/31(58%)	34/51(67%)	21/39(58%)	24/35(69%)	21/28(75%)	10/14(71%)
High IgM index (>0.079)	9/29(31%)	16/47(34%)	12/34(35%)	7/34(21%)	4/22(18%)	2/12(17%)
High IgA index (> 0.42)	2/26(8%)	7/29(24%)	5/29(17%)	2/23(9%)	4/14(29%)	2/11(18%)
High IgG synthesis* (>2.7mg/day)	20/31(65%)	40/51(78%)	29/39(74%)	26/35(74%)	23/28(82%)	12/14(86%)
Mean IgG synthesis* mg/day (SD)	10.3(12.2)	16.2(18.3)	12.3(17.1)	12.5(16.4)	13.5(12.9)	12.4(12)

* Calculated according to the Tourtellotte's formula, modified by the use of our own reference values.

Table 4. Cell count, oligoclonal bands and Ig indices (abnormal values/total number of samples) in CSF from MS patients as a function of clinical state

	Disease activity		
	relapses	slowly progressive	remission
High cell count (> 5/mm^3)	47/112(42%)^x	15/69(22%)^x	4/23(17%)^x
Oligoclonal bands	99/112(88%)	58/69(84%)	16/23(70%)
High IgG index (> 0.69)	70/112(62%)	48/69(70%)	13/23(56%)
High IgM index (> 0.079)	32/106(30%)	17/56(30%)	3/21(14%)
High IgA index (> 0.42)	17/78(22%)	6/47(13%)	3/16(19%)
High IgG synthesis (> 2.7 mg/day)	82/112(73%)	57/69(83%)	16/23(70%)
Mean IgG synthesis, mg/day (SD)	16.8(13.6)	19(20)	11.2(7.4)

^{x} Significant difference between patients in relapses vs patients in remission or with a slowly progressive disease ($p < 0.01$)

We looked for a correlation between cell counts, presence of oligoclonal bands, increase of Ig indices and interval between clinical onset and sampling (Table 3).

No significant difference was observed between patients with a short or long lasting disease. Several points must be underlined: (1) 29% of patients with a disease duration exceeding 10 years had yet a high CSF cell count; (2) the proportion of patients with CSF oligoclonal bands was remarkably constant whatever the disease duration (82 to 89%); (3) a high IgM index was observed in 37 out of 110 MS patients (34%) with a disease duration no longer than 5 years, and in 13 out of 68 patients (19%) with a disease exceeding 5 years; this difference, however, is not significant ($X^2 = 3.69$); (4) the mean IgG synthesis, in mg/day, was very similar in all sub-groups.

When the disease activity at the moment of sampling was taken into account, a high cell count was significantly more frequent in patients in relapse than in patients in remission or with a slowly progressive form of the disease ($p < 0.01$) (Table 4). The IgM index was more frequently increased in patients in relapses (32 out of 106 or 30%) or with a slowly progressive MS (17 out of 56 or 30%) than in patients in remission (3 out of 21 or 14%) but this difference was not statistically significant.

CONCLUSIONS

We have shown the occurrence of the local synthesis of the three main Ig isotypes within the CNS of MS patients. By comparison with the detection of oligoclonal bands, the determination of the IgG index is a rather insensitive method for the assessment of a humoral immune response within the CNS in MS. The IgA index calculated on total levels of IgA in CSF and serum is even less reliable for the detection of an intra-thecal production of IgA, as discussed above. Such a local synthesis of IgA is characterized by the release within the CSF of a high proportion of dimeric IgA. We failed to establish clear relationships between the local production of these Ig, and especially of IgM, and the clinical course of the disease.

It should be interesting to determine by longitudinal studies if relapses in a single patient are linked to an increase of the local IgM synthesis. This would be an argument for new or repetitive antigenic stimulations during exacerbations of the disease. Finally, it should be noted that the study of the humoral immune response at the level of the single B cell seems more informative than the determination of free CSF Ig (Henriksson et al.,1985).

ACKNOWLEDGEMENTS

We are thankful to Mrs. M.P. Van Antwerpen, M.A. Devulder and A. Dene-Wade for skillful technical assistance and to Mrs. Pee for competent editorial work. This work was supported by grants from the "Fonds de la Recherche Scientifique Médicale" (No 3.4529.79) and from the "Groupe belge d'Etude de la Sclérose en plaques".

REFERENCES

1. C.L. Cambiaso, A.E. Leek, F. De Steenwinkel, J. Billen and P.L. Masson. Particle Counting Immunoassay (PACIA). I. A general method for the determination of antibodies, antigens and haptens. J. Immunol. Methods. 18:33-40 (1977).

2. D.L. Delacroix and J.P. Vaerman. Influence of molecular size of IgA on its immunoassay by various techniques. III. Immunonephelometry. J. Immunol. Methods. 51:49-55 (1982a).
3. D.L. Delacroix, R. Meykens and J.P. Vaerman. Influence of molecular size of IgA on its immunoassay by various techniques. I. Direct and reversed single radial immunodiffusion. Mol. Immunol. 19:297-305 (1982b).
4. D.L. Delacroix, J.P. Dehennin and J.P. Vaerman. Influence of molecular size of IgA on its immunoassay by various techniques. II. Solid-phase radioimmunoassays. J. Immunol. Meth. 48:327-337 (1982c).
5. D.L. Delacroix, K.B. Elkon and J.P. Vaerman. IgA-size and IgA-subclass distribution in serum and secretions. Ann. N.Y. Acad. Sci. 409:812-814 (1983).
6. L.A. Hershey and J.L. Trotter. The use and abuse of the cerebrospinal fluid IgG profile in the adulta: practical evaluation. Ann. Neurol. 8:426-434 (1980).
7. A. Henriksson, S. Kam-Hansen and H. Link. IgM, IgA and IgG producing cells in cerebrospinal fluid and peripheral blood in multiple sclerosis. Clin. exp. Immunol. 62:176-184 (1985).
8. W.H. Kutteh, W.J. Koopman, M.E. Conley, M.L. Egan and J. Mestecky. Production of predominantly polymeric IgA by human peripheral blood lymphocytes stimulated in vitro with mitogens. J. Exp. Med. 152: 1424-1429 (1980).
9. W.H. Kutteh, S.J. Prince and J. Mestecky. Tissue origins of human polymeric and monomeric IgA. J. Immunol. 128:990-995 (1982).
10. E.C. Laterre (1965). Les protéines du liquide céphalo-rachidien à l'état normal et pathologique. Thèse, Arscia. Maloine, Paris.
11. M.A. Laurenzi, M. Marvra, S. Kam-Hansen and H. Link. Oligoclonal IgG and free light chains in multiple sclerosis demonstrated by thin-layer polyacrylamide gel isoelectric. Ann. Neurol. 8:241-247 (1980).
12. P. Livrea, M. Trojano, I.L. Simone, G.B. Zimatore, G. Lamontanara and R. Leante. Intrathecal IgG synthesis in multiple sclerosis: comparison between isoelectric focusing and quantitative estimation of cerebrospinal fluid IgG. J. Neurol. 224:159-169 (1981).
13. A. Lowenthal, A. Vansande and D. Karcher. The differential diagnosis of neurological diseases by fractionating electrophoretically the CSF gamma-globulins. J. Neurochem. 6:51-56 (1960).
14. P.L. Mason, C.L. Cambiaso, D. Collet-Cassart, C.G.M. Magnusson, C.B. Richards and C.J.M. Sindic. Particle Counting Immunoassay (PACIA). Meth. Enzymol. 74:106-139 (1981).
15. P.C. Montgomery and J.H. Pincus. Molecular restriction of anti-DNP antibodies induced by dinitrophenylated type III pneumococcus. J. Immunol. 111:42-51 (1973).
16. M. Oehmichen, D. Domasch and H. Withölter. Origin, proliferation and fate of cerebrospinal fluid cells. A review on cerebrospinal fluid cell kinetics. J. Neurol. 227:145-150 (1982).
17. J.E. Olsson and H. Link. Immunoglobulin abnormalities in multiple sclerosis. Relation to clinical parameters: exacerbations and remissions. Arch. Neurol. 28:392-399 (1973).
18. C.J.M. Sindic, C.L. Cambiaso, A. Depré, E.C. Laterre and P.L. Masson. The concentration of IgM in the cerebrospinal fluid of neurological patients. J. Neurol. Sci. 55:339-350 (1982).
19. C.J.M. Sindic, D.L. Delacroix, J.P. Vaerman, E.C. Laterre and P.L. Masson. Study of IgA in the cerebrospinal fluid of neurological patients with special reference to size, subclass and local production. J. Neuroimmunol. 7:65-75 (1984a).
20. C.J.M. Sindic, C.G.M. Magnusson, E.C. Laterre and P.L. Masson. IgE in the cerebrospinal fluid. J. Neuroimmunol. 6:319-324 (1984b).

21. C.J.M. Sindic. Cerebrospinal fluid proteins in diseases of the nervous system. Thesis. Nauwelaerts Printing, 3000 Leuven, Belgium. (1985).

22. E.J. Thompson, P. Kaufmann and P. Rudge. Sequential changes in oligoclonal patterns during the course of multiple sclerosis. J. Neurol. Neurosurg. Psych. 46:547-550 (1983).

23. E.J. Thompson and A. Vakaert. Free light chains in multiple sclerosis. Prot. Biol. Fl. 32:215-216 (1985).

24. G. Tibbling, H. Link and S. Öhman. Principles of albumin and IgG analyses in neurological disorders. I. Establishment of reference values. Scand. J. Clin. Lab. Invest. 37:385-390 (1977).

25. T.B. Tomasi, E.M. Tam, S. Saloman and R.A. Prendergast. Characteristics of an immune system common to certain external secretions. J. Exp. Med. 121:101-124 (1965).

26. W.W. Tourtellotte, A.R. Potvin, J.O. Fleming, K.N. Murthy, J. Levy, K. Syndulko and J.H. Potvin. Multiple sclerosis: measurement and validation of central nervous system IgG synthesis rate. Neurology. 30:240-244 (1980).

27. B. Vandvik. Oligoclonal IgG and free light chains in the cerebrospinal fluid of patients with multiple sclerosis and infectious diseases of the central nervous system. Scand. J. Immunol. 6:913-922 (1977).

28. E. Verjans, P. Theys, P. Delmotte and H. Carton. Clinical parameters and intrathecal IgG synthesis as prognostic features in multiple sclerosis. Part. I. J. Neurol. 229:155-165 (1983).

29. M.J. Walsh and W.W. Tourtellotte. Temporal invariance and clonal uniformity of brain and cerebrospinal IgG, IgA and IgM in multiple sclerosis. J. exp. Med. 163:41-53 (1986).

AUTOANTIBODIES TO NEURAL AND NON-NEURAL ANTIGENS IN MULTIPLE SCLEROSIS

Björn Ryberg

Department of Neurology, University of Lund
S-221 85 Lund, Sweden

Autoimmunity has long been thought to be involved in the pathogenesis of multiple sclerosis (MS). It is one of the dominating concepts in current MS research and provides a rationale for immunosuppressive treatment in this disease. However attractive this model may be,, it is still based on rather indirect evidence. Some support is provided by the histopathological findings, which include IgG capping on macrophages engaged in myelin breakdown (1) and the presence of the membrane attack complex of complement in the plaques (2). Although immunoregulatory disturbances may exist in MS, there is no convincing evidence for an antigen specific T cell mediated autoimmunity in this disease (3).

Various forms of experimental allergic encephalomyelitis (EAE), more or less similar to MS can be induced by crude CNS material (4) or purified neutral antigens, such as myelin basic protein (MBP) (5), gangliosides (6), and proteolipid apoprotein (7), but their relevance as models for MS remains unproven.

If pathology, cell mediated immunity, and EAE have not clearly documented autoimmunity in MS, some additional evidence comes from humoral factors of possible or proven immunoglobulin nature.

FUNCTIONALLY DEFINED FACTORS OF POSSIBLE IMMUNOGLOBULIN NATURE

Serum from patients with MS is often gliotoxic (8) and myelinotoxic (9) in vitro, and similar activity has been shown in MS CSF (10). The phenomenon is not specific for MS, but is found in many controls, most notably in ASL which is not characterized by primary demyelination. For many years it was believed that the in vitro myelinotoxic activity in MS is immunoglobulin mediated, but recent work has shown this only exceptionally to be true (11,12).

On the other hand, demyelination of the optic nerve in tadpoles after injection of MS CSF appears to be IgG mediated (13). The phenomenon is reported to be associated with the presence of oligoclonal IgG (14), but nothing is known about the antigen or antigens involved. In a phylogenetically less remote model sera from patients with MS and optic neuritis caused demyelination and oligodendroglial pathology more frequently than control sera when injected into the optic nerves of guinea pigs (15). Similar changes were induced by antisera to galactocerebroside (16), but the immunoglobulin or antibody nature of the human serum factor has not yet been demonstrated.

Probably unrelated to the demyelinating process, MS sera exhibit complement dependent, reversible neuroelectric blocking activity in mammalian CNS explants (17), but similar activity is found also in control sera (18). In an amphibian in vitro model, which appears more specific for demyelinating disease, the blocking activity seems to be IgG mediated (19). The factor is thought to act on the axon, but no antigen is identified. Neuroelectric blocking activity was not found in CSF (20).

IMMUNOLOGICALLY DEFINED FACTORS

In addition to these functional studies, there have been numerous more straightforward attempts to demonstrate autoantibodies to the CNS or to CNS constituents in MS. The results, which have been obtained by many different techniques, are contradictory (21-23). Particularly claims of autoantibodies to oligodendroglia have been challenged. A likely explanation for many of the inconsistencies is the unspecific affinity of normal human IgG or part of it to CNS structures, such as myelin, oligodendroglia, astroglia, neurons, fibroblasts and nuclear membranes (24-28). Some of the affinity to myelin and oligodendroglia may be mediated by myelin basic protein (MBP) (24,29). Because of problems of this kind, the existence in MS of autoantibodies to CNS antigens is not generally recognized.

In 1972 Laurell and Link reported complement-fixing antibodies to hydrosoluble brain proteins in 6 of 12 CSF from MS patients but not from controls (30). Working also with a complement fixation technique, I was unable to reproduce these findings. What I did find, however, was IgG antibodies to the water insoluble particulate fraction of CNS tissue, which contains essentially membranes and cytoskeleton (31,32). Antibodies reacting with crude brain homogenate were found in 88% of concentrated CSF samples, but only rarely in other neurological diseases or healthy controls. This difference is highly significant. Also in serum, where 40% of MS patients have detectable anti-brain antibodies, the difference to healthy controls is statistically significant (33). Some positive reactions are found in certain other conditions, particularly in the Guillain-Barré syndrome (GBS), where more than 70%, often in addition to antibodies to peripheral nerve, have complement-fixing antibodies to CNS antigens in the acute phase (34,35). Sera from patients with amyotrophic lateral sclerosis (ALS) are reported to be gliotoxic (8) and myelinotoxic (36) in vitro and to contain antibodies to myelin (37), MBP, and tubulin (38) detectable by immunofluorescence and immunoblotting. The lack of complement-fixing antibodies to brain homogenate in ALS patients is of great interest since it supports the specificity of the complement fixation assay (33).

Contrary to several other immunological methods the complement fixation technique does not seem to be significantly infuenced by the nonspecific affinity between IgG and CNS, and indeed seems to demonstrate a specific antigen-antibody reaction. This concept is supported by several observations (31-33,35,39):

1) The CSF and serum reactant in MS has been identified as IgG.
2) Positive reactions are practically found only in demyelinating diseases, such as MS and GBS.
3) Most control sera fail to give a positive reaction even undiluted.
4) There is no correlation between IgG level and antibody titers in MS samples.

5) The reaction is relatively disease specific even at a standardized IgG concentration.
6) CSF/serum ratios for IgG and anti-brain antibodies are not correlated.
7) Individual MS and GBS samples show different reaction patterns, indicating that several antibody specificities are involved.

The ability of the complement fixation method to differentiate between specific and non-specific binding of IgG to white matter membranes is illustrated by an experiment that is part of a pilot study made in collaboration with Göran Kronvall in 1978 (Fig.1). In a radioimmunoassay we measured the amount of IgG binding to a defined amount of white matter membranes by ^{125} I-labelled protein A. No difference in IgG binding in 3 MS sera and 3 control sera was found, although the MS sera had appreciable titers of complement-fixing antibodies to the same antigen preparation. In control experiments these antibodies bound to protein A, and should therefore be detectable by labelled protein A. Similar results were obtained in MS and control CSF. This study confirmed the nonspecific binding of immunoglobulins to white matter membranes and indicated that specific antibody contributes only a minor part of bound IgG, even in sera with relatively high titers against that target. In a ^{125} I-protein A microassay similar to ours, Steck and Regli (26) also found no difference in IgG binding to bovine oligodendroglia in sera from patients with MS and other neurological disorders, whereas sera from healthy controls showed lower binding.

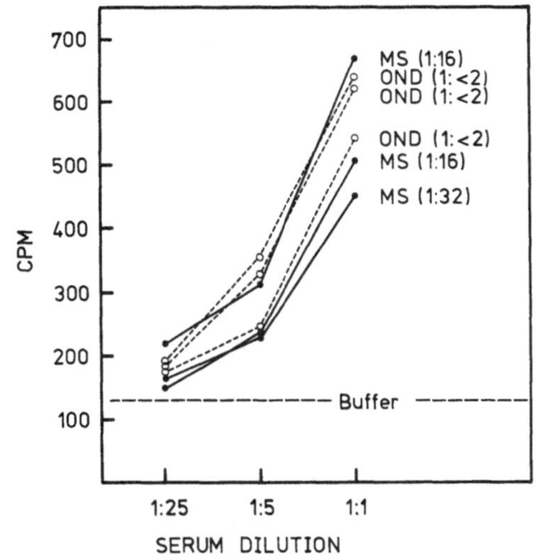

Fig.1. ^{125} I-protein A assay for IgG binding to human white matter membranes in sera from 3 MS patients (•——•) and 3 patients with other neurological diseases (OND) (o----o). Titers in the complement fixation assay against the same antigen are given in parenthesis. The radioimmunoassay was performed in plastic tubes by adding 5 mg (wet weight) human white matter membranes suspended in 100 µl PBS containing 0.25% gelatin and 0.1% Tween 20 to 50 µl dilutions of sera. After incubation for 30 min at room temperature the membranes were washed three times in 2 ml of the above buffer followed by incubation for another 30 min at room temperature with ^{125} I labelled staphylococcal protein A. The membranes were washed once in 2 ml buffer and the radioactivity of the pellets was measured (Ryberg & Kronvall 1978, unpublished results).

The reason why the complement fixation test does work where so many other tests have failed is not known. One explanation for its favourable signal to noise ratio could be that the conformational change in the IgG molecule, essential for the reaction with Clq (40), occurs only upon specific binding to antigen. Another explanation could be a less efficient spacing or arrangement of non-specifically bound IgG molecules (41). It would be desirable further to assess the antibody nature of immunoglobulins binding to nervous tissue by the use of F(ab')2 fragments. This, however, is not possible in the complement fixation assay, which is dependent on the Fc part of the molecule.

The CSF/serum ratio for anti-brain antibodies is often elevated compared to that of IgG, suggesting an intrathecal synthesis. In order to assess this, an antibody index equal to CSF/serum antibody titer: CSF/serum albumin was formed by analogy with the IgG index to compensate for a possible impairment of the blood brain barrier (42,43). A wide range of values was found indicating that anti-brain antibodies are produced on both sides of the blood-brain barrier. In MS the antibodies are to a great extent produced intrathecally, whereas in GBS extrathecal production dominates (Fig.2) (43). From these observations it is clear that the responsible immunologic aberration in MS is not limited to the CNS,

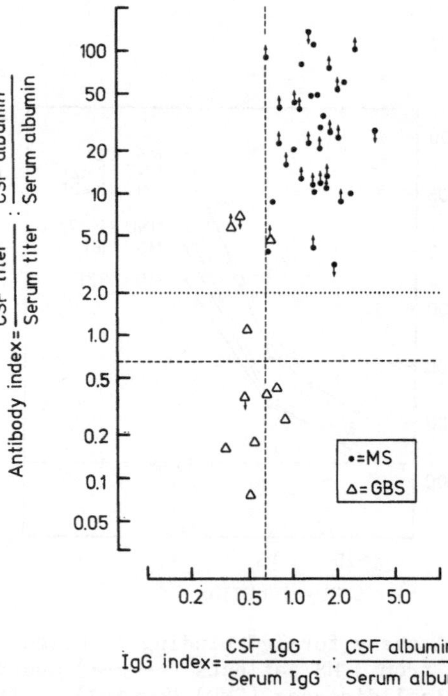

Fig.2. The relation between antibody index values for complement-fixing anti-brain antibodies and IgG index values in MS (•) and the Guillain-Barré syndrome (Δ) (Ryberg 1984). Where the antibody titer in CSF or serum was below the level of detection, maximum or minimum index values were calculated and the fact that the actual value may be lower or higher is indicated by an arrow. The dashed lines correspond to index values of 0.66, which is considered to represent the upper normal limit for the IgG index. The horizontal dotted line represents a provisional upper normal value of 2.0 for antibody index for IgG antibodies.

but often involves the extrathecal compartment. Longitudinal studies did not show significant titer changes in CSF or serum in relation to exacerbations, but in early MS there was a tendency for anti-brain antibodies to occur earlier in the CSF than in serum. This might reflect a progressive dissemination of the autoimmune process beyond the CNS (33,44).

The titers of the complement-fixing anti-brain antibodies in CSF and serum are to some extent correlated with a more malignant course and more pronounced invalidity in MS (33). Although they may be induced by the disease, it is tempting to speculate that these antibodies are involved in immunologically mediated damage to the CNS. Such damage could be effected by the antibodies themselves or by their interaction with complement, K-cells and phagocytic cells.

AUTOANTIGENS IN MS

Having established a method for the demonstration of anti-brain antibodies in MS, I hoped to be able to identify the reacting CNS antigen. This, however, turned out to be a formidable task. What was expected to be one antigen was indeed a host of antigens, some of them losing reactivity during attempts at isolation.

In occasional CSF and serum samples anti-brain reactivity could be traced to cerebroside and sulfatide (Fig.3), two glycolipids with rich representation in the CNS, including myelin and oligodendroglia (32). This was the first demonstration of antibodies to sulfatide in man. The hydrophilic carbohydrate moiety is the immunologically reactive part in both molecules (32). CSF titers but not serum titers against cerebroside are significantly elevated in MS compared with controls (45).

In other MS samples only a partial characterization of the components reacting with the complement-fixing anti-brain antibodies has been achieved (32). The characteristics of the involved antigens or antigen-like activities are summarized below:

1) Protein of intrinsic type in CNS myelin. Reacting epitope not carbohydrate. Not species specific (46).
2) Antigen associated with CNS myelin. Organ specific. Labile to heat. Not solubilized by saline or water. Nonlipid. Species restricted (not found in bovine brain).
3) Antigen equally distributed between grey and white matter. Organ specific. Labile to heat. Not solubilized by saline. Nonlipid.
4) Antigen present predominantly in grey matter and possibly present in some nonneural tissues. Labile to heat. Not solubilized by saline. Nonlipid.
5) Cerebroside (galactosylceramide). Relatively myelin specific.

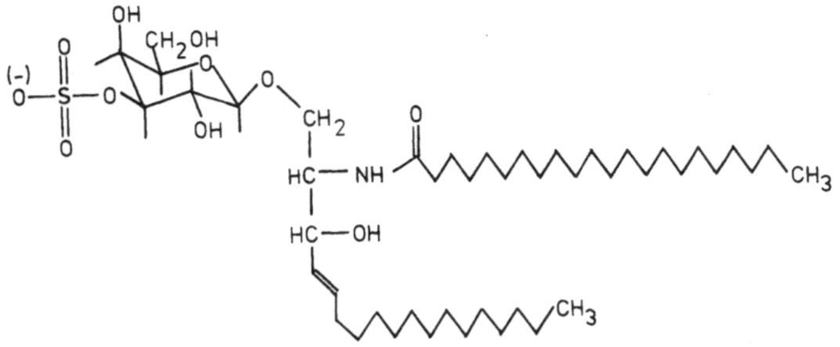

Fig.3. Sulfatide (galactosylceramide-3-sulfate).

6) Sulfatide (galactosylceramide-3-sulfate). Relatively myelin specific.
7) Cholesterol in combination with a variety of lipids with different degrees of polarity.

This list should be regarded as provisional, as future studies are expected to show further heterogeneity in some of the indicated specificities.

The litera
The literature is vast and results are very inconsistent. I was interested to know whether any of the MS related anti-brain antibodies I am studying is directed to this encephalitogenic antigen. In collaboration with Claude Jacque in Paris, I assayed antigenic activity in brain from Shiverer mice, which have a relatively selective deficiency of MBP, against a panel of MS amples representing different profiles of reactivity of neural antigens. No significant difference in antigenic titer was seen in Shiverer brain and control brain (47). This shows that antibrain reactivity is not dominated by antibodies to MBP in most MS samples. Although anti-MBP-antibodies may be detected by some techniques, other specificities of anti-brain antibodies seem to be more prevalent, and should attract interest as tools to find alternative encephalitogens and as potential mediators of autoimmune CNS damage.

In addition to antibodies to the two CNS glycolipids discussed above a humoral immune response to various gangliosides has been reported by several groups (48), but this finding is not disease specific. Ganliosides are claimed to be encephalitogenic (6). Antibodies to these glycolipids can experimentally induce epileptic seizures and other neurophysiological effects in vivo (49), and were found to have demyelinating effects in vitro (50).

Encephalitogenic properties have also been reported in proteolipid protein (7), but a RIA for antibodies to this antigen gave negative results in CSF from patients with MS and other neurological diseases (51). A similar assay for antibodies to myelin associated glycoprotein (MAG), however, showed slightly higher levels of binding in MS CSF than in control CSF (52).

Employing an immunoblotting technique Newcombe et al. (38) found IgM, IgG and IgA antibodies in MS directed to several CNS proteins, among which IgM antibodies to tubulin and MBP predominated. A similar antibody spectrum was found in other neurological diseases as well, including ALS and subacute sclerosing panencephalitis. Antibodies to other cytoskeletal constituents have been demonstrated in some MS sera (53) but, again, are not specific for demyelinating diseases. Antibodies of such specificity may explain some of the reactivity to smooth muscle found in occasional samples of MS CSF (54), and in serum from patients with MS and other conditions (55).

Antibodies to glial fibrillary acidic protein (GFAP) were found in CSF and serum from a patient with Devic's syndrome (56), but were looked for with negative results in CSF and serum in MS (55).

Antibodies to pituitary peptides, detectable by immunocytochemical techniques, have been reported in a third of MS sera (58). The reacting peptides have not yet been identified.

Serum and CSF from patients with several diseases of infectious and possible autoimmune nature, including MS, contain lymphocytotoxic and monocytotoxic antibodies (59,60). Most of these antibodies are cold-reacting, but as some of them are functional at 37°C, physiological effects are not unlikely (60).

Antinuclear antibodies were found more frequently in MS sera than in healthy controls (61). Also the closely related antibodies to DNA and RNA have been reported to occur more often in MS CSF and MS sera than in controls (62), but others have failed to confirm this (55).

Employing an ELISA, Vandenbark et al.(63) found increased binding to crude extracts of human brain in CSF IgG from many MS patients but also from other patient categories. The antibodies seemed to react with a number of, largely unidentified, antigens in brain from MS and other patients.

In experiments by Hukkanen et al.(64) MS CSF showed elevated binding of radiolabelled and solubilized white matter membrane glycoproteins from MS white matter but not from control brain. Also cytosol material from MS brain showed an elevated tendency to react with IgG from MS sera (65). The corresponding antigens do not seem to be conventional autoantigens, but may represent products of the demyelinating process or an infectious agent.

In spite of many unclear results, the impression gained from this brief overview is that MS is associated with an increased incidence of autoantibodies to several CNS antigens and possibly to some non-neural antigens, although a very limited number of anti-brain antibody specificities are found in the individual patients according to my own experience with the complement fixation technique. Together with the analogous finding of increased titers and intrathecal production of antibodies to several viruses in MS (66), this observation may reflect a preferential exposure of some auto- and heteroantigens, an impaired B cell control, or both.

REFERENCES

1. J.W. Prineas and J.S. Graham. Multiple Sclerosis: Capping of surface immunoglobulin G on macrophages engaged in myelin breakdown. Ann. Neurol. 10:149 (1981).
2. B.P. Bozsik, S. Komoly and A. Fazekas. The demonstration of membrane attack complex /MAC/ of complement by immunohistological methods. Ann. Immunol. hung. 24:267 (1984).
3. R.W. Baumhefner and W.W. Tourtellotte. Cellular immunology in multiple sclerosis. A review through 1984. In: "Concepts immunopathol," Vol.2, J.M. Cruse and R.E. Lewis, eds., Karger, Basel (1985).
4. E. Witebsky and J. Steinfeld. Untersuchungen über spezifische Antigen-funktionen von Organen. I. Mitteilung. Z. ImmunForsch. exp. Ther. 58:271 (1928).
5. S. Leibowitz and R.A.C. Hughes. Experimental allergic encephalomyelitis. In: "Immunology of the nervous system". J. Turk, ed., Edward Arnold, London (1983).
6. O. Cohen, B.A. Sela, M. Schwarz, N. Eschhar and I.R. Cohen. Multiple sclerosis-like disease induced in rabbits by immunization with brain gangliosides. Isr. J. Med. Sci. 17:711 (1981).
7. F. Cambi, M.B. Lees, R.M. Williams and W.B. Macklin. Chronic experimental allergic encephalomyelitis produced by bovine proteolipid apoprotein: Immunological studies in rabbits. Ann. Neurol. 13:303 (1983).
8. O. Berg and B. Källen. Gliotoxic effect of serum from patients with neurological diseases. Lancet. 1:1051 (1962).

9. M.B. Bornstein. A tissue culture approach to demyelinative disorders. Nat. Cancer Inst. Monog. 11:197 (1963).
10. G. Lamoureux and A.G. Borduas. Immune studies in multiple sclerosis. Clin. exp. Immunol. 1:363 (1966).
11. I. Grundke-Iqbal and M.B. Bornstein. Multiple sclerosis: Serum gamma globulin and demyelination in organ culture. Neurology. 30:749 (1980).
12. K. Bradbury, S.R. Aparicio, D.W. Summer, A. Macfie, P. Sagar, N.R. Griffin and C.C. Bird. Comparison of in vitro demyelination and cytotoxicity of humoral factors in multiple sclerosis and other neurological diseases. J. Neurol. Sci. 70:167 (1985).
13. T. Tabira, F.J. Wolfgram, H. DeF. Webster, S.H. Wray and D.E. McFarlin. Myelinotoxicity of CSF fractions from multiple sclerosis patients tested in an in vivo model. Neurology. 27:374 (1977).
14. L. Stendahl-Brodin, H. Link and K. Kristensson. Myelinotoxic activity on tadpole optic nerve of cerebrospinal fluid from patients with optic neuritis. Neurology. 29:882 (1979).
15. R.C. Sergott, M.J. Brown, R.M.D. Polenta, R.P. Lisak and D.H. Silberberg. Optic nerve demyelination induced by human serum: Patients with multiple sclerosis or optic neuritis and normal subjects. Neurology. 35:1438 (1985).
16. R.C. Sergott, M.J. Brown, D.H. Silberberg and R.P. Lisak. Antigalactocerebroside serum demyelinates optic nerve in vivo. J. Neurol. Sci. 64:297 (1984).
17. M.B. Bornstein and S.M. Crain. Functional studies of cultured brain tissues as related to "demyelinative disorders". Science. 148:1242 (1965).
18. F.J. Seil. Tissue culture studies of neuroelectric blocking factors. In: "Demyelinating disease". S.G. Waxman and J.M. Richie, eds. Raven Press, New York (1981).
19. C.L. Schauf and F.A. Davis. The occurrence, specificity and role of neuroelectric blocking factors in multiple sclerosis. Neurology. 28(2):34 (1978).
20. C.L. Schauf and F.A. Davis. Circulating toxic factors in multiple sclerosis: A perspective. In: "Demyelinating disease". S.G. Waxman and J.M. Ritchie, eds. Raven Press, New York (1981).
21. C.E. Lumsden. The clinical immunology of multiple sclerosis. In: "Multiple sclerosis -A reappraisal". 2nd edition, D. McAlpine, C.E. Lumsden and E.D. Acheson, eds. Churchill Livingstone. Edingburgh & London (1972).
22. J.A. Aarli and O. Tönder. "Immunological aspects of neurological diseases". S. Karger, Basel (1980).
23. S. Leibowitz and R.A.C. Hughes. Multiple sclerosis. In: "Immunology of the nervous system". J. Turk, ed. Edward Arnold, London (1983).
24. J.A. Aarli, S.R. Aparicio, C.E. Lumsden and O. Tönder. Binding of normal human IgG to myelin sheaths, glia and neurons. Immunology. 28:171 (1975).
25. U. Traugott, D.S. Snyder and C.S. Raine. Oligodendrocyte staining by multiple sclerosis serum is non-specific. Ann. Neurol. 6:13 (1979).
26. A.J. Steck and F. Regli. Oligodendrocyte-binding antibodies in multiple sclerosis: ^{125}I-protein A studies. Neurology. 30:540 (1980).
27. P.G.E. Kennedy and R.P. Lisak. Do patients with demyelinating disease have antibodies against human glial cells in their sera? J. Neurol. Neurosurg. Psychiat. 44:164 (1981).
28. B.I. Ma, B.S. Joseph, M.J. Walsh, A.R. Potvin and W.W. Tourtellotte. Multiple sclerosis and cerebrospinal fluid immunoglobulin binding to the Fc receptors of oligodendrocytes. Ann. Neurol. 9:37 (1981).
29. C.J.M. Sindic, C.L. Cambiaso, P.L. Masson and E.C. Laterre. The binding of myelin basic protein to the Fc region of aggregated IgG to immune complexes. Clin. exp. Immunol. 41:1 (1980).

30. A.B. Laurell and H. Link. Complement-fixing antibrain antibodies in multiple sclerosis. Acta Neurol. Scand. 48:461 (1972).
31. B. Ryberg. Complement-fixing antibrain antibodies in multiple sclerosis. Acta Neurol. Scand. 54:1 (1976).
32. B. Ryberg. Multiple specificities of antibrain antibodies in multiple sclerosis and chronic myelopathy. J. Neurol. Sci. 38:357 (1978).
33. B. Ryberg. Antibrain antibodies in multiple sclerosis. Relation to clinical variables. J. Neurol. Sci. 54:239 (1982).
34. S.C. Melnick. Thirty-eight cases of the Guillain-Barré syndrome: An immunological study. Br. Med. J. 1:368 (1963).
35. B. Ryberg, B. Hindfelt, B. Nilsson and J.E. Olsson. Antineural antibodies in Guillain-Barré syndrome and lymphocytic meningoradiculitis (Bannwarth's syndrome). Arch. Neurol. 41:1277 (1984).
36. D. Hughes and E.J. Field. Myelinotoxicity of serum and spinal fluid in multiple sclerosis: A critical assessment. Clin. exp. Immunol. 2:295 (1967).
37. R.P. Lisak, B. Zweiman and M. Norman. Antimyelin antibodies in neurological diseases. Immunofluorescent demonstration. Arch. Neurol. 32:163 (1975).
38. J. Newcombe, S. Gahan and M.L. Cuzner. Serum antibodies against central nervous system proteins in human demyelinating disease. Clin. exp. Immunol. 59:383 (1985).
39. B. Ryberg and G. Kronvall. Immunoglobulin characterization by bacterial absorption of antibrain antibodies in multiple sclerosis. Eur. Neurol. 20:374 (1981).
40. H. Metzger. The effect of antigen on antibodies: Recent studies. In: "Contemporary topics in molecular immunology," vol.2, R.A. Reisfeld and F.P. Inman, eds. Plenum Press, New York (1978).
41. D.R. Burton. Immunoglobulin G: Functional sites. Molecular Immunology. 22:161 (1985).
42. B. Ryberg. Intrathecal and extrathecal production of antibrain antibodies in multiple sclerosis. J. Neurol. Sci. 48:1 (1980).
43. B. Ryberg. Extra- and intrathecal production of antineural antibodies in Guillain-Barré syndrome. Evaluation by an antibody index. Neurology. 34:1378 (1984).
44. B. Ryberg. A longitudinal study of antibrain antibodies in multiple sclerosis. J. Neurol. Sci. 54:263 (1982).
45. J. Ruutiainen, M. Viljanen, A. Salmi and H. Frey. Galactocerebroside antibodies in serum and cerebrospinal fluid of multiple sclerosis and brain tumour patients. In: "Protides of the biological fluids", vol. 30, H. Peeters, ed. Pergamon Press, Oxford (1982).
46. B. Ryberg. Studies on complement-fixing antibrain antibodies in multiple sclerosis, Thesis, University of Lund, Lund, Sweden (1981).
47. B. Ryberg and C. Jacque. Are anti-brain antibodies in multiple sclerosis directed to myelin basic protein? Studies employing the Shiverer mouse mutant. Acta Neurol. Scand. 73:247 (1986).
48. R. Arnon, E. Crisp, R. Kelly, G.W. Ellison, L.W. Myers and W.W. Tourtellotte. Anti-ganglioside antibodies in multiple sclerosis. J. Neurol. Sci. 46:179 (1980).
49. S. Karpiak, Y.L. Huang and M.M. Rapport. Immunological model of epilepsy. J. Neuroimmunol. 3:15 (1982).
50. G.A. Roth, M. Röyttä, R.K. Yu, C.S. Raine and M.B. Bornstein. Antisera to different glycolipids induce myelin alterations in mouse spinal cord tissue cultures. Brain Res. 339:9 (1985).
51. J.L. Trotter. Studies on the role of myelin proteolipid protein in chronic progressive experimental encephalomyelitis and multiple sclerosis. Ann. Neurol. 14:115 (1983).
52. A. Wajgt and M. Gorny. CSF antibodies to myelin basic protein and to myelin-associated glycoprotein in intrathecal production of antibodies. Acta Neurol. Scand. 68:337 (1983).

53. S.A. McMillan and M. Haire. The specificity of IgG- and IgM-class smooth muscle antibody in sera of patients with multiple sclerosis and active chronic hepatitis. Clin. Immunol. Immunopathol. 14:256 (1979).
54. H.J. Nordal and B. Vandvik. Evidence of local synthesis of smooth-muscle antibodies in the central nervous system in isolated cases of multiple sclerosis and chronic lymphocytic meningoencephalitis. Scand. J. Immunol. 6:327 (1977).
55. T. Hyypiä, M. Viander, M. Reunanen and A. Salmi. Antibodies to nuclear and smooth muscle antigens in multiple sclerosis and control patients. Acta Neurol. Scand. 65:629 (1982).
56. C.H.J. Chou, F.C.H. Chou, W.W. Tourtellotte and R.F. Kibler. Devic's syndrome: Antibody to glial fibrillary acidic protein in cerebrospinal fluid. Neurology. 34:86 (1984).
57. J. Ruutiainen, J. Newcombe, A. Salmi, D. Dahl and H. Frey. Measurement of glial fibrillary acidic protein (GFAP) and anti-GFAP antibodies by solid phase radioimmunoassays. Acta Neurol. Scand. 63:297 (1981).
58. B. Langvad Hansen, G. Nörgaard Hansen, C. Hagen and P. Brodersen. Autoantibodies against pituitary peptides in sera from patients with multiple sclerosis. J. Neuroimmunol. 5:171 (1983).
59. A.L. Schochet, H.L. Weiner, J. Walker, K. McIntosh and P.F. Kohler. Lymphocytotoxic antibodies in multiple sclerosis. Clin. Immunol. Immunopathol. 7:15 (1977).
60. L. Rumbach, M.M. Tongio, J.M. Warter, C. Marescaux, S. Mayer and F. Rohmer. Lymphocytotoxic and monocytotoxic antibodies in the serum and cerebrospinal fluid of multiple sclerosis patients. J. Neuroimmunol. 3:263 (1982).
61. P. Dore-Duffy, J.O. Donaldson, B.L. Rothman and R.B. Zurier. Antinuclear antibodies in multiple sclerosis. Arch. Neurol. 39:504 (1982).
62. E. Schuller, N. Delasnerie and P. Lebon. DNA and RNA antibodies in serum and CSF of multiple sclerosis and subacute sclerosing panencephalitis patients. J. Neurol. Sci. 37:31 (1978).
63. A. Vandenbark, F. Van Rompey, D. Nijst, H. Heyligen and J. Raus. Cerebrospinal fluid antibodies detect brain antigens. In: "Immunological and clinical aspects of multiple sclerosis". R.E. Gonsette and P. Delmotte, eds. MTP Press Limited, Lancaster (1984).
64. V. Hukkanen, J. Ruutiainen, A. Salmi, M. Reunanen and H. Frey. Antibodies in cerebrospinal fluid to white matter glycoproteins in multiple sclerosis patients. Neurosci. Lett. 35:327 (1983).
65. J. Clausen. Serum antibodies against cytosol antigens in multiple sclerosis. J. Neurol. Sci. 60:205 (1983).
66. K.P. Johnson, B. Vandvik and E. Norrby. Immunological responses to viruses in multiple sclerosis: Humoral immunity. In: "Clinics in immunology and allergy", vol.2, No.2, B.H. Waksman, ed. W.B. Saunders Company Ltd, London (1982).

INTRATHECAL IgG (Gm) ALLOTYPES IN MULTIPLE SCLEROSIS

Jean-Michel Goust[1,2], Jean-Philippe Salier[1,3]
and Hans Link[4]

[1]Department of Basic and Clinical Immunology and Microbiology
[2]Department of Neurology, Medical University of South Carolina, Charleston, South Carolina 29425
[3]Unite INSERM U295, St. Etienne du Rouray, France
[4]Department of Neurology, Karolinska Institutet, Huddinge University Hospital, S-14186 Huddinge, Stockholm, Sweden

An elevation of intrathecal IgG was the first immunologic abnormality to be observed in Multiple Sclerosis (1). It is now well established that it represents an increased local synthesis by B lymphocytes whose persistent activation and differentiation in the CNS could result from a relative unresponsiveness of some of these B cells to suppression (2) and or from defective suppressor T cell functions (3-4). The oligoclonal pattern observed after isoelectric focusing of the CSF is an indicator of the restricted nature of the intrathecal and intraparenchymal immune response (4). However, this type of pattern, when found with purified antigen-specific normal IgG is constituted of a heterogenous population of IgG in each band (5). Thus, antigenic markers of IgG representing genetic markers of individual clones such as the Gm allotypes, would represent better indices of clonal restriction. We first observed that the frequency of the particular phenotype Gm 1,17,21 was higher than expected in MS in a population from the Western USA (6). This was subsequently confirmed in Australia (7) and Sweden (8). That this could represent an association due to the spread of the disease from Scandinavia is suggested by the fact that this was not observed in French population (9). Furthermore, allelic exclusion implies that in heterozygotes G1m(1) or G1m(3) allotypes or IgG1 are produced by distinct B cell subsets which are imbalanced in MS patients (10).

Paired CSF and serum samples obtained from clinically definite MS patients were studied. Gm phenotypes and haplotypes were determined from the array of allotypes found in the patient's serum by inhibition of hemagglutination as previously reported (6). The CSF sample was used to determine the concentrations of the IgG1 allotypes G1m(1) and G1m(3) by radioimmunoassay using anti-Gm human sera as previously described (10). More recently a rabbit antiserum specific for the IgG3 G3m(11) allotype was also used for the quantitation of this allotype (11).

Three populations of patients suffering from clinically definite MS were studied. The first included those individuals whose CSF and serum had been obtained through the National Research Bank, Los Angeles, CA.

The second group of patients was under the care of Dr. H. Link and was selected on the basis of the availability of several CSF-serum pairs obtained over a period of 2 to 4 years. The third group included individuals followed at the Neurological Clinic of the Hospital H. Mohdor, Creteil, France.

We previously showed (10) that, in heterozygous Gm^1/Gm^3 MS persons, the G1m(1) allotype of IgG1 was four times more abundant in the CSF than G1m(3). This observation did not establish that an intrathecal production of these allotypes actually occurred. It could have represented an under evaluation of the G1m(3) concentration. Indeed, this allotype is determined by the existence of an Arginine in position 214 in the CH1 domain of the IgG1 heavy chains. However, the expression of the epitope surrounding this amino acid is strongly influenced by the type of light chain attached to the whole IgG1 molecule so that the apparent G1m(3) concentration is higher with lambda chains than with kappa chains (12). Since an increased kappa/ lambda ratio has been reported in the CSF of up to 50% of the MS patients (13) this could have caused an underestimation of the true G1m(3) concentration. After the completion of our initial study (10), we obtained the concentrations of albumin and IgG in the serum and CSF of all the individuals entered in this study. In heterozygous Gm^1/Gm^3, the IgG1 G1m(1) constituted 68% of the total IgG, IgG1 G1m(3) being only 15.2%. Together these two allotypes of IgG1 constituted 84% of the total CSF IgG (Table 1). In Gm^3/Gm^3 homozygous the concentrations of IgG1 G1m(3) and of total IgG were very strongly correlated ($r=0.841$; $p<0.01$) and IgG1 G1m(3) represented all of the CSF IgG. Different results were observed in heterozygous Gm^1/Gm^3 in whom there was no relation ($r=0.17$) between IgG1 G1m(3) and total IgG concentrations, whereas a significant correlation was observed between G1m(1) and IgG concentrations ($r=0.746$; $p<0.05$). The most significant correlation in this group was between the total concentration of IgG1 allotypes (IgG1 G1m(1+3)) and total IgG ($r=0.824$; $p<0.01$). This strict correlation between allotype and total IgG concentrations establishes that the concentrations of IgG1 allotypes determined by radioimmunoassay are unbiased by technical artifacts.

Table 1. Relative Proportions of IgG and IgG1 Allotypes in the CSF of Homozygous Gm^3/Gm^3 and Heterozygous Gm^1/Gm^3 MS Patients (*)

A = Homozygous Gm^3/Gm^3 (16)

Total IgG 12.06 ± 0.41
IgG1 G1m(3) = 12.9 ± 4.0

B = HeterozygousGm^1/Gm^3 (10)

Total IgG = 12.09 ± 1.13
IgG1 G1m(1) = 8.26 ± 2.61
IgG1 G1m(3) = 1.84 ± 0.44
IgG1 G1m (1+3) = 10.15 ± 3.00 (**)

IgG1 G1m (1)/IgG = .68
IgG1 G1m (3)/IgG = .152
IgG1 G1m (1+3)/IgG = .84

(*) Data obtained with the population studied in Reference (10). All values are expressed in mg/ 1 ± SEM

(**) Addition of the IgG1 G1m(1) + IgG1 G1m(3) concentrations

Furthermore, it strengthens the previously described predominance of IgG1 amongst other IgG subclasses in the CSF of MS patients in whom it was found to constitute 80.6% to 82% of the total IgG (14,15) and that in Gm^3/Gm^3 individuals the totality of intrathecal IgG are IgG1. To further ascertain that these allotypes were actually synthesized intrathecally, an allotype index was calculated according to Tibling and Link (16) and compared to the CSF IgG index calculated in the same individual. The results (Table 2) demonstrate that both IgG1 allotypes are produced intrathecally. As expected, there was a strong correlation between the total IgG index and the IgG1 G1m(3) index in homozygous G1m(3), and between the IgG1 G1m(1) and IgG1m(1+3) indices and the IgG index in heterozygous Gm^1/Gm^3, in whom, however, the CSF IgG1 G1m(3) index was above 0.7 in only 4 individuals. Thus the quantitatively imbalanced representation of only one of the two possible allotypes of IgG1 observed in heterozygous is most likely due to a true intrathecal synthesis of IgG1 G1m(1) contrasting with a more seldom observed synthesis of IgG1 G1m(3). Thus, even though the CSF IgG Index does not represent a true synthetic rate (16), it is reasonable to assume that the basis for this phenomenon is a disproportionate increase in the lesions of the B cell clones committed to produce IgG1 G1m(1), associated to a relative exclusion of B cell clones producing IgG1 G1m(3). This is indeed probable as shown in a later study of allotype concentrations in the eluates of different plaques from several M.S. brains (17).

Table 2. Relations between CSF Allotypes Indices and CSF IgG Index

(A) Homozygous Gm^3/Gm^3 (16)

CSF Index = 0.988 ± 0.29
CSF IgG1 G1m Index(1) = 2.11 ± 0.65

Correlation between CSF IgG Index and CSF IgG1 G1m(3) Index: (r = 0.828; p<0.001)

(B) Heterozygous Gm^1/Gm^3 (10)

CSF IgG Index(1) = 0.976 ± 0.05
CSF IgG1 G1m(1) Index = 2.74 ± .77
CSF IgG1 G1m(3) Index = 0.64 ± 0.07
CSF IgG1 G1m(1+3) Index = 1.43 ± 0.30

Correlation between:
(a) CSF IgG Index and CSF IgG1 G1m(1) Index
r = 0.746 p<0.05
(b) CSF IgG Index and CSF IgG1 G1m(3) Index
r = 0.557 (n.s.)
(c) CSF IgG Index and CSF IgG1 G1m(1+3) Index
r = 0.828 p<0.001

Nevertheless, the study of a single sample does not establish the persistence of this phenomenon in a long-lasting disease. To determine this, a group of Swedish MS patients from whom serial serum and CSF samples had been collected over a period of two or three years, was studied. The results (Tables 3 and 4) establish that in Gm^1/Gm^3 heterozygous patients, the intrathecal synthesis of the IgG1 G1m(1) allotype dominates within the CSF, as indicated by the finding that the IgG1 G1m(1) Index was permanently higher than the IgG1 G1m(3) index in all patients at all points in time. However, an intrathecal synthesis of IgG1 G1m(3), indicated by an IgG1 G1m(3) Index > 0.70 was observed in 21/30 samples (40%), and present at some point in time in all but one patient but never exceeding the G1m(1) Index. Eventually intrathecal synthesis of IgG3 though

Table 3. Longitudinal study of CSF IgG Indices and CSF Allotypes Indices in heterozygous Gm^1/Gm^3 MS patients

Sample # year	Indices[1] IgG	G1m(1)	G1m(3)	G3m(11)	IgG1[2]	CSF IgG	IgG(Allo)[3]
Patient # 2							
1 1978	0.96	4.41	0.85*	0.42	3.13	6.0	10.29
2 1978	1.0	3.66	0.49	2.60*	2.40	7.8	9.575
3 1980	1.23	4.76	0.60	0.49	3.05	8.0	6.87
4 1980	1.06	4.20	0.89*	0.45	2.88	7.4	6.23
5 1982	1.13	3.43	0.48	0.13	2.14	6.8	5.86
Patient # 7							
1 1980	3.23	6.89	5.23*	0.63	6.16	10.4	10.8
2 1981	3.46	14.10	8.15*	1.04*	10.93	11.1	13.9
3 1981	3.11	10.10	5.0*	0.62	7.44	11.3	13.6
4 1982	3.50	5.68	3.24*	0.60	4.39	11.9	9.8

Patient # 8							
1 1980	1.9	11.0	0.28	0.37	6.13	12	16.5
2 1980	1.3	6.95	0.53	0.72	4.38	8.2	10.8
3 1980	1.45	6.09	0.67	2.19*	3.92	10.8	10.7
4 1981	1.75	7.28	0.70	0.21	2.10	15	16.25
5 1982	2.01	3.62	0.27	1.27*	2.25	14.4	9.1

(1) IgG Indices calculated according to Ref.16 CSF Alb, Serum Alb, CSF IgG and serum IgG were determined at the time of L.P. Gm allotype concentrations in the same samples were used to calculate the G1m(1), G1m(3) and G3m(11) Indices.

(2) The IgG1 Index was calculated using the sum of the IgG1 G1m(1) and IgG1 G1m(3) allotypes.

(3) IgG Allo = sum of the allotypes concentration: (IgG1, G1m(1) + IgG1 G1m(3) + IgG3 G3m(11)) in mg/dl.

The asterisk(*) denotes those CSF in which the IgG1 G1m(3) Index and/or the IgG3 G3m(11) Index is higher than 0.7.

Table 4. Longitudinal study of CSF IgG Indices and CSF Allotypes Indices in heterozygous Gm^1/Gm^3 MS patients

	Indices					CSF IgG	IgG(Allo)(3)
Patient # 9							
Sample # year	IgG (1)	G1m(1) (1)	G1m(3) (1)	G3m(11) (1)	IgG_1 (2)		
1 1981	1.21	3.72	2.15*	1.59*	3.18	5.6	6.5
2 1981	0.83	4.06	0.70	0.31	2.61	4.7	5.47
3 1981	1.30	4.32	0.60	0.50	2.71	6.4	6.8
4 1981	1.22	2.81	0.60	0.16	2.18	6.5	6.27
5 1982	1.23	3.94	0.53	0.43	2.43	6.9	7.06
Patient # 13							
1 1980	1.23	8.80	0.59	0.50	5.20	7.3	6.98
2 1980	1.82	5.10	1.76*	1.69*	3.90	10.4	7.94
3 1980	1.17	3.16	3.56*	1.40*	3.30	7.1	7.45
4 1981	1.0	4.93	1.11*	0.68	3.47	6.4	7.59

Patient # 16							
1 1981	1.28	2.50	1.24*	0.30	1.93	6.3	5.0
2 1981	0.92	2.55	0.74*	0.33	1.66	5.1	5.07
3 1981	1.27	3.29	1.84*	1.58*	2.61	6.6	6.6
4 1981	0.86	2.26	0.61	0.37	1.43	5.3	5.06
Patient # 18							
1 1976	1.33	6.80	0.39	0.20	3.15	5.0	4.74
2 1976	1.15	7.09	0.27	0.10	3.27	5.2	5.93
3 1977	1.45	5.00	0.34	0.47	2.44	5.4	3.67

Table legends same as for Table 3.

much lower than IgG1 synthesis, was sometimes observed since an IgG3 G3m(11) Index above 0.70 was found in 8 out of 30 (26%) of the CSF studied. The most striking feature of these data was the apparently independent fluctuation of all these Indices. Even if this might be somehow related to the activity of the disease, the small number of subjects and the relativity of the clinical criteria used to determine disease activity definitely preclude any conclusion.

At any rate, this excessive intrathecal production of IgG1 G1m(1) persists for years in heterozygous Gm^1/Gm^3 suggesting that once they have entered the CNS, these particular G1m(11) B-cell clones are maintained at a permanent level of differentiation. This observation agrees with the data of Walsh and Tourtellotte (18) and suggests that in MS patients IgG bands are truly "oligoclonal" not only because of their restricted physico-chemical characteristics, but also in the genetic restrictions evidenced by their CH region since at least 85% of the IgG should be IgG1 G1m(1) in Gm^1/ Gm^3 and Gm^1/Gm^1 MS patients and IgG1 G1m(3) in Gm^3/Gm^3 MS patients. The extent of this clonal restriction is also evidenced by the relative dominance of some IgG idiotypes which are found in the serum and the CSF of MS patients (19,20) where they constitute 24 to 33% of the CSF IgG (20). The association of these putative V gene products to the predominant gamma 1 gene products observed in our study, though not impossible, appears nevertheless unlikely, due to the random nature of the V - (D) - J recombinations (21) so that a large clonal heterogeneity could still exist within the restricted B cell population found in MS. The transient appearance of G1m(3) and/ or of G3m(11) production on this predominant G1m(1) production probably indicates the entry of new B cell clones in the CNS and could correspond to the appearance of new oligoclonal bands in an otherwise stable pattern as reported by Vartdal (22). This persistent IgG1 G1m(1) production could result from a preferential activation of this subset by autologous T cells and their products, driving this subset toward growth and differentiation (23) once it has been selected by the CNS. We previously suggested that the selection of the B cells may be achieved by way of an Ig-CH (allotype)-linked recognition unit on the B-cell membrane, which would be complementary to a structure expressed on the vascular endothelium of the blood-brain barrier (25), the selective egress from blood to CNS of IgG1 G1m(1) B cells in Gm^1/Gm^3 individuals leading to their relative depletion in the peripheral blood. A different recognition unit may be present in Gm^3/Gm^3 individuals whose circulating lymphocytes have been depleted of IgG1 G1m(3) producing B cells which have homed into the patient's CNS (25). The Gm phenotype does not by itself entirely determine the degree of intrathecal activation of these selected B-cell clones since the CSF IgG levels and CSF IgG indices of Gm^3/Gm^3 patients are not different from those of Gm^1/Gm^3 individuals. Gm^1/Gm^1 patients were too few to observe in this group the higher level of CSF IgG reported by Sandberg-Wollheim et al.(8). Once these allotype-restricted B cells have entered the CNS, their activation may be HLA restricted. Indeed, the quantitative expression of the Gm gene products may be influenced by the HLA-DR type of the individual, so that Gm^1/Gm^3, HLADR2(+) MS patients have higher levels of IgG1 G1m(1) and of total IgG in their CSF than Gm^1/Gm^3, HLADR2(-) patients. In contrast in Gm^3/Gm^3 patients, the presence of the HLADR2(+) was associated with CSF levels of IgG1 G1m(3) which were significantly lower than those found in Gm^3/Gm^3, HLADR2(-) individuals (25).

T lymphocytes which play a role in MHC-restricted B-cell activation, most likely use a different recognition unit to enter the CNS. It has been suggested that the T cells emigrating in an exudate use as recognition unit the MHC antigens expressed on the vascular side of the endothelium (26), where HLA-DR has been found in humans (27). The human T cells interacting with the non-polymorphic part of HLA-DR (class II-MHC antigens) bear the CD4 molecule (28), and have been found to infiltrate MS lesions (29). These CD4 cells, whose IL-2 production in response to class II-MHC antigens on autologous B cell lines exceeds that of normal T cells (30), could, once activated, perpetuate the intraparenchymal immune response in which Gm and MHC restrictions, determining the amplitude of the response, could influence the severity of the disease, as suggested in a recent study (31).

REFERENCES

1. E.A. Kabat, M. Glusman and V. Knaub. Quantitative estimation of the albumin and -globulin in normal and pathologic cerebrospinal fluid by immunochemical methods. Am. J. Med. 4:653 (1942).
2. J.M. Goust, P. Arnaud, E.L. Hogan. Defective regulation of IgG production in Multiple Sclerosis. Neurology. 32:228 (1982).
3. B.G.W. Arnasson, J.P. Antel, A.T. Reder. Immunoregulation in Multiple Sclerosis. Ann. N.Y. Acad. Sci. 436:133 (1985).
4. P.Y. Paterson, C.C. Whitacre. The enigma of oligoclonal immunoglobulin G in cerebrospinal fluid from Multiple Sclerosis patients. Immunol. Today. 2:111 (1981).
5. J.D. Rodwell. Heterogeneity of component bands in isoelectric focusing patterns. Anal. Biochem. 119:440 (1982).
6. J.P. Pandey, J.M. Goust, J.P. Salier and H.H. Fudenberg. Immunoglobulin G heavy chain (Gm) allotypes in Multiple Sclerosis. J. Clin. Invest. 67:1797 (1981).
7. D.N. Propert, C.C.A. Bernard and J. Simons. Gm allotypes and Multiple Sclerosis. J. Immunogen. 9:359 (1982).
8. M. Sandberg-Wollheim, L.G. Baird, M.S. Schanfield, M.H. Knopper, K. Youker and T.G. Tachovsky. Association of CSF IgG concentrations and immunoglobulin allotypes in Multiple Sclerosis and optic neuritis. Clin. Immunol. Immunopathol. 31:212 (1984).
9. R. Sesboue, M. Daveau, J.D. Degos, C. Martin-Mondiere, L. Rivat-Peran, A. Coquerel, J.M. Goust and J.P. Salier. IgG(Gm) allotypes and Multiple Sclerosis in a French population. Clin. Immunol. Immunopathol. 37:145 (1985).
10. J.P. Salier, J.M. Goust, J.P. Pandey and H.H. Fudenberg. Preferential synthesis of the G1m(1) allotype of IgG1 in the central nervous system of Multiple Sclerosis patients. Science. 213:1400 (1981).
11. J.P. Salier, H. Sarvas, H.M. Reisner, A.C. Wang. and H.H. Fudenberg. Quantitative studies of Gm allotypes. III. Some effects of IgG aggregation in radioimmunoassays using human IgM and rabbit IgG anti-Gm antibodies. Mol. Immunol. 16:217 (1979).
12. J.P. Salier, C. Rivat, L. Rivat, C. Bastard, G. Virella, H.H. Fudenberg and A.C. Wang. Quantitative studies of Gm allotypes. IV. Quantitative variations of G1m(3) antigenicity in relation to light chain type and VK subgroup. Mol. Immunol. 17, 229 (1980).
13. H. Link and O. Zetterval. Multiple Sclerosis: disturbed kappa/lambda light chains ratio of immunoglobulin G in cerebrospinal fluid. Clin. Exp. Immunol. 6:435 (1970).
14. K. Eickhoff, W. Kaschka, F. Skvaril, L. Theilkaes and R. Heipertz. Determination of IgG subgroups in cerebrospinal fluid of Multiple Sclerosis patients and others. Acta Neurol. Scandinav. 60:277 (1979).
15. W.P. Kaschka, L. Theilkaes, K. Eickhoff and F. Skvaril. Disproportionate elevation of the immunoglobulin G1 concentration in cerebrospinal fluid of patients with Multiple Sclerosis. Inf. Immun. 26:933 (1979).
16. A.K. Lefvert and H. Link. IgG production within the central nervous system: a critical review of proposed formulae. Ann. Neurol. 17:13 (1985).

17. J.P. Salier, P. Glynn, J.M. Goust and M.L. Cuzner. Distribution of latent IgG(Gm) allotypes in plaques of Multiple Sclerosis brains. Clin. Exp. Immunol. 54:634 (1983).
18. M.J. Walsh and W.W. Tourtellotte. Temporal invariance and clonal uniformity of brain and cerebrospinal fluid IgG, IgA, IgM in Multiple Sclerosis. J. Exp. Med. 163:41 (1986).
19. T.G. Tachovski, M. Sandberg-Wollheim and L.G. Baird. Characterization of anti-idiotypic antibodies produced against MS CSF and detection of cross-reactive idiotypes in several MS CSF. J. Immunol. 129, 764 (1982).
20. L.M. Nagelkerken, M. Van Zoonen-Van Exel, H.K. Van Wallbeck, S.C. Aalberse and T.A. Out. Analysis of cerebrospinal fluid and serum of patients with Multiple Sclerosis by means of anti-idiotypic antisera. J. Immunol. 128:1102-1106 (1982).
21. T. Honjo. Immunoglobulin genes. In: "Annual Review of Immunology". Ann. Rev. Inc. Pub. 499 (1983).
22. F. Vartdal and B. Vandvik. Multiple Sclerosis: Subclasses of intrathecally synthesized IgG and measles and varicella zoster virus IgG antibodies. Clin. Exp. Immunol. 54:641 (1983).
23. T. Kishimoto. Factors affecting B cell growth and differentiation. In: "Annual Review of Immunology". Ann. Rev. Pub. 133 (1985).
24. J.M. Goust and J.P. Salier. Imbalance in recruitment of IgG(Gm) allotypes producing B cell subsets from blood to brain in Multiple Sclerosis. Cell. Immunol. 88:551 (1984).
25. J.P. Salier, C. Martin-Mondiere, R. Sesboue, M. Daveau, J.M Goust, A. Govaerts, E. Schuller and J.D. Degos. HLA-DR-dependent variation of intrathecal IgG1(Gm) allotype synthesis in Multiple Sclerosis. J. Immunol. 134:1551 (1985).
26. M. Skoskiewicz, R.B. Colvin, E. Schneeberger and P.S. Russell. Widespread and selection induction of major-histocompatibility complex-determined antigens in vivo by gamma-interferon. J. Exp. Med. 162: 1645 (1985).
27. S.L. Hauser, A.K. Bhan, F.H. Gilles, C.F. Hoban, E.L. Reinherz, S.F. Schlossman and H.L. Weiner. Immune histochemical staining of human brain with monoclonal antibodies that identify lymphocytes, monocytes and the Ia antigen. J. Neuroimmunol. 197 (1983).
28. E.W. Biddison, P.E. Rao. M.E. Talle, G. Goldstein and S. Shaw. Possible involvment of the OKT4 molecule in T-cell recognition of class II HLA antigens. J. Exp. Med. 156:1065 (1982).
29. U. Traugott, E.L. Reinherz and C.S. Raine. Multiple Sclerosis: Distribution of T cell, T cell subsets and Ia positive macrophages in lesions of different age. J. Neuroimmunol. 4:201 (1983).
30. S.J. Verselis and J.M. Goust. CD4 T cell activation in Multiple Sclerosis. J. Neuroimmunol. (submitted).
31. J.P. Salier, R. Sesboue, C. Martin-Mondiere, M. Daveau, P. Cesaro, B. Cavelier, A. Coquerel, L. Legrand, J.M. Goust and J.D. Degos. Combined influences of Gm and HLA phenotypes upon Multiple Sclerosis susceptibility and severity. J. Clin. Invest. (In press).

Gm ALLOTYPES IN MULTIPLE SCLEROSIS

D.E. Bulman[1], J.P. Pandey[2],
and G.C. Ebers[3]

[1]Department of Clinical Neurological Sciences, University of Western Ontario
[2]Department of immunology, University of South Carolina Charleston, South Carolina
[3]Department of Clinical Neurological Sciences, University Hospital, University of Western Ontario, P.O. Box 5339 London, Ontario, Canada N6A 5A5

INTRODUCTION

It has recently become clear that genetic factors play an important role in susceptibility to MS and ideed, they may be necessary for the development of the disease. This has been shown most clearly in a Canadian population-based study of twins which demonstrated a high concordance rate in identical pairs and a ten-fold lower concordance rate in fraternal twins and siblings (Ebers, et al., submitted for publication). Furthermore, strong evidence implicates the immune system in the pathogenesis of the disease. This includes the recent development of animals models in which tissue injury is clearly mediated by T-lymphocytes. These models appear to closely parallel the human disease.

The pathology of MS is consistent with immunologically mediated damage. As well, the high frequency of oligoclonal banding in MS CSF supports immunological stimulation as part of the MS process. Since several aspects of immune responsiveness are under genetic control, it would seem profitable to study genetic markers associated with immune responsiveness in patients with MS.

There are numerous levels at which the immune response may be genetically controlled. The most obvious of these constitute the Class II major histocompatibility determinants present on the surface of macrophages. These molecules, in conjunction with antigen, are recognized by antigen specific T-cells. In mice and other species these molecules may function as immune response (IR) genes and determine responsiveness or lack of responsiveness to discrete antigenic determinants.

Studies in MS have shown clearly that MS is associated with the HLA-A3, B7,DR2 haplotype, at least in European populations (reviewed in McDonald, 1986; Ebers 1984). This has led to the expectation that MS is determined by a gene in linkage disequilibrium with the DR2 antigen as part of the above haplotype. However, studies of multiplex families have given ambiguous results for linkage to DR2 (Ebers et al., 1983). Loose linkage has been implied by these data. This poses a conundrum since loose linkage would be inconsistent with the substantial population association, at least for European derived peoples, unless some form of selection is postulated. Possible explanations for these data include disease heterogeneity (i.e. HLA-linked and unlinked cases which as of yet are undistinguishable), or epistasis (i.e. interaction of linked and/or unlinked genes to produce overall susceptibility). The possible existence of a second gene (or others) unlinked to HLA (Ho, et al, 1982; Ebers, 1983) has led to the examination of other loci putatively associated with immune responsiveness.

Variable (V) region genes in humans are encoded on chromosome 14 and may potentially be responsible for IR gene effects. Therefore, markers linked to these genes seem appropriate for study in MS patients and their families. The Gm system constitutes a series of very tightly linked immunoglobulin (Ig) heavy chain allotypic markers in close proximity to Ig V regions. The exact recombination fractions have yet to be accurately defined; such data could be influenced by the possibly high recombination rates within the V region area.

At least three reports have suggested a modest association between MS and Gm ^{1,17,21} (Pandey et al., 1981; Propert et al., 1982; Sandberg-Wollheim, 1984). This has been interpreted to mean that a gene(s) linked to Gm has played an important role in MS susceptibility. On the basis of the above considerations and these early reports, we have studied Gm allotypes in MS patients and controls to try to confirm the reported population association. Furthermore, multiplex families have been studied to evaluate the notion that a Gm linked susceptibility gene exists.

METHODS

a) Non Familial MS: One hundred and fifty-eight caucasian MS patients from Southwestern Ontario with clinically definite (Schumacher et al., 1968) or laboratory supported probable disease (Poser et al., 1984) were studied.
b) Controls consisted of 89 neurologically normal caucasians from the same geographically defined area as the MS cases.
c) Fifty-nine multiplex MS families comprising 509 individuals were typed for Gm and genotype frequencies were derived.
d) Gm allotyping was performed by Dr. J. Pandey using standard techniques (Vyas et al., 1968) without knowledge of affection status or familial relationships. Discrepancies in pedigree data were resolved by retyping.
e) Genotype frequencies for Gm1, Gm2 and Gm3 were calculated using the computer program Allotype (Morton et al., 1983).
f) Linkage analysis was performed using the computer program COMBIN (McLean et al., 1984).

RESULTS

The frequencies of Gm phenotypes in non-familial MS and control cases are seen in Table 1.

Linkage analysis using COMBIN showed that the maximum likelihood score was obtained with the model of no linkage with equal coupling frequencies. (Bulman et al., submitted for publication).

Table 1. Percentage distribution of Gm phenotypes in Multiple Sclerosis Patients (n=153)[a] and Normal controls (n=84)[a].

Gm Phenotype	MS Patients	Normal Control	X^2	P
1,17,21	5.23	3.57	.066	>0.75
1,2,17,21	3.92	5.95	.151	>0.50
1,2,3,17,5,13,21	12.42	17.86	.900	>0.25
1,3,17,5,13,21	27.45	25.00	.065	>0.75
3,5,13	50.98	47.62	.129	>0.25
Total	100.00	100.00		

[a] Three MS patients and 5 controls could not be definitively typed, were therefore not included into these totals.

The distribution of Gm genotypes in the 59 multiplex families in the affected and unaffected family members is seen in Table 2.

Table 2. Affection by Gm Allotype. Upper Number in Each Cell is Absolute Number of Cases. Lower Number is Row Percentage.

	GM GENOTYPE					
Affection	11	12	13	23	33	Total
Normal	29	2	118	13	229	391
	7.4	0.5	30.2	3.3	58.6	76.8
MS	8	2	32	5	71	118
	6.8	1.7	27.1	4.2	60.2	23.2
Total	37	4	150	18	300	
	7.3	.8	29.5	3.5	58.9	509

DISCUSSION

The available evidence suggests that MS susceptibility is determined by HLA-linked and unlinked loci (Ho et al., 1982; Ebers et al., 1983). Earlier reports in small MS patient samples suggested an association between MS and the Gm ^{1,17,21} allotype (Pandey et al., 1981; Propert et al., 1982; Sandberg-Wollheim et al., 1984). This has made Gm a candidate marker for the hypothesized HLA-unlinked locus (loci). The results presented here are similar to those reported elsewhere (Sesboue et al., 1985). The data do not support an association since the Gm ^{1,17,21} frequency was found to be the same in MS patients and controls.

Furthermore, the linkage study in a large number of multiplex families and the results of a smaller study reported by Haile et al., (1985) seem to clearly indicate that MS susceptibility is not linked to Gm. Nevertheless, the data from Gm studies have suggested to us a possible explanation for some of the population associations in MS.

Steinberg's Atlas of Gm allotypes (Steinberg and Cook, 1981) shows that the frequency of Gm ^{1,17,21} follows a definite north/south cline. Frequencies in Northern European populations approximate 30% gradually declining to 15% in Southern Europe. This cline is reminiscent of the well known north/south gradient for multiple sclerosis itself and raises the possibility that the modest Gm association reported, reflects a population stratification effect. It is not impossible that ethnicity differences between MS patients and their controls account for some of the population associations described in MS. This would obviate the implication that each of the associations signifies yet another susceptibility gene linked to the marker locus.

It is interesting that in a population which ethnically is relatively uniform, such as that of Southwestern Ontario, no association was found. The linkage study not surprisingly failed to support the hypothesis of a Gm-linked MS susceptibility gene and it would seem important that other markers be studied. However, because the recombination fraction between Gm and V-region genes has not been defined, the use of restriction fragment length polymorphisms for the V region should be employed to fully evaluate the role of V region genes in MS susceptibility. Such studies are in progress.

The realization that Gm allotype frequencies follow geographical clines has led us to re-evaluate the geographical distribution of MS which has been widely assumed to reflect the influence of an obscure environmental factor. We have shown (Ebers and Bulman, 1986) in the United States Veterans data (Kurtzke, 1979), which has unique ascertainment virtues, that the geographic distribution of MS can be explained at least as well on a genetic basis. Highly significant correlations were found when the rate of MS in each state was compared to that percentage of the population within the state which was of Northern European background. The largest correlations were found for peoples of Scandinavian ancestry.

It may well be that there exists no specific MS agent but rather that the triggering of the MS process resembles the situation in post-infectious encephalomyelitis or post-infectious polyneuritis where numerous specific inciting agents can be readily identified. Among these triggers no common thread exists except the association with a discrete immunological stimulus, usually a viral infection or an immunization.

We doubt the validity of migration studies which, according to some investigators, have supported the existence of a specific environmental agent. Our main objection is that migrants are highly selected and may not be representative of the country from which they originate. For example, migrants from Israel cannot be assumed to have the same rate of MS in Western Europe as the indigenous population. If this is assumed, the argument becomes circular because one has already concluded that environment and not genetic susceptibility is responsible for the development of the disease.

In summary, the frequency of Gm allotypes were not found to be altered in MS patients as compared to controls. Evidence against linkage of Gm susceptibility to MS was shown with the study of multiplex families. Gm allotype frequencies, however, do illustrate geographical clines recalling the worldwide distribution of MS. We propose that the prevalence of MS on a global basis reflects the distribution of ethnic migrations and the stratification of susceptibility genes. Further work is needed to confirm this suggestion and further to characterize the genetic nature of MS susceptibility.

ACKNOWLEDGEMENTS

The authors wish to acknowledge Brenda Bass for excellent editorial assistance and Carole Sutherland for typing the manuscript.

REFERENCES

1. G.C. Ebers, D.E. Bulman, A.D. Sadovnick, D.W. Paty, S. Warren, W. Hader, T.J. Murray, T.P. Seland, P. Duquette, T. Gray, R. Nelson, M. Nicolle and D. Brunet. A population based study of multiple sclerosis twins. Submitted for publication.
2. G.C. Ebers and D.E. Bulman. The geography of MS reflects genetic susceptibility. Neurol. (Suppl.1). 36(4):108 (1986).
3. G.C. Ebers, N. Morten and D.W. Paty. Segregation and linkage analysis of HLA typing in familial MS. Neurol. 33 No 4(2):180 (1983).
4. R.W.C. Haile, A. Goldstein, L. Field and M.L. Marazita. A linkage analysis of Gm locus and multiple sclerosis. Genet. Epidemiol. 2:29-34 (1985).
5. H.Z. Ho, J.L. Tiwari, R.W. Haile, P.I. Terasaki and N.E. Morton. HLA-linked and unlinked determinants of multiple sclerosis. Immunogenet. 15:509-17 (1982).
6. J.F. Kurtzke, G.W. Beebe and J.E. Norman. Epidemiology of multiple sclerosis in US veterans: III. Migration and the risk of MS. Neurol. 35:672-78 (1979).
7. C.J. Maclean, N.E. Morton and S. Yee. Combined analysis of genetic segregation and linkage under an oligogenic model. Computer Biomed. Res. 17: 471-80 (1984).
8. W.I. McDonald. The mystery of the origin of multiple sclerosis. J. Neurol. Neurosurg. Psychiat. 49: 113-23 (1986).
9. N.E. Morton, D.C. Rao and M.M. Lalouel. Methods in Genetic Epidemiology. S. Karger, Switzerland (1983).
10. J.P.Pandey, J.M. Goust, J.P. Salier and H.H. Fudenberg. Immunoglobulin G heavy chain (Gm) allotypes in multiple sclerosis. J. Clin. Invest. 67: 1797-800 (1981).
11. C.M. Poser, D.W. Paty, L. Scheinberg, W.I. McDonald, F.A. Davis, G.C. Ebers, K.P. Johnson, W.A. Sibley, D.H. Silberberg and W.W. Tourtellotte. New diagnostic criteria for multiple sclerosis. Guidelines for Research Protocols. In: "The Diagnosis of Multiple Sclerosis", C.W. Poser, ed. Thieme-Stratton Inc., New York (1984).
12. D.N. Propert, C.C.A. Denard and M.J. Simons. Gm allotypes and multiple sclerosis. J. Immunogenet. 9: 359-61 (1982).
13. M. Sandberg-Wollheim, L.G. Baird, M.S. Schanfield, M.H. Knoppers, K. Youker and T.G. Tachovsky. Association of CSF IgG concentrations and immunoglobulin allotypes in multiple sclerosis and optic neuritis. Clin. Immunol. Immunopath. 31: 212-21 (1984).
14. G.A. Schumacher, G. Beeber, R.F. Kibler, L.T. Kurland, J.F. Kurtzke, F. McDowell, B. Nagler, W.A. Sibley, W.W. Tourtellotte and T.L. Willmon. Problems of experimental trials of therapy in MS: Report of the panel on the evaluation of experimental trials in MS. Ann. NY Acad. Sci. 122: 552-68 (1986).
15. R. Sesboue, M. Daveau, J.D. Degos, C. Martin-Mondrere, J.M. Goust, E. Schuller, L. Rivat-Peran, A. Coquerel, M. Dujardin and J.P. Salier. IgG (Gm) allotypes and multiple sclerosis in a french population: Phenotype distribution and quantitative abnormalities in CSF with respect to sex, disease severity and presence of intrathecal antibodies. Clin. Immunol. Immunopath. 37: 143-53 (1985).

16. A.G. Steinberg and G.E. Cook. The distribution of the Human Immunoglobulin Allotypes. Oxford Monographs on Medical Genetics. Oxford University Press, Oxford.

17. G.N. Vyas, H.H. Fudenberg, H.M. Pretty and E.R. Golder. A new rapid method for genetic typing of human immunoglobulins. J. Immunol. 100: 274-9 (1968).

THE INTRATHECAL ANTIBODY PRODUCTION IN MULTIPLE SCLEROSIS: NONSENSE VERSUS DISEASE-RELATED ANTIBODIES

Walter Gerhard[1], Dale McCreedy[1], Magnhild Sandberg[2] and Hilary Koprowski[1]

[1]The Wistar Institute of Anatomy and Biology, Philadelphia PA 19104
[2]The Department of Neurology, University of Lund, Sweden

INTRODUCTION

The production of restricted immunoglobulin (Ig) subpopulations by intrathecally localized B cells is the most frequent laboratory finding in multiple sclerosis (MS) patients. Numerous studies have been conducted in the past to elucidate the potential pathogenetic relevance of this intrathecal Ig production (for review see ref.1). In brief, the following observations were made: 1) Intrathecally produced antibodies display many different specificities and, to date, no single specificity (e.g. antiviral, anti-self component) characteristic for all MS patients has been defined. The types of antiviral antibody specificities comprised among the intrathecally produced antibodies seems to depend on the general immune status of the MS patient group under study. 2) Although the intrathecally produced Ig's are present, by definition, at higher relative concentration (compared to total Ig or albumin) in CSF, they are present at higher absolute concentration in serum. 3) There is no obvious relationship between specificity or extent of intrathecal Ig production and clinical course of disease. 4) Neither idiotypic nor spectrotypic analysis has revealed an Ig subpopulation common to MS patients. 5) Ig eluted form distinct plaques of an individual MS brain comprise spectrotypes that are unique for each plaque. 6) Intrathecal antibody production to irrelevant bystander antigens can be observed in experimental model systems and also in MS patients. Based on these findings, it has been proposed that the intrathecal Ig production is an epiphenomenon of the disease, resulting exclusively from the random recruitment of circulating B cells into the intrathecal compartment where they are stimulated, by locally active mitogenic factors, to antibody secretion. Accordingly, the specificities of the intrathecally produced antibodies are thought to have no relation to the disease process, i.e. they are "non-sense" antibodies (2). This hypothesis is difficult to reconcile, however, with observations indicating a remarkable stability in the composition of intrathecally produced Ig within individual patients over several years of disease (3-9).

Even if one accepts that the majority of intrathecally produced antibodies derive from randomly recruited and non-specifically activated B cells, it remains possible that a minor portion of the intrathecal antibody production is "disease-related", i.e. results from stimulation of B cell subsets by antigens present in or released from the developing plaque. We have tried to test this possibility as follows: Anti-idiotypic hybridoma antibodies were generated to CSF-Ig of MS patients and were then used to monitor the concentration of individual Ig-subpopulations in serum and CSF in the course of the disease. In one patient, who was in chronic progressive phase of disease, an Ig-subpopulation was found to be produced intrathecally at more or less invariant concentration over the entire 7 year observation period (4). In a second patient, who displayed a relapsing form of disease, we monitored three distinct Ig-subpopulations and found that one was only transiently synthesized by intrathecal B cells while the other two were produced, in some relation to the clinical course of disease, over the entire 5 year observation period (5). In the following, we report observations made on this patient during two additional years of disease in which the patient experienced another exacerbation. Additionally, we have determined the albumin concentration in all paired CSF/serum samples to assess extent of intrathecal Ig production over the entire observation period.

MATERIALS AND METHODS

Reagents and Assays

The concentration of total Ig and of idiotypically defined Ig-subpopulations in serum and CSF were determined by radioimmunoassay (RIA) as described previously (5). Albumin concentration in serum and CSF was determined by RIA as follows: Affinity-purified rabbit-anti-human-albumin was diluted 1/1000 in 0.02 M NaCl and 0.05 ml samples were adsorbed overnight into wells of polyvinyl plastic plates. The wells were then blocked by incubation with 1% bovine serum albumin in phosphate buffered saline (PBS-1% BSA). The wells were incubated for 4 hours with 0.025 ml of iodinated human albumin (20 000 cpm/well) and 0.025 ml of CSF or serum samples diluted in PBS-1% BSA, washed and the radioactivity bound to wells measured. The dilution of the testsample giving 50% inhibition of 125-I-albumin binding was determined and used as relative measure for the albumin concentration in the test sample. Ig-index and idiotype(Id)-index were calculated according to the formula:

(CSF - Ig / serum - Ig) / (CSF - Alb. / serum - Alb.)

CSF and Serum Specimens

Paired CSF and serum samples were obtained from a male MS patient. The history of this patient has been described previously (5). In brief, the patient was admitted to the hospital with symptoms of leftsided optic neuritis in February of 1978. By March 1978, dissemination of symptoms became apparent and spinal fluid obtained during this period revealed an increased Ig-index and oligoclonal bands. After a generally very active disease phase during 1978, the patient recovered sufficiently to perform parttime and later fulltime work. Several exacerbations occurred between 1979 to 1985 (see also Fig.1), the latest in November, 1984. The patient was given three ACTH treatments (indicated by arrows in Fig.1) during the course of disease.

All anti-idiotypic antibodies were generated against CSF-Ig obtained in April 1978.

RESULTS

Total Intrathecal Ig Production in Course of Disease

Intrathecal Ig production was assessed as outlined in the Materials and Methods section by determination of the Ig-index in paired CSF/serum samples. Ig-index values exceeding 0.66 are considered abnormal and indicative of intrathecal Ig production. As shown in Fig.1, considerable variations in extent of intrathecal Ig production occurred in the course of disease. On the basis of the presently analysed samples, it seems that the intrathecal Ig production occurred in several waves of declining intensity in the course of disease. It is possible that the wave-like pattern of intrathecal Ig production is related to the ACTH treatment.

CSF obtained in March 1978 two months after onset of clinically overt disease was used for production of four murine anti-idiotypic (anti-Id) hybridoma antibodies. The four anti-Id's were shown to recognize three distinct Ig-subpopulations which, toghether, constituted approximately 5% of the total CSF-Ig of the March 1978 CSF sample. These Ig-subpopulations are referred to in the following as ID-19, ID-40 and ID-97.

Longitudinal Analysis of Intrathecal Synthesis of ID's

The Id-indices were computed as the Ig-index except that ID concentrations in CSF and serum were used instead of total Ig concentration. Before considering in detail the behaviour of individual ID's (Fig.2), two general points are noteworthy: 1) Most of the Id-indices greatly exceed the total Ig-index in the same paired CSF/serum sample. This is because the total Ig-index provides a measure of the average intrathecal production of all Ig-subpopulations, some displaying higher and others lower indices than the total Ig. For example, an ID-index which is 10 times greater than the Ig-index indicates a 10 times more preferential intrathecal production of the given Ig-subpopulation compared to the total Ig (of which the ID may only be a small fraction). 2) Fig.2 shows also the total Ig-indices (asterisk). However, for better comparison, the Ig-indices are plotted as multiples of 10. Thus, an ID-index which coincides with an Ig-index mark indicates 10 times more preferential intrathecal production of the given ID compared to total Ig.

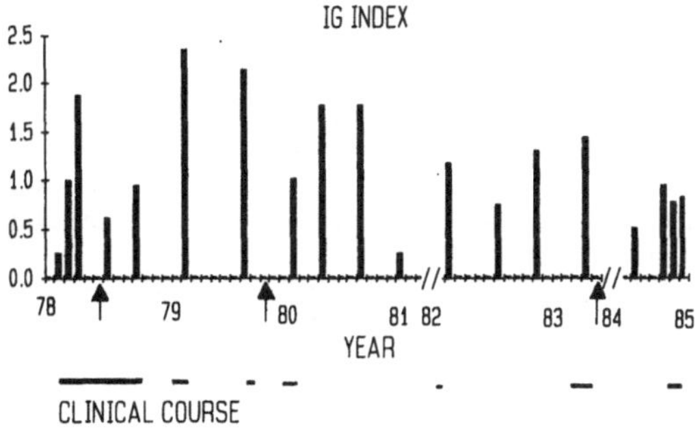

Fig.1. Variations in total intrathecal Ig production in the course of disease. Total Ig and albumin in paired CSF/serum samples was determined by RIA. The Ig index was computed according to formula given in Materials and Methods section. Arrows indicate ACTH treatment. Exacerbations are indicated as horizontal bars below the x-axis.

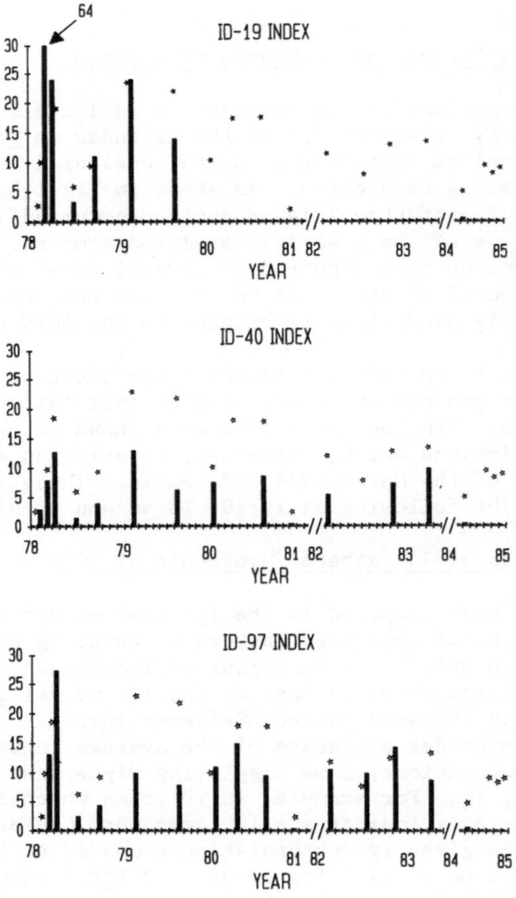

Fig.2A. Variations in intrathecal production of an idiotypically defined Ig-subpopulation (ID-19). The ID-indices (vertical bars) were computed according to same formula as the Ig-indices except that solely the given ID concentrations in CSF and serum were taken into account. The total Ig indices are indicated, on a 10 fold enlarged scale, by asteriks.

Fig.2B. Variations in intrathecal production of an idiotypically defined Ig-subpopulation (ID-19). The ID-indices (vertical bars) were computed according to same formula as the Ig-indices except that solely the given ID concentrations in CSF and serum were taken into account. The total Ig indices are indicated, on a 10 fold enlarged scale, by asteriks.

Fig.2C. Variations in intrathecal production of an idiotypically defined Ig-subpopulation (ID-19). The ID-indices (vertical bars) were computed according to same formula as the Ig-indices except that solely the given ID concentrations in CSF and serum were taken into account. The total Ig indices are indicated, on a 10 fold enlarged scale, by asteriks.

Accordingly, ID-19 (fig.2A) displayed very preferential intrathecal synthesis during two consecutive waves of intrathecal Ig production but then disappeared. ID-40 (Fig.2B) participated in the intrathecal Ig-synthesis up to 1983, though in a somewhat erratic fashion. For example, it could be detected in the CSF samples of February and September of 1980 but not in CSF of May 1980 in spite of considerable intrathecal Ig production at that point in time. ID-40 could not be detected during the last exacerbation (November/December, 1984). ID-97 (Fig.2C) participated strongly in the intrathecal Ig production throughout the disease except for the last exacerbation.

Concentration of ID's in Serum

Fig.3 shows the previously determined ID levels (5) in serum including the most recent samples of 1984 and 1985. The plots have been manipulated, as follows, to facilitate comparison of the ID concentrations: The ID concentrations determined by competition RIA are dependent upon the sensitivity of the given ID-assay. These assays can not be standardized directly because purified ID-preparations are not available. However, based on the concentration of total Ig and ID's in the March 1978 CSF sample and the finding that anti-ID-19, anti-ID-40 and anti-ID-97 precipitated 1.3%, 1.5% and 2.4% of the total Ig from that CSF sample, we estimate that 1) the anti-ID-97 assay is roughly three times more sensitive than the anti-ID-19 and anti-ID-40 assays and 2) the anti-ID-97 assay is roughly 10 times and the anti-ID-19 and anti-ID-40 assays roughly 3 times more sensitive than the total Ig assay. These differences have been taken into account in the plots shown in Fig.3. which, accordingly, indicate the ID concentrations as fractions of the total Ig. It can be seen that the relative ID concentrations in serum fluctuate roughly in parallel to the fluctuations observed in ID-indices in CSF. Overall, their relative concentration is slowly declining.

DISCUSSION

There is no doubt that significant Ig production by intrathecally localized B cell subpopulations occurs in most MS patients. What remains still unresolved, however, is the question of the mechanism(s) responsible for induction of this intrathecal B cell response. There are two alternative explanations: 1) B cells, after being randomly recruited into the inflammatory foci of the CNS, are non-specifically activated by local mitogenic stimuli. 2) B cells, again following random recruitment into the CNS, are activated in an antigen-specific manner, be it by cognate interaction with antigen-specific helper T cells or through bystander activa-

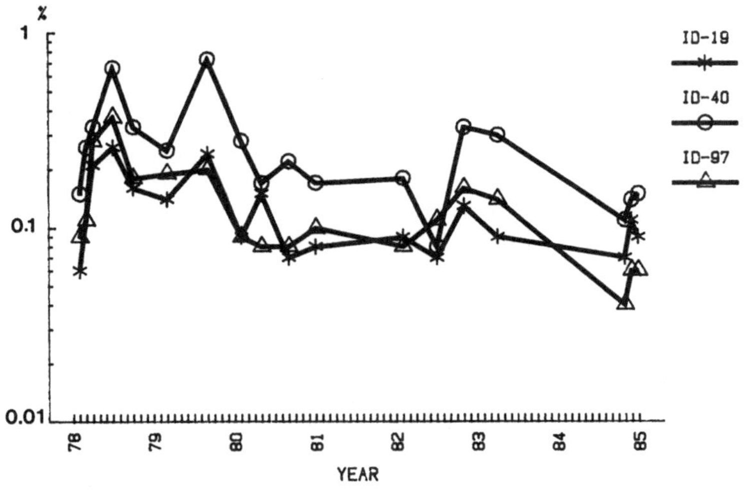

Fig.3. Variations in ID concentration in serum. The ID concentrations are expressed as percent of total serum Ig.

tion following recognition of the given antigen in the CNS. Distinction between these mechanisms is important because, in the former case, the intrathecally produced Ig's provide no clues as to the possible nature of the antigen(s) involved in the disease process (i.e. they are "nonsense antibodies") while in the latter case relevant information may be derived from specificity analyses of the intrathecally produced Ig's. Of course, it is possible also that both mechanisms of stimulation take place, some B cells being activated in a non-specific and others in an antigen-specific manner. In this case it would be useful if one could differentiate "nonsense" from potentially "disease-related" antibodies.

The two hypotheses make slightly different predictions: Mitogenic activation predicts that the composition of the intrathecally produced Ig's reflects primarily the composition of the circulating B cell pool at the time of recruitment of lymphocytes into the CNS and, accordingly, may (but does not necessarily have to) change from one exacerbation to the other. By contrast, antigen-specific stimulation predicts the repetitive activation of the same B cell subpopulation(s), largely independent of its (their) concentration in the circulating B cell pool at the time of recruitment. In our analysis of three individual Ig subpopulations we found that one (ID-19) participated strongly in two and the other (ID-40 and ID-97) in four consecutive waves of intrathecal Ig-production which occurred at intervals of approximately one year. Although this behaviour is not necessarily incompatible with mitogenic activation, it does agree better with an antigen-specific stimulation mechanism, particularly in the case of ID-97 secreting B cells which, judging from the low concentration of ID-97 in serum, may constitute only a minor portion of the total B cell pool during most stages of the disease. In this context, it is noteworthy that one out of 52 MS patients tested contained an Ig subpopulation in serum which crossreacted idiotypically with ID-97. So far, our attempts to define the antigen-specificity of ID-97 (or ID-19 and ID-40) have been unsuccessful.

None of the Ig subpopulations analysed here were detectable in CSF obtained during and shortly after the last exacerbation in November/December 1984. However, we tested CSF samples only at a 1/3.3 dilution and, since the total intrathecal Ig production is extremely modest during this last exacerbation, these ID's may have gone undetected even if they still constituted a significant portion of the total intrathecal Ig production during this stage of the disease.

Each of the three Ig subpopulations exhibited ID-indices that greatly exceeded the total Ig-indices, indicating highly preferential intrathecal synthesis (compared to total Ig). Nevertheless, as observed in other studies (8,10) the absolute concentration of these Ig subpopulations was always higher in serum and their level in serum showed fluctuations that paralleled roughly the fluctuations in intrathecal synthesis. During the first peak of intrathecal synthesis (March and April 1978), for example, ID-19, ID-40 and ID-97 were present on average at 8-, 25- and 14-fold higher absolute concentration in serum than in CSF. These findings are not incompatible, however, with the idea that significant intrathecal antigen-specific stimulation occurred. We have previously found, for example, that mice inoculated intracerebrally with Sendai virus (approx. 90% of the inoculum is thought to escape into extrathecal compartments during inoculation), exhibit a clear intrathecal antibody response yet, the intrathecal antiviral antibody titers remain consistently (except for antibodies of IgA isotype) 100 or more fold lower than the serum antibody titers (11). Thus, antigen may be more effective in inducing an extrathecal than an intrathecal immune response and release of some antigen into the extrathecal compartment during initial exacerbation may lead to the concomitant induction of a significant extrathecal immune response. In addition, one must keep in mind the possibility that antibodies may be removed selectively from CSF if they are directed to antigens present at high concentration in CNS. We have shown, for example, that the titers of passively transferred antiviral antibodies in CSF of intracerebrally infected mice depends on the reactivity of the antibodies with the infecting virus, i.e. the titer of a virus-reactive antibody is initially reduced relative to a non-reactive antibody (12), presumably because the virus-reactive antibodies tend to adsorb (and thus become removed from CSF) to the viral determinants expressed in the CNS.

In conclusion, our findings are compatible with (but do not prove) the idea that part of the intrathecal antibody response in MS patients may result from an antigen-specific rather than a non-specific (mitogenic) stimulation of certain B cell subpopulations in the course of disease.

ACKNOWLEDGEMENTS

This work was supported by grant NS 11036 from the National Institutes of Health, grant R6851 from the National Multiple Sclerosis Society and by the Swedish Medical Research Council (project No.386-19X-06265-053) and the Alfred Österlund Foundation.

REFERENCES

1. P.Y. Paterson and C.C. Whitacre. The enigma of oligoclonal immunoglobulin G in cerebrospinal fluid from multiple sclerosis patients. Immunol. Today, June :111 (1981).
2. D.H. Mattson, R.P.Roos and B.G.W. Arnason. Isoelectric focusing of IgG eluted from multiple sclerosis and subacute sclerosing panencephalitis brains. Nature. 287:335 (1980).
3. L.G. Baird, T.G. Tachovsky, M. Sandberg-Wollheim, H. Koprowski and A. Nisonoff. Identification of a unique idiotype in cerebrospinal fluid and serum of a patient with multiple sclerosis. J. Immunol. 124:2324 (1980).
4. W. Gerhard, A. Taylor, Z. Wroblewska, M. Sandberg-Wollheim and H. Koprowski. Analysis of a predominant immunoglobulin population in the cerebrospinal fluid of a multiple sclerosis patient by means of an anti-idiotypic hybridoma antibody. Proc. Natl. Acad. Sci. USA. 78:3225 (1981).
5. W. Gerhard, A. Taylor, M. Sandberg-Wollheim and H. Koprowski. Longitudinal analysis of three intrathecally produced immunoglobulin subpopulations in an MS patient. J. Immunol. 134:1555 (1985).
6. J.E. Olsson and K. Nilsson. Gamma globulins of CSF and serum in multiple sclerosis: Isoelectric focusing on polyacrylamide gel and agarose electrophoresis. Neurology. 29:1383 (1983).
7. J.P. Salier, P. Glynn, J.M. Goust and M.L Cuzner. Distribution of nominal and latent IgG (Gm) allotypes in plaques of multiple sclerosis brain. Clin. Exp. Immunol. 54:634 (1983).
8. G.C. Ebers. A study of CSF idiotypes in multiple sclerosis. Scand. J. Immunol. 16:151 (1982).
9. M.J. Walsh and W.W. Tourtellotte. Temporal invariance and clonal uniformity of brain and cerebrospinal IgG, IgA and IgM in multiple sclerosis. J. Exp. Med. 163:41 (1986).
10. L.M. Nagelkerken, M.Z. van Exel, H.K. van Walbeek, R.C. Aalberse and T.A. Out. Analysis of cerebrospinal fluid in serum of patients with multiple sclerosis by means of anti-idiotypic antisera. J. Immunol. 128: 1102 (1982).

11. W. Gerhard, Y. Iwasaki and H. Koprowski. The central nervous system associated immune response to parainfluenza virus in mice. J. Immunol. 120:1256 (1978).
12. P.C. Doherty and W. Gerhard. Breakdown of the blood-cerebrospinal fluid barrier to immunoglobulin in mice injected intracerebrally with neurotropic influenza A virus. J. Neuroimmunol. 1:227 (1981).

ANALYSIS OF THE HUMAN ANTI-MYELIN ASSOCIATED GLYCOPROTEIN IgM-SYSTEM WITH ANTI-IDIOTYPIC ANTIBODIES

Andreas J. Steck and Nicole Page

Laboratory of Neurobiology, Department of Neurology
Centre Hospitalier Universitaire Vaudois, 1011 Lausanne
Switzerland

INTRODUCTION

Numerous studies have described monoclonal IgM antibodies with apparent specificity for myelin associated glycoprotein (MAG) in association with a chronic demyelinating neuropathy which occurs in a population of patients with monoclonal B-cell proliferation (monoclonal gammopathy of undetermined significance or Waldenström macroglobulinaemia) (1,2,3). Although the pathogenesis of this neuropathy is still poorly understood, these findings suggest that it is an antibody-mediated autoimmune neuropathy.

A remarkable feature of the human monoclonal IgM anti-MAG antibodies is their species and site specificity: they bind strongly to human, primate, bovine, cat, dog and guinea-pig myelin, but not to rat or mouse myelin (4). The presently available biochemical data suggest that the monoclonal IgM reacts with the carbohydrate moiety of MAG and not with the polypeptide backbone (5,6). This view has been strengthened by the finding that the anti-MAG antibodies cross-react with a peripheral nerve glycolipid (5). Recent immunochemical studies disclosed some details of the nature of the antigenic determinant on this glycolipid, which appears to be a sulfated complex carbohydrate with five sugar residues (7). Preliminary work on the characterization of the oligosaccharide binding the anti-MAG antibodies on MAG has also been reported (8).

Although one could assume that the anti-MAG antibodies all react with the same antigenic determinant, this opinion has been challenged by several lines of evidence. Blocking experiments have revealed differences between individual anti-MAG IgM (9,10). The reactivity of the HNK-1 mouse monoclonal antibody with MAG (11) has lead to studies of the reaction of a series of human anti-MAG antibodies with NK-cells. Considerable variation in the reactivity of the human anti-MAG IgM was found with NK cells 12.

Immunoglobulins contain unique structures in their heavy and light chains that impart to them the property of specificity. Monoclonal antibody molecules, such as these displaying anti-MAG activity, bear a structure restricted to a single light-chain type and to a particular variable region that may be unique to each patient. These structures or antigenic determinants are called idiotypes (id) and the antibodies that are directed against them are termed anti-idiotypic (id) antibodies (13). In order to further analyse the id present on the anti-MAG IgM, several groups, including our own, have used both polyclonal and monoclonal anti-id antibodies. The work we discuss here will review the results obtained in our laboratory with monoclonal anti-id antibodies, suggesting that the set of id among the anti-MAG IgM is heterogenous. As we shall see, the application of these anti-id antibodies has also revealed the presence of naturally occurring anti-id antibodies in the sera of some of these patients. The functional role of these anti-id antibodies as well as their potential use in therapy is discussed.

The human anti-MAG IgM system displays a degree of heterogeneity

To search for shared id in human anti-MAG IgM antibodies, we screened the sera of 20 patients with two different mouse monoclonal anti-id antibodies. The characterization of these antibodies has been described in previous publications (14,15). An important feature of these monoclonal anti-id antibodies is that they appear to be directed against the combining site of the IgM, since they inhibit the interaction between the anti-MAG IgM and MAG. In Table 1, we show that each anti-id antibody reacted uniquely with its autologous IgM and not with other monoclonal proteins from a total of 20 IgM, 10 of which had anti-MAG activity. Using id-specific polyclonal antisera, Khan reported also that there was no evidence of id cross-reactivity between different MAG-binding IgM monoclonal proteins (16). In similar experiments, however, Evans et al. (17) and Seligmann et al. (3) identified some degree of cross-reaction which may indicate the presence of a weak dominant id or a framework structure overrepresented in this group of patients with anti-MAG antibodies. In interpreting these data, however, one should appreciate that the nature of the id expressed by these novel human autoantibodies has not yet been characterized. Furthermore, the relationship between id and binding specificity of immunoglobulin is indeed a complex one. Thus, for example, a drastic change in id but not antigen-binding specificity of an antibody can occur by single aminoacid substitution (18). Thus, the absence of id sharing in the patients described here may therefore reflect a certain degree of genetic diversity of the immunoglobulin variable regions without affecting antigen binding specificity or may reflect minor differences in the fine specificity of the MAG binding IgM between different patients.

Studies of naturally occurring anti-id antibodies

Evidence for naturally occurring anti-id antibodies or auto-anti-id antibodies was derived from experiments based on a site consumption assay, where wells coated with a patient's anti-MAG IgM were incubated with a labelled mouse monoclonal anti-id antibody in the presence of various concentrations of the patient's IgG fraction. Such an assay using the monoclonal anti-id antibody R9DB2 is shown in Fig.1. The results revealed that patient SA IgG fraction inhibited the binding of labelled R9DB2 to its id-IgM, whereas control IgG fraction did not. Similar results were found with patient CR IgG fraction and the anti-id antibody A8F2 (14 and Fig.4). Again the binding of A8F2 to its id-IgM was inhibited by the patient's IgG fraction, suggesting that in each case, the IgG fraction contained antibodies to the anti-MAG IgM. These natural anti-id antibodies seemed to be only present in the autologous IgG fraction, since IgG fractions from other patients with anti-MAG IgM or control IgM did not have any effect.

Table 1. Reaction of monoclonal anti-id antibodies to neuropathy associated IgM monoclonal protein.

Patients	anti-MAG activity	Reaction with A8F2	Reachtion with R9DB2
Bl.P.	+	-	-
D.J.	-	-	-
BA.P.	-	-	-
C.R.	+	+	-
B.A.	-	-	-
K.A.	+	-	-
Hug H.	-	-	-
V.A.	+	-	-
M.A.	+	-	-
J.E.	+	-	-
N.S.	-	-	-
Mc C.	-	-	-
W.	-	-	-
J.	-	-	-
M.M.	-	-	-
P.G.	-	-	-
F.E.	+	-	-
S.A.	+	-	+
P.H.	+	-	-
H.C.	+	-	-

Anti-MAG activity was assayed by the immunoblot technique as previously described (1). Reaction with the anti-id antibodies A8F2 and R9DB2 was tested using microwells coated with patient's serum (1:20), then incubated with A8F2 or R9DB2 (1:1000) and finally with ^{125}I-F(ab')$_2$ fragment anti-mouse Ig (50.000 cpm). A8F2 was raised against the IgM monoclonal protein of patient C.R., R9DB2 was raised against the IgM monoclonal protein of patient S.A.

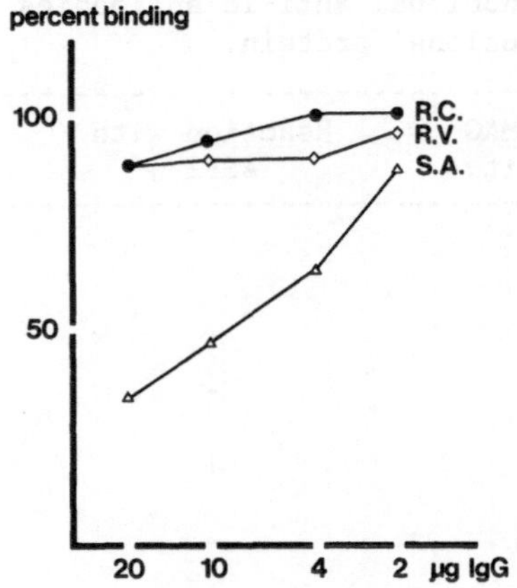

Fig.1. Competition assay demonstrating inhibition of binding of ^{125}I-R9DB2 to SA IgM on microwell plates. ^{125}I-R9DB2 was added in the presence of various cencentrations of SA IgG (△), control IgG (◇) and IgG (•) from patient CR. CR and SA are patients with monoclonal anti-MAG antibodies. R9DB2 is a mouse monoclonal anti-id antibody reacting with SA IgM.

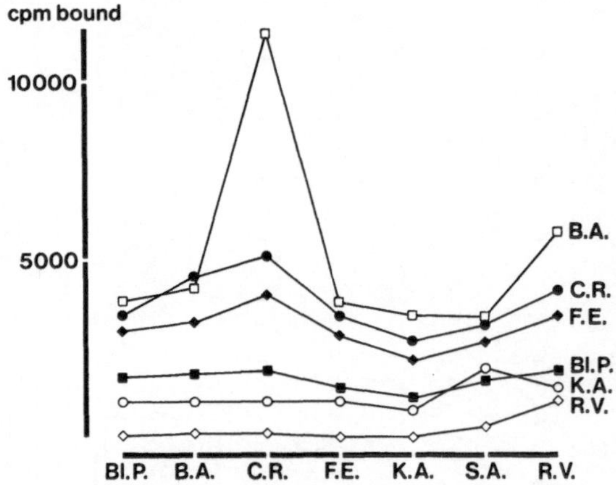

Fig.2. Binding of various IgG fractions to autologous or homologous monoclonal or polyclonal IgM on microwells. IgM components were isolated from the serum of the patients by Ultrogel ACA 34 (LKB) column chromatography and IgG components were further separated by protein-A sepharose (Pharmacia) column chromatography. Plates were coated with IgM (10 µg/ml) and incubated with IgG fractions (0.3 mg/ml). Bound IgG were counted after incubation with ^{125}I-protein A. C.R., F.E., Bl.P and K.A. are patients with monoclonal IgM anti-MAG antibodies; B.A. is a patient with a monoclonal IgM without anti-MAG activity; and R.V., has no monoclonal protein.

This approach has, however, an obvious drawback in that it requires the availability of a specific anti-id antibody for each individual patient to look for evidence of a more general anti-id response in patients with anti-MAG antibodies. To overcome the limitation of this method, we turned to a direct binding test where isolated IgG fractions from various patients were tested for their reactivity towards autologous or homologous IgM fractions. Using this direct binding test, we found that in none of the patients, except BA, was there binding to autologous or homologous IgM fraction (Fig.2). The interaction between BA IgG and CR IgM appears idiotypic because binding was also observed against the F(ab')2 fragment of CR IgM (data not shown). We were also unable to show any evidence of reactivity of IgG fractions from patient CR or SA, previously shown to contain auto-anti-id as revealed by a competition assay with monoclonal anti-id antibodies.

In order to elucidate the nature of the reactivity of BA IgG to CR IgM, we performed inhibition studies. The results of a competition assay showed that the binding of CR IgM to MAG was completely inhibited in the presence of BA IgG, whereas addition of KA IgG or CR IgG had no effect (Fig.3). The next step was to look for a competition between A8F2, the monoclonal anti-id antibody, and BA IgG for binding to CR IgM. Although CR IgG inhibited the binding of A8F2 to CR IgM, BA IgG as well as control IgG had no effect (Fig.4). Taken together these results would suggest the presence of anti-id antibody activity to CR IgM in BA IgG fraction, which is clearly different from that revealed indirectly by A8F2. But it should be noted that in none of the patients studied so far have we found evidence of antibodies reacting directly with their autologous monoclonal IgM components. It appears therefore that circulating anti-id antibodies in sufficient level to be detected by their direct reactivity are not part of the immune response in patients with monoclonal anti-MAG IgM. Such a low incidence of anti-id antibodies to monoclonal immuno-globulins is not surprising. Lindström and Williams found no evidence of anti-id antibodies in 136 patients with monoclonal proteins (19). Among the reasons accounting for this finding, one should mention that it is possible that anti-id are undetectable because they are fixed and cleared by the id. Alternatively patients with high concentrations of circulating id may display a degree of tolerance at the level of B-cells that may result in suppression of the anti-id response.

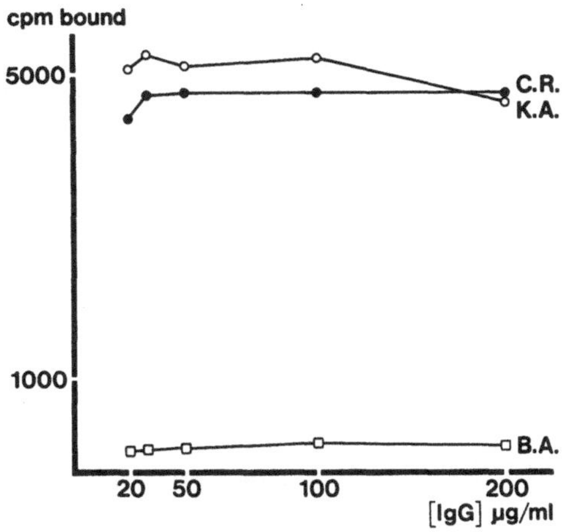

Fig.3. Inhibition of CR ^{125}I-IgM to MAG by IgG fractions. Microwell plates were coated with an extract enriched in MAG (25). CR ^{125}I-IgM was incubated with various dilutions of IgG fractions from patients with monoclonal IgM anti-MAG antibodies (C.R. and K.A.) and from a patient with a monoclonal IgM without anti-MAG activity (B.A.).

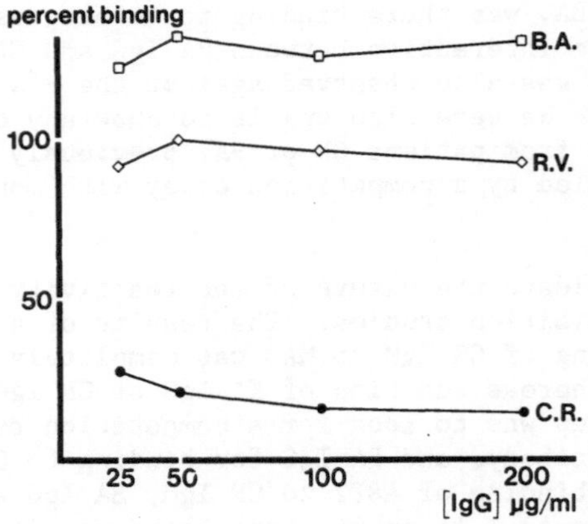

Fig.4. Inhibition of ^{125}I-A8F2 to CR IgM on microwell plates. ^{125}I-A8F2 was added in the presence of various dilutions of IgG fractions to wells coated with CR IgM (0.1 mg/ml). CR is a patient with a monoclonal anti-MAG IgM, BA is a patient with a monoclonal IgM without anti-MAG activity and RV has no monoclonal protein. A8F2 is a mouse monoclonal anti-id antibody reacting with CR IgM.

Anti-id antibodies as potential therapeutical agents

In cases of polyneuropathy associated with paraproteinaemia, if the antibody can be shown to react with nervous tissue and a pathogenic role is suspected, the rational approach to therapy is to try to reduce serum antibody levels. This can be achieved using immunosuppressive drugs and plasmapheresis. In the case of neuropathy with antibodies to MAG, intensive plasmapheresis results in a lowering of the total IgM level, but within one or two weeks of discontinuing treatment, there is a rebound effect and the serum IgM returns to pre-treatment levels (2,20). It has been shown also that plasmapheresis effectively, although probably transiently, reduces IgM deposits in nerve (21). Most studies of the effect of plasmapherisis have observed little or no objective clinical improvement, but one study has reported objective improvement in 7 out of 9 patients (22). A degree of resistance to plasmapheresis is to be expected in view of the malignant character of the monoclonal IgM production. An attractive therapeutic target is the surface immunoglobulin of the anti-MAG-B-cell clone. In this respect anti-id antibodies appear particularly well suited for the treatment of B-cell neoplasm. Anti-id antibodies do not only react, as we have shown, with the secreted antibody but also with B-cells having the same antigenic specificity. Several attempts have been made to modulate the immune response by anti-id therapy (23). Antigen specific suppression leading to the deletion of a particular id has been reported in experimental models. In man it has been reported that repeated injection of a monoclonal antibody specific for the id of a B-cell lymphoma was effective in inducing biological and clinical improvement (24). Such a strategy should be applicable in patients with monoclonal IgM antibodies to MAG. Since the titer of id-protein may be particularly high in serum, plasmapheresis or cytostatic treatment may be needed before specific immunotherapy with anti-id antibodies is initiated. A search for a common idiotype in human anti-MAG IgM would also be important because it would circumvent the need for a different anti-id reagent for each individual patient.

ACKNOWLEDGEMENTS

We are indebted to Dr. N.R. Ling, University of Birmingham, U.K., for kindly providing one of the anti-idiotype antibodies used in this study. We are grateful to Mrs. Geneviève Perruisseau for expert laboratory assistance and to Mrs. L. Ohayon for preparing the manuscript. This study was supported by grants from the Swiss National Science Foundation and from the Swiss Multiple Sclerosis Society.

REFERENCES

1. A.J. Steck, N. Murray, C. Meier, N. Page and G. Perruisseau. Demeyelinating neuropathy and monoclonal IgM antibody to myelin associated glycoprotein. Neurology (N.Y.) 33: 19-23 (1983).
2. C. Melmed, D. Frail, I. Duncan, P. Braun, D. Danoff, M. Finlayson and J. Stewart. Peripheral neuropathy with IgM Kappa monoclonal immunoglobulin directed against myelin-associated glycoprotein. Neurology 33: 1397-1405(1983).
3. M. Seligmann, J.C. Brouet, K. Dellagi and C. Schmitt. Antibody activities of human monoclonal immunoglobulins with special reference to monoclonal IgM in patients with peripheral neuropathy. In: "Autoimmunity" R.S. Schwartz, ed. Raven Press, New York (in press).
4. A.J. Steck, N. Murray, M. Vandevelde and A. Zurbriggen. Human monoclonal antibodies to myelin associated glycoprotein. J. Neuro-Immunol. 5: 145-156 (1983).
5. A.A. Ilyas, R.H. Quarles, T.D. MacIntosh, M.J. Dobersen, B.D. Trapp, M.C. Dalakas and R.O. Brady. IgM in human neuropathy related to paraproteinaemia binds to a carbohydrate determinant in the myelin-associated glycoprotein and to a ganglioside. Proc. Natl. Acad. Sci. 81: 1225-1229 (1984 a).
6. M.E. Shy, T. Vietorisz, E. Nobile-Orazio and N. Latov. Specificity of human IgM M-protein that bind to myelin-associated glycoproteins: peptide mapping, deglycosylation and competitive binding studies. J. Immunol. 133: 2509-2512 (1984).
7. K.H. Chou, A.A. ILyas, J.E. Evans, R.H. Quarles and F.B. Jungalwala. Structure of a glycolipid reacting with monoclonal IgM in neuropathy and with HNK-1. Biochem. Biophys. Res. Commun. 128: 1, 383-388 (1985).
8. M.E. Shy, C.A. Gabel, E. Vietorisz and N. Latov. Characterization of oligosaccharides that bind to anti-myelin associated glycoprotein M proteins. Annals Neurol. 18: 129 (1985).
9. A.J. Steck and N. Murray. Monoclonal antibodies to myelin associated glycoprotein reveal antigenic structures and suggest pathogenic mechanisms. Springer Semin. Immunopathol. 8: 29-43 (1985).
10. K. Dellagi, P. Duponey, J.C. Brouet, A. Billecoq, D. Gomez, J.P. Clauvel and M. Seligmann. Waldenström macroglobulinaemia and peripheral neuropathy: a clinical and immunological study of 25 patients. Blood. 62: 280-285 (1983).
11. K.C. McGarry, S.L. Helfand, H. Quarles and J.C. Roder. Recognition of myelin associated glycoprotein by the monoclonal antibody HNK-1 (Leu-7). Nature. 306: 376-378 (1983).
12. K. Dellagi and J.C. Brouet. Antigen shared between myelin and NK-cells. Lancet 1: 1244 (1984).
13. N.K. Jerne. The generative grammar of the immune system. The EMBO Journal. 4: 847-852 (1985).
14. N. Page, N. Murray, G. Perruisseau and A.J. Steck. A monoclonal anti-idiotypic antibody against a human monoclonal IgM with specificity for myelin associated glycoprotein. J. Immunol. 134: 3094-3099 (1985).

15. N. Murray, N. Page and A.J. Steck. The human anti-myelin associated glycoprotein IgM system. Annals Neurol. (in press) (1986).
16. S.N. Kahn. Human monoclonal IgM autoantibodies with restricted antigenic specificity for myelin. Express unrelated idiotypes. J. Neurol. Sci. 69: 161-170 (1985).
17. S.W. Evans, N.P. Gregson, S.L. Leibowitz and N.R. Ling. Investigation of the idiotypic determinants of IgM monoclonal proteins associated with neuropathy. Clin. Exp. Immunol. 57: 621-625 (1984).
18. A. Radbruch, S. Zaiss, C. Kappen, M. Brüggemann, K. Beyreuther and K. Rajewsky. Drastic change in idiotypic but not antigen-binding specificity of an antibody by a single amino-acid substitution. Nature. 315: 506-508 (1985).
19. F.D. Lindström and R.C. Williams. Serum anti-immunoglobulins in multiple myeloma and benign monoclonal gammopathy. Clin. Immunol. Immunopathol. 3: 503-513 (1975).
20. A.J. Steck, C. Meier, M. Vandevelde and F. Regli. Polyneuropathies et gammapathies: une forme avec anticorps anti-glycoproteine MAG. Rev. Neurol.(Paris). 140: 1: 28-36 (1984).
21. C. Meier, K. Roberts, A. Steck, C. Hess, E. Milani and I. Tschopp. Polyneuropathy in Waldenström's macroglobulinaemia: reduction of endoneurial IgM deposits after treatment with chlorambucil and plasmapheresis. Acta Neuropathol.(Berl.) 401: 297-307 (1984).
22. K. Lassoued, K. Dellagi, J.C. Brouet, J.P. Clauvel, A. Bussel and M. Seligmann. Effects of plasma exchange in nine patients with peripheral neuropathy and monoclonal IgM directed to myelin-associated glycoprotein. Plasma ther. Transf. Technol. 6: 449-452 (1985).
23. I.M. Roitt, D.K. Male, G. Guarnotta. L.P. de Carvalho, A. Cooke, F.C. Hay, P.M. Lydard and Y. Thanavala. Idiotypic networks and their possible exploitation for manipulation of the immune response. Lancet. 1: 1041-1045 (1981).
24. R.A. Miller, D.G. Maloney, R. Warnke and R. Levy. Treatment of B-cell lymphoma with monoclonal anti-idiotype antibody. N. Engl. J. Med. 306: 517-522 (1982).
25. R.H. Quarles and C.F. Pasnak. A rapid procedure for selectively isolating the major glycoprotein from purified rat brain myelin. Biochem. J. 163: 635-637 (1977).

IDIOTYPES IN THE IMMUNE RESPONSE TO MEASLES VIRUS

J. Gheuens

Laboratory of Neuropathology, Born Bunge Stichting
Universitaire Instelling Antwerpen
B-2610 Wilrijk, Belgium

INTRODUCTION

Like isotypes and allotypes, idiotypes are serologically defined antigenic determinants of immunoglobulins (Nisonoff et al., 1975). Unlike allotypes and isotypes, idiotypes are individually specific to a given immunoglobulin. They are expressed by the V-region (often on the H- and L-chain combined) and can often be localized in the antigen binding site (Capra and Kehoe, 1975). Idiotypes have also been found on B-cells, and regulatory and effector T-cells. There is a large repertoire of idiotypes, and usually many different idiotypes are expressed in an antigen-specific immune response. However, in some immune responses a large fraction of the antibodies expresses the same idiotype; this is then called a cross-reacting idiotype. Idiotype expression is genetically controlled, and inbred animals sometimes express identical cross-reacting idiotypes upon challenge with a given antigen (Urbain et al., 1981).

Idiotypes play an important role in immunoregulation. More specifically, they allow specific cell recognition among regulatory T-cells, effector-T cells and B-cells. A model of idiotype-specific immunoregulation, termed the network theory, has been proposed by Jerne (1974). The network hypothesis has been very influential, and there are now many experimental data supporting the concept of an immune system organized as an idiotypic network (Bona, 1981: Golub, 1980; Raff, 1977; Urbain et al., 1981). Inherent to all concepts of idiotype-specific immunoregulation, is that idiotypes are recognized by the immune system in which they are expressed. In other words, idiotypes break the rule that "self" is not immunogenic in physiological conditions, and they give rise to anti-idiotype. A possible explanation for this is that the immune system does not effectively express most of its idiotypes at the time tolerance is acquired, because of lack of B-cell expansion in the absense of antigen.

There are two main interests in studying idiotypes related to multiple sclerosis (MS). One is to identify cross-reacting idiotypes specific to the disease. Such idiotype could serve as disease marker. It could also lead to identification of an MS specific antigen. The second interest stems from the role of idiotypes in immunoregulation. It is perceived that MS patients have some form of disturbed immunoregulation. This is apparent from the observed changes in lymphocyte subpopulations, the restricted heterogeneity of immunoglobulins, and perhaps also from the increased anti-viral antibody titers reported in the patients (McFarlin and McFarland, 1982).

In the present work, measles virus was chosen as a model to study the possible role of idiotypes in anti-viral immune responses. An assembled measles virus contains 6 structural peptides, 2 of which are expressed on the surface, the hemagglutinin (HA) and the fusion protein (F1). Two are associated with the genome (ss-RNA), the nucleocapsid (NC) and the major phosphorylated protein (P). The matrix (M) protein is located just under the envelope of the virus. There is also a large RNA polymerase (L). Each of these polypeptides can be immunogenic (Hall et al., 1979, Trudgett et al., 1980) and therefore, the immune response against measles virus is very complex and heterogeneous.

This complexity makes the study of idiotypes difficult, because of the large repertoire involved. Therefore, monoclonal antibodies directed against individual measles polypeptides were used in this work (Table 1). The monoclonal antibodies were raised in BALB/c mice after immunization with the Edmonston strain of measles virus. Initially, the idiotypes of three monoclonal antibodies directed against three different epitopes of the viral HA were defined using syngeneic antisera. The possible role of idiotypes in the immune response to measles virus, and some concepts of the network theory were studied using these reagents. Next, monoclonal antibodies to measles HA, as well as to P and NC were used to analyse the human antibody response against individual epitopes of the virus.

IDIOTYPES OF MONOCLONAL ANTIBODIES TO MEASLES HA

The idiotypes of 3 different monoclonal antibodies against the HA of measles (C2, V17 and B2) were defined by raising syngeneic antisera (in BALB/c mice) after immunization with monoclonal antibody-KLH conjugates (Gheuens et al., 1981). After such immunization, high titered anti-idiotypic antisera were obtained, as demonstrated with appropriate controls. In these case of C2 and B2, anti-idiotype could inhibit the binding between the idiotype-bearing antibody and the HA, indicating binding site idiotype. The syngeneic antiserum against the V17 anti-HA monoclonal antibody did not inhibit its binding to the HA, probably indicating a framework idiotype.

There was no cross-reaction among the idiotypes on the three anti-HA monoclonal antibodies, that were shown to be directed against different epitopes of HA (Rammohan et al., 1983). A limited idiotypic cross-reaction was observed between the C2 monoclonal antibody and polyclonal anti-Edmonston BALB/c serum. There was no idiotypic cross-reaction between the mouse anti-HA monoclonal antibodies and human anti-measles positive sera.

These results indicated that syngeneic anti-idiotype could be raised against monoclonal anti-measles antibodies, and that, as expected, there was little evidence of cross-reacting idiotype (Gheuens et al. 1981).

EFFECT OF ANTI-IDIOTYPE ON THE BIOLOGICAL ACTIVITY OF ANTI-HA ANTIBODIES

Because the tree anti-HA monoclonal antibodies C2, V17 and B2 inhibited hemagglutination by the virus and could neutralize measles, it was examined if the anti-idiotypic antisera could inhibit these biological activities.

Anti-idiotype was therefore added to hemagglutination inhibition mixtures, consisting of Rhesus erythrocytes, measles antigen and anti-HA monoclonal antibody in appropriate concentrations. The anti-idiotype to C2 and B2 inhibited hemagglutination inhibition. Anti-idiotype to the V17 monoclonal antibodies had no effect on V17 hemagglutination inhibition.

Corresponding results were obtained in experiments in which anti-idiotype was added to virus neutralization tests with C2, V17 and B2 monoclonal antibody. The neutralization tests were plaque assays with 100 plaque forming units of virus and fixed amount of monoclonal antibody resulting in 50% virus neutralization. It was observed that anti-idiotype to the C2 and B2 monoclonal antibodies could inhibit virus neutralization by the antibody, whereas the anti-idiotype to V17 could not.

These results suggested that, should anti-idiotype occur in a normal immune response against a pathogenic virus, it may interfere with the biological function of the antiviral antibody, apart from its role in immunoregulation. It is conceivable that such effect on the anti-viral antibody activity could interfere with pathogenesis (Gheuens et al., 1981).

EVIDENCE FOR AN INTERNAL IMAGE OF MEASLES HA IN AN ANTI-IDIOTYPE RESPONSE

The network theory proposes that each antibody expresses an idiotype that will give rise to anti-idiotypic antibody, which in itself will express an idiotype that will raise anti-idiotype and so forth. Idiotype expressing antibody can be referred to as Ab1, anti-idiotype as Ab2 and anti-anti-idiotype as Ab3. In the network theory, some particular properties of these successive populations of antibodies were proposed. For instance, a subpopulation of Ab3 would present an identical idiotype as the Ab1, but not have its antigen binding properties. This set of antibodies was termed "the non-specific parallel set". Another idea was that, because of the conformational complementarity of antigen and antigen binding site, and because idiotypes are often binding site associated, the binding site of a subpopulation of the Ab2 would conformationally resemble an epitope on the antigen. The Ab2 was said to present an "internal image" of the antigen (Jerne, 1974).

A series of experiments were done to assess if anti-idiotype presented an internal image of measles HA. First, the effect of anti-idiotype on infection with measles virus was examined as follows. Vero-cells were first incubated with different amounts of anti-idiotype or appropriate controls, and then with 100 plaque forming units of Edmonston measles virus. A standard plaque assay was then performed.

It was observed that anti-idiotype to C2 and V17 could significantly inhibit measles infection, and somewhat surprisingly, anti-idiotype to B2 could not. This phenomenon was reproducible, not due to virus neutralization and specific for measles virus: vesicular stomatitis virus infection of Vero-cells could not be inhibited by anti-idiotype sera to monoclonal antibodies against measles HA.

A possible explanation for these results is that the anti-idiotypic antisera (Ab2) contained a population of antibodies that expressed an internal image of measles HA. This could then compete with the HA for binding to the cell receptor for the virus, and inhibit viral infection.

It was then examined if human sera containing anti-measles antibodies, would bind to the internal image in the BALB/c Ab2. To assess this, affinity purified anti-idiotype (Ab2) to C2, V17 and B2 anti-HA was coated on plastic plates, and incubated with human serum known to contain anti-measles antibodies. After washes, the plates were incubated with radiolabeled anti-human immunoglobulins.

A result was termed positive if the binding of a human serum to Ab2 was at least two times higher than binding to control BALB/c immunoglobulin. The sera from 3 normal adults, 4 multiple sclerosis patients, 8 subacute sclerosing panencephalitis patients and 1 infant prior to measles immunization were tested. This latter serum did not bind to any of the Ab2's. All but one of the other human sera bound to the C2 Ab2, four bound to the V17 Ab2, and none bound to the B2 Ab2. Most significantly, these results agreed with those of the previous experiment, in the sense that the C2 and V17 Ab2 possibly expressed internal image, but B2 Ab2 did not.

HUMAN SERUM ANTIBODY TO DEFINED EPITOPES OF MEASLES VIRUS

Compared to the immune response against a hapten, an anti-viral immune response is extremely complex and heterogeneous, and associated with a large idiotype repertoire. This complexity leads to questions on the repertoire of the anti-measles immune response. Such questions have particular importance in MS because of the restricted charge heterogeneity of gammaglobulins, or oligoclonal reaction observed in this condition.

Restricted heterogeneity of gammaglobulins is not specific to MS; it is found in other neurological conditions, albeit often less pronounced, in a smaller fraction of the patients and often transient compared to MS. It is pronounced in infections that are accompanied by an intense immune response, such as neurosyfilis, trypanosomiasis, subacute sclerosing panencephalitis (SSPE), progressive rubella encephalitis). It is also found in serum of experimentally immunised animals. Its molecular basis is not well understood. As the normal heterogeneity of immunoglobulins is predominantly determined by the extent of the V-region repertoire, it is only logical to assume restricted expression of V-region repertoire as the explanation of restricted charge heterogeneity of immunoglobulins. In SSPE, some experimental evidence has supported this. On the other hand, predominant expression of certain L-chain types and H-chain classes have been described in MS (Lowenthal et al., 1984).

It is not known if the restricted charge heterogeneity of immunoglobulins in SSPE is associated with a restricted anti-measles antibody repertoire. In order to study the anti-measles antibody repertoire, it was examined if the epitopes defined by monoclonals anti-measles antibodies after immunization of BALB/c mice with a killed laboratory strain of measles virus were immunogenic in man after infection.

The following method was used. A known amount of a BALB/c anti-measles monoclonal antibody was reacted with measles antigen coated plastic plates, in the presence of serial dilutions of SSPE serum. After washing, the plates were incubated with radiolabelled anti-mouse immunoglobulin. If the presence of SSPE serum reduced the binding of the monoclonal antibodies to the antigen, this was thought to indicate that the SSPE serum contained antibodies against the same epitope of measles as defined by the monoclonal antibodies. The dilution of human serum producing 50% inhibition of radioactive binding was called the titer, and expressed in log 2 units. With this method, 27 serum samples from 8 SSPE patients were analysed against 3 different anti-HA, 2 anti-P and 2 anti-NC monoclonal antibodies (Table 1), as well as against polyclonal BALB/c anti-measles serum.

Following results were obtained (Fig.1). First, SSPE serum could inhibit the binding of BALB/c anti-measles serum to measles virus, indicating similarities among the different antibody repertoires. All SSPE patients had antibody against the C2, V17 and B2 epitopes of HA. This in-

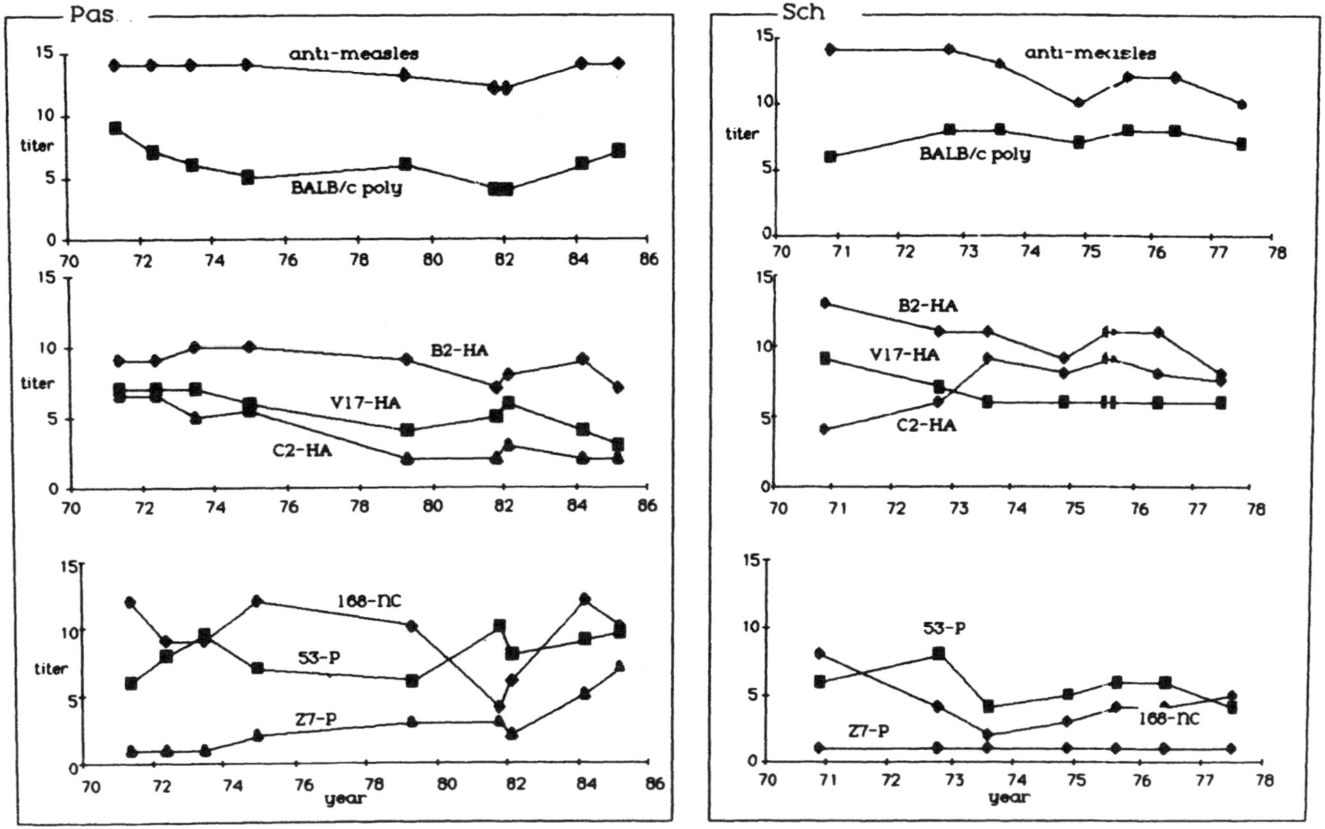

Fig.1. Serum antibody titers to defined epitopes of measles virus in 2 SSPE patients; 9 samples from 14 years of disease were available in patient Pas..., 7 samples from 7 years of disease in patient Sch...; the top panel shows anti-measles antibody titers in solid-phase radioimmunoassay, and the SSPE serum titers producing 50% inhibition of binding of polyclonal BALB/c anti-measles serum to measles antigen; the middle and bottom panels show SSPE serum titers against defined epitopes of measles virus (see text and Table 1 for explanation).

dicated some homology of repertoire among different SSPE patients. It is also significant that the B2 and V17 epitopes are known to be lacking from the hamster neurotropic strain (HNT) HA (Rammohan et al., 1983).

Table 1. Monoclonal antibodies to measles virus

Name	Polypeptide	Epitope
79XIC2 (C2)	hemagglutinin	C2-HA
79XVV17 (V17)	hemagglutinin	V17-HA
80IIIB2 (B2)	hemagglutinin	B2-HA
81153 (53)	P-peptide	53-p
81I153 (153)	P-peptide	153-p
83VIIZ7 (Z7)	P-peptide	Z7-p
81I168 (168)	nucleocapsid	168-NC

Note: all monoclonal antibodies were raised in BALB/c mice after immunization with Edmonston strain of measles virus; all were produced in the Neuroimmunology Branch (Chief: Dr. D.E. McFarlin), NINCDS, NIH, Bethesda, Md., USA.

None of the SSPE patients had antibody against the 153 epitope of the P-peptide, indicating a clear difference among men and mice anti-measles repertoires. The patients had different titers against the 53-P and 168-NC epitopes. In addition, these titers fluctuated markedly in the course of the disease. (Fig.1.)

From these results the following can be concluded. Some epitopes of measles virus, as defined by specific monoclonal antibodies, appeared to be recognized by SSPE patients. There appeared to be partial homology of anti-measles antibody repertoire among mice after measles immunisation and humans after infection, and homology among different SSPE patients. Particular here is that the SSPE patients had antibody to epitopes known to be lacking on the HA of the neurotropic HNT strain. This means that they had been exposed to these epitopes. This could indicate that the virus has become defective, and neurotropic, only after infection. It could also indicate that the defective character of the HA in HNT plays no role in neurotropism in SSPE.

Lastly, although overall anti-measles antibody titers fluctuated very little in the course of the disease, there were pronounced changes in antibody titers to serologically defined individual epitopes. It is not clear if this reflects changing exposure to these epitopes, but it does indicate active immunoregulation. The anti-measles antibody response in SSPE therefore seems to be dynamically regulated, as one would expect a normal immune response to be.

CONCLUSION

The possible role of idiotype and anti-idiotype in the immune response to measles virus was studied using monoclonal anti-measles antibodies. It was shown that anti-idiotype can specifically interfere with the biological activity of idiotype-expressing antibody. This implies that if auto-anti-idiotype occurs in the course of an immune response to virus, it could have a role in pathogenesis, apart from its role in immunoregulation. In addition, results were obtained that suggested the occurrence of an internal image of an epitope on measles HA in an anti-idiotype response. This supported a concept of the network theory. Lastly, analysis of serum antibody to defined epitopes of measles virus in SSPE patients indicated homologies of antibody repertoire among different patients, as well as dynamic immunoregulation.

ACKMNOWLEDGEMENTS

J.G. was recipient of a Forgarty Research Fellowship in the Neuroimmunology Branch (Chief: Dr. D.E. McFarlin), NINCDS, NIH, Bethesda, Md. (USA), and later of a Senior Research Assistant Fellowship of the National Fund for Scientific Research (Belgium) in the Laboratory of Neurochemistry (Prof. Dr. A. Lowenthal), Born-Bunge Stichting, University of Antwerp (Belgium) during part of this work.

REFERENCES

1. C. Bona. Regulation of clonal expression through immune network (limited network model). Compend. Immunol. 2: 223 (1981).
2. J.D. Capra and J.M. Kehoe. Hypervariable regions, idiotypy and antibody-combining sites. Adv. Immunol. 20: 1 (1975).
3. J. Gheuens, D.E. McFarlin, K.W. Rammohan and W.J. Bellini. Idiotypes and biological activities of murine monoclonal antibodies against the hemagglutinin of measles virus. Infect. Immun. 34: 200 (1981).
4. E.S. Golub. Idiotypes and the network hypothesis. Cell. 22: 641 (1980).
5. W.W. Hall, R.A. Lamb and P.W. Choppin. Measles and subacute sclerosing panencephalitis proteins: Lack of antibodies to the matrix protein with subacute sclerosing panencephalitis. Proc. Natl. Acad. Sci. USA. 76: 2047 (1979).
6. A. Lowenthal, R. Crols, E. De Schutter, J. Gheuens, D. Karcher, M. Noppe and A. Tasnier. Cerebrospinal fluid proteins in neurology. Int. Rev. Neurobiol. 25: 95 (1984).
7. D.E. McFarlin and H.F. McFarland. Multiple sclerosis, pts. 1 & 2. N. Engl. J. Med. 307: 1183-1246 (1982).
8. A. Nisonoff, J.R. Hopper and S.B. Spring. "The antibody molecule". Academic Press, New York (1975).
9. M. Raff. Immunological networks. Nature. 265: 205 (1977).
10. K.W. Rammohan, H.F. McFarland, W.J. Bellini, J. Gheuens and D.E. McFarlin. Antibody-mediated modification of encephalitis induced by hamster neurotropic measles virus. J. Inf. Dis. 147: 546 (1983).
11. A.G. Trudgett, W.J. Bellini and D.E. McFarlin. Antibodies to the structural polypeptides of measles virus following acute infection and in SSPE. Clin. Exp. Immunol. 39: 652 (1980).
12. J. Urbain, C. Wuilmart and P.A. Cazenave. Idiotypic regulation in immune networks. Contemp. Top. Mol. Immunol. 8: 113 (1981).

MONOCLONAL AND OLIGOCLONAL IMMUNOGLOBULIN M IN THE CEREBROSPINAL FLUID

P. Gallo, F. Bracco, S. Morara and B. Tavolato

Department of Neurology, University of Padova
Via Giustiniani 5, I-35128 Padova, Italy

SUMMARY

To detect monoclonal and oligoclonal IgM in serum and cerebrospinal fluid, we used anion-exchange chromatography followed by agarose IEF, double immunofixation and peroxidase staining. Since the native pentameric IgM molecules did not migrate in the gel, the reduction in the monomeric form was necessary. In three CSF samples from patients with IgM benign monoclonal gammopathy it was possible to detect the M-component. In one neurosyphilis CSF an intrathecal synthesis of IgM was demonstrated. In six CSF from patients with MS, we failed in detecting IgM monoclonal bands.

INTRODUCTION

Quantitative and qualitative abnormalities of humoral immunity, reflecting an intrathecal synthesis of immunoglobulins, can be demonstrated in cerebrospinal fluid (CSF) from patients with multiple sclerosis (MS). An increased IgG-index is found in about 70% of patients, while the IgM-index appears elevated in about 50% (1). Among the qualitative (i.e. electrophoretic) findings, the presence of IgG oligoclonal bands can be demonstrated in up to 95% of MS CSF. These are IgG characterized by a restricted heterogeneity and are thought to be the expression of IgG synthesis by a few clones of B lymphocytes segregated within the central nervous system (CNS). IgM oligoclonal bands have also been demonstrated in MS CSF (2). From an immunological point of view, this may be the most important finding. In fact, the presence of IgM having restricted heterogeneity may indicate: 1) the presence of few lymphocyte clones elaborating a primary response against a "recent antigen" located within the CNS, 2) a continuous stimulation by an "active" antigen within a "persistent" infection. However, our experience leads us to question the possibility of a valid and reliable demonstration of IgM oligoclonal bands either in concentrated or in native CSF by means of conventional techniques such as IEF in agarose gel.

In fact, the physico-chemical characteristics of the pentameric IgM molecule (very high molecular weight, wide hydrodynamic radius, complex stereochemical structure) constitute limiting factors for studies on gel systems. Moreover, the amplification techniques commonly used for the detection of IgM in unconcentrated CSF (i.e. peroxidase staining, avidin-biotin-peroxidase complex, peroxidase-anti-peroxidase) may be the source of unspecific staining.

The following report describes the results of a preliminary study on CSF IgM by means of anion-exchange chromatography followed by agarose isoelectric focusing.

MATERIAL AND METHODS

Samples

3 paired CSF and serum samples from patients with IgM benign monoclonal gammopathy, 6 paired CSF and serum samples from patients with multiple sclerosis as well as one paired CSF and serum sample from a patient with neurosyphilis were included in this pilot study. The native CSF specimens (from 10 to 15 ml) were concentrated by ultrafiltration using Minicon B15 chambers. Adjustment of the sera protein concentrations was performed by dilution with 0.15 M NaCl.

Anion-exchange chromatography

The separations were performed on the fast protein liquid chromatography (FPLC) system (Pharmacia, Fine Chemicals, Uppsala, Sweden) which consists of a LCC-500 liquid chromatography controller, two P-500 pumps, a MV-7 valve, a UV-1 single path monitor, a REC-482 two channel recorder, and a FRAC-100 fraction collector. The system was equipped with a Mono-Q column HR 5/5 (Pharmacia). The start buffer was 0.025 M phosphate buffer, pH 6.7, and the eluting buffer was 0.3 M phosphate buffer, pH 6.5. The buffers were titrated to the respective pH with HCl and degassed. Prior to application on the column (via a 0.5 ml loop) the samples were diluted 1:5 with start buffer and filtered through a sterile 0.22 µn disposable filter (Millipore). The anion-exchange chromatography was performed in a two-steps gradient a follows: 100% start buffer in the first 12 ml, 50% start buffer +50% eluting buffer during the following 12 ml, 100% eluting buffer in the next two ml (25th and 26th ml) and finally 4 ml of 100 start buffer. The total gradient volume was 30 ml (see Fig.1), the flow rate was 2.0 ml/min, the absorbance of the eluate was measured at 280 nm and the collection of the fractions was volume based (i.e. 2 ml volume). After every run, the column was washed with 1 ml of 70% acetic acid and 3 ml 2M NaCl via a reversed direction flow. Quantification of IgG and IgM in the corresponding fractions was carried out by nephelometry.

```
METHOD NO. 2

 0.0 CONC %B     0.0
 0.0 ML/MIN     2.00
 0.0 CM/ML      1.00
 0.0 PORT.SET    6.1
 0.0 VALVE.POS   1.2
12.0 CONC %B     0.0
12.0 CONC %B    50.0
24.0 CONC %B    50.0
24.0 CONC %B     100
26.0 CONC %B     100
26.0 CONC %B     0.0
30.0 CONC %B     0.0
30.0 PORT.SET    6.0
```

Fig.1. Double-step anion-exchange program. Flow rate: 2ml/min, Chart speed 1 cm/ml. Total gradient volume: 30 ml. For explanation see the text.

Agarose isoelectric focusing (AIEF)

Isoelectric focusing of the native samples and the anion-exchange chromatography fractions was performed on 0.8 agarose home-made gel plates with ampholine pH 3.5-10.0 (LKB, Bromma, Sweden). AIEF was followed either by Coomassie BB staining as previously described (Kostulas and Link) or by specific immunofixations on nitrocellulose membrane. This was done as follows: after IEF and transfer of proteins to nitrocellulose membrane, a first immunofixation with rabbit anti-human IgG (IgA, IgM) was followed by a second immunofixation with swine anti-rabbit Ig peroxidase conjugated. The CSF and serum samples as well as the IgG-containing fractions were studied in the native state, while material from the IgM-containing fractions was run natively as well as after mild reduction with B-mercaptoethanol (Sigma Chemical Co., USA), which reduced the pentameric IgM molecules to the monomeric forms.

Isogel was from FMC Corp., Marine Colloids D.V. Rockland, USA. Coomassie BB 250-R was from Sigma Chemical Co., St. Louis, USA. Nitrocellulose membranes BA 85, No 401193 were from Schleicher and Schüll, Dassel, FRG. Antisera were from Dako Glostrup, Denmark.

RESULTS

Fig.2 shows the double-step anion-exchange chromatography profiles of a serum (continuous line) and a CSF (dotted line) from a patient with an IgG BMG. The same amount of IgM was loaded onto the column, i.e. 0.5 mg of IgM (the CSF had an IgM concentration of 58 mg/l, so 10 ml of CSF were used in this case). The chromatography profiles showed three main peaks: the first peak eluted within the first 4 ml, was the IgG-containing peak, while the last one, eluted between the 26th and the 29th ml of the gradient, was the IgM-containing peak. As previously described (4) duplicate separations and nephelometry assay showed high run to run reproducibility. No IgM at all was detected in the IgG-containing fractions, neither was IgG found in the IgM fractions, which usually contained traces of albumin.

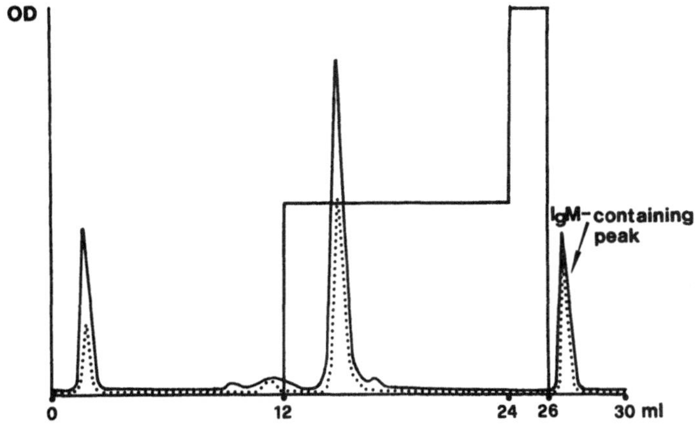

Fig.2. Double-step anion-exchange profiles of the serum (continuous line) and the CSF (dotted line) from a patient with IgM monoclonal gammopathy. The total gradient volume (30 ml) is indicated in the X axis, the optical density (280 nm) in the Y axis.

Fig.3 shows a Coomassie stained agarose IEF of the fractions collected from an anion exchange separation of an IgM myeloma serum. The IgG-containing peak was run in position 1, the IgM-containing peak was run either in the native form (position 9) as well as after mild reduction with B-mercaptoethanol (position 10). The IgG pattern is clearly seen to come out in the first fraction while the IgM paraprotein is clearly seen in the last fraction. The IgM migrated in the gel as quite broad band near the application point. This was the result we had with all the IgM monoclonal components (more than 20 serum samples) run on AIEF. The mild reduction with B-mercaptoethanol (in the experiment of Fig.3: 5.0 μg of purified IgM + 0.08 M B-mercaptoethanol in a final volume of 100 μl), that reduces the pentameric IgM in monomeric IgM without producing free light chains, showed a spectrum of several bands migrating in a restricted pH range (Fig.4). This pattern was similar to that displayed an IEF by the IgG paraproteins.

Applying this method (anion exchange chromatography-mild reduction of the IgM containing fraction-agarose IEF-specific immunofixation-amplification and staining by the avidin-biotin-peroxidase complex), we detected an IgM pattern in neurosyphilis CSF, which was different from that of the correspondent serum, suggesting an intrathecal synthesis of oligoclonal IgM. In the six MS CSF studied, we were not able to detect any intrathecal synthesis of IgM.

DISCUSSION

We have been working for four years about CSF IgM with quite frustrating results. We noticed that the pentameric IgM molecules do not enter completely and move extremely slowly in the agarose IEF gels. Usually they migrate as a broad band not far from the application point. We tried several concentrations of agarose and mixtures of agarose and acrylamide (5) but the results were always the same.

Even the IgM monoclonal gammopathies migrate as a single broad band near the application point while they should fractionate into a spectrum of bands, since they undergo the same post-synthetic charge displacement as IgG monoclonal gammopathies do. Only in few IgM myeloma was it possible to detect some faint IgM bands migrating to a little more alkaline re-

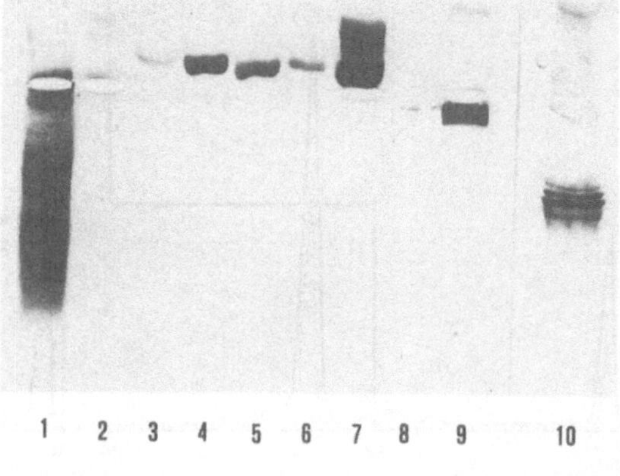

Fig.3. Agarose IEF followed by Coomassie BB staining of the fractions collected from an anion-exchange chromatography of an IgM myeloma serum. The IgM-containing peak was run in the native form (9) as well as after mild reduction (10).

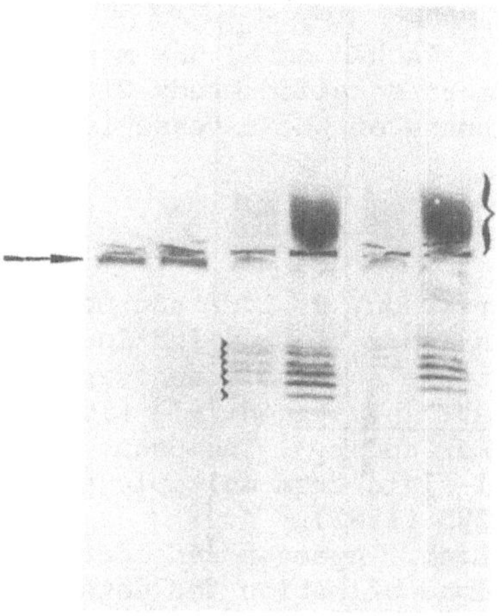

Fig.4. Nitrocellulose membrane immunostained with double-immunofixation and peroxidase staining.
1) Native serum and CSF from a patient with IgM/K M-component;
2) and 3) the same samples after reduction. The arrow indicates the band of native pentameric IgM paraprotein; the arrow heads indicate the monomeric IgM with monoclonal aspects. The bracket indicates the polyclonal IgM pattern.

gion than the main broad IgM band. In our opinion, these bands were made up of monomeric IgM molecules. After mild reduction with B-mecaptoethanol all the IgM paraproteins showed a spectrum of several closely spaced bands quite similar to that showed by the IgG paraproteins.

Concerning to the CSF, the normal IgM concentration is between 100 and 200 µg/l and it increases up to 1.0 µg/l in MS CSF. This amount is still too low to be detected in unconcentrated CSF by the most sensitive amplification systems today available, even by the avidin-biotin-peroxidase complex staining technique.

The CSF concentration is a real source of unspecific staining. When the CSF was concentrated up to 50-100 fold, we noticed the frequent unspecific staining of bands belonging to the IgG oligoclonal patterns or to the free light chains pattern. The CSF IgG concentration increased the risk of unspecific stainings clearly showing that they were in part due to the amount of IgG loaded onto the gel.

It seemed clear to us that the demonstration of a real monoclonal or oligoclonal IgM pattern was not possible simply by means of IEF of the native CSF and serum.

To avoid the unspecific staining due to the IgG pattern, the anion-exchange fractionation of the serum and CSF was performed as above described. This method allowed the complete separation of IgG from IgM as shown in Fig.3. The mild reduction with B-mercaptoethanol was clearly another important step.

The negative results we had on MS CSF might be explained with the low amount of CSF used. A more detailed study with larger volumes of CSF from patients in the active phase of the disease is undergoing in our lab.

REFERENCES

1. P. Forsberg, A. Henriksson, H. Link and Ohman. Reference values for CSF-IgM, CSF-IgM/s-IgM ratio and IgM-index and its application to patients with multiple sclerosis and septic meningoencephalitis. Scand. J. Clin. Lab. Invest. 44:7-12 (1984).
2. G. Keir, R.W.H. Walker and E.J. Thompson. Oligoclonal immunoglobulin M in cerebrospinal fluid from multiple sclerosis patients. J. Neurol. Sci. 57:281-285 (1982).
3. V. Kostulas and H. Link. Agarose isoelectric focusing of unconcentrated CSF and radioimmunofixation for detection of oligoclonal bands in patients with multiple sclerosis and other neurological diseases. J. Neurol. Sci. 54:117-127 (1982).
4. P. Gallo, A. Sidén and B. Tavolato. Anion exchange chromatography and isoelectric focusing of serum immunoglobulins. Prot. Biol. Fluids, in press (1986).
5. D.E. Jackson, C.A. Skandera, C.A. Owen, E.T. Lally and P.L. Montgomery Isoelectric focusing of IgA and IgM in composite acrylamide-agarose gel. J. Immunol. Methods. 36:315-324 (1980).

SPECIFICITY OF OLIGOCLONAL IgG IN CHRONIC RELAPSING EAE IN GUINEA PIGS

Pankaj D. Mehta and Bruce A. Patrick

NY State Institute for Basic Research in Developmental Disabilities, Staten Island, NY 10314

INTRODUCTION

The sensitization of young strain 13 guinea pigs with homologous spinal cord in complete Freund's adjuvant and killed mycobacterium tuberculosis has been shown to result in a relapsing experimental allergic encephalomyelitis (R-EAE) in about 65% of the animals injected (1). In these animals, demyelinating lesions develop in brain, spinal cord and optic nerves over the course of the disease, and become more extensive with each recurring episode. These results are consistent with those seen in multiple sclerosis (2). Several investigators have reported the presence of oligoclonal IgG bands in cerebrospinal fluid (CSF), serum and brain extracts of R-EAE animals (3-7). The object of the present work was to determine the specificity of oligoclonal IgG from CSF and serum obtained sequentially from individual R-EAE animals during the course of the disease.

Specificity of oligoclonal IgG in chronic relapsing EAE

The presence of antibodies to myelin components in CSF and sera from chronic R-EAE guinea pigs have been shown by a number of investigators using enzyme-linked immunosorbent assay or radio-immunoassay. It is well established that a low level of antibodies to myelin basic protein (MBP) are present in sera from animals sacrified during acute EAE, whereas the titers are significantly increased during or after the first relapse (7-9). Similar results were obtained in a number of sera collected during the course of the disease from individual animals. Overall, CSF had 50-100 fold lower titers than those seen in matching serum. Antibody titers to proteolipid apoprotein were also found in sera from these animals, however, the titers were 25-50 times lower than those of anti-MBP antibodies (10). Investigators (8-9) also showed the presence of low titers of anti-lipid antibodies in sera from these animals during or shortly after the first relapse. Recent studies of Glynn et al. (11) suggest that in most chronic R-EAE animals circulating antibodies bind more avidly to peptide epitopes expressed by MBP-lipid complexes than MBP in aqueous solution.

Although the above methods show the presence of antibody to specific proteins or lipids, they are unable to show if the antibody activity is associated with polyclonal or oligoclonal IgG. In contrast, imprint electroimmunofixation (12) does not allow a precise quantitation of specific antibody, but is sensitive enough to demonstrate the antibody activity of oligoclonal or polyclonal IgG against suspected antigens. In support of this, the method has been successfully applied to determine the association of viral or bacterial antibodies with oligoclonal IgG in CSF and serum of patients with SSPE (12-13) and progressive rubella panencephalitis (14).

Because most of the oligoclonal IgG in both acute and chronic R-EAE sera could not be absorbed with CNS antigens as shown in immunofixation after electrophoresis, investigators concluded that the bands may not be relevant to the disease process (15). Recently, the specificity of oligoclonal IgG in sera from chronic relapsing EAE guinea pigs was determined by using imprint electroimmunofixation (16). The response of oligoclonal IgG to spinal cord and mycobacterium tuberculosis appeared to be equal in animals sacrified during first remission and in those sacrified after recovery from acute EAE. In contrast, in animals sacrified during or after the first relapse, the oligoclonal IgG seems to be directed predominantly against spinal cord (Fig.1). In imprint electroimmunofixation, the oligoclonal IgG specific to spinal cord did not react with guinea pig liver and kidney. In addition, activity to spinal cord could be removed from sera by absorption with spinal cord but not with kidney or liver. Our studies also showed that sera from R-EAE animals collected during or after the first relapse, have oligoclonal IgG specific to MBP and proteolipid apoprotein. The band patterns specific to these proteins differ in number,

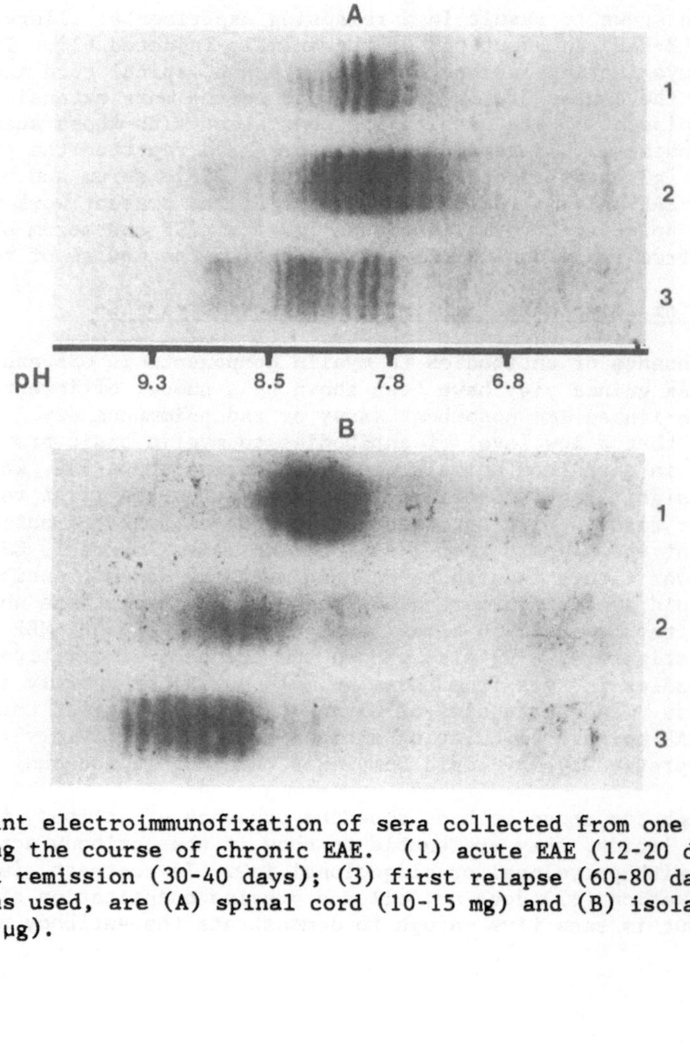

Fig.1. Imprint electroimmunofixation of sera collected from one guinea pig during the course of chronic EAE. (1) acute EAE (12-20 days); (2) first remission (30-40 days); (3) first relapse (60-80 days). Antigens used, are (A) spinal cord (10-15 mg) and (B) isolated MBP (100 µg).

intensity and isoelectric point from sera of individual animals during different episodes of the disease. Overall, the oligoclonal IgG specific to MBP was stronger than that seen with proteolipid apoprotein. The specificity of MBP specific bands was confirmed by showing a lack of reactivity against histone and lysozyme. When the sera were absorbed with total myelin proteins prior to imprint electroimmunofixation, a few oligoclonal IgG bands specific to spinal cord antigens were still seen. The data suggest that the oligoclonal IgG in part is directed against myelin lipids.

CSF from a few R-EAE animals when examined against myelin proteins, had patterns identical to those seen in matching sera. However, the overall intensity of CSF oligoclonal IgG was weaker in CSF than that of sera, due to their lower IgG level.

Specificity of oligoclonal IgG in MS

The specificity of the major portion of oligoclonal IgG in MS is not known. However, in most MS patients, evidence of the intrathecal IgG synthesis to a number of viruses as well as the presence of anti-brain antibodies in their CSF (17-18) have been reported. It is possible that the greater number of oligoclonal IgG bands are not directed against any specific set of antigens but represent a general activation of B-cell clones during attacks of MS (19).

Employing imprint electroimmunofixation, investigators (20) showed antibodies to a number of viruses in CSF of MS, but the antibody activity was associated more with polyclonal IgG than oligoclonal IgG. Thus, the specificity of a major portion of oligoclonal IgG in CSF of MS is still unaccounted for. We, as well as others, were unable to show association of anti-myelin proteins antibody activity with oligoclonal IgG in CSF of MS. Although the presence of antibodies to glycolipids in CSF of MS has been reported (21), it is not clear if the activity is associated with the oligoclonal IgG.

SUMMARY

Although our studies show that oligoclonal IgG in chronic R-EAE guinea pigs possess antibody activity to myelin proteins and lipids, it is not clear whether these antigens are targets of the oligoclonal IgG response or if the immune response against these antigens is a secondary phenomena that develops only as the disease progresses. There was no correlation between the occurrence of relapses and demyelination with the humoral immune response against myelin proteins. Since a number of studies indicate the presence of myelin lipid antibodies during or after the first relapse, and impairment of blood-brain-barrier in chronic R-EAE guinea pigs, circulating antibodies either to myelin lipids or MBP-lipid complexes could be responsible for CNS demyelination.

ACKNOWLEDGEMENT

This work was supported by the National Institutes of Health Grant # NS-14406.

REFERENCES

1. H.M. Wisniewski and A.B. Keith. Chronic relapsing allergic encephalomyelitis: an experimental model of multiple sclerosis. Ann. Neurol. 1:144 (1977).

2. H.M. Wisniewski, H. Lassmann, G. Schuller-Levis, P.D. Mehta and R.E. Madrid. Pathogenesis of perivenous and demyelinating encephalomyelitis and its relevance for multiple sclerosis research. In: "Multiple Sclerosis; Present and Future", G. Scarlato and W.B. Matthews, eds. Plenum Press, New York. p.1. (1984).
3. P.D. Mehta, H. Lassmann and H.M. Wisniewski. Immunologic studies of chronic relapsing EAE in guinea pigs. Similarities to multiple sclerosis. J. Immunol. 127:334 (1981).
4. T.K. Olsson, K. Kristensson, J. Leijon and H. Link. Demonstration of serum IgG antibodies against myelin during the course of relapsing experimental allergic encephalomyelitis in guinea pigs. J. Neurol. Sci. 54:359 (1982).
5. P. GLynn, D. Weedon, J. Edwards, A.J. Suckling and M.L. Cuzner. Humoral immunity in chronic relapsing experimental autoimmune encephalomyelitis. J. Neurol. Sci. 57:369 (1982).
6. D. Karcher, H. Lassmann, A. Lowenthal, K. Kitz and H.M. Wisniewski. Antibodies restricted heterogeneity in serum and cerebrospinal fluid of chronic relapsing experimental allergic encephalomyelitis. J. Neuroimmunol. 2:93 (1982).
7. B. Schwerer, G.B. Schuller-Lewis, P.D. Mehta, R.E. Madrid and H.M. Wisniewski. Cellular and humoral immune response to MBP during the course of chronic relapsing EAE. Prog. Clin. Biol. Res. 146:187 (1984).
8. H. Lassmann, G. Suchanek, K. Kitz, H. Stemberger, B. Schwerer and H. Bernheimer. Antibodies in the pathogenesis of demyelination in chronic relapsing EAE. Prog. Clin. Biol. Res. 146:165 (1984).
9. T. Tabira and M. Endoh. Humoral immune response to myelin basic protein, cerebroside and ganglioside in chronic relapsing EAE of guinea pigs. J. Neurol. Sci. 67:201 (1985).
10. M. Endoh, T. Tabira and T. Kunishita. Antibodies to proteolipid apoprotein in chronic relapsing experimental allergic encephalomyelitis. J. Neurol. Sci. 73:31 (1986).
11. P. Glynn, D. Weedon and M.L. Cuzner. Chronic experimental autoimmune encephalomyelitis. Circulating autoantibodies bind predominantly determinants expressed by complexes of basic protein and lipids of myelin. J. Neurol. Sci. 73:111 (1986).
12. H.J. Nordal, B. Vandvik and E. Norrby. Demonstration of electrophoretically restricted virus-specific antibodies in serum and cerebrospinal fluid by imprint electroimmunofixation. Scand. J. Immunol. 7:381 (1978).
13. F. Vartdal, B. Vandvik and E. Norrby. Viral and bacterial antibody response in multiple sclerosis. Ann. Neurol. 8:248 (1980).
14. B. Vandvik, M.L. Weil, E. Norrby and M. Grandien. Progressive rubella panencephalitis: local synthesis in brain of oligoclonal virus-specific IgG antibodies and homogneous free light chains in the central nervous system. Acta Neurol. Scand. 57:53 (1978).
15. C.C. Whitacre, D.H. Mattson, E.D. Day, D.J. Petersen, P.Y. Paterson, R.P. Roos and B.G.W. Arnasson. Oligoclonal IgG in rabbits with experimental allergic encephalomyelitis non-reactivity of the bands with sensitizing neural antigens. Neurochem. Res. 7:1209 (1982).
16. P.D. Mehta, B.A. Patrick and H.M. Wisniewski. Specificity of oligoclonal IgG bands in sera from chronic relapsing experimental allergic encephalomyelitis guinea pigs. J. Immunol. 134:2338 (1985).
17. B. Ryberg. Multiple specificities of antibrain in multiple sclerosis and chronic myelopathy. J. Neurol. Sci. 38:357 (1978).
18. M.K. Gorny, Z. Wroblewska, D. Pleasure, S.L. Miller, A. Waijgt and H. Koprowski. CSF antibodies to myelin basic protein and oligodendrocytes in multiple sclerosis and other neurological diseases. Acta Neurol. Scand. 67:338 (1983).

19. P.Y. Paterson and C.C. Whitacre. The enigma of oligoclonal immunoglobulin G in cerebrospinal fluid from multiple sclerosis patients. Immunol. Today. 2:111 (1981).
20. F. Vartdal and B. Vandvik. Multiple sclerosis: electrofocused "bands" of oligoclonal CSF IgG do not carry antibody activity against measles, varicella-zoster or rotaviruses. J. Neurol. Sci. 54:99 (1982).
21. T. Endo, D.D. Scott, S.S. Stewart, S.K. Kundy and D.M. Marcus. Antibodies to glycosphingolipids in patients with multiple sclerosis and EAE. 132:1793 (1984).

EPITOPES OF MYELIN BASIC PROTEIN: THE DETECTION OF IMMUNOREACTIVE MYELIN BASIC PROTEIN IN BODY FLUIDS

John N. Whitaker and Renga I. Vasu

From the Departments of Neurology and Cell Biology and Anatomy at the University of Alabama at Birmingham and from the Neurology and Research Services of the Birmingham VA Medical Center
Department of Neurology, University of Alabama at Birmingham, University Station, Birmingham, AL 35294

INTRODUCTION

The loss of myelin from the central nervous system (CNS) lesions of multiple sclerosis (MS) has provided a rationale for the analysis of cerebrospinal fluid (CSF) and other body fluids for myelin components. The detection of such components offers a laboratory approach to verifying and monitoring disease activity and in determining what range or type of myelin components may gain access to the immune system and possibly stimulate cellular or humoral autoimmunity.

MBP-LIKE MATERIAL IN CSF

Beginning with the observation by Johnson and Herndon (1970), who detected myelin debris in CSF sediment from individuals with damaged CNS myelin, a number of investigators have utilized an immunochemical assay of CSF to look for myelin basic protein (MBP), a protein restricted to CNS and peripheral nervous system (PNS) myelin (reviewed in Whitaker & Snyder, 1982). MBP comprises 30% of CNS myelin proteins and has been extensively analyzed because of its capacity to induce experimental allergic encephalomyelitis in susceptible animals (Carnegie & Moore, 1980; Norton, 1981). The studies reporting on the detection of MBP-like material in CSF of MS patients have differed in certain technical details but all have some uniformity in demonstrating that MBP-like material can be detected by immunochemical means but without disease specificity in the CSF of individuals following acute CNS myelin damage (Biber et al., 1981; Burgisser et al., 1981; Carson et al., 1978; Cohen et al., 1976; Cohen et al., 1980; Delasalle et al., 1982; Massaro et al., 1985; Ohta et al., 1980; Thompson et al., 1985; Warren et al., 1983; Warren & Catz, 1985; Whitaker, 1977; Whitaker et al., 1980a). Although this material is presumably MBP or a fragment thereof, the material detected has never been validated by biological means or chemical purification. Thus, the reference to this immunoreactivity as MBP-like is more appropriate and expresses the caution which should be taken until total validation is available.

FEATURES OF MBP-LIKE MATERIAL IN CSF

Attempts to elucidate the properties of MBP in CSF have consisted of determining size (Bashir & Whitaker, 1980a; Carson et al., 1978; Karlsson & Alling, 1984; Sunderland & McPherson, 1980), epitopes (Biber et al., 1981; Cohen et al., 1980; Whitaker, 1977; Whitaker et al., 1980a) or the parallelism of dilution of CSF MBP-like material with MBP (Burggisser et al., 1982; Palfreyman et al., 1978). Although a large form of MBP has been reported to be present in the CSF of MS patients (Carson et al., 1978; McPherson & Catz, 1985), two investigations of the gel filtration of MBP-like material in CSF cross-reactive with MBP peptide 45-89 (Bashir & Whitaker, 1980) or MBP (Karlsson & Alling, 1984) have demonstrated a spectrum of sizes of MBP-like material in CSF with larger forms predominating in CSF from persons with cerebral infarction and smaller forms existing in CSF from persons with acute phase MS. Studies of the epitopes of MBP present have shown the dominant epitope present, was MBP peptide 45-89 (Whitaker, 1977), especially an epitope toward the carboxyl-terminal of the peptide (Whitaker et al., 1980b). Although antigenic material cross-reactive with bovine MBP peptide 89-169 has been reported to be present in CSF (Biber et al., 1981), the report has not been confirmed (Whitaker et al., 1980b; Whitaker, 1984). The dilutional analysis of CSF MBP-like material has demonstrated a moderate non-parallelism with MBP (Burgisser et al., 1982; Palfreyman et al., 1978).

In seeking to detect by immunochemical means MBP-like material in body fluids, it has been noted that the antisera used are highly variable in terms of the amount of MBP-like material detected and in the ability to detect it all. Many antisera which react specifically and in high affinity with MBP fail to detect MBP-like material in CSF. The investigations reported from this laboratory have emphasized the importance of using a fragment of MBP as the radioligand with the fragment most successfully employed as that of human MBP peptide 45-89, cleaved from the intact molecule of 170 residues by limited pepsin digestion (Whitaker, 1977) or treatment with cathepsin D (Whitaker et al., 1980). Past (Whitaker, 1977) and recent (Whitaker et al., 1986; Gupta et al., 1986) studies have shown the greater utility of immunoassays using this radioligand. With an immunochemical analysis of the reaction with a variety of MBP peptides, it has been shown that with the radioligand of human MBP peptide 45-89 the carboxyl half of this peptide is the site which bears the epitope most critical to the detection of MBP-like material in CSF and that those antisera which detect the highest amounts of MBP-like material react with the carboxyl decapeptide of 80-89 (Whitaker et al., 1986). This peptide has the sequence of threonine-glutamine-aspartic acid-glutamic acid-asparagine-proline-valine-valine-histidine-phenylalanine. Shorter fragments with deletion of the carboxyl-terminal phenylalanine show no reactivity, those peptides with a deleted threonine at position 80 show very little and those with the addition of up to six carboxyl-terminal residues to MBP peptide 80-89 beyond the phenylalanine at position 89 show no reactivity. Those residues with amino terminal extensions still react but often less well. These observations indicate that the epitope in MBP peptide 80-89 is likely to involve the entire decapeptide presumably in a conformation that is necessary for simulation with the MBP-like material in CSF. It should be noted that the recognition of this decapeptide's importance came only after the correct sequence of this decapeptide was defined (Gibson et al., 1984). Previously, an incorrect assignment of sequence was followed in synthesizing MBP peptides with glutamine and aspartic acid assigned to residues 83-84 when it should have been glutaminic acid and asparagine. This difference may have a marked influence on the reactivity of antisera with MBP peptide 80-89 (Whitaker, 1984; Whitaker et al., 1986). The identification of human MBP 45-89 as containing the major epitope is in agreement with studies performed on the size of the immunoreactive material in CSF of MS patients (Bashir and Whitaker, 1980; Karlson & Alling, 1984).

MBP-LIKE MATERIAL IN OTHER BODY FLUIDS

The presence of MBP-like material in CSF implies that this material should be found in some form in other body fluids such as blood and urine. It is likely that material released into the CSF might also reach the blood directly from brain or spinal cord. In fact, MBP-like material has been reported in blood of humans after CNS damage (Palfreyman et al., 1979) and normally in rats in the neonatal period (Fujinami et al., 1978); however, validation of this MBP-like material as MBP or MBP peptides is not available. The clearance of MBP-like material from body fluids has a possible role in allowing the MBP-like material to reach and stimulate the immune system and also has relevance to what form the MBP-like material in urine and perhaps blood might have. In a series of investigations it has been shown that the kidney is responsible for the clearance of human MBP peptide 45-89 (Bashir and Whitaker, 1980b) and that different renal proteinases are responsible for the degradation of this peptide. The human kidney contains renal proteinases which can degrade human MBP peptide 45-89 which differ from the proteinases present in the kidneys of other species (Whitaker et al., 1982; Whitaker & Heinemann, 1983a; Whitaker & Heinemann, 1983b). Utilizing this experimental data, it was inferred that MBP-like material, probably in the form of small MBP peptides, might be found in urine if the appropriate reagents were available.

Studies on the epitopes in the carboxyl-terminal region of MBP peptide 45-89 has previously shown that this region of the MBP molecule had interesting characteristics as to its epitope features. Most notably, the carboxyl-terminal portion appears to have different potential conformations that may exist (Whitaker et al., 1980b) or not exist in the intact molecule (Whitaker et al., 1977). This implied that at least two, and possibly more, epitopes were present in this decapeptide of MBP. A number of antisera have been screened for their ability to detect MBP-like material in urine, and recently one antiserum, a rabbit antiserum directed against the carboxyl-terminal portion of bovine MBP peptide 43-88 (the same region as human MBP peptide 45-89) detects MBP-like material in urine. The assay employed is similar to that used for CSF with human MBP peptide 45-89 as the radioligand but a different antiserum is required for the detection of urinary MBP-like material. None of the antisera yet examined can detect MBP-like material in both CSF and urine. The characterization of the epitope of MBP-like material in urine has helped to clarify the basis for this distinction. The epitope of MBP peptide 45-89 recognized by the antiserum detecting MBP-like material in urine also reacts with epitope in the decapeptide of human MBP 80-89; however, this epitope is not present in intact MBP ans seems to be shifted more toward the carboxyl-terminal of the decapeptide (Whitaker et al., 1985). Thus, it reacts better with MBP peptides 81-89 and 82-89 than does the antiserum detecting MBP-like material in CSF. The features of this antiserum detecting urinary MBP-like material are similar to those mentioned above for the antisera reacting with a novel or neo-antigen of MBP not present in the intact molecule (Whitaker et al., 1977).

In studies still continuing, the features of the MBP-like material in urine have been further characterized (Whitaker et al., 1985). The material in the urine is resistant to boiling for 10 minutes, behaves on gel filtration as a molecule of about 1,000 daltons and has been partially purified by HPLC which should provide a means for its isolation and characterization.

MONOCLONAL ANTIBODIES TO HUMAN MBP PEPTIDE 80-89

In concert with these studies of polyclonal reagents and the characterization of the epitopes of MBP in CSF and urine, studies have also been performed to analyze the epitopes of MBP in the carboxyl-terminal region of MBP peptide 45-89 with murine monoclonal antibodies (Price et al., 1986). These studies have shown, similar to results with polyclonal reagents, that the variety of epitopes of MBP is much greater than might be anticipated. Three custom synthesized MBP peptides, bovine MBP peptide 79-88, human MBP peptide 80-89, and human MBP peptide 82-91, were used to produce four murine monoclonal antibodies that were selected on the basis of reaction in a solid phase radioimmunoassay with human MBP. The monoclonal antibodies were compared with respect to antigen specificity against intact MBP and 10 overlapping MBP peptides. One monoclonal antibody recognized an epitope near the amino-terminus of bovine MBP peptide 79-88. A second monoclonal antibody was directed towards an epitope that is more reactive in human MBP peptide 45-89 than in intact MBP, but is not recognized in any of the small MBP peptides examined. The third monoclonal antibody detected an epitope near the middle of human MBP peptide 80-89, whereas the fourth monoclonal antibody reacted with the C-terminal portion of human MBP peptide 82-91. Epitopes recognized in solid phase assays were sometimes not detected by the same monoclonal antibody in a fluid phase double antibody radioimmunoassay. These results demonstrated the multiplicity of potential epitopes in a dodecapeptide of MBP and do not support the concept of a single, dominant epitope in the region of MBP peptide 80-89. Monoclonal antibodies of high affinity ultimately may furnish an alternative to the use of polyclonal anti-MBP reagents in immunoassays of MBP-like material in body fluids.

SUMMARY

One of the dominant epitopes of MBP-like material detected in human CSF and urine is from the C-terminal region of human MBP peptide 45-89. As reflected by the immunochemical features of MBP recognized by the antisera utilized, the form of MBP peptide-like material in the CSF and urine is different, presumably a result of proteolysis in the kidney during the clearance process. These results indicate that at least a portion of the ten residues of human MBP 80-89 is likely to reach the immune system. Results of studies with polyclonal and monoclonal reagents illustrate the variety of epitopes present in small regions of the MBP molecule and the critical nature of these epitopes both for immunoassays and, possibly, for the detection of immune response against such small peptides.

REFERENCES

1. R.M. Bashir and J.N. Whitaker. Molecular features of immunoreactive myelin basic protein in cerebrospinal fluid of persons with multiple sclerosis. Ann. Neurol. 7:50-57 (1980).
2. R.M. Bashir and J.N. Whitaker. Metabolism of a peptide of human myelin basic protein in the rabbit. Neurology (Minneapolis). 30:1184-1192 (1980).
3. A. Biber, D. Englert, D. Dommasch and K. Hempel. Myelin basic protein in cerebrospinal fluid of patients with multiple sclerosis and other neurological diseases. J. Neurol. 225:231-236 (1981).
4. P.H. Burgisser, J.M. Mathieu, N. DeTribolet and E. Gautier. Dosage de la proteine basique de la myeline dans le liquide cephalo-rachidien au cours d'affections neurologiques. Schweiz med. Wschr. 112:643-647 (1982).

5. P.R. Carnegie and W.J. Moore. Myelin basic protein. In: "Proteins of the Nervous System", 2nd edition. R.A. Bradshaw and D.M. Schneider, eds. Raven, New York. (1980).
6. J.H. Carson, E. Barbarese, P.E. Braun and T.A. McPherson. Components in multiple sclerosis cerebrospinal fluid that are detected by radioimmunoassay for myelin basic protein. Proc. Nat. Acad. Sci. 75: 1976-1978 (1978).
7. S.R. Cohen, R.M. Herndon and G.M. McKhann. Myelin basic protein in cerebrospinal fluid as an indicator of active demyelination. Radioimmunoassay of myelin basic protein in spinal fluid. An index of active demyelination. N. Engl. J. Med. 295:1454-1457.
8. S.R. Cohen, B. Jubelt, B.R. Brookw, R.M. Herndon and G.M. McKhann. A diagnostic index of active demyelination: Myelin basic protein in cerebrospinal fluid. Ann. Neurol. 8:25-31 (1980).
9. A. Delasalle, C. Jacque, J. Drouet, M. Raoul, J.C. Legrand and F. Cesselin. Radioimmunoassay of the myelin basic protein in biological fluids, conditions improving sensitivity and specificity. Biochimie. 62:159-165 (1980).
10. R.S. Fujinami, P.Y. Paterson, E.D. Day and V.A. Varitek. Myelin basic protein serum factor: An endogenous neuroantigen influencing development of experimental allergic encephalomyelitis in Lewis rats. J. Exp. Med. 148:1716-1721 (1978).
11. B.W. Gibson, R.D. Gilliom, J.N. Whitaker and K. Biemann. Amino acid sequence of human myelin basic protein peptide 45-89 as determined by mass spectrometry. J. Biol. Chem. 259:5028-5031 (1984).
12. M.K. Gupta, C. Johnson, J.N. Whitaker and H. Goren. Measurement of human MBP fragment (45-89) in CSF: A more sensitive indicator of demyelination than MPB. Ann. Neurol. In press.(1986).
13. A.R. Massaro, F. Michetti, A. Laudisio and P. Bergonzi. Myelin basic protein and S-100 antigen in cerebrospinal fluid of patients with multiple sclerosis in the acute phase. Ital. J. Neurol. Sci. 6:53-56 (1985).
14. W.T. Norton. Formation, structure and biochemistry of myelin. In: "Basic Neurochemistry", 3rd edition, G.J. Seigel, R.W. Albers, B.W. Agranoff and R.T. Katzman, eds. Little, Brown and Co., Boston. (1981).
15. M. Ohta, F. Matsubara, T. Konishi and H. Nishitani. Radioimmunoassay of myelin basic protein in cerebrospinal fluid and its clinical application to patients with neurological diseases. Life Sciences. 27:1069-1974 (1980).
16. J.W. Palfreyman, S.G.T. Thomas and J.C. Ratcliffe. Radioimmunoassay of human myelin basic protein in tissue extract, cerebrospinal fluid and serum and its clinical application to patients with head injury. Clin. Chim. Acta. 82:259-270 (1978).
17. J.W. Palfreyman, R.V. Johnston, J.G. Ratcliffe, D.G.T. Thomas and C.D. Forbes. Radioimmunoassay of serum myelin basic protein and its application to patients with cerebrovascular accidents. Clin. Chim. Acta. 92:403-409 (1979).
18. J.O. Price, J.N. Whitaker, R.L. Vasu and D.W. Metzger. Multiple epitopes in a dodecapeptide of myelin basic protein determined by monoclonal antibodies. J. Immunol. 136:2426-2431 (1986).
19. S.M. Sunderland and T.A. McPherson. Big basic protein: Detection in normal and MS brains as well as in CSF from MS patients. Clin. Res. 28:700A (1980).
20. A.J. Thompson, J. Brazil, C. Feighery, A. Whelan, J. Kellet, E.A. Martin and M. Hutchinson. CSF myelin basic protein in multiple sclerosis. Acta Neurol. Scand. 72:577-583 (1985).
21. K.G. Warren, I. Catz and T.A. McPherson. CSF myelin basic protein levels in acute optic neuritis and multiple sclerosis. Can. J. Neurol. Sci. 10:235-238 (1983).

22. K.G. Warren and I. Catz. The relationship between levels of cerebrospinal fluid myelin basic protein and IgG measurements in patients with multiple sclerosis. Ann. Neurol. 17:475-480 (1985).
23. J.N. Whitaker. Myelin encephalitogenic protein fragments in cerebrospinal fluid of persons with multiple sclerosis. Neurology. 27: 911-920 (1977).
24. J.N. Whitaker. Indicators of disease activity in multiple sclerosis. Studies of myelin basic protein-like materials. Ann. NY Acad. Sci. 436:140-150 (1984).
25. J.N. Whitaker, R.P. Lisak, R.M. Bashir, O.H. Fitch, J.M. Seyer, R. Krance, J.A. Lawrence, L.T. Ch'ien and P. O'Sullivan. Immunoreactive myelin basic protein in the cerebrospinal fluid in neurological disorders. Ann. Neurol. 7:58-64 (1980a).
26. J.N. Whitaker, C.H.J. Chou, F.C.H. Chou and R.F. Kibler. Molecular internalization of a region of myelin basic protein. J. Exp. Med. 146:317-333 (1977).
27. T.A. McPherson and I. Catz. A double antibody radioimmunoassay for myelin basic protein in cerebrospinal fluid. Clin. Biochem. 18: 297-299 (1985).
28. J.N. Whitaker and D.S. Snyder. Myelin components in the cerebrospinal fluid in disease affecting central nervous system myelin. Clinics Allergy Immunol. 2:469-482 (1982).
29. J.N. Whitaker, M.A. Heinemann and B.G. Uzman. The renal degradation of myelin basic protein peptide 43-88 by two enzymes in different subcellular fractions. Biochem. J. 201:543-553 (1982).
30. J.N. Whitaker and M.A. Heinemann. Species comparison of renal proteolytic activity for myelin basic protein peptide 43-88. Comp. Biochem. Physiol. 74B:445-448 (1983a).
31. J.N. Whitaker and M.A. Heinemann. The degradation of human myelin basic protein peptide 43-88 by human renal neutral proteinase. Neurology. 33:744-749 (1983b).
32. J.N. Whitaker, O.F. Smith, R. Vasu and M.A. Heinemann. Immunoreactive myelin basic protein-like material in the urine: Development and characterization of the immunoassay. Ann. Neurol. 18: 129 (1985).
33. J.N. Whitaker, M. Gupta and O.F. Smith. Epitopes of immunoreactive myelin basic protein in human cerebrospinal fluid. Ann Neurol. In press (1986).

ANALYSIS OF IMMUNE COMPLEXES IN MULTIPLE SCLEROSIS

Patricia Coyle

Department of Neurology, Health Sciences Center, T-12-020
SUNY at Stony Brook, Stony Brook, NY 11794

Immune complexes were purified from multiple sclerosis spinal fluid using polyethylene glycol precipitation or column chromatography. Both techniques detected complexes when conventional assay (the Raji cell assay) was negative. Complexed IgA and IgM were frequent findings along with IgG complexes. These complexes were present in sufficient quantity to examine by gel electrophoresis and silver stain; intact and dissociated complexes could be compared. Future studies should permit immune complexes from different patients to be examined for common components.

INTRODUCTION

Multiple sclerosis (MS) is a disease of unknown etiology. The two leading theories as to its pathogenesis postulate either a viral infection of brain (1), or an autoimmune attack against an unknown brain antigen (Ag) (2). In both infectious and autoimmune disorders, circulating immune complexes (IC) are formed and contain diagnostically important Ag and antibody (Ab). The analysis of components of dissociated IC could prove quite useful in learning more about MS. Numerous studies have now documented that IC are indeed present in MS cerebrospinal fluid (CSF) (3-13), but the levels are frequently low. And few studies have reported successful isolation and characterization of IC components. In earlier work using the Raji cell assay, we found low levels of complexes in the CSF of 50% of MS patients experiencing an exacerbation. By absorbing, then eluting and dissociating the complexes from the Raji cell surface, we could detect complex components which included IgG and IgA, herpes simples type I Ag and Ab, myelin basic protein Ag and Ab, and glycolipid Ab. There are potential problems with using this assay to isolate IC however. The Raji cell is a transformed lymphocyte and therefore anti-lymphocyte Abs (which have been reported in MS patients) could interfere with the assay. The assay will detect only complement-fixing complexes. Finally, the isolation technique of eluting bound complexes from the Raji cell surface also removes cell components; this makes electrophoretic studies on the isolated IC very difficult. For theses reasons we have been looking at alternative methods to purify and probe the CSF IC found in MS patients.

MATERIALS AND METHODS

Subjects

CSF was collected from 15 patients with definite MS (14), and 14 patients with a variety of other neurological disorders (OND) including headache, benign intracranial hypertension, trauma, stroke or TIA, and seizure disorder. CSF was kept frozen at -70°C until use.

Polyethylene glycol (PEG) precipitation

IC were precipitated from CSF by adding 0.9 ml of CSF to 0.9 ml of 7% PEG in phosphate buffered saline (PBS). After an overnight incubation at 4°C, the CSF was centrifuged at 8,320 g for 15 minutes. The pellets were then washed twice with 0.75 ml of 3.5% PEG and resuspended in 0.9 ml of PBS.

Column chromatography

CSF was fractionated by chromatography on Sephadex G200 (Pharmacia Fine Chemicals, New Jersey) on 1.5 x 100 cm columns (Econo-columns, Bio-Rad, New York).

The column was equilibrated with PBS and calibrated with standards (Gel filtration calibration kit, Pharmacia Fine Chemicals, New Jersey). Immunoglobulin standards were run to determine where IgM, monomeric IgA, and monomeric IgG eluted. All fractionations were carried out by loading the columns with 1.5 ml of CSF. The flow rate was maintained at 10 to 15 ml/hr and 1.5 ml fractions were collected.

Raji Cell Assay

A modified microELISA assay was used to detect IC as previously reported (15). Levels were read from a standard curve in µg/ml aggregated human globulin (AHG)-equivalent.

Immunoglobulin determination

IgG, IgA and IgM were measured in the PEG precipitates and G200 fractions using a microELISA assay as previously reported (16). This assay detects concentrations as low as 1 ng/ml.

Electrophoresis

IC were analysed by SDS-polyacrylamide gel electrophoresis (SDS-PAGE). G200 fractions containing IC were concentrated 20 times by overnight lyophilization. PEG precipitates were used without further concentration. For non-reducing gels samples were brought up in 46% sucrose, 3% SDS with 0.7% bromophenol blue, and incubated at 37°C for 15 minutes. For reducing gels samples were brought up in 1.5% dithioerythritol, 2% SDS, 0.8M Tris HLC 15% glycerol with 0.7% bromophenol blue, and incubated at 100°C for 5 minutes. Samples were then run on 5% stacking gels and 7% or 9% separating gels as previously reported (17).

Silver Stain

Silver-staining of gels was carried out according to Guevera, et al. (18). This technique uses ethanol washes and ammoniacial silver hydroxide.

RESULTS

IC were precipitated from CSF using PEG, and the immunoglobulin content measured (Fig.1). In order to determine the normal range, 5 control CSF were run and the mean plus 3 standard deviation values calculated for each immunoglobulin class (IgG = 72 ng/ml; IgA = 13.5 ng/ml; IgM = 18.1 ng/ml). Results above these cutoffs were considered indicative of IC. Based on that calculation, 8 of 15 MS and 1 of 14 OND spinal fluids contained IgG complexes; 1 MS and 1 OND contained IgA complexes; and 7 MS and 4 OND contained IgM complexes.

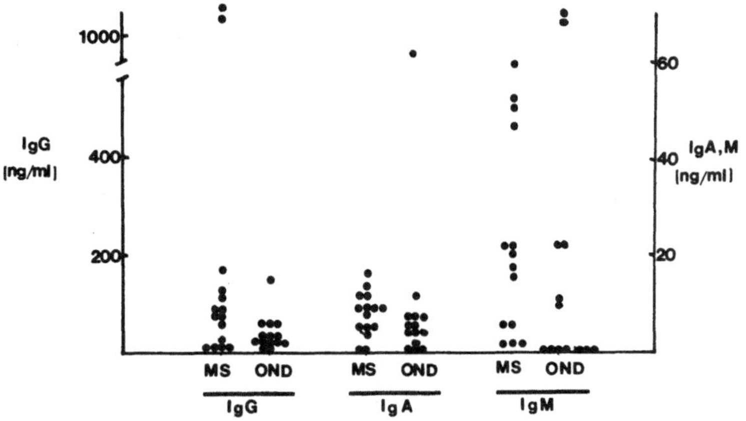

Fig.1. Complexes were precipitated from 15 MS and 14 OND spinal fluids using PEG. IgG, IgA and IgM were measured in the PEG precipitates by ELISA and expressed in ng/ml. (IgM was measured in 14 MS samples).

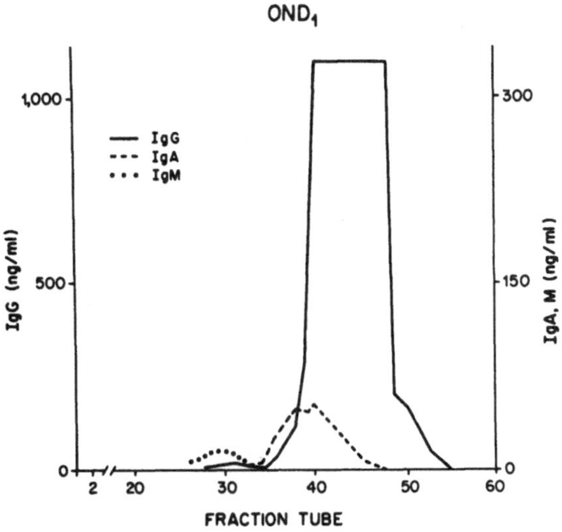

Fig.2. CSF (1.5 ml) was fractionated by G200 column chromatography. Sixty tubes containing 1.5 ml were collected and IgG, IgA and IgM measured in each fraction tube. A representative patient (OND1) is shown. CSF immunoglobulins were detected in fractions identical to where immunoglobulin standards eluted. No evidence for IC was found in this sample.

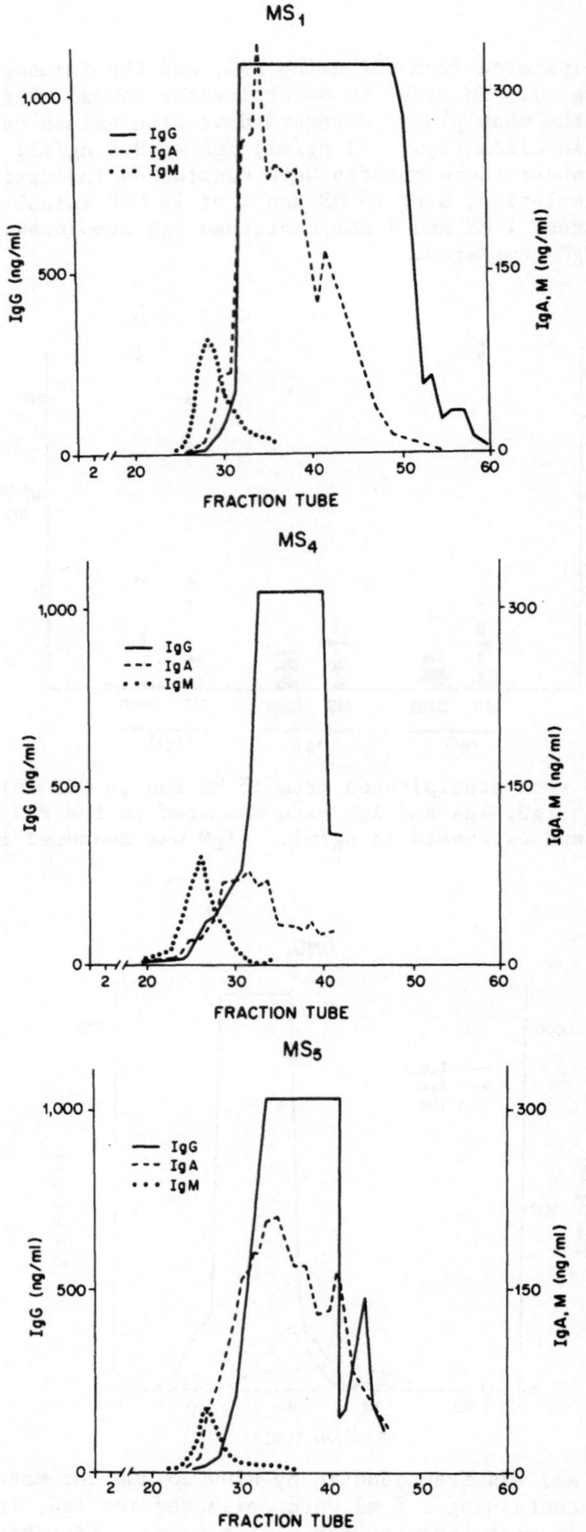

Fig.2. G200 CSF fractions from 3 MS patients (MS1,MS4,MS5) are shown. All had evidence of complexed IgG and IgA, eluting from the column much earlier than monomeric standards.

Five MS and 5 OND spinal fluid samples were then run on G200 columns and the fractions collected and assayed for IgG, IgA and IgM. A representative OND spinal fluid is shown in Fig.2. Monomeric IgG began to be detected in significant amounts at tube 37; IgA was detected a little earlier. IgM was found in very low quantities beginning at tube 25. In the 5 OND samples run, none showed evidence of complexed IgG and only one had complexed IgA (IgA detected in tubes 26-42, OND 5; data not shown). All of the MS spinal fluids showed evidence of IC on column chromatography. Three samples (Fig.3) contained both complexed IgG and IgA. MS2 showed evidence for complexed IgG and MS3 had complexed IgA (Fig.4). When the various methods for detecting CSF complexes were compared, it was clear that IC were present in CSF even when the Raji cell assay was negative (Table 1).

Table 1. CSF IC results using three assays

Subjects	G200	PEG	Raji[a]
MS1	IgG, IgA	IgG, IgM	12
MS2	IgG	IgG	--
MS3	IgA	IgM	7
MS4	IgG, IgA	IgG	--
MS5	IgG, IgA	IgG, IgA, IgM	--
OND1	--	--	--
OND2	--	--	--
OND3	--	--	--
OND4	--	ND[b]	--
OND5	IgA	--	--

[a] Expressed as ug/ml AHG equivalent.
[b] ND = not done.

In order to determine whether IC were present in quantities sufficient to detect by electrophoresis, the G200 fractions containing IgG complexes from patient MS2 were pooled, concentrated, then run on SDS-PAGE. In addition to a high molecular weight band (280-295K) at the top of the gel, there was a single band detected at a molecular weight of 220K which was clearly heavier than monomeric IgG (data not shown). PEG-precipitated IC from patient MS3 (which appeared to contain IgM complexes) were run, reduced and unreduced (Fig.5). Besides a band at the top of the gel (280K) there was a single band weighing 225K. After reduction 3 bands were noted: a 76K band (which co-migrated with mμ heavy chain), a dense 65K band, and a 55K band (Fig.5). No low molecular weight bands were detected.

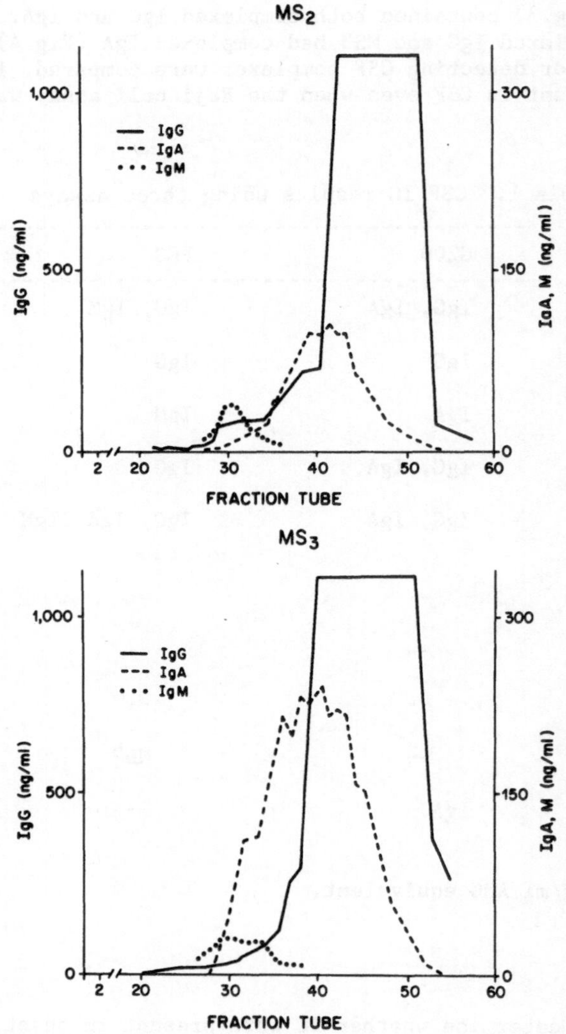

Fig.4. G200 CSF fractions from 2 MS patients are shown. Patient MS2 shows evidence of IgG complexes (tubes 28-34); patient MS3 shows evidence of IgA complexes (tubes 28-34).

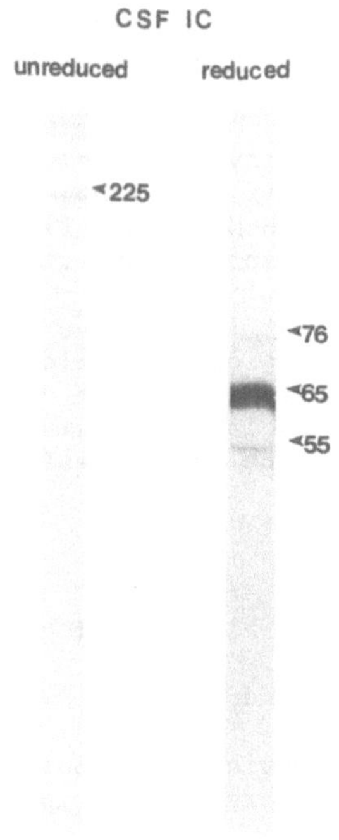

Fig.5. PEG-precipitated IC from patient MS3 were run on SDS-PAGE. The unreduced gel shows a band at the top (280K) and a single band within the gel (225K). After reduction 3 bands are present: a 76K band that co-migrated with mu chain, a dense 65K band and a 55K band.

DISCUSSION

In the present study two different techniques were used to purify CSF IC: PEG precipitation and G200 column chromatography. By combining both complementary approaches, evidence for complexes could be found in 11 of 15 MS spinal fluids as compared to 4 of 14 OND spinal fluids. Conventional assays which use binding properties tend to exclude whole classes of IC. These alternative techniques, which depend only on molecular sizing, detected complexes in CSF even when the sensitive Raji cell assay was negative. Thus IC may actually be present in MS spinal fluid at an even higher frequency than previous studies had indicated. This would be consistent with the notion that the MS disease process is active even when there is no overt evidence for disease flareup.

The real significance of finding IC in MS spinal fluid lies in the possibility of analysing the components of the complexes. The primary Ag target of attack in MS is not known. It could be a brain component, or even a latent viral agent that cross-reacts with a normally sequestered brain component and thus triggers an autoimmune attack. The identification of this Ag would permit us to design Ag-specific immunosuppressive treatment for MS, as well as being a major step in elucidating the etiology of MS.

Our preliminary studies on a small number of samples suggests that the analysis of CSF IC with current available techniques is very possible. Both the PEG and G200 methods provided a sufficient concentration of IC to analyse by ELISA and electrophoresis. Non-reducing and reducing gels permit identification of discrete complexes and their dissociated components, with molecular weight sizing. This allows comparison of IC from different patients with the goal of identifying a common Ag. The finding of very frequent IgA and IgM complexes in MS spinal fluid was an unexpected one; the Raji cell assay had detected mainly IgG complexes. Preliminary work suggests the IgM complexes may involve monomers rather than pentamers. With regard to the IgA complexes, we are now examining the possibility that polymeric IgA is present in MS spinal fluid. Polymeric IgA might suggest a link to a mucosal Ag such as an extrinsic virus (19).

In summary, it appears that IC may be a very frequent occurrence in MS spinal fluid. Current technology now allows the components of these IC to be characterized. Future studies on the dissociated complexes from a number of patients may help to clarify their significance in MS, and may ultimately offer insight into the pathogenesis of this puzzling disease.

REFERENCES

1. R.T. Johnson. The possible viral etiology of multiple sclerosis. Adv. Neurol. 13: 1 (1975).
2. D.E. McFarlin, H.F. McFarland. Multiple Sclerosis. NEJM 307: 1183-1246 (1982).
3. H. Deicher, H.M. Zu Schwabedissen, B. Baruth, U. Patzold and P. Haller. CSF Immune Complexes in Multiple Sclerosis. Experimentor. 35: 1249 (1979).
4. P.K. Coyle,B.R. Brooks, R.L. Hirsch, S.R. Cohen, P.O'Donnel, R.T. Johnson and J.S. Wolinsky. CSF lymphocyte populations and immune complexes in active multiple sclerosis. Lancet. 2: 229 (1980).
5. G. Glikmann, S.E. Svehag, E. Hansen, O. Hansen, S. Husby, H. Nielsen and C. Farrell. Soluble immune complexes in CSF patients with multiple sclerosis and other neurological diseases. Acta Neurol. Scandinav. 61: 333 (1980).
6. U. Patzold, P. Haller, B. Baruth, W. Liman and H. Deicher. Immune complexes in multiple sclerosis: relation to clinical pattern. J. Neurol. 222: 249 (1980).
7. T. Arnadottir, R. Kekomaki, G.A. Lund, M. Reunanen and A.A. Salmi. Circulating immune complexes in patients with multiple sclerosis. J. Neurol. Sci. 55: 273 (1982).
8. A. Salmi, B. Ziola, M. Reunanen, I. Julkunen and O. Wagner. Immune complexes in serum and CSF of multiple sclerosis patients and patients with other neurological diseases. Acta Neurol. Scandinav. 66: 1 (1982).
9. W. Wallen and J.L. Woyciechowska. CSF immune complexes in MS: association with activity of disease but not with antibody to myelin or certain viruses (abstract). Neurology. 32: A 147 (1982).
10. G.A. Lund, T. Arnadottir, V. Hukkanen, M. Reunanen and A. Salmi. Characterization of immune complexes in multiple sclerosis by an antigen-specific immune complex radioimmunoassay. J. Neuroimmunol. 4: 253 (1983).
11. A. Wajgt, M.K. Gorny and R. Jenek. The influence of high-dose prednisone medication on autoantibody specific activity and on circulating immune complex level in CSF of multiple sclerosis patients. Acta Neurol. Scandinav. 68: 378 (1983).
12. P.K. Coyle. CSF immune complexes in multiple sclerosis. Neurology. 35: 429 (1985).
13. R.A. Rudick, J.M. Bidlack and D.W. Knutson. Multiple sclerosis CSF immune complexes that bind Clq. Arch. Neurol. 42: 856 (1985).
14. C.M. Poser, D.W. Paty, L. Scheinberg, W.I. McDonald, F.A. Davis, G.C. Ebers, K.P. Johnson, W.A. Sibley, D.H. Silberberg and W.W. Tourtellotte. New diagnostic criteria for MS: guidelines for research protocols. Ann. Neurol. 13: 227 (1983).

15. P.K. Coyle, N. Banks and S.E. Schutzer. A micro-ELISA Raji cell assay to detect immune complexes. J. Immunol. Methods. 74: 191 (1984).
16. P.K. Coyle and Z. Procyk-Dougherty. MS immune complexes: an analysis of component antigens and antibodies. Ann. Neurol. 16: 660 (1984).
17. P.K. Coyle and C. Johnson. Optimal detection of oligoclonal bands in CSF by silver stain. Neurology. 33: 1510 (1983).
18. J. Guevara, D.A. Johnston, L.S. Ramagali, B.A. Martiñ, S. Capetillo and L.V. Rodriguez. Quantitative aspects of silver deposition in proteins resolved in complex polyacrylamide gels. Electrophoresis. 3: 197 (1982).
19. A.N. Ponzi, C. Merlino, A. Angeretti and R. Penna. Virus-specific polymeric IgA antibodies in serum from patients with rubella, measles, varicella, and herpes zoster virus infection. J. Clin. Microbiol. 22: 505 (1985).

THE DETECTION OF BRAIN ANTIGENS WITHIN THE CIRCULATING IMMUNE COMPLEXES OF PATIENTS WITH MULTIPLE SCLEROSIS

Jacqueline Friedman, Daniel Buskirk and John B. Zabriskie

Department of Bacteriology and Immunology, Rockefeller University, New York, New York 10021

INTRODUCTION

In spite of intensive efforts by a large number of laboratories, the etiology as well as the pathogenic mechanisms involved in the disease multiple sclerosis (MS) remain unknown. Epidemiological data would suggest an event that occurs early in life and which might be associated with exposure to an infectious agent (Lumsden 1972).

Among the many hypotheses entertained with respect to this disease has been the concept that the tissues of MS patients share antigenic determinants with certain viral antigens. The outline of events leading to pathological damage are thus conceptualized as follows: The genetically susceptible individual is exposed to one of these agents early in life and is left with clones of immune cells with specificity both for viral antigens and antigenic components of brain tissue. A second and much later non-specific event triggered perhaps by such diverse factors as a second viral infection, stress our trauma, permits the passage of these cells and/or antibodies through the blood brain barrier to the target organs. Implicit in this concept is that there is no need for persistance of virus at the time of the disease onset and that the "cross reaction" may only be "one-way" (i.e. involving only a part of the viral antigen which reacts with brain tissue or conversely).

While there have been many studies of anti-brain antibodies in MS individuals (Rastogi et al., 1979; Ryberg 1978; Clausen 1983), the complexity of the antigens involved and the questions of specificity of these antibodies in MS prompted us to look at the possibility that relevant brain antigens might be present in the circulating immune complexes of these patients and that these antigens might be cross-reactive with viral antigens. Our present data indicates that immune complexes do contain brain antigens and that these antigens are cross reactive with certain measles virus components. Both the nature and the specificity of these findings lend support to the theory of a prior viral infection early in life may play an important role in the pathogenesis of multiple sclerosis.

METHODS

Patients

Patients were chosen from among those followed in the multiple sclerosis inpatient and outpatient program at Rockefeller University. Diagnosis was based on the history of the illness, physical examination and the presence of oligoclonal bands in the cerebrospinal fluid. The pattern and degree of patients' pathology did not correlate with the level of immune complexes detected in their sera by the assays used.

Preparation of Immune Complexes

A serum fraction enriched in immune complexes was prepared essentially according to the method of Creighton et al., 1973 and assayed by the Clq method of Coyle et al., 1980 or by the Raji cell assay (kindly performed by Dr. N.K. Day at the Memorial Sloan-Kettering Cancer Research Institute, New York).

Preparation of Antisera to Human Immune Complexes

Samples of each immune complex preparation were aliquoted into 500 µg of protein mixed with 1.5:1 vol. of Bacto Freund's incomplete adjuvant (D. Feo Laboratories, Detroit, Mi) and injected both intramuscularly and intradermally into rabbits weekly for 8 weeks. The rabbits were bled 3 weeks after the final injection and gamma globulin fraction were isolated by standard techniques.

Preparation of Brain Antigen

Brain cytosols were prepared by mechanically disrupting equal amounts of fresh autopsy brain tissue (10-15 grams) in .15 M phosphate buffered saline (PBS) at pH 7.0. Following centrifugation, the supernatant fluid (saline extract) was concentrated and dialyzed in PBS and stored in aliquots at -70°C until use. A KCl extract of this material was prepared by resuspending the brain pellet after saline extraction in 100 cc of 3 M KCl and stirring gently for 24 hours at 4°C. The suspension was then centrifuged at 17,000 RPM for 30 minutes and the supernatant collected (KCL extract). This was repeated for three extractions.

Glycoprotein enriched brain preparations of MS and normal brain tissue were prepared according to the method of Rastogi et al., 1979.

Crossed immunoelectrophoresis (CIE)

Antisera to MS immune complexes were tested for their response to brain antigens by CIE after one dimensional "rocket" electrophoresis ascertained the optimal ratio of antigens to antibodies. CIE was conducted as described (Weeke 1975). Tandem CIE was performed by placing two antigens in separate wells 8 mm apart in the first dimension as described (Weeke 1975).

Immunoblotting

Anti-immune complex antisera were tested for reactivity to brain and viral antigens by the immunoblotting technique as described by others (Blake et al., 1984).

Co-precipitation of viral antigens

Reactivity of anti-immune complex serum to measles antigens was assayed by the coprecipitation technique described by Hall and Choppin (1979). Measles infected vero cells were cultured in medium containing methionine S^{35} to internally label the viral antigens. The antigens were solubilized in RIPA buffer and incubated with the appropriate antiserum. The reactive mixture was then centrifuged with protein-A Sepharose beads and after removal of the beads the coprecipitated material was subjected to SDS Page gel electrophoresis.

Enzyme-linked immunosorbent assay (ELISA)

The ELISA assay for antibody binding to brain and viral antigen was carried out according to the method of Engrall and Perlmann (1974) with the following modification: Microtiter plates (Falcon Labware, Oxnard, CA) were coated with the appropriate antigens diluted in 0.1M tris buffer pH 9.8 overnight at room temperature. After serial washing in a buffer containing 0.01 M Tris 0.05% BRIJ detergent (Pierce Chemical Co., Rockford, IL) and 0.15 M NaCl, the appropriate antibody was diluted in the buffer and placed in the microtiter wells for 2 hours at 37°C. After washing, alkaline phosphatase-coupled antibody was applied and the reaction was quantitated on a Titer Tek Multi-scanner at 405 NM. The results were expressed as the experimental reading after subtraction of antibody and antigen control values.

Immunofluorescence Technique

The indirect immunofluorescence technique was carried out essentially as described by Zabriskie et al., 1970.

Cytotoxity Assay

This standard cytotoxicity assay was carried out according to the method of Terasaki et al., 1978 using a known panel of lymphocytes containing haplotype antigens from the HLA-A, B, C and Dr loci.

RESULTS

Immunoelectrophoresis Experiments

To determine if immune complexes in MS patients contained brain antigens, cytosols of MS brain and normal brain samples were placed in antigen wells in quantities of 20 μg and 10 μg and subjected to rocket immunoelectrophoresis against antiserum to MS immune complexes. As seen in Fig.1, both MS and normal brain reacted with the serum to form multiple precipitin arcs.

As a control, antisera made to immune complexes from rheumatic fever and glomerulonephritis patients were similarly tested against brain antigens and no precipitation arcs appeared. This indicated that human serum proteins, including gamma globulins, were not responsible for the reactions observed with the anti-MS immune complex rabbit serum. Additionally, when human IgG was used as an antigen run in tandem on the same slide with MS brain extract against anti-MS complex sera, no band of identity was precipitated between the two antigens, indicating that the possible presence of IgG in the brain tissue was not responsible for the peaks elicited (see Fig.2).

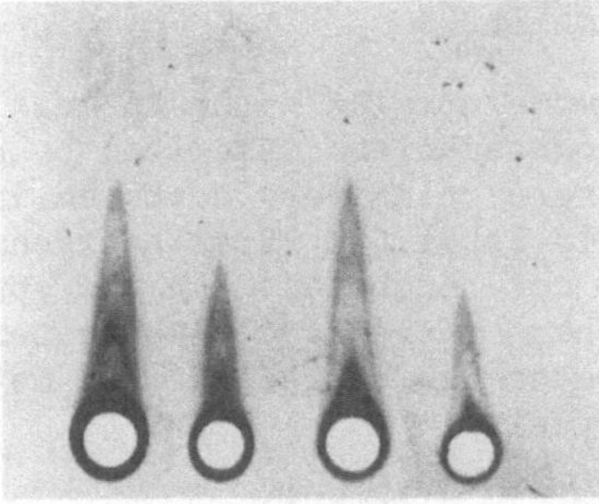

Fig.1. "Rocket" electrophoresis technique using MS and non MS brain cytosols: Lane A = 20 µgs MS extract, Lane B = 10 µgs MS extract, Lane C = 20 µgs non MS extract, Lane D = 10 µgs non MS extract. Antiserum was a rabbit anti-MS complex serum. Note extra precipitin arcs in Lanes A and B not seen in Lanes C and D.

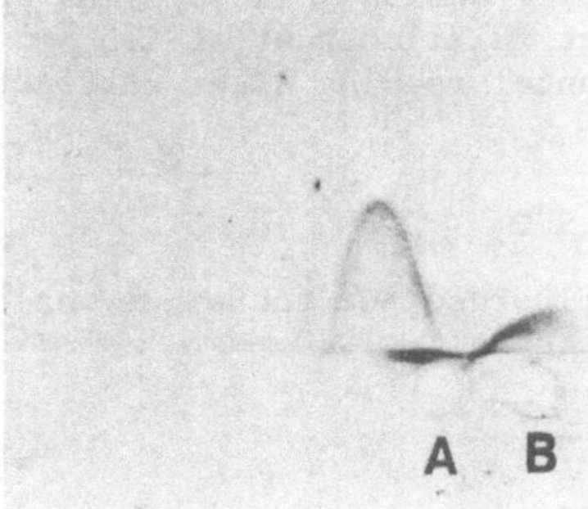

Fig.2. Tandem immunoelectrophoresis experiment with a KCl extract of MS brain (Lane A) and a human gamma globulin preparation (Lane B) seen in tandem against a rabbit anti MS complex serum. Note the lack of any identity of the precipitin arcs between the wells.

In order to more clearly differentiate the reactions between anti-MS complex sera and brain antigens, two-dimensional crossed immunoelectrophoresis was conducted using the same antigens. As noted in Fig.3, additional peaks appeared at the cathodic end of the slide containing the MS glycoprotein eluates. Similar results were obtained with saline extracts of normal and MS brain tissue.

Detection of Reactivity to Brain Antigens by the ELISA Method

As a further verification of the findings on immunoelectrophoresis, MS and normal brain were assayed for reactivity against anti-MS immune complex sera in the ELISA assay. As seen in Table 1, when cytosol and four KCl extracts of normal and MS brains were incubated with a rabbit antiserum to MS complexes, different degrees of reactivity were produced. The single MS cytosol gave a clear reactivity above normal cytosol, and a significant difference was noted between two of four samples of MS KCl extracts as compared to normal KCl extracts.

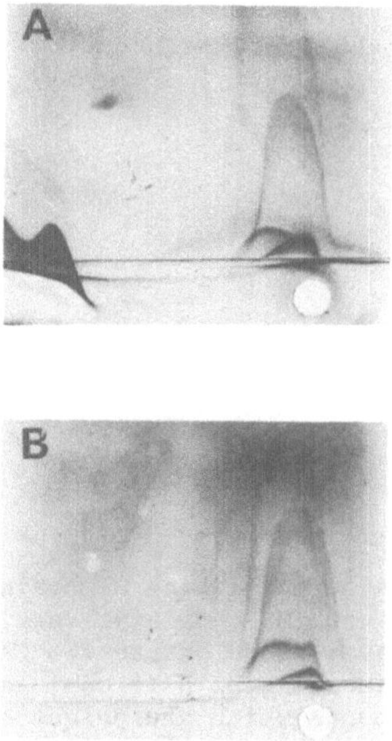

Fig.3. Crossed immunoelectrophoresis (CIE) experiments utilizing MS and non MS Con A sepharose eluates. Note presence of two prominent peaks seen in the MS brain eluate (arrow) not seen in the non MS brain eluate (bottom).

Immunoblotting Experiments

To further define the brain antigens reactive to anti-MS complex sera, MS and normal brain cytosols were electrophoresed on SDS gels and immunoblotted against 3 anti-MS immune complex sera. As seen in Fig.4, multiple reactive bands were common to both MS and normal brain extracts. However, this experiment elicited reactions to MS brain which were not present in normal tissue as well as bands seen with normal tissue but not MS extracts.

Table 1. ELISA results utilizing various MS and non MS brain extracts and a rabbit serum to MS complexes

Extract	Number*	Extract Dilutions	
		1/100	1/1000
MS Cytosol	1	1.697	1.429
MS KCl ext.	1	.565	.725
MS KCl ext.	2	.445	.153
MS KCl ext.	3	--	1.472
MS KCl ext.	4	--	1.003
NL Cytosol	1	.547	.593
NL KCl ext.	1	.314	.196
NL KCl ext.	2	.448	.043
NL KCl ext.	3	--	.603
NL KCl ext.	4	--	1.142
Measles ext.		--	.394
Vero Cell Control		--	.118

* Numerals refer to different MS and non-MS brain extracts.
Dotted line refers to not done.

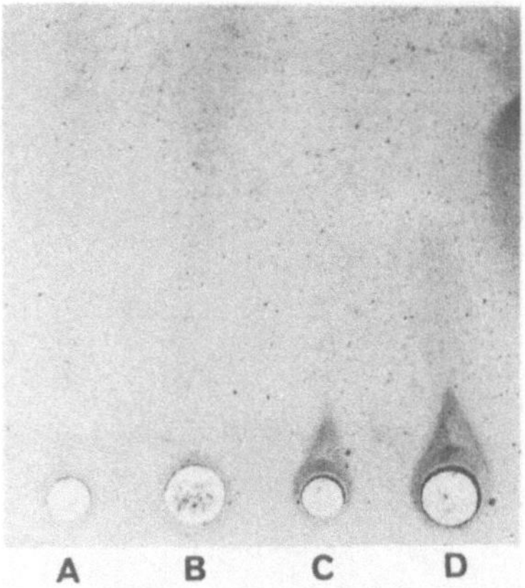

Fig.4. Immunoblotting technique utilizing MS brain extracts and non MS extracts and rabbit anti MS complexes sera. Lanes A-C three different rabbit sera against MS extracts. Lanes E-G same three sera against non MS extracts. Lane D is conjugated serum control. Note appearance of bands which are unique to MS brains as well as bands only seen in non MS extracts.

Viral studies

In order to ascertain if antisera to immune complexes reacted with viral antigens or brain antigens cross-reactive with viral, "rocket" immunoelectrophoresis was conducted using anti-MS complex serum and measles antigens cultured in a vero cell line. As noted in Fig.5, a reactive peak was elicited against the measles antigens (lanes C,D), whereas no peak was seen over the wells containing vero cell control without measles antigen (A,B).

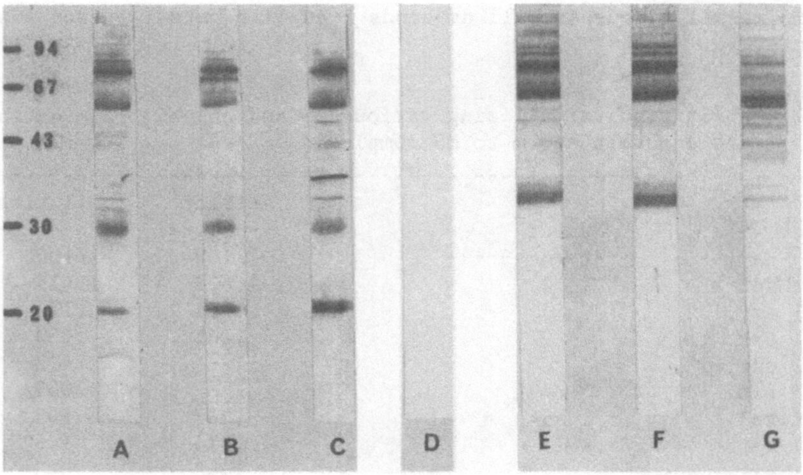

Fig.5. Rocket immunoelectrophoresis reacting rabbit anti-MS immune complex serum against measles virus cultured in vero cells. Note the reactivity of wells C and D containing measles antigens in contrast to wells A and B containing vero cell pack controls.

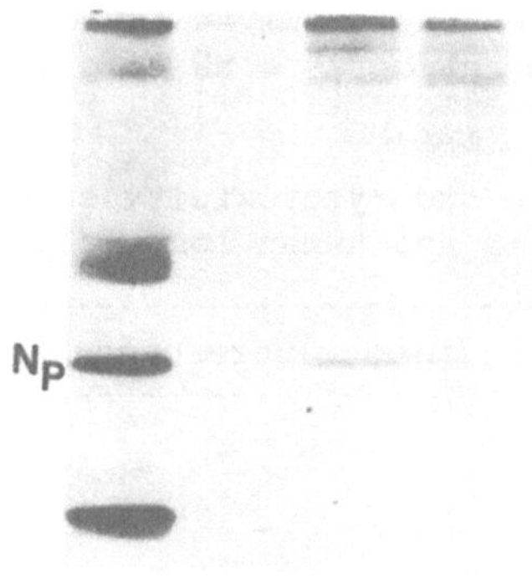

Fig.6. A Co-precipitation radioautograph experiment in which a Methionine S^{35} labelled measles preparation is first mixed with two different anti MS complex rabbit sera (C and D), co-precipitated with protein A sepharose beads and then run on SDS PAGE gels and developed radioautographically. Note the presence of a line of reaction in lanes C and D which is of the same molecular weight as the measles nucleocapsid (Np) antigen. Lane A is known human serum reacting against the major bands of measles protein. Lane B is pre-immune rabbit serum.

A more specific assay of this phenomenon utilized the co-precipitation technique and auto-radiography. After coprecipitation and electrophoresis on an SDS gel, an autoradiograph of the gel showed a band suggesting reactivity to the nucleocapsid (NP) measles antigen (see Fig.6, lanes C & D). In contrast, pre-immune serum gave no reaction (lane B). Lane A contained the standard of measles antigens.

To determine the specificity of the measles response as compared to other viral antigens immunoblotting experiments were conducted utilizing anti-MS complex serum against Sendai virus cultured in vero cells. Vero control cells and those with Sendai virus elicited no response with the anti-immune complex serum whereas vero cells infected with measles produced 3 bands.

As a further verification of the reactivity to measles antigens, rabbit antiserum to pooled MS complexes were tested in the ELISA assay against an extract of a measles infected vero cell line and the uninfected vero cell control. As seen in Table 1 wells containing the measles extract gave an average optical density of .394 compared to the optical density of .118 of the wells containing extracts of the uninfected vero cells.

Determination of Anti-Lymphocyte Antibodies in Anti MS Complex Sera

In order to validate the finding that the antisera to MS immune complexes were reactive to brain tissue, it was necessary to rule out the possibility that lymphocyte membrane antigens possibly trapped within the MS immune complexes were responsible for the observed cross-reactivity with brain antigen as previously suggested by others in SLE patients (Bluestein and Zvaifler, 1976). First, mononuclear cell preparations isolated by the Ficoll-Hypaque technique were tested for reactivity to four anti-immune complex sera using the indirect immunofluorescence technique described above. No reactivity was detected in the indirect immunofluorescence assay. A second assay used was the standard cytotoxicity technique against a panel of lymphocytes containing 33 known Dr and HLA specificities. With the exception of one serum at low dilution, no positive reaction was produced with the antisera to MS complexes.

Table 2. Immunofluorescence and cytotoxicity studies with rabbit anti-immune complex sera and human mononuclear cell populations

	Immunofluorescence*	Cytotoxicity**
Rabbit # 1 (anti MS)	-	-
Rabbit # 2 (anti MS)	-	-
Rabbit # 3 (anti MS)	-	+
Rabbit # 4 (anti MS)	-	-
Rabbit # 5 (acute AGN)	-	-
Rabbit # 6 (anti ARF)	-	-

* Indirect immunofluorescence was carried out with mononuclear cell preparations of MS patients.

** Standard cytotoxity assay carried out on a panel of lymphocytes of 33 known Dr and HLA specificities.

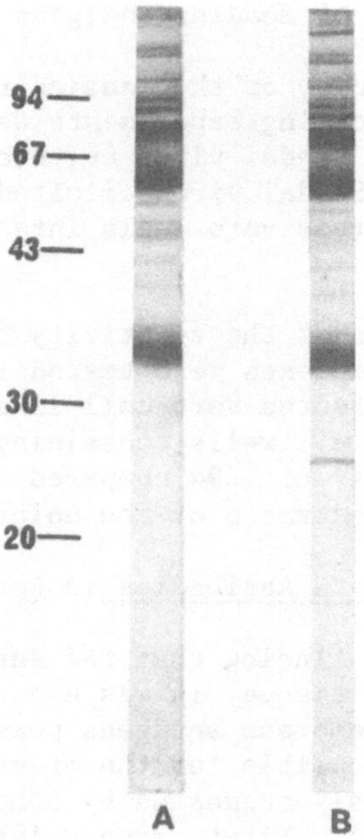

Fig.7. Immunoblotting experiment using rabbit anti MS complex sera and MS brain extracts. Lane A is the serum absorbed with a mononuclear cell preparation obtained from an MS patient. Lane B is the unabsorbed control. Note disappearance of only one band at 25,000 daltons (Land A) after the absorption.

Finally, rabbit anti-MS complex serum was absorbed with whole peripheral blood mononuclear cells from MS and non-MS controls. The antiserum was retested by immunoblotting against MS brain tissue. As seen in Fig.7, only one band at 25,000 daltons was lost post absorption (lane A) as compared to the unabsorbed control (lane B). Thus, lymphocyte membrane antigens cross-reactive to brain antigens do not appear to be a major factor in the observed reactivity of anti-immune complex sera to brain antigens.

<u>Myelin Associated Antigens, Gangliosides, and Cerebrosides</u>

As MS is defined as a demyelinating disease, myelin antigens (kindly provided by Dr. George Hashim, St. Luke's Hospital, New York) were tested for antigenicity against MS immune complex serum. Preparation of human and rabbit myelin basic protein elicited no reactivity in the CIE assay. However, the purified lipophilin (proteolipid) component of myelin described by Hashim (1980) did react in CIE (Fig.8).

DISCUSSION

Elevated levels of circulating complexes have been noted in the sera and CSF of MS patients. However, investigators differ with respect to whether or not the complexes are related to disease activity (Noronha et al., 1981; Tachovsky et al., 1970). The disagreement noted among these authors may in reality reflect the chronic and intermittent course of the disease. Unlike classical acute immune complex mediated diseases, the effect of the circulating complexes in MS patients may exert their influence over years. In addition, the size of the complex, antigenic charge and antigen/antibody ratio may all be important factors in the actual pathological damage exerted by these complexes (Lahita et al., 1980).

Our present studies indicate that circulating complexes obtained from MS patients do indeed contain brain antigens within the complex and that some of these brain antigens cross-react with components of the measles virus. The specificity of the reaction was attested to by the fact that rabbit sera prepared against non-MS complexes did not exhibit any reactivity to these brain antigens. While others (Hauser et al., 1983) have detected anti-lymphocyte antibodies in MS patients, our lymphocyte studies virtually excluded lymphocytic antigens as a major component of our complexes.

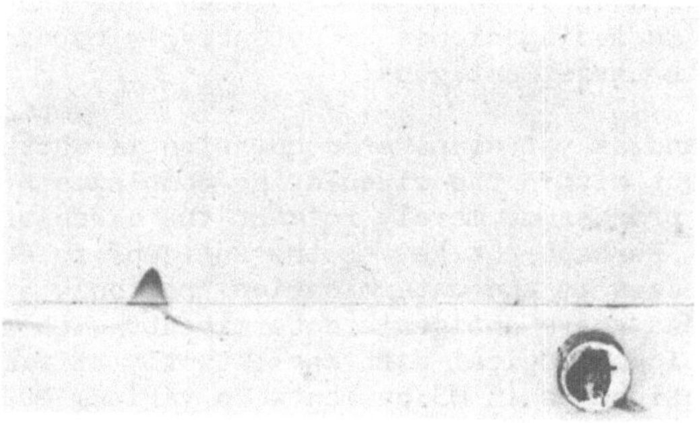

Fig.8. CIE experiment utilizing a human brain lipophilin preparation against a rabbit anti-MS immune complex serum. Note the presence of a prominent precipitin arc and the similarity in migration pattern of this arc and the one seen in Figures 3 and 4.

The exact nature of the brain antigens detected by these rabbit anti-immune complex sera remains unknown. Using partially purified preparations of human myelin, at least some of these antigens detected by our anti-immune complex sera were similar to the myelin associated glycoprotein, Wolfgram protein (unpublished data) and lipophilin or proteolipid proteins described by others (Newcombe et al., 1985; Hashim et al., 1980). In contrast, myelin basic protein (M.W. 20,000) does not appear to be a major reactive antigen within the complex.

The question of whether or not our anti immune complex sera detected brain antigens unique to MS patients remains unresolved. Using the CIE technique, it appeared that certain extra precipitin arcs were seen when MS brain cytosol was employed and these results were confirmed in our ELISA assay. However, our immunoblotting experiments failed to reveal any clear cut differences between MS and non-MS brain cytosols. The use of more purified brain antigens from MS and non-MS tissue will hopefully resolve this issue.

Perhaps most relevant to the disease process was our observation that our anti-immune complex rabbit sera reacted with components of the measles virus, particularly the nucleocapsid antigen. The specificity of the reaction was evident in that non-infected vero cells as well as Sendai infected vero cells (a related paramyxovirus) gave no reaction, indicating that the observed binding was not secondary to a non-specific viral activation of cellular elements.

At least two interpretations of these results are possible. The first hypothesis is that there are latent viral infections including measles occuring in MS patients and that the circulating complexes contain these viral antigens. While this concept is supported by some researchers (Coyle and Procsk-Dougherty 1984), others (Haase 1983; Raine et al., 1977) have been unsuccessful in detecting any viral antigen or the viral genome in MS brain tissue.

The alternative hypothesis and one favoured by us is that measles viral antigens either share antigenic determinants with brain antigens or carry host antigens within their viral envelopes. Precedents for this explanation can be found in the studies by Rastogi et al., (Rastogi et al., 1979) who suggested that there was a cross-reaction between brain and viral antigens. The question of whether or not host proteins could be encoded within the viral envelope of various viruses has also received attention recently (Armstrong et al., 1984).

Viewed in the context of the disease process itself, these cross-reactive antigens (or host proteins incorporated into the virus envelope) would be capable of including clones of potentially cytotoxic T cells with specificity for brain target antigens.

The difficult and as yet unanswered question is whether or not the brain antigens present within the circulating complexes are directly relevant to the disease process or merely reflect the circulating "flotsam" of prior brain damage. Perhaps the key to the antigens relevant to initiating the disease process is the determination that only a specific population of brain antigens share antigenic determinants with a virus. Viewed in the context of epidemiological data consistantly affirming the presence of high titers of antibodies in MS patients to various envelope viruses (Norrby et al., 1974) these findings support the concept that viruses capable of incorporating host brain antigens or cross-reactive with these antigens might initiate a chronic immune response. Thus the further definition of these antigenic relationships will be needed to resolve these important questions concerning the specificity of the brain antigen present in MS complexes.

REFERENCES

1. M.A. Armstrong, K.B. Fraser and P.V. Shirodaria. Recognition of host-membrane antigens in the envelope of measles virions. Interviology. 21:210-220 (1984).
2. M.S. Blake, K.H. Johnston, G.J. Russell-Jones and E.C. Gotschlich. A rapid sensitive method for detection of alkali phosphatase conjugated anti-antibodies on western blots. Anal. Biochem. 136:175-179 (1984).
3. H.G. Bluestein and N.J. Zvaifler. Brain reactive lymphocytoxic antibodies in the serum of patients with systemic lupus erythematosis. J. Clin. Invest. 57:509 (1976).
4. Clausen J. Serum antibodies against cytosol antigens in multiple sclerosis. J. Neurol. Sci. 60:205-216 (1983).
5. P.K. Coyle and Z. Procyk-Dougherty. Multiple sclerosis immune complexes: an analysis of competent antigens and antibodies. Ann. Neurol. 16:660-667 (1984).
6. D.W. Creighton, P.H. Lambert and P.A. Miesca. Detection of antibodies and soluble antigen antibody complexes by precipitation with polyethylene glycol. J. Immunology. 111:1219-1227 (1973).
7. E. Engrall and P. Perlmann. Enzyme-linked immunoabsorbent assay (ELISA). Immunochemistry. 8:874-879 (1971).
8. A.T. Haase. Detection of virus genes and their products in chronic neurological diseases. Presented at the MS Workshop, Woodshole, Massachusetts, April 7-10 (1983).
9. W.W. Hall, R.H. Lamb and P.W. Choppin. Measles and subacute sclerosing panencephalitis virus proteins: lack of antibody to the M protein in patients with subacute sclerosing panencephalitis. PNAS. 79:2047-2051 (1979).
10. G.A. Hashim, D.G. Wood and M.A. Moscarello. Myelin lipophilin-induced demyelinating disease of the central nervous system. Neurochem. Res. 5:1137-1145 (1980).
11. S.L. Hauser, E.L. Reinherz, C.J. Hogan, S.F. Schossman and H.L. Weiner.(1983). Immunoregulatory T-cells and lymphocytotoxic antibodies in acute multiple sclerosis: weekly analysis over a six month period. Ann. Neurol. 13:418-425 (1975).
12. S. Jacobson, G.T. Nepom, J.R. Richert, W.E. Biddison and H.F. McFarland. Identification of a specific HLA DR2 Ia molecule as a restriction element for measles virus-specific HLA class II-restricted cytotoxic T cell clones. J. Exp. Med. 161:263-268 (1985).
13. R.G. Lahita, A.B. Gottlieb, D. Koffler and H.C. Kunkel. Immunological alterations in SLE. In: "Streptococcal Diseases and the Immune Response". Eds. S.E. Read and J.B. Zabriskie. Academic Press, N.Y. p. 477.
14. C. Lumsden. The clinical immunology of multiple sclerosis. In: "Multiple Sclerosis - A reappraisal" 2nd edition. (D. McAlpine, C.E. Lumsden and E.D. Acheron Eds.) Churchill Publishers, Edingborough, London. 512-21 (1980).
15. H.A. Newcombe, S. Graham and M.L. Cuzner. Serum antibodies against central nervous system proteins in human demyelinating disease. Clin. Exp. Immunol. 59:383-390 (1985).
16. E. Norrby, H. Link and J.E. Olsson. Comparison of antibodies against different viruses in cerebrospinal fluid and serum sample from patients with multiple sclerosis. Infect. Immunol. 10:688-694 (1974).
17. A.B.C. Noronha, J.P. Antel, R.P. Roos and M.E. Madof. Circulating complexes in neurologic disease. Neurology. 31: 1402-1407.

18. H.S. Panitch, D.A. Hafler and K.P. Johnson. Antibodies to myelin basic protein in multiple sclerosis: clinical correlations. Neurology. 28:394 (1978).
19. C.S. Raine, J.W. Prineas, R.D. Sheppard, M.B. Bornstein and M. Dubois-Dalcq. Immunocytochemical studies for the localization of measles antigens in multiple sclerosis plaques and measles virus-infected CNS tissue. J. Neurol. Sciences. 33: 13-20 (1977).
20. S.C. Rastogi, J. Clausen, H. Offner, G. Konat and T. Fog. Partial purification of MS specific brain antigens. Acta Neurol. Scandinav. 59:281-296 (1979).
21. B. Ryberg. Multiple specificities of antibrain antibodies in multiple sclerosis and chronic myelopathy. J. Neurol. Sci. 38:357-382 (1978).
22. T.G. Tachovsky, H. Koprowski, R.P. Lisak. A.M. Theofilopoulos and F.J. Dixon. Circulating immune complexes in multiple sclerosis and other neurological diseases. Lance. 2:997-999 (1976).
23. P.I. Terasaki, D. Bennoco, M.S. Park, G. Ozturk and Y. Iwaki. Microdroplet testing for HLA A,B,C and D antigens. Am. J. Clin. Pathol. 69:103-120 (1978).
24. B. Weeke. In: "A Manual of Quantitative Immunoelectrophoresis". N.H. Axelsen, J. Kroll, B. Weeke, eds. Universites Forlaget, Oslo. 47-64 (1973a).
25. B. Weeke. In: "A Manual of Quantitative Immunoelectrophoresis". N.H. Axelsen, J. Kroll, B. Weeke, eds. Universites Forlaget, Oslo. 57-64 (1973b).
26. J.B. Zabriskie, K.C. Hsu and B.C. Seegal. Heart-reactive antibody associated with rheumatic fever: characterization and diagnostic significance. Clin. and Exp. Immunol. 7: 147-159 (1970).

REACTIVITY OF IMMUNE COMPLEX PREPARATIONS FROM MULTIPLE SCLEROSIS PATIENTS WITH ANTISERA AGAINST MULTIPLE SCLEROSIS BRAIN WHITE MATTER

Veijo Hukkanen[1] and Tom H. Stahlberg[2]

Departments of Virology[1] and Medical Microbiology[2]
University of Turku, Kiinamyllynkatu 13, SF-20520 Turku
Finland

The presence of circulating immune complexes (ICs) in multiple sclerosis (MS) has been confirmed in numerous studies, although their pathogenetic role has not been thoroughly elucidated. The antigen in the ICs in MS has not been defined, although in previous studies the lipid nature of the antigen has been suggested. In the present study we have analysed the possible presence of white matter protein antigens in the ICs prepared from sera or cerebrospinal fluid (CSF) of MS patients and their matched controls with other neurological diseases. IC fractions were prepared from two MS sera and one control serum by protein A-Sepharose affinity chromatography and from one MS serum, one MS CSF and one control serum by Clq affinity chromatography. The MS specimens were previously found positive in a Clq binding radioimmunoassay test (sera: 5.7, 7.0 and 13.2 SD units in assay, CSF: 15.9 SD units) while the control patients had values less than 2 SD units. The IC fractions were electrophoresed in polyacrylamide gradient gels, transferred to nitrocellulose and probed with rabbit antisera against MS brain white matter or control brain white matter. Preimmunization sera and an antiserum against human serum components were used as controls. The anti-MS-white matter serum reacted with polypeptide bands with MWs of 67 000, 100 000 and 120 000. The 67 000 protein is assumed to be albumin, contaminating the original immunization antigen as well as the IC preparations. The nature of the higher MW bands is more unclear, although they might again be normal serum/CSF components. The results do not exclude the presence of lipid brain antigens in MS ICs.

INTRODUCTION

Circulating immune complexes (ICs) have been detected in patients with multiple sclerosis (MS) (Tachovsky et al., 1976; Jacque et al., 1977; Goust et al., 1978; Coyle et al., 1980; Salmi et al., 1982; Arnadottir et al., 1982). The relationship between the clinical status of the patient and the amount of ICs seems to be unclear (Tachovsky et al., 1976., Coyle et al., 1980; Arnadottir et al., 1982; Dasgupta et al., 1982), although in an antigen-specific immunoassay test fluctuation has been found in the IC amounts coinciding with exacerbations (Lund et al., 1983). The studies on ICs in MS have been performed using differing methods, which affects comparison of the results (Salmi et al., 1982; Araga et al., 1984).

The antigen in the ICs in MS has not been defined. There are reports suggesting that the antigen in the ICs is a lipid, but not a protein (Jacque et al., 1977; Lund et al., 1983). In a previous study we have demonstrated antibodies in MS cerebrospinal fluid (CSF) to white matter (WM) glycoproteins (Hukkanen et al., 1983). The myelin breakdown in MS may also be preceded by a loss of a glycoprotein around some plaques (Itoyama et al., 1980; Prineas et al., 1984). The involvement of WM glycoproteins in the immunological attack against myelin in MS would suggest for their presence in the immune complexes during active myelin breakdown.

In this report we have studied the possible presence of white matter protein components in the immune complexes in MS by immunoblotting the isolated IC fractions from MS and control patients with rabbit antisera against MS and control brain white matter.

MATERIALS AND METHODS

Preparation of the Immune Complex Fractions

Immune complexes were prepared from three MS sera (5.7, 7.0 abd 13.2 SD units in IC radioimmunoassay; Lund et al., 1983), one MS CSF (15.9 SD units) and two sera from patients with headache and vertigo (below 2 SD units). The control patients were age- and sex-matched with two of the MS patients.

ICs were prepared from two of the MS sera and one control serum by protein A-Sepharose affinity chromatography. The procedure was modified from the method of Chenais et al. (1977). One ml of each of the sera with 5.7 and 7.0 SD units of IC and of one control serum were separately subjected to gel filtration in a Sephacryl S-400 column (Pharmacia, Sweden) in 0.1 M Tris, pH 8.0 and 0.5 M NaCl. The monomeric IgG peak was omitted and the macroglobulin fraction further subjected to protein A-Sepharose CL-4B (Pharmacia, Sweden) affinity chromatography. The fractions eluted with 0.1 M acetic acid/0.9% NaCl were neutralized with triethanolamine, dialyzed against 10 mM Tris, pH 6.8 and concentrated for electrophoresis.

ICs from the remaining specimens were isolated by Clq affinity chromatography. Human Clq was prepared from blood of three male volunteer donors according to the method described by Yonemasu and Stroud (1971) with modifications presented by Svehag and Burger (1976). Fifty ml of the pooled serum was subjected to dialysis against 0.026 M EDTA, pH 7.5, the precipitate dissolved in 0.020 M Na-acetate, pH 5.0, containing 0.75 M NaCl and 0.010 M EDTA, dialysed against 0.060 M EDTA, pH 5.0 and the precipitate dissolved in 0.005 M phosphate buffer, pH 7.5 containing 0.75 M NaCl and 0.010 M EDTA, and dialysed against 0.035 M EDTA, pH 7.5. The final precipitate was dissolved to 0.020 M Na-acetate pH 7.5, containing 0.75 M NaCl and 0.010 M EDTA. The Clq preparation was concentrated and loaded onto a Sephacryl S-400 column in 0.010 M Tris, pH 8.0 and 0.5 M NaCl. Fractions showing strongest reactivity with rabbit anti-human Clq serum (Boehringer, West Germany) in a standard EIA test were pooled and used for coupling to CNBr-activated Sepharose 4B (Pharmacia, Sweden) according to the manufacturer's recommendations. All the steps were performed at +4°C. The serum and CSF specimens for the IC preparation were adsorbed to the Clq-Sepharose in 0.1 M Tris, pH 8.0, the column washed with 0.1 M Tris, pH 8.0 and 0.5 M NaCl and the immune complexes eluted with 3 M NaSCN in 0.1 M Tris, pH 8.0. The IC fractions were then dialysed against 0.010 M Tris, pH 6.8 and concentrated for electrophoresis.

Electrophoresis and Immunoblotting

The IC preparations were electrophoresed in 8.0-18.0 % polyacrylamide gradient gels with 2.6% cross-linking. The stacking gel was 5%. After electrophoresis the proteins were transferred to nitrocellulose (0.22 μm, Schleicher and Schuell, West Germany) in an electroblotting apparatus with cooling (LKB, Sweden). The nitrocellulose filter was stained with toluidine blue and cut to appropriate slices which were then destained and saturated overnight with 5% non-fat dry milk in phosphate-buffered saline, pH 7.4 (PBS). The slices representing each IC preparation were then incubated for 3h at +37°C with the appropriate antisera diluted 1:50 in PBS containing 5% sheep serum, 0.5% bovine serum albumin and 0.1% Tween-20. The slices were washed with PBS/0.3 % Tween-20 and incubated with peroxidase-conjugated antibody against rabbit IgG (Orion Diagnostica, Finland) diluted 1:500 in the same buffer as the primary antibody. After an incubation of 1 h at +37°C the slices were washed as above and the bound antibody detected using 3-amino-9-ethyl-carbazole as substrate. As a control, 10 μl of normal human serum was electrophoresed and treated with the rabbit anti-WM sera. Also the IC preparations were probed with rabbit antiserum against human serum components (Boehringer, West Germany).

The rabbit antisera were prepared as described previously (Hukkanen et al., 1982) by injecting successively 0.5-1.0 mg of a surface me fraction of white matter in Freund's incomplete adjuvant to rabbits. The MS and control WM rabbit both received seven injections of the appropriate antigen. The reactivities of the antisera with the WM proteins have been described (Hukkanen et al., 1982).

RESULTS

The anti-MS WM rabbit serum showed some limited reactivity with normal human serum components with MWs of 67 000 and less (Fig.1, lane 2 and Fig.2, lane 3). The preimmunization serum did not react (Fig.1, lane 1, Fig.2, lane 2). The preparations from patients with other neurological diseases reacted also wery slightly with the anti-MS-WM rabbit serum: a band with MW of 67 000 was observable in the preparation made by Clq affinity column (Fig.2, lane 6) while the fraction prepared by protein A-Sepharose did not react with the anti-MS serum (Fig.2, lane 9). A clear reactivity was, however, observed when using an antiserum against human serum proteins (Fig.2, lanes 4 and 7). An MS serum IC fraction prepared by Clq column showed very low reactivity with the anti-normal WM serum (Fig.2, lane 12), whereas the use of anti-MS WM serum revealed a band with MW of 67 000 (Fig.1, lane 4, Fig.2, lane 14). The corresponding preimmunization sera gave never reactions with the IC fractions (Fig.1, lane 3, Fig.2, lanes 5,8,11 and 13). The MS CSF specimen, subjected to the Clq-Sepharose chromatography, showed similar reactivity as the MS serum ICs above (Fig.1, lanes 5 and 6). Both of the MS serum ICs prepared by protein A-Sepharose affinity chromatography contained proteins that reacted with the anti-MS WM serum, showing bands with MWs of 67 000, 100 000 and 120 000 (Fig.1, lanes 8 and 10). The preimmunization sera did not react (Fig.1, lanes 7 and 9).

DISCUSSION

The multiple sclerosis patients do have elevated rates of circulating immune complexes at some timepoint during the course of the disease. While some studies indicate a correlation of the IC amounts with the disease activity (Coyle et al., 1980; Dasgupta et al., 1982; Lund et al., 1983), others present controversial results (Tachovsky et al., 1976; Arna-

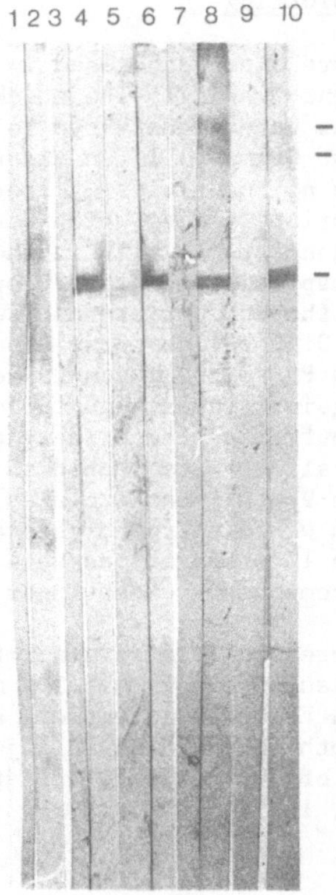

Fig.1. Immunoblot of IC preparations electrophoresed in 8-18% polyacrylamide gels and probed with antiserum against MS brain white matter membrane proteins. The antisera were preimmunization serum (lanes 1, 3, 5, 7 and 9) and hyperimmune serum against MS brain white matter (lanes 2, 4, 6, 8 and 10). The specimens were normal human serum (lanes 1 and 2), MS serum ICs prepared by Clq affinity chromatography (3 and 4), MS CSF ICs prepared as in 3 and 4 (5 and 6) and two separate specimens of MS serum ICs prepared by protein A affinity chromatography (lanes 7 - 10). The horizontal lines on the right, indicate the bands with MWs of 120 000, 100 000 and 67 000, from top to bottom.

dottir et al., 1982). Variation in amount of the immune complexes in relation to the clinical status might be a part of the immunoregulatory processes of the patient (see Salmi et al., 1982) or it might just reflect increased tissue destruction by immune mechanisms. In the latter case, the ICs are expected to contain myelin components that are antigenic in MS.

The brain antigen in the immune complexes is not well characterized. There are reports suggesting a lipid nature of the antigen (Jacque et al., 1977; Lund et al., 1983). The results of the present study do not indicate any specific brain protein antigen as a part of the immune complexes. The rabbit antisera raised against multiple sclerosis and control white matter did contain antibodies against white matter proteins with MWs of 22 300, 24 500, 45 700, 53 400, 58 000, 63 000, 69 000, 79 600, 86 500, 111 000 and 138 000, some of which are glycoproteins (Hukkanen et al., 1982). They reacted also strongly with purified human basic protein but not with galactocerebroside (Hukkanen et al., 1982). The major myelin protein antigens would thus be detected by use of these antisera. The major reactive protein in MS ICs with MW of 67 000 is expected to be serum albumin, that has copurified with the MS ICs. It must have been present in the immunization antigen, because the preimmune sera did not react with this component. It is, however, difficult to explain its over-representation in MS membranes as compared with control brain membranes, because the membrane fractions have been extensively washed with buffer during preparation. Another controversy arises from the fact shown in Fig.1, lane 2, where an overloaded human serum specimen showed less reactivity with the anti-MS sera than did the ICs. The 67 000 Dalton band comigrates with serum albumin in electrophoresis. The two high molecular weight proteins in MS serum ICs are perhaps also serum proteins, although the control experiment with human serum components does not show any reactive bands of this molecular weight. In an experiment using polyethylene glycol precipitation of ICs Jacque et al. (1977) have also analysed electrophoretically the ICs of MS patients and found a protein pattern resembling the plasma protein profile. This is in agreement with the present results, which again suggest that the antigens in MS ICs are lipids or lipid-associated.

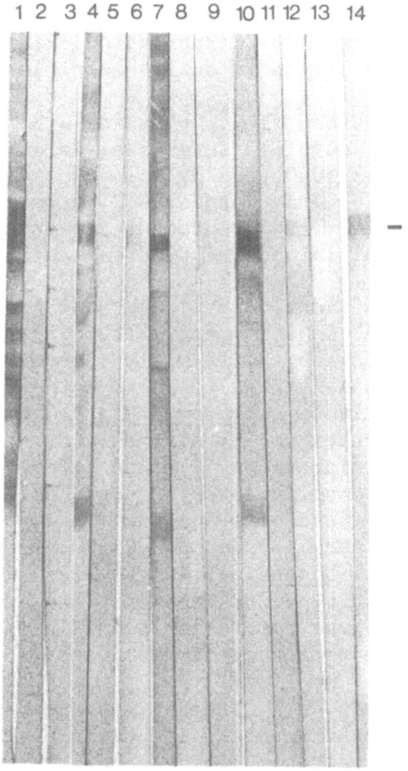

Fig.2. Immunoblot of IC preparations electrophoresed in 8-18% polyacrylamide gels and blotted with antisera against normal and MS brain white matter proteins. The antisera were rabbit antiserum against human serum components (lanes 1, 4, 7 and 10), preimmune (11) and hyperimmune serum against normal brain WM proteins (12) and preimmune (lanes 2, . 8 and 13) and hyperimmune serum against MS brain WM proteins (lanes 3, 6, 9 and 14). The specimens were normal human serum (1-3), control patient serum ICs prepared by Clq chromatography (4-6), control patient serum ICs prepared by protein A chromatography (7-9) and MS serum ICs prepared by Clq chromatography (10-14). The horizontal line on the right indicates the band with MW of 67 000.

ACKNOWLEDGEMENT

Dr. Timo Veromaa, Department of Medical Microbiology, University of Turku, is acknowledged for the rabbit antiserum against human serum.

REFERENCES

1. S. Araga, H. Irie and K. Takahashi. Conglutinin microtiter plate ELISA system for detecting circulating immune complexes. J. Neuroimmunol. 6:161 (1984).
2. T. Arnadottir, R. Kekomäki, G.A. Lund, M. Reunanen and A.A. Salmi. Circulating immune complexes in patients with multiple sclerosis. A longitudinal study of serum and CSF by Clq and platelet binding tests. J. Neurol. Sci. 55:273 (1982).
3. F. Chenais, G. Virella, C.C Patrick and H.H. Fudenberg. Isolation of soluble immune complexes by affinity chromatography using staphylococcal protein A-Sepharose as substrate. J. Immunol. Meth. 18:183 (1977).
4. P.K. Coyle, B.R. Brooks, R.L. Hirsch, S.R. Cohen, P. O'Donnell, R.T. Johnson and J.S. Wolinsky. Cerebrospinal-fluid lymphocyte populations and immune complexes in active multiple sclerosis. Lancet. ii:229 (1980).
5. M.K. Dasgupta, K.G. Warren, K.V. Johny and J.B. Dossetor. Circulating immune complexes in multiple sclerosis: Relation with disease activity. Neurology. 32:1000 (1982).
6. J.M. Goust, F. Chenais, J.E. Carnes, C.G. Hames, H.H. Fudenberg and E.L. Hogan. Abnormal T cell subpopulations and circulating immune complexes in the Guillain-Barré syndrome and multiple sclerosis. Neurology. 28:421 (1978).
7. V. Hukkanen, A. Salmi and H. Frey. Membrane protein antigens in multiple sclerosis. J. Neuroimmunol. 3:295 (1982).
8. V. Hukkanen, J. Ruutiainen, A. Salmi, M. Reunanen and H. Frey. Antibodies in cerebrospinal fluid to white matter glycoproteins in multiple sclerosis patients. Neurosci. Lett. 35:327 (1983).
9. Y. Itoyama, N.H. Sternberger, H. deF. Webster, R.H. Quarles, S.R. Cohen and E.P. Jr. Richardson. Immunocytochemical observations on the distribution of myelin-associated glycoprotein and myelin basic protein in multiple sclerosis lesions. Ann. Neurol. 7:167 (1980).
10. C. Jacque, P. Davous and N. Baumann. Circulating immune complexes and multiple sclerosis. Lancet. ii:408 (1977).
11. G.A. Lund, T. Arnadottir, V. Hukkanen, M. Reunanen and A. Salmi. Characterization of immune complexes in multiple sclerosis by an antigen-specific immune complex radioimmunoassay. J. Neuroimmunol. 4:253 (1983).
12. J.W. Prineas, E.E. Kwon, N.H. Sternberger and V.A. Lennon. The distribution of myelin-associated glycoprotein and myelin basic protein in actively demyelinating multiple sclerosis lesions. J. Neuroimmunol. 6:251 (1984).
13. A. Salmi, B. Ziola, M. Reunanen, I. Julkunen and O. Wagner. Immune complexes in serum and cerebrospinal fluid of multiple sclerosis patients and patients with other neurological diseases. Results of 4 different immune complex assays. Acta Neurol. Scand. 66:1 (1982).
14. S.E. Svehag and D. Burger. Isolation of Clq-binding immune complexes by affinity chromatography and desorption with a diaminoalkyl compound. Acta Path. Microbiol. Scand. Sect. C. 84:45 (1976).

15. T.G. Tachovsky, R.P. Lisak, H. Koprowski, A.N. Theofilopoulos and F.J. Dixon. Circulating immune complexes in multiple sclerosis and other neurologcial diseases. Lancet. ii:997 (1976).
16. K. Yonemasu and R.M. Stroud. Clq: Rapid purification method for preparation of monospecific antisera and for biochemical studies. J. Immunol. 106:304 (1971).

LONGITUDINAL AND CROSS SECTIONAL STUDIES OF MYELIN BASIC PROTEIN AND ANTI-MYELIN BASIC PROTEIN IN THE CEREBROSPINAL FLUID OF MULTIPLE SCLEROSIS PATIENTS

Kenneth G. Warren and Ingrid Catz

From the Division of Neurology, Department of Medicine
University of Alberta and the Department of Laboratory
Medicine, University of Alberta Hospital, Edmonton
Alberta, Canada, T6G 2G3

In 1983 Dasqupta et al. (1) reported the existence of myelin basic protein (MBP) containing immune complexes in the sera of multiple sclerosis (MS) patients. Since a hallmark of MS is elevated intrathecal IgG synthesis (2-5) and because there are increased levels of myelin basic protein and anti-myelin basic protein in the cerebrospinal fluid (CSF) of patients with active disease (5,6), the major purpose of our recent research has been to determine whether there is a relationship between free and bound forms of MBP in MS patients with active disease.

Levels of the free and bound forms of MBP and anti-MBP have been determined in longitudinal studies of patients with the acute form of MS, progressing disease, or with relapsing-progressive disease. In addition, the correlation coefficients between the free and bound forms of MBP and anti-MBP have been determined in two cross sectional studies of 80 patients with exacerbations and in 100 patients with progressing disease. The effect of high (160 mg/day) and mega (2000 mg/day) doses of intravenously administered methylprednisolone on the titers of free MBP and anti-MBP in MS patients with exacerbations has also been determined (7).

LONGITUDINAL CASE STUDIES

Case 1: Progressive multiple sclerosis (Fig.1)

This 28 year old male with the progressing form of multiple sclerosis (8) had 14 CSF analyses over a period of 83 weeks. Bound levels of MBP and anti-MBP are shown to be persistently higher than the corresponding free values in such patients. A close relationship of the titers of bound MBP and anti-MBP is illustrated in this patient. The high titers of bound anti-myelin basic protein and relatively low titers of free anti-myelin basic protein result in consistently low free/bound ratios.

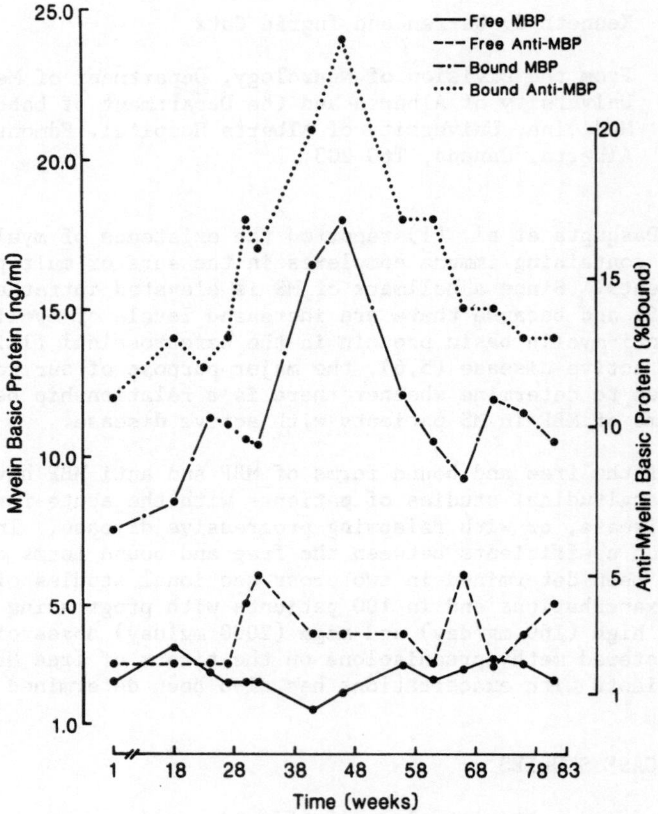

Fig.1. Longitudinal study of progressing multiple sclerosis.

Case 2: Acute multiple sclerosis (Fig.2)

The acute form of MS is characterized by a rapid downhill course resulting in premature death occurring within two years from the onset of the disease (8). The above 46 year old male with this syndrome had 16 CSF analyses over a period of 35 weeks. In contrast to the patient with progressing disease (Fig.1) this patient shows persistently higher levels of free MBP and anti-MBP relative to the bound forms. At the seventh CSF analysis the patient showed modest clinical improvement which correlated with a drop in the free proteins, but he again rapidly deteriorated and died shortly after the final CSF analysis. This longitudinal study suggests a high correlation between free forms as well as bound forms of MBP and anti-MBP. In this form of very active MS the free/bound anti-myelin basic protein ratio is consistently above unity.

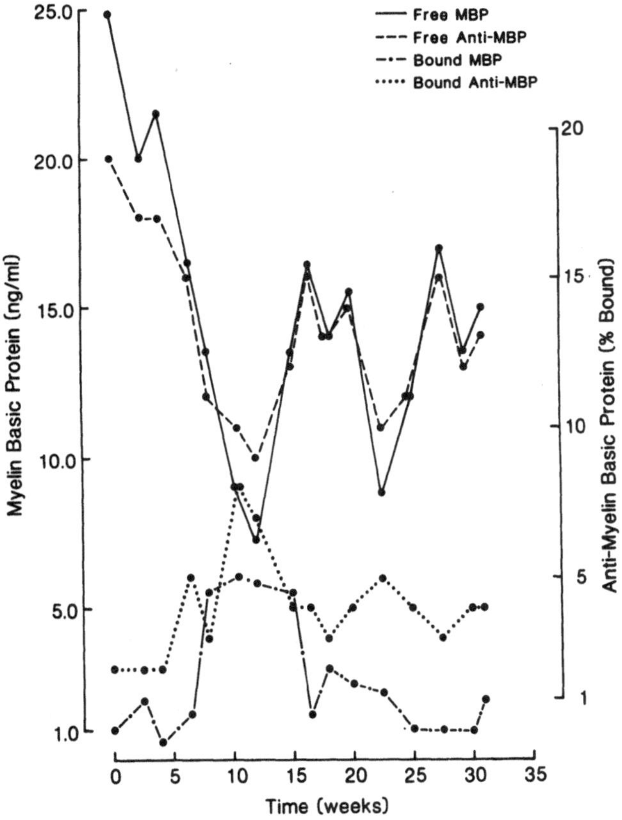

Fig.2. Longitudinal study of acute multiple sclerosis.

Case 3: Relapsing-progressing multiple sclerosis (Fig.3)

Free and bound levels of MBP and anti-MBP are illustrated in a 26 year old male with the relapsing-progressing form of MS (8), who had 22 CSF analyses over a period of 118 weeks. During periods of acute relapse (weeks 1 and 64-68) free levels of MBP and anti-MBP were higher than the bound fractions. Conversely, during the progressive phases (weeks 21-46 and 72-118) the bound fractions were higher than free levels. The close relationship between the two free and the two bound molecules is illustrated. The sinusoidal patterns of free and bound MBP and anti-myelin basic protein correlates with clinical profiles and is not random. The relapse phases are associated with an elevated free/bound anti-myelin basic protein ratio which exceeds unity, while the progressive phase does not.

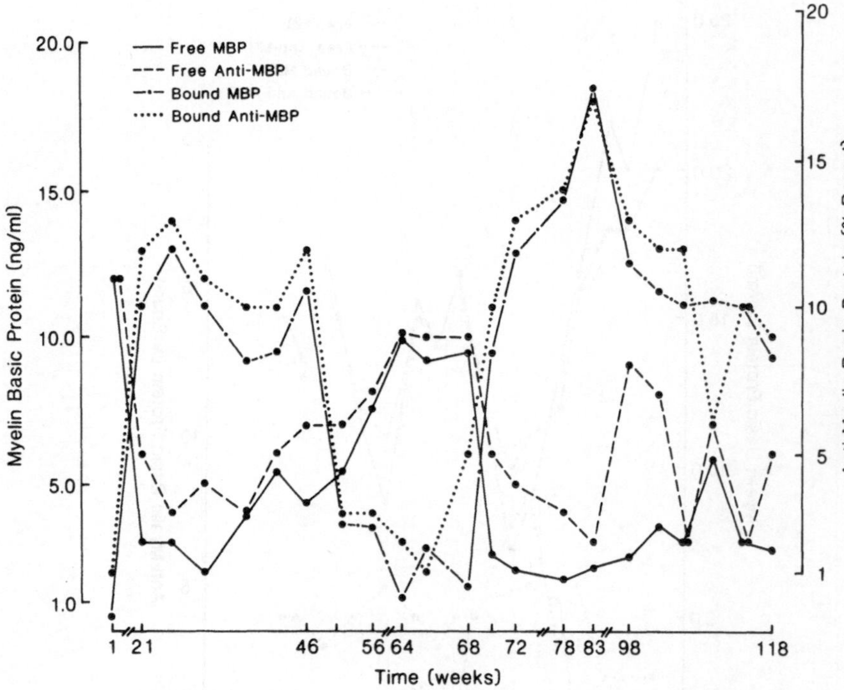

Fig.3. Longitudinal study of relapsing-remitting multiple sclerosis.

CROSS SECTIONAL STUDIES

1: Multiple sclerosis exacerbations (Fig.4)

Free and bound forms of anti-myelin basic protein and myelin basic protein were determined in 80 MS patients with exacerbations (Fig.4). In these patients the levels of free proteins were significantly higher than bound forms. The correlation coefficient between free anti-myelin basic protein and free myelin basic protein (r_F) was 0.95, and there was also a high correlation between the bound fractions ($r_B = 0.87$).

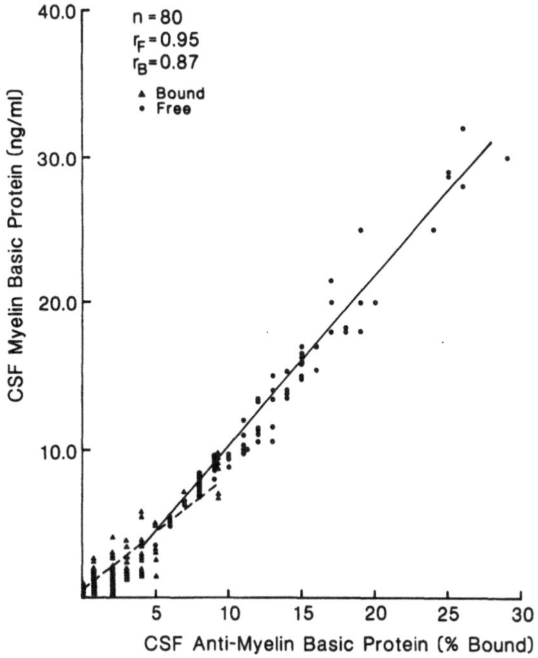

Fig.4. Cross sectional study of multiple sclerosis exacerbations (80 patients).

2: Progressive multiple sclerosis

In 100 patients with progressing disease bound levels of CSF anti-myelin basic protein and myelin basic protein exceeded the free forms (Fig.5). The correlation coefficient between bound anti-myelin basic protein and bound myelin basic protein (r_B) in this group was 0.93, while the correlation coefficient between the alternate free forms (r_F) was 0.71. Bound forms of these molecules were consistently quantitatively greater than free forms. Generally low levels of bound anti-MBP correlated with low levels of bound MBP and conversely higher titers of bound anti-MBP correlated with high titers of bound MBP. Rarely, exceptions such as relatively high levels of bound anti-MBP was associated with relatively low levels of bound MBP (◉), or the titer of bound anti-MBP may be associated with disproportionately high levels of bound MBP (⊡).

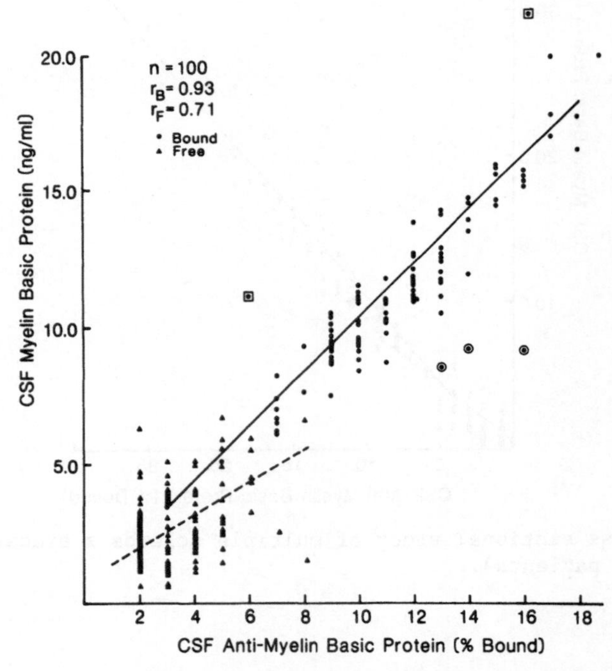

Fig.5. Cross sectional study of chronic progressing multiple sclerosis (100 patients).

3: The effect of methylprednisolone on cerebrospinal fluid myelin basic protein and anti-myelin basic protein levels

Titers of myelin basic protein (Fig.6) and anti-myelin basic protein (Fig.7) may be affected by medications used to treat MS patients. If MS patients with exacerbations are managed for 10 days with bed rest only [A] CSF MBP and anti-MBP does not significantly change. Administration of intravenous ACTH (60 units per day) [B] causes minimal change in MBP and no change in anti-MBP titers after 10 days. However, treatment of such patients with intravenous methylprednisolone in either high (160 mg per day) [C] or mega (2000 mg. per day) [D] doses causes a significant drop in both CSF MBP and anti-MBP titers. Anti-MBP was not totally eliminated from the CSF by methylprednisolone administered in either the high or mega dose quantities.

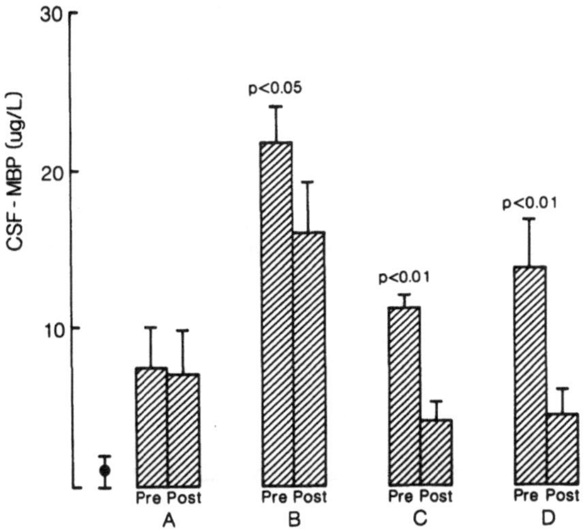

Fig.6. Effect of methylprednisolone on CSF myelin basic protein in MS exacerbations:

A = non-treated control group

B = intravenous ACTH 60 units/day x 10 days

C = "high" dose methylprednisolone 160 mg/day x 10 days

D = "mega" dose methylprednisolone 2000 mg/day x 10 days

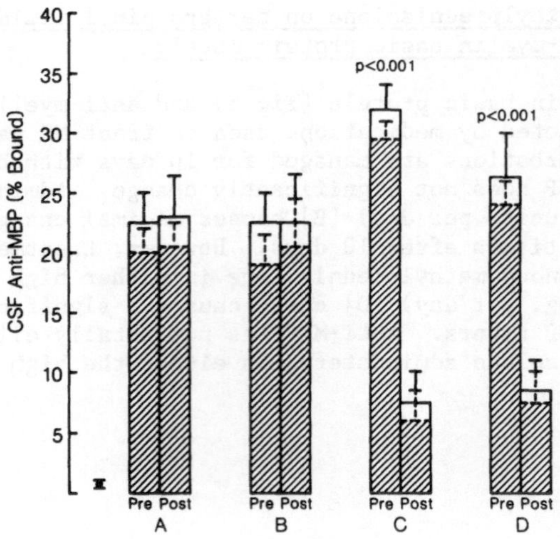

Fig.7. Effect of methylprednisolone on CSF anti-MBP in MS exacerbations:

Hatched area: free anti-MBP (pre acid hydrolysis)
Total area : total anti-MBP (post acid hydrolysis)
White area : bound anti-MBP

A = non-treated control group
B = intravenous ACTH 60 units/day x 10 days
C = "high" dose methylprednisolone 160 mg/day x 10 days
D = "mega" dose methylprednisolone 2000 mg/day x 10 days

CONCLUSION

Myelin basic protein and anti-myelin basic protein levels in the cerebrospinal fluid of multiple sclerosis patients are valuable indicators of disease activity and they can be used to monitor the effect of putative therapies. Neither MBP nor anti-MBP in free or bound form is present in the CSF of MS patients in clinical remission. MS exacerbations are characterized by markedly elevated levels of free MBP and anti-MBP and lower quantities of bound forms. The clinical severity of the exacerbations correlates with the quantity of MBP and anti-MBP. The progressive phase of MS is characterized by relatively high quantities of MBP and anti-MBP in bound forms along with normal or relatively low quantities of the free forms. The existence of anti-MBP in the CSF of MS patients with active disease suggests that it may be involved in the pathogenesis of the disease process. Anti-MBP accounts for only a proportion of intrathecally synthesized IgG of MS patients with active disease and for none of the IgG of the patients in remission. This suggests that the intrathecally synthesized IgG arises from more than one clone of lymphocytes and that MS is associated with multiple immune phenomena.

ACKNOWLEDGEMENTS

We would like to thank all MS patients from Nothern Alberta who participated in this project. Financial support for this research was provided by MS benefactors including Mr. and Mrs. Philip May and Friends of MS Patient Care and Research Clinic, Edmonton, Alberta, Mr. Clifford Geese,

Mrs. E. Laforge and the Tegler Foundation, Edmonton, Alberta, Mrs. G. Gerth and friends, Barrhead, Alberta and the Multiple Sclerosis Society of Canada, Alberta Division. Special thanks to Ms. Verona Jeffrey for excellent technical support and to Dr. D. Carroll, Mrs. D. Olmstead, Mrs. J. Christopherson and Mrs. P. Shaw who assisted with the clinical care of MS patients.

We are grateful to Dr. Harold Jacobs for his support and encouragement.

REFERENCES

1. M.K. Dasgupta, I. Catz, K.G. Warren, T.A. McPherson, J.B. Dossetor and P.R. Carnegie. Myelin basic protein: A component of circulating immune complexes. Can. J. Neurol. Sci. 10:239-243 (1983).
2. E.A. Kabat, M. Glusman and V. Knaub. Quantitative estimation of the albumin and gamma globulin in normal and pathologic cerebrospinal fluid by immunochemical methods. Am. J. Med. 4:653-662 (1948).
3. H. Link and G. Tibbling. Principles of albumin and IgG synthesis in neurological disorders. II. Evaluation of IgG synthesis within the central nervous sytem in multiple sclerosis. Scand. J. Clin. Lab. Invest. 37:397-401 (1977).
4. W.W. Tourtellotte and B. Ma. Multiple sclerosis: The blood brain barrier and the measurement of De Novo central nervous system IgG synthesis. Neurology (NY). 28:76-83 (1978).
5. K.G. Warren and I. Catz. The relationship between levels of cerebrospinal fluid myelin basic protein and IgG measurements in patients with multiple sclerosis. Ann. Neurol. 17:475-480 (1985).
6. K.G. Warren and I. Catz. Diagnostic value of cerebrospinal fluid anti-myelin basic protein in multiple sclerosis patients. Ann. Neurol. In press. (1986).
7. K.G. Warren, I. Catz, V.M. Jeffrey and D.J. Carroll. Effect of methylprednisolone on CSF IgG parameters, myelin basic protein and anti-myelin basic protein in multiple sclerosis exacerbations. Can. J. Neurol. Sci. 13:25-30 (1986).
8. D. McAlpine, C.E. Lumsden and E.D. Acheson. Multiple sclerosis: cause and prognosis. In multiple sclerosis: a reappraisal. Edinburgh & London, Churchill Livingstone. pp. 214. (1972).

DETECTION OF FREE AND BOUND FORMS OF ANTIBODIES TO MYELIN BASIC PROTEIN IN THE CEREBROSPINAL FLUID OF PATIENTS WITH MULTIPLE SCLEROSIS

Ingrid Catz and Kenneth G. Warren

From the Department of Laboratory Medicine, University of Alberta Hospital and the Division of Neurology, 9-101 Clinical Science Building, Department of Medicine, University of Alberta, Edmonton, Alberta, Canada T6G 2G3

Myelin basic protein (MBP) is a component of central nervous system (CNS) myelin. It has attracted considerable scientific interest because of its role in experimental allergic encephalomyelitis. Initially we observed that free (unbound) MBP is elevated in the cerebrospinal fluid (CSF) of multiple sclerosis (MS) patients with exacerbations (1,2). Subsequently, immune complexes containing MBP were identified in the serum and CSF of MS patients (3,4). Consequently, the purpose of our present research has been to detect whether there are antibodies to MBP in free and bound forms in the CSF of multiple sclerosis patients and if they correlate with disease activity.

METHODS

Patient population

Anti-MBP levels were determined in 146 MS patients and 112 controls. All MS patients had clinically definite disease (5). This group consisted of 33 patients in remission (R), 20 patients with clinically stable disease (S), 47 with progressing MS (P) and 46 experiencing exacerbations (E). All patients in remission were asymptomatic at the time of the study. Patients with stable disease had residual deficits but were not clinically deteriorating on a year to year basis while those with progressing disease were getting clinically worse on a monthly or yearly basis. All patients with exacerbations had experienced acute development of one or more neurological symptoms with associated signs which persisted for a minimum period of 24-48 hours, and they were all studied within 1-15 days from the onset of the attack. The control group of 112 patients consisted of 44 with psychoneurosis (N), 32 having myelograms for degenerative disc disease and 36 with miscellaneous neurological diseases exclusive of MS.

Intrathecal IgG synthesis

Matched CSF and serum samples were obtained from all patients. IgG and albumin levels were immediately determined by standard immunonephelometric techniques. Intrathecal IgG synthesis was estimated by the Link-Tibbling IgG Index (6) and by Tourtellotte's empirical formula for daily rate of CNS IgG synthesis (7). All remaining specimens were stored in aliquots in polypropylene tubes at -40°C within one hour of collection. All assays were performed without any knowledge of the clinical status of the patients.

Anti-myelin basic protein

Anti-MBP levels were determined in the CSF by a solid phase radioimmunoassay before and after acid hydrolysis in order to dissociate possible preformed immune complexes (8,9). Values obtained before hydrolysis represent the free circulating antibody (F anti-MBP), while post hydrolysis values represent the total amount of anti-MBP (T anti-MBP) present. Bound (B) fractions were calculated by subtracting the F from the corresponding T value. The antibody binding was measured at a CSF IgG concentration of 0.010 g/l (1 mg/dl). Microtiter plates (Immulon™, Dynatech, Alexandria, Virginia, USA) were coated with 10 µg/ml (100 µl/well) human MBP (h MBP) (10,11). Staphylococcus A Protein (Staph A Prot) was iodinated by the method of Hunter and Greenwood (12).

CSF acid hydrolisis: 100 µl CSF were acidified to pH=3 (1N acetic acid) for one hour at room temperature and then the pH was raised to neutral.

Anti-MBP assay: Aliquots of 100 µl diluted CSF (0.010 g IgG/l) before and after acid hydrolysis were incubated in MBP coated wells. After two hours at RT, the plates were inverted and the wells rinsed 5 times with 0.5% Tween 20 in borate buffered saline (BBS) pH=8.2; 0.1 ml of goat anti-human IgG (Fc specific) (Myles-Yeda Ltd.) diluted 1:100 with 0.5% Tween/BBS was then added and incubation continued at RT for one hour. Wells were rinsed and 0.1 ml of I^{125} Staph A Prot containing 30,000 cpm were added. One hour later wells were rinsed, separated and individually counted. Results were expressed as percent binding (%B). Four positive and two negative controls were used in each assay. Interassay variability (CV) at three different levels of 5, 10 and 20%B for 25 sets of duplicates was 3.0, 4.0 and 5.0 respectively, while interassay variability (CV) of the above controls done in quadruplicate over 10 different assays was 4.0, 5.0 and 7.0 respectively. Blanks were performed with each sample to determine nonspecific adherence uncoated wells. The nonspecific binding (< 1%) was subtracted from the matched counts of samples.

Validation of Anti-MBP Assay: When CSF samples with initially high IgG and anti-MBP values were serially diluted, anti-MBP levels paralelled IgG concentrations. Absorption of CSF anti-MBP, before and after acid hydrolysis, to MBP resulted in complete elimination of both F and T anti-MBP from samples that initially had high titers.

After calculating F/B ratios, means and standard deviations were calculated for each of the 3 anti-MBP fractions (F, T and B) as well as the F/B ratios in all groups of controls and MS patients. Results obtained in patients with psychoneurosis were accepted as baseline normal values.

Student's test was used to determine intergroup statistical differences for anti-MBP and F/B ratios in MS patients versus controls.

RESULTS

Intrathecal IgG synthesis

In this study 146 patients with clinically definite multiple sclerosis were compared with 112 controls. Intrathecal IgG synthesis estimated by the IgG Index (6) and daily rate of CNS IgG synthesis (7) was determined in all clinical groups in order to confirm their characteristic increase in the MS population. Forty-four patients with psychoneurosis and 32 with degenerative disc disease had normal values for both IgG index and daily IgG synthesis. In 36 patients with neurological diseases exclusive of MS, these values were slightly higher due to grossly abnormal results from 3 patients, one with subacute sclerosing panencephalitis and 2 (of 8) patients with post-infectious encephalomyelitis. All multiple sclerosis patients had an increased IgG index and daily IgG synthesis regardless of their clinical subgroup with highest values observed in those with chronic progressive disease. These estimates of intrathecal IgG synthesis were judged to be typical of these clinical groups (2) and confirmed the diagnostic accuracy of these patients.

Anti-myelin basic protein (Fig.1)

In 44 patients with psychoneurosis total anti-MBP was 1.5 ± 1.1 with corresponding free and bound values of 0.4 ± 0.3 and 1.2 ± 1.0 respectively. These values were considered normal. Similar results were observed in the group of patients with degenerative disc disease. Patients with neurological diseases other than MS had somewhat increased values of CSF anti-MBP in the bound form due to the same 3 patients with increased intrathecal IgG. Although MS patients in remission had an increased intrathecal IgG synthesis, none of these patients had detectable levels of anti-MBP in their CSF. Their values were identical to those of the control group of patients with psychoneurosis, All MS patients with stable disease had increased CSF anti-MBP in bound form. Highest levels of total CSF anti-MBP were recorded in the group of patients with chronic progressing disease. Similar to the group with stable disease, all patients with progressing MS had increased bound CSF anti-MBP but some (29 of 47) had also increased free antibody levels. Conversely, all 46 MS patients with exacerbations had increased levels of free CSF anti-MBP and only 16 of these patients had increased titers of bound antibody.

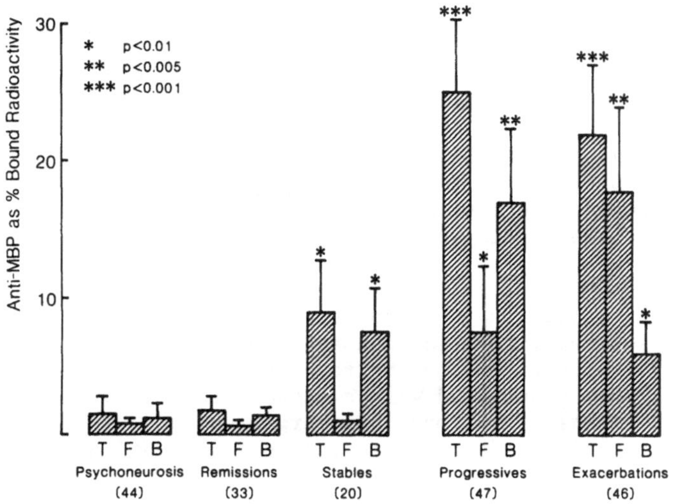

Fig.1. Total (T), free (F) and bound (B) CSF anti-MBP in a group of control patients (44 with psychoneurosis) and in four clinical subgroups of MS patients: 33 in complete clinical remission, 20 in a stable phase of the disease, 47 with progressing MS and 46 with exacerbations.

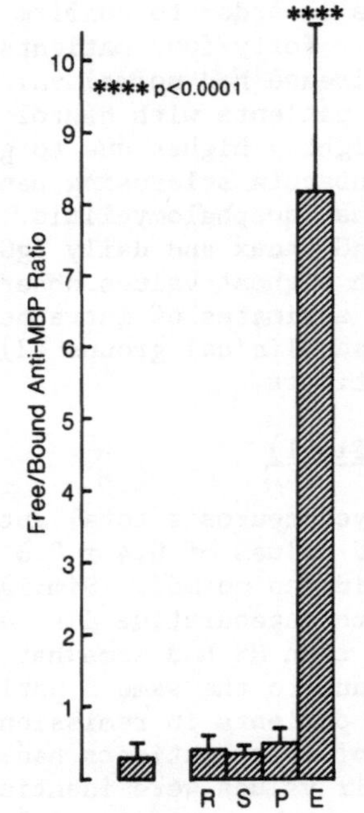

Fig.2. The free/bound anti-MBP ratio in four MS clinical subgroups (R,S,P,E)
R = complete clinical remission
S = stable phase of disability
P = progressing neurological deterioration
E = exacerbations

The free to bound anti-MBP ratio was dramatically elevated above 1.0 ($p < 0.0001$) only in MS patients experiencing exacerbations (Fig.2).

CONCLUSION

Free and bound forms of antibodies to MBP can be detected in the CSF of MS patients by a solid phase RIA. These antibodies are found only in MS patients with active disease. Although MS patients in remission may have increased intrathecal IgG synthesis, they do not have anti-MBP antibodies in their CSF. Bound anti-MBP antibodies are prevalent in MS patients with chronic progressing disease while free forms are predominant in patients with acute relapses. Antibodies to MBP are intrathecally produced (8).

Anti-MBP antibodies may be involved in the pathogenesis of MS. Acute clinical relapses are likely to be associated with a sudden "pulse" of large quantities of anti-MBP per narrow unit of time whereas progressive disease is probably associated with a steady state of synthesis of relatively lower quantities of antibody per larger unit of time; the incipience of anti-MBP antibodies and their regulation are undetermined.

ACKNOWLEDGEMENTS

We would like to thank all MS patients from Northern Alberta who participated in this project. This research was supported in part by Mr. and Mrs. Philip May and the Friends of Multiple Sclerosis Patient Care and Research Clinic, Edmonton, Alberta; Mrs. E. Laforge and the Tegler Foundation, Edmonton, Alberta; a special contribution from Mrs. G. Gerth and friends, Barrhead, Alberta and the Multiple Sclerosis Society of Canada (Alberta Division). Special thanks to Ms. Verona Jeffrey for excellent technical support, to Dr. D. Carroll, Mrs. P. Shaw and Mrs. J. Christopherson who helped with the clinical care of MS patients and to Drs. R. Blum and J. Miller who kindly provided samples from control patients. We are very grateful to Dr. Harold Jacobs for his constant support and encouragement.

REFERENCES

1. K.G. Warren, I. Catz and T.A. McPherson. CSF myelin basic protein in optic neuritis and multiple sclerosis. Can. J. Neurol. Sci. 10:235-238 (1983).
2. K.G. Warren and I. Catz. The relationship between levels of cerebrospinal fluid myelin basic protein and IgG measurements in patients with multiple sclerosis. Ann. Neurol. 17:475-480 (1985).
3. M.K. Dasgupta, I. Catz, K.G. Warren, T.A. McPherson, J.B. Dossetor and P.R. Carnegie. Myelin basic protein: A component of circulating immune complexes in multiple sclerosis. Can. J. Neurol. Sci. 10(4): 239-243 (1983).
4. P.K. Coyle. CSF immune complexes in multiple sclerosis. Neurology. 35:429-432 (1985).
5. G.A. Schumacher, G. Beebe, R.E. Kibler, L.T. Kurkland, J.F. Kurtzke, F. McDowell, B. Nagler, W.A. Sibley, W.W. Tourtellotte and T.L. Willman. Problems of experimental trials of therapy in multiple sclerosis. Ann. NY Acad. Sci. 122:552-568 (1965).
6. G. Tibbling, H. Link and S. Ohlman. Principles of albumin and IgG analyses in neurological disorders. I. Establishment of reference values. Scand. J. Clin. Lab. Invest. 37:385-390 (1977).
7. W.W. Tourtellotte. On cerebrospinal fluid IgG Quotients in MS and other diseases. A review and new formula to estimate the amount of IgG synthesized per day by the central nervous system. J. Neurol. Sci. 10:279-304 (1970).
8. I. Catz and K.G. Warren. Intrathecal synthesis of autoantibodies to myelin basic protein in the cerebrospinal fluid of multiple sclerosis patients. Can. J. Neurol. Sci. 13:21-24 (1986).
9. R.F. Bashir and J.N. Whitaker. Molecular features of immunoreactive myelin basic protein in cerebrospinal fluid of persons with multiple sclerosis. Ann. Neurol. 7:50-57 (1980).
10. G.E. Diebler, R.E. Marteson and M.W. Kies. Large scale preparation of myelin basic protein from central nervous tissue of several mammalian species. Prep. Biochem. 2:139-165 (1972).
11. R.E. Marteson, V. Luthy and G.E. Diebler. Cleavage of rabbit myelin basic protein by pepsin. J. Neurochem. 36:58-68 (1981).
12. W.M. Hunter and F.C. Greenwood. Preparation of I^{131} labelled human growth hormone of high specific activity. Nature. 195:495 (1962).

IMMUNOGLOBULINS: NEW APPROACHES FOR THEIR EVALUATION IN MULTIPLE SCLEROSIS

Hans Link, Slavenka Kam-Hansen and Annemarie Henriksson

Department of Neurology, Karolinska Institute, Huddinge University Hospital, S-141 86 Huddinge, Stockholm, Sweden

INTRODUCTION

An abnormal intra-blood-brain barrier (BBB) B-cell response as reflected by elevated concentration of IgG and appearance of oligoclonal IgG bands in cerebrospinal fluid (CSF) is the most frequently observed and undisputed immune abnormality demonstrable in patients with multiple sclerosis (MS), despite the fact that application of many, often highly sophisticated methods has made it possible to outline a great number of derangements of immune variables and regulation (for review see ref.1). Studies of this abnormal intra-BBB immune response have for many years focused on IgG. In recent years, evidence has been presented that intra-BBB production of IgM is common in patients with MS (2-4), while intra-BBB synthesis of IgA is infrequent (5). Since various factors may have an influence on the concentrations of free Ig demonstrable in CSF (Table 1) and the extent to which these factors are involved in patients with MS as compared to controls is not known, it can be questioned whether demonstrable aberrations of concentrations of free Ig are really representative for existing derangements of B-cell function. Of the different factors given in Table 1, local synthesis by CSF lymphocytes is probably quantitatively of low-grade importance in comparison with the two other mechanisms included in the 'afferent axis'. The mechanisms on the 'efferent axis' have hitherto mostly been neglected in discussions of Ig concentrations in CSF. Greatly elevated activities of the peptidase leucyl-B-naphthylamide (6) and of acid and neutral proteinases (6,7) have been reported in CSF from patients with MS. To what extent these abnormal enzyme activities influence Ig levels in CSF is not known. Little is also known about consumption of Ig and antibodies at targets but it may be anticipated that this mechanism has substantial influence on concentrations in CSF of Ig of the various classes, and of specific antibodies (reviewed in ref.8). Consumption at target can be exemplified by our observation that water-soluble CNS extracts obtained from guinea pigs with chronic relapsing experimental allergic encephalomyelitis (r-EAE) did not contain measurable amounts of IgG antibodies against myelin when examined by a sensitive enzyme-linked immunosorbent assay (ELISA) while the same assay revealed high concentrations of such antibodies in supernatants from short-term (18 h) cultures of CNS and meningeal lymphocytes obtained from the same animals (9).

Table 1. Factors influencing concentrations of free Ig and antibodies in CSF

Afferent axis	Efferent axis
Transudation via blood-brain-barrier	Clearance
Local production within CNS and meninges	Metabolism
Local synthesis by CSF lymphocytes	Differences in half-life (IgG 25 days; IgA 6 days; IgM 5 days) (ref.43)
	Proteolysis
	Consumption at target

It can thus be anticipated that studies performed directly on CSF lymphocytes (CSF-L) in comparison with peripheral blood lymphocytes (PBL) will give information in addition to that available from determinations of concentrations of free Ig or antibodies in CSF. In this paper, we present results from our laboratory regarding enumeration of Ig-secreting cells in CSF and peripheral blood by applying an indirect hemolytic plaque-forming cell assay, and a new method adopting culture of CSF-L and PBL directly in antigen-coated microtitre plates followed by determination of antibodies present in culture supernatants by ELISA directly in the plates. The data indicate that studies of B-cell responses on cellular level are more sensitive and reveal a more diversified immune response within the CNS as well as systemically in comparison with measurements of concentrations of free Ig.

Immunoglobulin producing cells in CSF and peripheral blood

By modifications of the hemolytic plaque assay originally described by Jerne and Nordin (10) including use of protein-A coated erythrocytes, it became possible to enumerate cells producing Ig of different classes in body fluids (11). The principle of the assay rests in the ability of staphylococcal protein-A to bind Fc regions of IgG subclasses. Coupling of protein-A to sheep red blood cells (SRBC) with chromium chloride and subsequent admixture of these target cells with class-specific antisera with complement and lymphocytes allow development of plaque-forming cells secreting Ig of any particular class depending on specificity of antiserum used (Fig.1). The method was originally employed in the murine system but soon also for studies of human cells (12-15).

Modification of the protein-A plaque assay for 20×10^3 mononuclear cells has allowed enumeration of Ig-producing cells in CSF and, in parallel, peripheral blood from patients with MS, aseptic meningo-encephalitis (AM) and controls (16-19). There is no evidence that normal CSF contains Ig producing cells (18), but larger groups of subjects need to be examined to settle this question. Table 2 presents data for IgG, IgM and IgA producing cells in each of 37 patients with MS (18,19).

In CSF, 33 (89%) of these 37 MS patients had elevated (>2) numbers of cells producing IgG, 21 (57%) IgM and 26 (70%) IgA. As expected, IgG producing cells predominated in 27 of the patients but, surprisingly, IgM predominated in 6 and IgA in 3 while one patient had the same number of IgG and IgA producing cells in CSF.

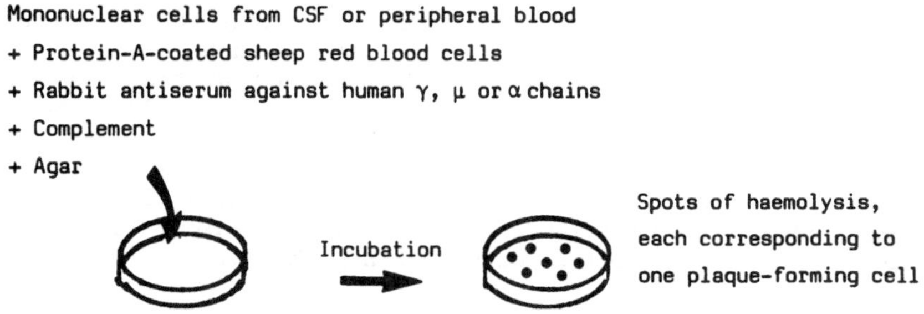

Fig.1. Principles of protein A plaque assay.

A correlation was found between numbers of IgM producing cells in CSF and CSF IgM index, while no such correlation was observed for IgG or IgA. In fact, altogether 28 of the 37 patients had in their CSF elevated numbers of cells producing Ig of a certain class in presence of normal value of corresponding CSF Ig index. This discrepancy was most frequently observed for IgA, since no less than 22 patients had elevated numbers of IgA producing cells in CSF and normal CSF IgA index.

It is also apparent from Table 2 that higher numbers of IgG producing cells/20 x 10^3 cells were present in CSF compared to peripheral blood in the majority of MS patients. Furthermore, 16 patients had higher numbers of IgM and 7 IgA producing cells in CSF.

In peripheral blood, significantly higher numbers of cells producing IgG, IgM and IgA were found in the 37 patients with MS when compared with results obtained in 27 healthy controls. As expected, IgA producing cells predominated in both groups.

Subgrouping of the patients according to Goust et al. (20) into those with active (13 patients) and stable (24 patients) MS did not reveal any differences for Ig producing cells.

Taken together, the CSF data are expected as far as IgG is concerned. For IgA, the results are unexpected. Only a minority of MS patients display evidence for intra-BBB IgA synthesis when CSF IgA concentration is presented as CSF IgA/total protein ratio (21,22) or CSF IgA index (5,23). On the other hand, one investigation disclosed higher CSF IgA levels expressed as % of CSF total protein in 22 MS patients during exacerbations in comparison with remissions (24). Among the 31 patients presented in Table 2 who were examined for CSF IgA index, only one had an increased value, while 23 of these 31 patients had elevated numbers of IgA producing cells in CSF. The conclusion can therefore be drawn that intra-BBB production of IgA is common in MS although not detectable by conventional determination of CSF IgA levels. This conclusion is further corroborated by the recent observation of oligoclonal IgA bands in CSF - also reflecting intra-BBB IgA synthesis - in 16 of 20 randomly selected patients with MS (25). This observation needs, however, confirmation from other laboratories.

Analysis of correlation between numbers of cells producing Ig of a certain class and corresponding CSF Ig index as a measure of level of free Ig in CSF may allow speculations regarding representativity of CSF cells in relation to cells present in nervous system lesions. The positive correlation observed between numbers of Ig producing cells in CSF of all 3 classes and the corresponding CSF Ig index values in patients during the acute phase of AM (17) might indicate that both variables mirror fairly well an inflammatory process which is localized mainly to the immediate vicinity of the subarachnoidal space. The lack of such correlations in MS for IgG and IgA might, on the other hand, indicate that the intra-parenchymatous IgG and IgA synthesis is not well reflected in CSF. The positive correlation observed in MS for IgM might allow one to anticipate that an IgM response is demonstrable in CSF especially in MS patients who - as patients with AM - have infiltrates of mononuclear cells close to the subarachnoidal space. The observation that cells containing   chains are mostly rare in MS brains (26) favours this hypothesis.

Table 2. Numbers of plaque-forming cells (PFC) per 20 x 10^3 lymphocytes from peripheral blood and CSF in 37 patients with multiple sclerosis. Underlined figures denote specimens where the corresponding CSF Ig index was abnormally high. Asterisk refers to specimens where corresponding CSF Ig index was not determined (Henriksson, 1986).

Patient No.	Mononuclear cells in CSF x 10^6/L	IgG PFC Blood	IgG PFC CSF	IgA PFC Blood	IgA PFC CSF	IgM PFC Blood	IgM PFC CSF
1	21.5	4	45	11	5	10	2
2	17	6	593	17	2	2	14
3	19	7	4	68	10	10	3*
4	13.5	11	21	17	1	4	25*
5	7	9	71	30	11	2	1
6	16	20	151	135	34	14	1
7	14	14	39	57	18	4	2
8	5	10	106	32	94	6	0
9	23.5	2	314	10	10*	0	0
10	11	20	0	105	4	9	19
11	7	8	79	41	24	6	14
12	6.5	4	86	10	10	1	7
13	19.5	7	80	12	1	8	2
14	13.6	10	16	28	36	0	10*
15	16.5	8	1	25	3	4	2
16	9.5	16	281	95	83*	23	26
17	22.5	19	161	25	14	6	4
18	12.5	13	58	25	18	4	4
19	5.5	12	10	16	10	4	4
20	7	6	0	8	3	3	12
21	51	14	143	39	5	3	8
22	30.5	4	520	3	4*	0	7
23	38	19	858	95	60	27	71
24	3.5	18	54	26	0	4	0*
25	7	10	215	15	31	3	307
26	2.5	18	234	10	24	2	24
27	14	7	8	8	13	17	77
28	3.5	8	14	0	0*	3	0
29	6	12	122	28	34	0	18
30	13	5	299	14	1*	15	4
31	2.5	14	122	26	48	12	2
32	3.5	7	96	17	0	3	2
33	12.5	19	0	20	1	2	8
34	19.5	2	184	15	0*	3	1
35	6	9	243	25	2	6	0
36	10.5	8	89	21	0	0	0
37	5.5	26	102	61	26	5	0

The demonstration of intra-BBB IgM and/or IgA synthesis in a majority of patients with MS underlines the need for future studies of CSF IgM and CSF IgA regarding antibody specificities. Among 28 MS patients recently examined, IgM antibodies against one or more of 3 different viruses examined were found in serum in 43% and in CSF in 14% (27). Thus, MS may be accompanied by a systemic IgM response against one or more viruses. No evidence was, however, obtained for intra-BBB production of the viral IgM antibodies examined in this study.

Demonstration of intra-blood-brain barrier synthesis of specific antibodies

Methods demonstrating semiquantitative and qualitative abnormalities have been used to demonstrate intra-BBB production of specific antibodies. The former include determination of CSF/serum ratio for Ig class-specific antibody in question related to CSF/serum ratio of reference antibody such as adenovirus which are present in most subjects; a 4-fold or higher difference between these ratios is considered to reflect intrathecal synthesis (28). This principle has been used for demonstration in MS of intra-BBB production of IgG antibodies against various viruses, and it has been documented by this means that individual MS patients may produce within their brain antibodies against more than one virus (29). Alternatively, a CSF antibody index may be calculated, e.g. CSF acetylcholine receptor (AChR) antibody index equal to (CSF/serum AChR IgG antibody): (CSF/serum albumin) (30). This index compensates for influence due to serum antibody levels as well as BBB damage. Elevated values therefore reflect intra-BBB production of the antibody in question. This principle has been employed inter alia for evaluation of intra-BBB synthesis in MS and controls of IgG antibodies against oligodendrocytes (31).

Qualitative changes indicative of intra-BBB antibody production have been obtained by separation of CSF and corresponding serum by electrophoresis or isoelectric focusing (IF) followed by analysis of separated IgG for antibody specificities. The latter has been performed by either immunofixation with antigen-containing agarose gel plates and autoradiography (32), or transfer of separated proteins to nitrocellulose membrane loaded with specific antigen followed by visualization of antigen-antibody complexes on the membrane by immunoperoxidase staining (33), and supplementary avidin-biotin amplification to increase sensitivity (34). The latter procedure (Table 3) has been utilized recently to identify IgG antibodies against myelin basic protein (MBP). In fact, 8 of 26 patients with MS (31%) displayed oligoclonal IgG antibodies against MBP in CSF but not in corresponding serum, reflecting intra-BBB production (Fig.2) (34).

These various methods have revealed intra-BBB synthesis of IgG antibodies against various viruses, bacterial components and/or autoantigens in a majority of patients with MS. It is, however, generally considered that these antibodies represent only a minor part of the IgG produced within the brain (for review see ref.1, 35). Furthermore, antibodies under examination in MS up to present time have rarely had relation to oligoclonal IgG bands irrespective if demonstrated by electrophoresis or IF. However, the intra-BBB-produced IgG antibodies are still monoclonal or oligoclonal, migrating as one or more bands within the background polyclonal IgG (Fig.2). Since bands corresponding to the specific antibody can not be demonstrated in the patient's serum, it must be concluded that a highly restricted number of clones of B-cells are activated within the CNS-CSF compartment and transformed into plasma cells which secrete the antibody in question. The mechanism behind this B-cell activation is unknown, as is the role of intra-BBB produced antibodies in the pathogenesis of MS. None of the antibodies examined up to present time seems to be specific for MS. Thus, simultaneous occurrence of different viral anti-

Table 3. Procedure for demonstration of oligoclonal IgG bands (left part) and IgG antibodies against human myelin basic protein (MBP) (right part) in CSF and serum

Agarose isoelectric focusing of CSF and corresponding serum	
CSF and serum with IgG concentrations of 20-30 mg/l in 10 ul.	CSF and serum with IgG concentrations of 100 mg/l in 10 μl.
transfer of separated proteins to nitrocellulose membrane	transfer of separated antibodies to nitrocellulose membrane coated with MBP and blocked with bovine serum albumin
blocking of remaining free protein-binding sites on membrane with bovine serum albumin	binding of antibodies to MBP on the membrane
Visualization of IgG or IgG antibodies against MBP by incubation of membrane with 1. Rabbit anti-human IgG Fc (primary antibody); 2. Biotinylated goat anti-rabbit IgG (secondary antibody); 3. Avidin-biotin-peroxidase complex -Peroxidase staining with 3-amino-9-ethylcarbazole as substrate -Visual inspection and comparison of band patterns	

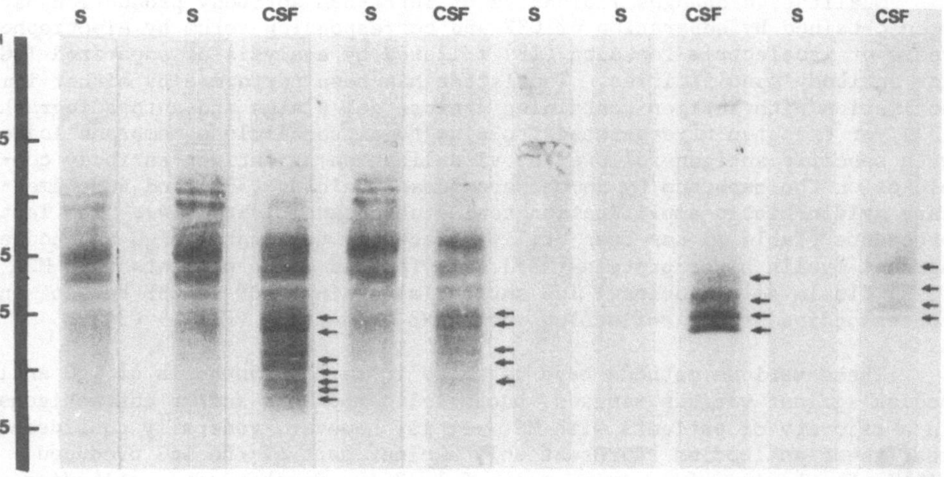

Fig.2. Patterns from agarose isoelectric focusing (AIF), transfer of separated proteins to nitrocellulose membrane, immunoenzyme labelling and avidin-biotin amplification for detection of IgG in unconcentrated CSF and corresponding serum (S) (1-5), and from AIF, immunoblotting and avidin-biotin amplification for demonstration of IgG antibodies against myelin basic protein (MBP; 6-10). 2-3 and 7-8 correspond to S and CSF from one patient with MS, 4-5 and 9-10 to S and CSF obtained one year later from the same patient. Arrows in 3 and 5 denote oligoclonal IgG bands, in 8 and 10 bands of IgG antibodies against MBP 1 and 6 correspond to pooled blood donor serum (From ref. 34).

bodies has been observed in CSF from patients with cerebrovascular disease and oligoclonal bands in CSF (36), while antibodies against MBP have been demonstrated in e.g. subacute sclerosing panencephalitis (37).

An alternative approach to analysis of intra-BBB-cell response is examination of antibody production on the cellular level. A procedure developed by Forsberg et al. (38-40) makes possible analysis of antibody production per 0.5 x 10^5 CSF-L or PBL. Shortly, the procedure consists of cultivation of cells directly in ELISA plates for 18 h (Fig.3). Applying ELISA for measurements of antibodies present in the culture supernatants, positive absorbance values correspond to amount of antibodies of a given class. An absorbance ratio for e.g. virus specific antibodies produced by CSF-L and PBL can be calculated. If >1, it indicates that antibody production at CSF-L level is higher than corresponding extra-BBB antibody production as measured at PBL level.

This procedure has yielded new information about the intra-BBB immune response in infectious nervous system diseases. Among patient groups examined, all 10 with herpes zoster with usual symptoms from the skin and peripheral sensory nerves but no symptoms from the CNS, were found to have CSF-L with the capacity to produce specific IgG antibodies at an even higher degree than the corresponding number of PBL (Fig.4). Calculating antibody indices which are based on measurements by ELISA or free antibodies in CSF and serum and which in an indirect way may indicate intra-BBB antibody production, only 3 of these 10 patients were found to be positive. These observations clearly indicated that 1) ordinary herpes zoster is accompanied by a pronounced intra-BBB immune response and, 2) in vitro analysis of antibody production on the cellular level (cell-ELISA) is more sensitive than determination of free antibodies in CSF and serum. Similar discrepancies indicating high sensitivity, specificity and reliability of

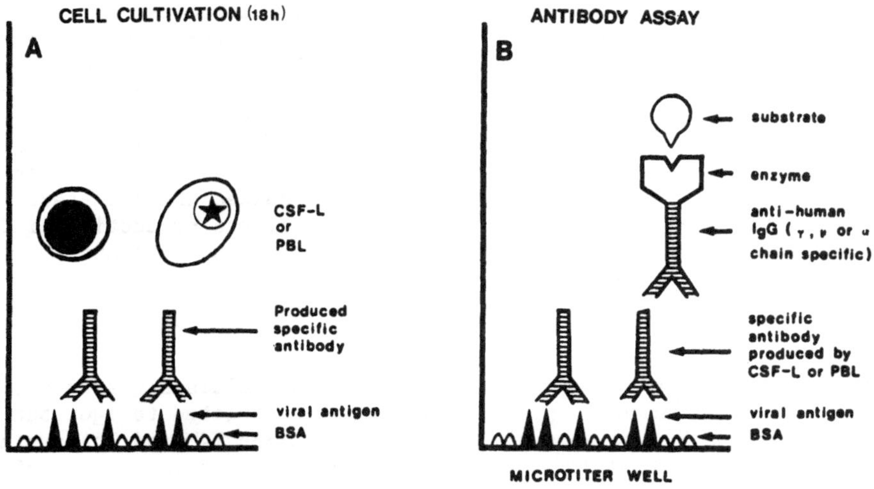

Fig.3. Principles for detection of antibody production by mononuclear cells isolated from CSF (CSF-L) and peripheral blood (PBL) cultivated in antigen-coated wells of microtiter plates (A). Specific antibodies of different classes produced during 18 h of culture were detected by adding heavy chain specific anti-human Ig conjugated with enzyme = alkaline phosphatase. After further incubation, substrate = p-nitrophenyl phosphate in diethanolamine buffer was added (B). After further incubation, absorbance was measured in a photometer.

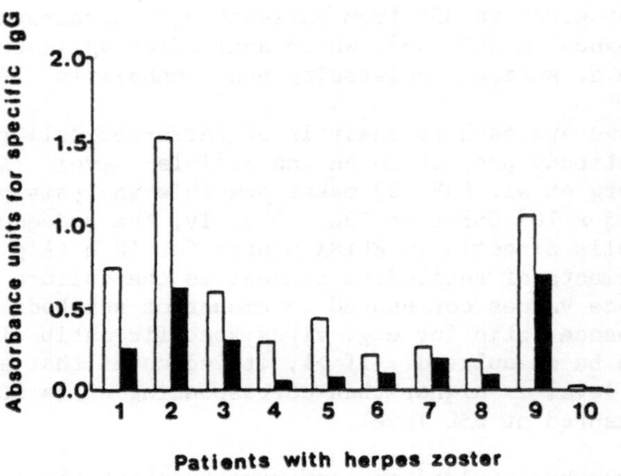

Fig.4. Absorbances of IgG antibodies against varicella zoster virus produced by lymphocytes in CSF (unfilled bars) and peripheral blood (filled bars) of 10 patients with herpes zoster. Experiments were done with 10^5 (patient No. 1-6) or 5×10^4 (patient No. 7-10) lymphocytes.

this 'cell-ELISA' were found in mumps meningitis and herpes simplex encephalitis, and it may be a useful diagnostic tool in CNS infections (39,40). This assay should also be of value in definition of the intra-BBB antibody response in MS. It must be remembered that quantitation of free antibodies - and of free Ig - in body fluids reflects remnents of a situation that occurred days or weeks ago, while 'cell ELISA' enables analysis of the immune status at the time when the specimens are drawn.

Having registered negative results on examination of 47 consecutive Swedish MS patients' CSF and serum regarding IgG antibodies against HTLV-I when analysed by ELISA using commercial HTLV-I antigen-coated microtitre plates, we adopted the more sensitive 'cell-ELISA' to analyse production of IgG antibodies against HTLV-I by CSF-L, PBL and bone marrow cells from 7 patients with MS (41). The rationale of these studies has been the recent observation of elevated titers of antibodies against this human retrovirus in some of American and Swedish MS patients tested (42). For 'cell-ELISA' we utilized commercial HTLV-I virus coated ELISA plates. Even this highly sensitive technique did not reveal the production of IgG antibodies against HTLV-I by lymphocytes from any of the patients.

SUMMARY

Enumeration of cells secreting Ig of different classes has revealed that the intra-BBB immune response in MS is not restricted to IgG, but that a majority of MS patients also display intra-BBB IgM and IgA synthesis. The latter is not demonstrable by conventional determinations of free IgA levels in CSF. For all three main Ig classes, enumeration of Ig producing cells by a protein-A plaque assay has been found to be more sensitive compared to determination of CSF Ig, even when expressed as corresponding index values. Many reasons may be responsible for the discrepancy noticed between numbers of Ig producing cells and levels of corresponding Ig, including binding of free Ig to target and accentuated turn-over of free Ig as a result of proteolytic enzymes. Patients with MS have in peripheral blood elevated numbers of IgG, IgM and IgA producing cells, despite normal concentrations in serum of corresponding Ig, indicating that B-cell response in MS is not restricted to the brain but systemic as well.

A new method - 'cell-ELISA' constituting 18 h culture of 10^5 CSF-L and PBL in specific antigen coated ELISA plates followed by measurement of IgG antibodies bound to antigen - revealed intra-BBB B-cell response which was more pronounced than corresponding extra-BBB response, in 10 consecutive patients with ordinary herpes zoster, while conventional ELISA revealed intra-BBB production of specific IgG antibodies in only 3 of the patients. 'Cell-ELISA' is recommended for analysis of intra-BBB production of specific antibodies in MS. Preliminary studies of CSF-L, PBL and bone marrow lymphocytes from patients with MS in HTLV-I coated ELISA plates have, however, revealed negative results, as have our search for HTLV-I IgG antibodies in MS CSF and serum by conventional ELISA.

ACKNOWLEDGEMENTS

The author's studies presented in this review have been supported by the Swedish Medical Council (grant No. 3381).

REFERENCES

1. A.T. Reder and B.G.W. Arnason. Immunology of multiple sclerosis. In: "Handbook of Clinical Neurology, Vol.3 (47): Demyelinating diseases". J.C. Koestler, ed. Elsevier Science Publishers B.V., Amsterdam (1985).
2. A.C. Williams, E.S. Mingioli, H.F. McFarland, W.W. Tourtellotte and D.E. McFarlin. Increased CSF IgM in multiple sclerosis. Neurology. 28:996 (1978).
3. C.J.M. Sindic, C.L. Cambiaso, A. Depre, E.C. Laterre and P.L. Masson. The concentrations of IgM in the cerebrospinal fluid of neurological patients. J. Neurol. Sci. 55:339 (1982).
4. P. Forsberg, A. Henriksson, H. Link and S. Öhman. Reference values for CSF-IgM, CSF-IgM/S-IgM ratio and IgM index, ands its application on patients with multiple sclerosis and aseptic meningoencephalitis. Scand. J. Clin. Lab. Invest. 44:7 (1984).
5. C.J.M. Sindic, D.L. Delacroix, J.P. Vaerman, E.C. Laterre and P.L. Masson. Study of IgA in the cerebrospinal fluid with special reference to size, subclass and local production. J. Neuroimmunol. 7:65 (1984).
6. U.K. Rinne and P.J. Riekkinen. Esterase, peptidase and proteinase activities of human cerebrospinal fluid in multiple sclerosis. Acta Neurol. Scand. 44:156 (1968).
7. M.L.Cuzner, A.N. Davison and P. Rudge. Proteolytic enzyme activity of blood leucocytes and cerebrospinal fluid in multiple sclerosis. Ann. Neurol. 4:337 (1979).
8. H. Link, S. Kam-Hansen and A. Henriksson. Studies on B-lymphocyte function in multiple sclerosis. In: "Multiple sclerosis. Present and future". G. Scarlato adn W.B. Matthews, eds. Plenum Press, New York and London (1984).
9. T. Olsson, A. Henriksson and H. Link. In vitro synthesis of immunoglobulins and autoantibodies by lymphocytes from various body compartments during chronic relapsing experimental allergic encephalomyelitis. J. Neuroimmunol. 9:293 (1985).
10. N.K. Jerne and A.A. Nordin. Plaque formation in agar by single antibody-producing cells. Science. 140:405 (1963).
11. E. Gronowicz, A. Coutinho and F. Melchers. A plaque assay for cells secreting Ig of a given type or class. Europ. J. Immunol. 6:588 (1976).
12. A.G. Bird and S. Britton. A new approach to the study of human B lymphocyte function using an indirect plaque assay and a direct B cell activator. Immunol. Rev. 54:41 (1979).

13. A. Freijd and T. Kunori. Spontaneous plaque-forming human lymphocytes detected with the protein-A plaque assay. Scand. J. Immunol. 11:283 (1980).
14. L. Hammarström, C.I.E. Smith, D. Pettersson, H. Mellstedt and G. Holm. The protein-A plaque assay: a new system for detection of cells secreting a given idiotype. J. Immunol. 124:140 (1980).
15. A.S. Fauci and H.M. Moutsopoulos. Polyclonally triggered B cells in the peripheral blood and bone marrow of normal individuals and in patients with systemic lupus erythematosus and primary Sjögren's syndrome. Arthr. Rheum. 24:577 (1981).
16. A. Henriksson, S. Kam-Hansen and R. Andersson. Immunoglobulin-producing cells in CSF and blood from patients with multiple sclerosis and other inflammatory neurological diseases enumerated by Protein-A plaque assay. J. Neuroimmunol. 1:299 (1981).
17. P. Forsberg and S. Kam-Hansen. Immunoglobulin-producing cells in blood and cerebrospinal fluid during the course of aseptic meningoencephalitis. Scand. J. Immunol. 17:531 (1983).
18. A. Henriksson, S. Kam-Hansen and H. Link. IgM, IgA and IgG producing cells in cerebrospinal fluid and peripheral blood in multiple sclerosis. Clin. Exp. Immunol. 62:176 (1985).
19. A. Henriksson. Immunoglobulin producing cells in nervous sytem diseases. Acta Neurol. Scand. 73, Suppl. 104:1-109 (1986).
20. J.M. Goust, E. Hogan and P. Arnaud. Abnormal regulation of IgG production in multiple sclerosis. Neurology. 32:228 (1982).
21. H. Link and R. Müller. Immunoglobulins in multiple sclerosis and infections of the nervous system. Arch. Neurol. 25:326 (1971).
22. E.S. Mingioli, W. Strober, W.W. Tourtellotte, J.N. Whitaker and D.E. McFarlin. Quantitation of IgG, IgA and IgM in the CSF by radioimmunoassay. Neurology. 28:991 (1978).
23. L. Stendahl-Brodin and H. Link. Relation between benign course of multiple sclerosis and low-grade humoral immune response in cerebrospinal fluid. J. Neurol. Neurosurg. Psych. 43:102 (1980).
24. J.E. Olsson and H. Link. Immunoglobulin abnormalities in multiple sclerosis. Relation to clinical parameters: exacerbations and remissions. Arch. Neurol. (Chic.) 28:392 (1973).
25. L.M.E. Grimaldi, R.P. Roos, E.A. Nalefski and B.G.W. Arnason. Oligoclonal IgA bands in multiple sclerosis and subacute sclerosing panencephalitis. Neurology. 35:813 (1985).
26. M.M. Esiri. Multiple sclerosis - a quantitative and qualitative study of immunoglobulin-producing cells in the central nervous system. Neuropathol. Appl. Neurobiol. 6:9 (1980).
27. F. Chiodi, V.A. Sundqvist, H. Link and E. Norrby. Viral IgM antibodies in serum and cerebrospinal fluid in patients with multiple sclerosis and controls. Acta Neurol. Scand., in press (1986).
28. E. Norrby, H. Link and J.E. Olsson. Measles virus antibodies in multiple sclerosis. Comparison of antibody titers in cerebrospinal fluid and serum. Arch. Neurol. 30:285 (1974).
29. E. Norrby, H. Link, J.E. Olsson, M. Panelius, A. Salmi and B. Vandvik. Comparison of antibodies against different viruses in cerebrospinal fluid and serum samples from patients with multiple sclerosis. Infect. Immun. 10:688 (1974).
30. S. Kam-Hansen, O. Abramski and H. Link. CSF acetylcholine receptor antibody index in myasthenia gravis and controls. Acta Neurol. Scand. 65, Suppl. 90:143 (1982).
31. A. Steck and H. Link. Antibodies against oligodendrocytes in serum and CSF in multiple sclerosis and other neurological diseases. ^{125}I-protein-A studies. Acta Neurol. Scand. 69:81 (1984).
32. H.J. Nordal, B. Vandvik and E. Norrby. Demonstration of electrophoretically restricted virus-specific antibodies in serum and cerebrospinal fluid by imprint electroimmunofixation. Scand. J. Immunol. 7:381 (1978).

33. R. Dörries and V. Ter Meulen. Detection and identification of virus-specific, oligoclonal IgG in unconcentrated cerebrospinal fluid by immunoblot technque. J. Neuroimmunol. 7:77 (1984).
34. M. Cruz, T. Olsson, J. Ernerudh,B. Höjeberg and H. Link. Immunoblot detection of IgG antimyelin basic protein antibodies in CSF of multiple sclerosis patients after isoelectric focusing. Submitted. (1986).
35. B. Roström. Specificity of antibodies in oligoclonal bands in patients with multiple sclerosis and cerebrovascular disease. Acta Neurol. Scand. 86:1-84 (1981).
36. B. Roström, H. Link, M. Laurenzi, S. Kam-Hansen, E. Norrby and B. Wahren. Viral antibody activity of oligoclonal and polyclonal immunoglobulins synthesized within the central nervous system in multiple sclerosis. Ann. Neurol. 9:569 (1981).
37. H.S. Panitch, C.J. Hooper and K.P. Johnson. CSF antibody to myelin basic protein: measurement in patients with multiple sclerosis and subacute sclerosing panencephalitis. Arch. Neurol. 37:206 (1980).
38. P. Forsberg, A. Fryden and S. Kam-Hansen. Production of specific antibodies by CSF lymphocytes in patients with herpes zoster. Lancet. I:404 (1984).
39. P. Forsberg. Studies on immunoglobulins and specific antibodies in central nervous sytem infections. Acta Neurol. Scand. 73, Suppl. 105:1-76 (1986).
40. P. Forsberg, S. Kam-Hansen and A. Fryden. Production of specific antibodies by CSF lymphocytes in patients with herpes zoster, mumps meningitis and HSV encephalitis. Scand. J. Immunol., in press.
41. F. Lolli, S. Fredrikson, S. Kam-Hansen and H. Link. Studies on HTLV-I antibodies in multiple sclerosis. Submitted.
42. H. Koprowski, E.C. Defreitas, M.E. Harper, M. Sandberg-Wollheim, W.A. Sheremata, M. Robert-Guroff, C.W. Saxinger, M.B. Feinberg, F. Wong-Staal and R.C. Gallo. Multiple sclerosis and human T-cell lymphotropic retroviruses. Nature. 318:154 (1985).
43. L.E. Hood, I.L. Weissman, W.B. Wood and J.H. Wilson. "Immunology" 2nd Ed. The Benjamin Cummings Publishing Company Inc., Menlo Park (1984).

FREE LIGHT CHAINS OF IMMUNOGLOBULINS IN MULTIPLE SCLEROSIS: A PUTATIVE INDEX OF THE INTRATHECAL HUMORAL IMMUNE RESPONSE

Richard A. Rudick

Department of Neurology and Center for Brain Research
University of Rochester School of Medicine and Dentistry
Box 605 Strong Memorial Hospital, Rochester, New York 14642

INTRODUCTION

One of the most consistent features of multiple sclerosis (MS) is a demonstrably exaggerated intrathecal humoral immune response (1). Immunoglobulin G (IgG) has been shown to be selectively increased in MS CSF (2) and has restricted subclass (3), Gm allotype (4), idiotype (5), light chain (6,7) and charge (8) characteristics compared with IgG in autologous blood. Two-dimensional electrophoresis studies have shown that the restricted IgG electrophoretic spectrotypes seen in individual patients remain remarkably constant over long time intervals (9). Taken together, this evidence that CSF IgG has sharply restricted characteristics suggests that the humoral immune response is predominantly localized in the CNS and is selective rather than entirely nonspecific.

The ratio of IgG-containing kappa light chains (IgG) to IgG-containing lambda light chains (IgG) has been shown to be increased in CSF but not serum of MS patients (10,11), suggesting preferential intrathecal synthesis of IgG . Free kappa and lambda light chains (i.e. light chains not covalently bound to functional immunoglobulin molecules) have been demonstrated in MS CSF both by immunoassays (12,13,14) and immunoelectrophoresis techniques (14,15,16,17), suggesting asynchronous light and heavy chain synthesis, probably due to humoral immune activation.

The studies summarized here focused on these free light chains in MS CSF and suggests: 1) CSF free light chains originate from intrathecal synthesis rather than from degradation of IgG; 2) free kappa and lambda chains are neutral to anodal in charge, displaying electrofocusing spectrotypes distinctly different from whole IgG from the same CSF sample; 3) free light chains account for a significant proportion of total intrathecal antibody synthesis in MS; 4) CSF free kappa chains are present in increased concentrations in 90% of MS patients, are relatively specific for MS, and correlate with the presence of clinically-silent brain lesions seen by magnetic resonance imaging (MRI) in patients with possible MS.

METHODS

Patients

Patients were evaluated clinically by an observer unaware of the results of CSF analysis, and assigned to one of 4 groups as shown in Table 1. Group 1 consisted of 84 patients with definite MS by Poser Criteria (18). Group 2 consisted of 39 patients with possible MS by Rose Criteria (19). Eighteen of these patients had monosymptomatic optic neuritis and 7 progressive myelopathy without clinical evidence of disseminated disease. Group 3 consisted of 40 patients with culture-established infections of the types listed in the Table. Group 4 consisted of 29 individuals with neurologic disease other than infections or MS as listed in the Table. The miscellaneous group include single patients with multiple infarct dementia, ceroid lipofuscinosis, IgA Gammopathy, seizure disorder, chronic inflammatory polyneuropathy, and dementia of uncertain etiology.

Table 1. Patients included in this study

GROUP 1	MULTIPLE SCLEROSIS		84
GROUP 2	POSSIBLE MULTIPLE SCLEROSIS		39
	Optic neuritis	18	
	Myelopathy	7	
	Other	14	
GROUP 3	INFECTIONS OF CNS		40
	Viral	15	
	Bacterial	21	
	Fungal	4	
GROUP 4	OTHER NEUROLOGIC DISEASES		29
	Systemic lupus	3	
	Neuropathy	2	
	Disc disease	13	
	Normal volunteers	5	
	Misc (one each--see text)	6	

Processing of CSF

Samples of CSF were collected within 1 hr of the LP, processed promptly, and stored at -70°C. CSF samples were routinely evaluated as follows: IgG and albumin were measured by electroimmunodiffusion (20) and total protein was measured (21). Samples were concentrated and analysed Samples were concentrated and analysed by electrophoresis in agarose gels to detect oligoclonal bands (OCB) (22) by an observer who was unaware of the clinical date. Total and differential cell counts were performed.

Sodium dodecyl sulfate polyacrylamide gel electrophoresis (SDS-PAGE)

SDS-PAGE was performed using 1.5 x 120 mm slab gels (23), consisting of 8% or 10% acrylamide. Samples of CSF were concentrated by ultrafiltration to a final IgG concentration of 2-3 mg/ml. Samples containing 20 μg IgG were then solubilized in Laemmli sample buffer containing 2% SDS and, when appropriate, 2-mercaptoethanol (5% w/v) prior to electrophoresis at 150 v at ambient temperature.

Isoelectric focusing (IEF)

IEF was carried out in 0.5 mm agarose slab gels containing pH gradients from 3.5-9.5. Samples were concentrated to 1-5 µg/ml IgG or light chains, applied to the gel surface, and separated at 15 watts to a maximum of 1500 volts. Gels were focused for 60 minutes at maximum voltage, after which protein was blotted to nitrocellulose.

Immunoenzyme staining

Proteins separated by SDS-PAGE were eluted into nitrocellulose sheets (24) by electrophoresis overnight at a constant current of 100 mA. IEF gels were blotted to nitrocellulose by overlaying the gel with weighted nitrocellulose for 1 hour. Nitrocellulose strips were fixed for 30 min in 25% isopropanol and 10% acetic acid before staining with appropriate antibody preparations. After fixing the protein bound to the nitrocellulose sheets, unreacted sites were blocked with 3% bovine serum albumin (BSA) in 1.5% NaCl in 50 mM TRIS. Blots were then reacted with biotinylated antibody, washed and reacted with horseradish peroxidase conjugated to avidin. After extensive washing, the blots were developed with 0.05% diaminobenzidine containing 0.01% hydrogen peroxide.

Gel filtration

Concentrated samples of CSF were separated by gel filtration in a 2.5 cm x 100 cm column packed with Sephadex G-200. Fractions containing whole IgG were pooled separately from fractions containing free light chains, were concentrated and studied by isoelectric focusing as described above.

Radioimmunoassays (RIAs)

The RIAs for free kappa and lambda chains were described previously (25). Briefly, the assays were competitive-binding fluid-phase RIAs. The primary antisera (Dako, Copenhagen) were raised in rabbits by immunization with pooled Bence-Jones kappa or lambda chains followed by extensive absorbtion with whole IgG, leaving primarily antibodies specific for "free" light chains (ie the antibodies reacted preferentially with free kappa or lambda chains relative to whole IgG). A pool of 10 Bence-Jones kappa or lambda chains was assessed for purity by SDS-PAGE and used both to develop standard curves and as radioligands following labelling with ^{125}I by the Chloramine T method (26). Antibodies were reacted with standard proteins or CSF in the presence of radioligand in a final volume of 500 µl prior to precipitation with staphylococcal protein A. The sensitivity of both assays was 0.05 µg/ml and the between and within assay variability under 10%. The specificities of the assays for free compared with bound light chains were adequate to measure free kappa chains in whole CSF or serum samples, and free lambda chains in whole CSF samples (25). The results of the kappa chain assay were found to be unaffected by as many as 10 freeze-thaw cycles, or by storage at 4° or 20° for one week.

RESULTS

SDS-PAGE and immunoblot studies (Fig.1, Table 2)

CSF samples were studied by immunoblot analysis of SDS-PAGE gels to determine the presence and nature of low-molecular weight immunoglobulin bands (27). Eighteen MS patients and 14 Group-4 controls were studied in this fashion. The total quantity of IgG (20 μg) applied to the gels was normalized and CSF samples were run in SDS but without reducing agents. Control serum IgG studied in this fashion was restricted to a single broad band at an apparent molecular weight (mw) of approximately 150 kd. In the initial series of experiments, an antiserum reactive with human immunoglobulins that was class and light chain isotype nonspecific revealed lowmolecular weight bands at 20-25 kd and at 40-50 kd molecular weight in addition to whole IgG in the expected location (Fig.1A). Each MS sample contained low molecular weight immunoglobulin bands; none of the control samples had similar bands. The low molecular weight bands in MS CSF were shown to react with antibodies specific for kappa chains and lambda chains, but not with antibodies specific for gamma chains (Fig.1B). CSF samples containing low-molecular-weight immunoglobulin bands were treated with 2-mecaptoethanol prior to separation by SDS-PAGE. This reducing agent resulted in a loss of staining at 40-50 kd mw and a shift to 20-25 kd mw, suggesting that the 40-50 mw staining represented dimers of the lower molecular weight bands (data not shown).

Samples of CSF from two MS patients were depleted of IgG and free light chains by immuno-absorption with solid-phase anti-human immunoglobulin antibodies. These IgG-depleted CSF samples were then used to treat CSF samples from 3 control patients to determine if MS CSF contained some factor(s) capable of "generating" free light chains from whole IgG. The control CSF samples were then studied by SDS-PAGE followed by immunoblot analysis. Treating control CSF samples in this fashion failed to generate free light chains from whole IgG in the control CSF.

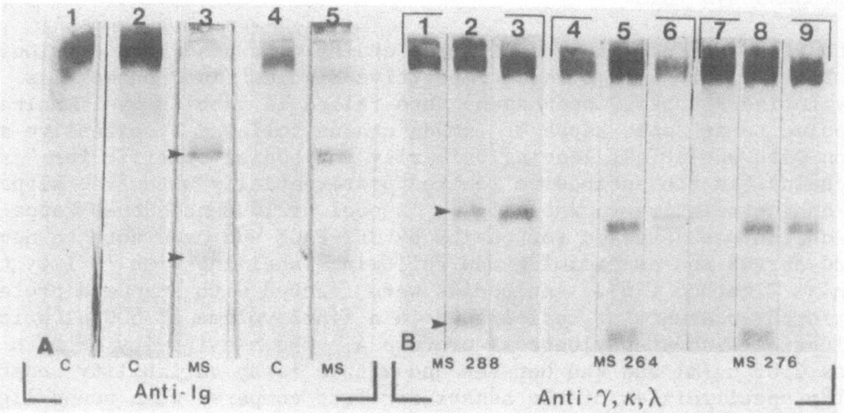

Fig.1. Nitrocellulose strips stained for human immunoglobulins (A) or for specific heavy or light chains (B). CSF was concentrated, separated by SDS-PAGE, blotted to nitrocellulose and probed for low molecular weight immunoglobulin material (arrows). Fig.1A. 10% polyacrylamide gel. All strips were stained with an antiserum reactive with light and heavy chains. Lanes 1,2,4: Control patients. Lanes 3,5: MS patients. Note low molecular weight bands (arrow heads) with apparent kD of 20-25 and 40-50. Fig.1B. Nitrocellulose strips from 8% polyacrylamide gel. Lanes 1,4,7 were stained with anti-gamma chain antibodies; 2,5,8 with anti-kappa chain antibodies; 3,6,9 with anti-lambda chain antibodies. Note free kappa and lambda chains (arrow heads) but absence of free gamma chains.

Table 2. Summary of SDS-page immunoblot analysis

	MS (n=14)	CONTROLS (n=14)	COMMENTS
Low MW IgG bands	8/8	0/14	Bands were detected with antiserum to whole IgG
Kappa dimers	10/10	ND	
Kappa monomers	8/10	ND	Bands were
Lambda dimers	10/10	ND	detected with
Lambda monomers	3/10	ND	specific antisera
Free gamma chain	0/10	ND	
Bands reduced with 2-mercaptoethanol	2/2	NA	Suggests dimers of light chain were reduced to monomers
Light chains "released" by treatment with MS CSF	NA	0/3	Controls CSF was incubated with IgG-depleted CSF from MS patients (see text)

ND: not done
NA: not applicable

These studies suggested that free monomers and dimers of light chains of IgG were commonly present in MS CSF. The light chains were likely derived from synthesis and release of unbound light chains rather than from degradation of whole IgG, since free heavy chains were absent and MS CSF failed to "release" free light chains in control CSF.

Charge characteristics of free light chains (Fig. 2-4)

Studies were performed to determine the charge characteristics of free light chains in MS CSF in order to assess charge heterogeneity and for comparison with charge characteristics of whole IgG in the same CSF samples. For these experiments, CSF samples from 9 MS patients were fractionated by chromatography in Sephadex G-200 columns. Figure 2 illustrates a typical experiment. The figure shows the OD280 profile of CSF together with the elution profile of a mixture of Bence-Jones proteins labelled with ^{125}I. The presence of free light chains in the lower molecular weight fractions was confirmed by RIA. The IgG fractions were pooled separately from those containing free light chains. Samples of IgG fractions and light chains fractions were then concentrated and separated in 0.5 mm agarose slab gels containing pH gradients from 3.5-9.5. Proteins were then blotted to nitrocellulose strips, which were stained with antisera specific for kappa, lambda, or gamma chains. In each experiment, unfractionated CSF and unfractionated serum were run as controls. Fig.3 illustrates a typical result, while Fig.4 summarizes the findings. For purposes of analysis, the pH gradients were divided into 3 regions: I - 3.5-6.0; II - 6.1-7.9; III - 8.0-10.0. Fig.3 shows that the alkaline bands of IgG present in whole CSF (lane 3) were also present in the IgG fractions from the column (lane 4). Highly alkaline bands were absent in serum as expected (lane 2). Free kappa chains (lane 6) were more anodal and fewer in number than IgG (lane 5). Free lambda chains (lane 8) were similarly more anodal and more restricted in heterogeneity than IgG (lane 7).

Fig.4. summarizes the results from 9 patients. As is evident from Fig.4, the total number of bands of free light chains was less than the number of IgG bands, and the free light chains were considerably more anodal. There were an average of 13 bands of whole IgG (0% in region I, 63% in region II, and 37% in region III); 8.5 bands of free kappa chains (12% in region I, 79% in region II, and only 9% in region III); and an average of 7.5 bands of free lambda chains (20% in region I, 80% in region II, and 0% in region III).

This study suggests that: 1) free light chains in MS CSF are heterogeneous in charge, suggesting that they are polyclonal in origin; 2) CSF free light chains are neutral to anodal in charge compared with whole IgG from the same CSF sample, suggesting that either the free light chains in CSF are genetically distinct from light chains incorporated into IgG, or that gamma chains contribute the predominant alkaline charge to CSF IgG; and 3) free light chains do not contribute significantly to the alkaline OB pattern observed in MS CSF.

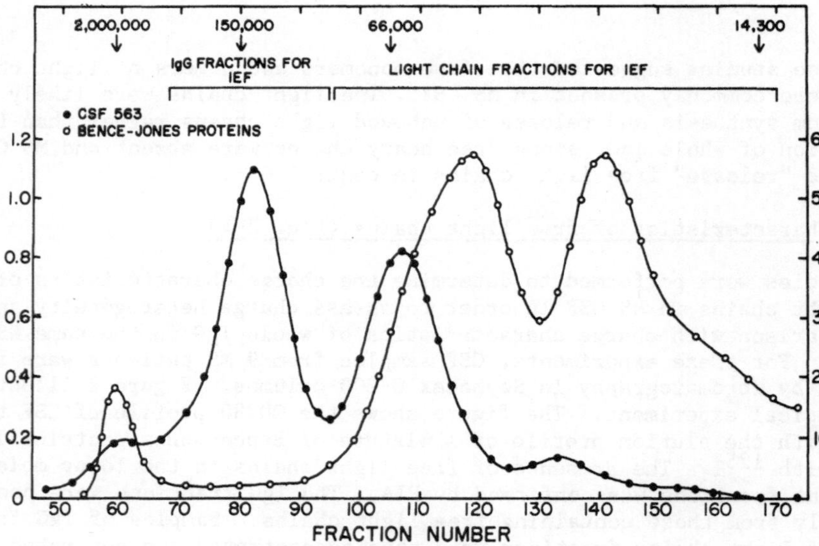

Fig.2. Preparative gel filtration profile of CSF and molecular weight markers. CSF was concentrated and chromatographed in 2.5 x 100 cm Sephadex G-200 column. Fractions containing IgG were pooled separately from fractions containing free light chains for subsequent isoelectric focusing.

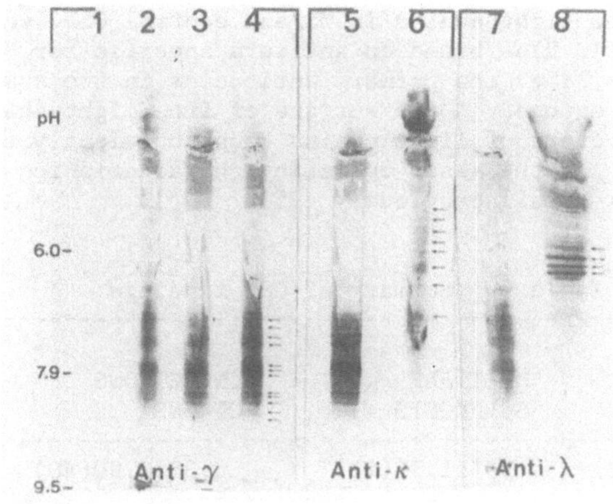

Fig.3. Nitrocellulose blots from IEF gels stained for gamma chains (1-4), kappa chains (5-6), or lambda chains (6-7). Lane 1: light chain fractions; Lane 2: whole serum; Lane 3: whole CSF; Lane 4: IgG fractions; Lane 5,6: IgG fractions, light chains fractions stained for kappa chains; Lane 7,8: IgG fractions, light chain fractions stained for lambda chains. Lane 4 shows cathodal mobility of whole IgG, lane 6 shows relatively anodal mobility of free kappa chains, and lane 8 shows relatively anodal mobility of free lambda chains.

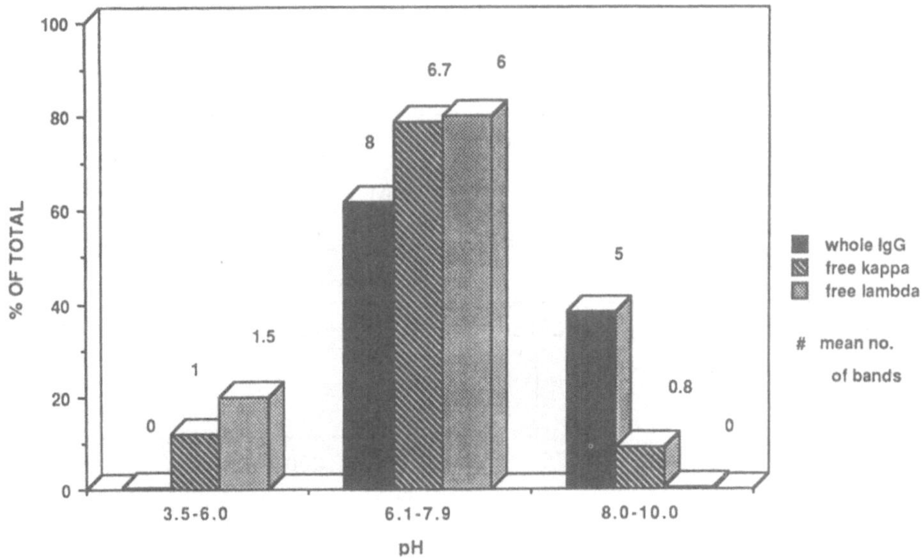

Fig.4. Distribution of charge on whole IgG, free kappa chains and free lambda chains. Note that 15-20% of free light chains focus at pH < 6.0, while only 4% of free kappa chains focus at pH > 8.0.

Immunoassays

To quantify free light chains in MS and control CSF, we developed sensitive and specific RIAs based on antisera specific for "free" but not "bound" light chains, i.e. the primary antibodies in the assays recognized hidden determinants exposed on the surface of free light chains but buried in the tertiary structure of light chains bound covalently to heavy chains. The details of the assay operating characteristics were described above and in greater detail previously (25).

Table 3. Summary of CSF findings

	MULTIPLE SCLEROSIS	INFECTIONS OF CNS	OTHER NEUROLOGIC DISEASES
Free kappa chains (μg/ml)	1.55±1.75(82)*	0.35±0.80(40)	0.07±0.08(25)
	p<.0001		
	p<.0001		
Free lambda chains (μg/ml)	1.02±1.10(51)	0.67±0.92(33)	0.50±0.35(17)
	p =.14		
	p = .06		
Free kappa:Free lambda	2.85±4.79(51)	0.40±0.32(33)	0.18±0.13(17)
	p<.01		
	p = .03		
Free kappa:Albumin ($x\ 10^{-4}$)	106±116(66)	4.4±4.3(31)	3.7±2.9(23)
	p<.0001		
	p<.0001		
IgG:Albumin ($x\ 10^{-2}$)	86±65(66)	23±10(30)	22±8(23)
	p<.0001		
	p<.0001		
IgG (mg %)	12.8±11.2(76)	12.1±17.1(36)	4.8±4.5(29)
	P = .73		
	p<.01		

* Mean ± 1 Std Dev (# Tested)

Table 3 summarizes the results of testing the patients listed in Table 1. MS patients had significantly higher levels of free kappa chains (MS - 1.55 μg/ml; vs infections - 0.35 μg/ml; vs other neurologic diseases - 0.07 μg/ml), free kappa/free lambda ratio (2.85 vs 0.40 vs 0.18); free kappa/albumin ratio (106 x 10^{-4} vs 4.4 x 10^{-4} vs 3.7 x 10^{-4}). Absolute differences between groups were less marked for free lambda chains, IgG, or IgG/albumin ratio, although they were significantly different for the latter parameter.

Ninety percent of the MS patients had kappa chain levels above 0.25 μg/ml, the upper limit of normal defined by the ond group, while only 23% of the patients with infections and 8% of other neurologic diseases had abnormally high levels.

In MS patients, the level of free kappa correlated with the level of whole IgG (regression analysis, r = 0.80) but not well with the IgG synthesis rate (r = 0.61), the IgG index (r = 0.36), or the CSF to serum albumin ratio (r = 0.20). The level of free lambda chains correlated poorly with IgG (r = 0.23). In contrast, free lambda chains correlated well with the IgG concentration in patients with infections (r = 0.80), but kappa chains correlated with IgG poorly in this group (r = 60), suggesting that the IgG response in MS is predominantly IgG , while the IgG response in infections may be predominantly IgG .

Elevated kappa chains correlated with brain lesions by MRI in patients with monosymptomatic optic neuritis (28). In patients with definite MS, the level of free kappa chains was independent of the duration of disease or the presence of remissions, but was higher in patients with MRI lesions (mean 1.66 μg/ml vs 1.05 μg/ml), oligoclonal bands (mean 2.02 μg/ml vs 0.42 μg/ml), and visual evoked potential abnormalities (mean 1.67 μg/ml vs 0.59 μg/ml).

Thus, a selective elevation of free kappa chains in CSF was a consistent and relatively specific abnormality in the MS patients, correlated with brain lesions by MRI, and appeared to have considerable diagnostic value in patients with possible MS.

DISCUSSION

Our studies focused on free kappa and lambda light chains in CSF from MS patients and controls. We found that MS CSF consistently contained free kappa and lambda chains dimers and less commonly monomers, but never contained free heavy chains. Compared with IgG from the same CSF samples, free light chains were somewhat more restricted in charge heterogeneity and considerably less cathodal. Finally, RIA data showed that free kappa chains were increased in MS CSF to a much greater degree than were free lambda chains, and this pattern was relatively specific for MS when compared with infections or other neurological disorders.

The origin of the free light chains is likely to be from intrathecal synthesis rather than from degradation of whole antibody. First, free heavy chains were never observed as would be expected if whole IgG were degraded. Second, free light chains were predominantly in the form of dimers; monomers should have been relatively concentrated if their presence resulted from diffusion from blood. Third, the CSF to serum ratio of free kappa chains was markedly elevated when compared to reference proteins (data not shown, see reference 27 for discussion), and in some instances exceeded 1.0. Finally, there was no relationship between the level of CSF free kappa chains and CSF total protein or the ratio of CSF albumin to serum albumin concentrations. Thus the concentration of free kappa chains was independent of measures that reflect the integrity of the blood-brain barrier.

The exact cell population(s) responsible for synthesis of free light chains is less certain. Cells in CSF, which probably reflect the parenchymal cell population to some extent, have been found to be "activated" by use of flow cytometry techniques (29). Most of these cells appear to be T-lymphocytes bearing receptors for the monoclonal antibody OKT4, but a substantial proportion of activated cells do not bear T-lymphocyte markers (30). Some of these unidentified cells are probably of the B-lymphocyte lineage. Ia^{+} cells, which include mature B cells, have been observed in MS brain at the edge of plaques and in perivascular loci (31). Such activated mature B cells may secrete both free light chains and whole IgG. This likelihood is supported by evidence for increased intrathecal synthesis of whole IgG in MS[2], and by the selective synthesis of both IgG [10] and free kappa chains as reported here.

It is also possible, however, that free light chains in MS derive from immature, defective, or even malignant B-lymphocytes . For example, pre-B cells derived from human fetal liver synthesize free light chains (32), as do malignant pre-B lymphocytes (33), lymphocytes derived from patients with hypogammaglobulinemia (34), and malignant B-cells of patients with multiple myeloma or chronic lymphocytic leukemia (35). The possibility of defective or transformed B-lymphocytes that has been postulated to occur in MS (36) has not been ruled out by the studies reported here.

It seems most likely that free light chains represent the activity of an intensely stimulated mature B cell population, and therefore may reflect the intensity of the underlying immune response. In the MS patients included in this study, free light chains accounted for a significant proportion of the intrathecal immunoglobulin synthesis, being approximately 6% of the whole IgG in relative molar concentration. This may be explained by a more rapid rate of light chain relative to heavy chain synthesis resulting in the release of both intact immunoglobulin molecules and free light chains. Experimental evidence in support of this concept has been reported (37, 38, 39). Additional descriptive studies have documented excess free light chains in blood of patients with a variety of conditions characterized by increased synthesis of immunoglobulins such as benign monoclonal gammopathy (35) and systemic dysimmune diseases (40). Thus, the presence of free light chains may be an accurate index of an ongoing intrathecal humoral immune response in MS. To the extent that the severity of disease relates to the intensity of this response, measures of free light chains may be potentially useful for predicting progression. Further studies will be required to assess this important issue.

Although the cause of selective kappa chain synthesis is unclear, several possibilities seem plausible. First, the nature of the immunological stimulus may influence the light chain isotype of the induced antibodies. Thymus-dependent antibody responses may preferentially evoke an immunoglobulin-kappa (Ig) response (41), while thymus-independent antigens induce a predominant immunoglobulin-lambda (Ig) response (42). The IgG response to thymus-dependent antigens may require T-lymphocyte participation (43). Thus, light chain isotype predominance may be determined by the nature of the antigenic stimulus. Alternatively, kappa chain predominance may be caused by genetic factors. For example, SJL mice express low levels of lambda light chains due to the presence of a regulatory gene (44). Finally, selective kappa chain expression may be associated with selective expression of heavy chain isotypes (3) or allotypes (4), which have been reported in MS CSF. This phenomenon has been demonstrated in mice (45) and humans (46).

Partly because the cause of kappa predominance is unclear, the biological significance of free kappa chain synthesis in MS is also uncertain. It seems unlikely, however, that free light chains are themselves pathogenic. Free light chains from antibodies of known specificity have been shown to bind antigen with extremely low affinities (47, 48, 49), and although Bence Jones proteins may be pathogenic to renal tubular epithelial cells, the intracellular concentration within the CNS seems unlikely to approach than in the renal tubule of myeloma patients.

The principal practical significance of this observation is the potential diagnostic value of the measurement of free kappa chains (25). Most IgG assays suffer from their nonspecificity. For example, oligoclonal bands have been observed in a variety of patients with diseases other than MS (50, 51), and various quantitative measures of IgG have likewise been noted to be nonspecific (52, 53), compared with our findings. Analyses of the relative value of various methods for IgG analysis, including free kappa chains, will require that multiple assays be used to test the same CSF samples. Such studies are currently ongoing. Our studies to date, however, suggest that the finding of increased CSF levels of free kappa chains is relatively specific for MS.

ACKNOWLEDGEMENTS

Supported by US PHS grant numbers NS00791 & NS20303. The excellent technical assistance of Christina Brown and Martha Miller is gratefully acknowledged.

REFERENCES

1. R.A. Rudick. Humoral immunity in multiple sclerosis: Clinical and investigative aspects. Sem. Neurol. 5:107-116 (1985).
2. W.W. Tourtellotte, A.R. Potvin and J.O. Fleming. Multiple sclerosis: Measurement and validation of central nervous system IgG synthesis rate. Neurology. 30:240-244 (1980).
3. B. Vandvik, J.B. Natvig and D. Wiger. IgG1 subclass restriction of oligoclonal IgG from cerebrospinal fluids and brain extracts in patients with multiple sclerosis and subacute encephalitides. Scan. J. Immunol. 5:427-436 (1976).
4. J.P. Salier, J.M. Goust, J.P. Pandey and H.H. Fudenberg. Preferential synthesis of the G1m(1) allotype of IgG1 in the central nervous system of multiple sclerosis patients. Science. 213:1400-1402 (1981).
5. T.G. Tachovsky, M. Sandberg-Wollheim and L.G. Baird. Rabbit anti-human CSF IgG. I. Characterization of anti-idiotype antibodies produced against MS CSF and detection of cross-reactive idiotypes in several MS CSF. J. Immunol. 129:764-770 (1982).
6. H. Link and R. Muller. Immunoglobulins in multiple sclerosis and infections of the nervous system. Arch. Neurol. 25:326-344 (1971).
7. F. Bollengier, P. Delmotte and A. Lowenthal. Biochemical findings in multiple sclerosis. III. Immunoglobulins of restricted heterogeneity and light chain distribution in cerebrospinal fluid of patients with multiple sclerosis. J. Neurol. 212:151-158 (1976).
8. K.P.Johnson, S.C. Arrigo, B.J. Nelson and A. Ginsberg. Agarose electrophoresis of cerebrospinal fluid in multiple sclerosis. Neurol. 27:173-191 (1977).
9. M.J. Walsh, W.W. Tourtellotte, J. Roman and W. Dreyer. Immunoglobulin G, A, and M -Clonal restriction in multiple sclerosis cerebrospinal fluid and serum - Analysis by two-dimensional electrophoresis. Clin. Immunol. Immunopath. 35:313-327 (1985).

10. H. Link and O. Zetterval. Multiple sclerosis: Disturbed kappa: Lambda chain ratio of immunoglobulin G in cerebrospinal fluid. Clin. Exp. Immunol. 6:435-438 (1970).
11. J.E. Olsson and H. Link. Immunoglobulin abnormalities in multiple sclerosis. Arch. Neurol. 28:392-399 (1973).
12. F. Bollengier, A. Lowenthal and W. Henrotin. Bound and free light chains in subacute sclerosing panencephalitis and multiple sclerosis serum and cerebrospinal fluid. J. Clin. Chem. Clin. Biochem. 13: 305-310 (1975).
13. F. Bollengier, N. Rabinovitch and A. Lowenthal. Oligoclonal immunoglobulins, light chain ratios and free light chains in cerebrospinal fluid and serum from patients affected with various neurological diseases. J. Clin. Chem. Clin. Biochem. 16:165-173 (1978).
14. D.H. Matson, R.P. Roos, J.E. Hopper and B.G.W. Arnason. Light chain composition of CSF oligoclonal IgG bands in multiple sclerosis and subacute sclerosing panencephalitis. J. Neuroimmunol. 3:63-76 (1982).
15. B. Vandvik. Oligoclonal IgG and free light chains in the cerebrospinal fluid of patients with multiple sclerosis and infectious diseases of the central nervous system. Scand. J. Immunol. 6:913-922 (1977).
16. M.A. Laurenzi, M. Mavra, S. Kam-Hansen and H. Link. Oligoclonal IgG and free light chains in multiple sclerosis demonstrated by thin-layer polyacrylamide gel isoelectric focusing and immunofixation. Ann. Neurol. 8:241-247 (1980).
17. J.M. Perini, J. Lebas, P. Roussel and G. Biserte. Evidence for heterogeneous or incomplete immunoglobulins in oligoclonal CSF studied by electroimmunofixation. Clin. Chim. Acta. 96:205-214 (1979).
18. C.M. Poser, D.W. Paty, L. Scheinberg, W.I. McDonald, F.A. Davis, G.C. Ebers, K.P. Johnson, W.A. Sibley, D.H. Silberberg and W.W. Tourtellotte. New diagnostic criteria for multiple sclerosis: Guidelines for research protocols. Ann. Neurol. 13:227-232 (1983).
19. A.S. Rose, G.W. Ellison, L.W. Myers and W.W. Tourtellotte. Criteria for the clinical diagnosis of multiple sclerosis. Neurol. 26(2): 20-22 (1976).
20. W.W. Tourtellotte, B. Tavolato, J.A. Parker and P. Comiso. Cerebrospinal fluid electroimmunodiffusion. An easy, rapid, sensitive, reliable, and valid method for the simultaneous determination of immunoglobulin-G and albumin. Arch. Neurol. 25:345-350 (1971).
21. O.H. Lowry, N.J. Rosenbrough, A.L. Far and R.J. Randall. Protein measurement with Folin phenol reagent. J. Biol. Chem. 193:265-275 (1951).
22. K.P. Johnson, S.C. Arriogo, B.J. Nelson and A. Ginsberg. Agarose electrophoresis of cerebrospinal fluid in multiple sclerosis. Neurol. 27:273-191 (1977).
23. V.K. Laemmli and M. Favre. Maturation of head of bacteriophage-T4 1. DNA packaging events. J. Mol. Biol. 80:575-579 (1973).
24. H. Towbin, T. Staehelin and J. Gordon. Electrophoretic transfer of proteins from polyacrylamide gels to nitrocellulose sheets: Procedure and some applications. Proc. Natl. Acad. Sci. USA. 76:4350-4354 (1979).
25. R.A. Rudick, A. Pallant, J.M. Bidlack and R.M. Herndon. Free kappa chains in multiple sclerosis spinal fluid. Ann. neurol. In press.
26. P.J. McConhahey and F.J. Dixon. A method of trace iodination of protein for in vivo studies. Int. Arch. Allergy Appl. Immunol. 29:185-189 (1966).
27. R.A. Rudick, D.M. Peter, J.M. Bidlack and D.W. Knutson. Multiple sclerosis: Free light chains in cerebrospinal fluid. Neurol. 35: 1443-1449 (1985).

28. R.A. Rudick, L. Jacobs, P. Kinkle and W. Kinkle. Analysis of free kappa light chains in CSF of patients with monosymptomatic optic neuritis. Correlation with nuclear magnetic resonance imaging findings. Arch. Neurol. In press.
29. A. Noronha, D.P. Richman and B.G.W. Arnason. Detection of in vivo stimulated cerebrospinal fluid lymphocytes by flow cytometry in patients with multiple sclerosis. N. Engl. J. Med. 303:713-717 (1980).
30. A. Noronha, D.P. Richman and B.G.W. Arnason. Multiple sclerosis: activated cells in cerebrospinal fluid in acute exacerbations. Ann. Neurol. 18:722-725 (1985).
31. U. Traugott, E.L. Reinherz and C.S. Raine. Multiple sclerosis. Distribution of T cells, T cell subsets, and Ia-positive macrophages in lesions of different ages. J. Neuroimmunol. 4:201-221 (1983).
32. A.C. Hannam-Harris and J.L. Smith. Free immunoglobulin light chain synthesis by human foetal liver and cord blood lymphocytes. Immunol. 43:417-423 (1981).
33. A.C. Hannam-Harris, J. Gordon and J.L.Smith. Immunoglobulin synthesis by neoplastic B lymphocytes: Free light chain synthesis as a marker of B cell differentiation. J. Immunol. 125:2177-2181 (1980).
34. J. Gordon and J.L. Smith. Free immunoglobulin light chain synthesis by lymphocytes from patients with hypogammaglobulinaemia. Clin. Exp. Immunol. 34:288-294 (1978).
35. F. Dammaco and J. Waldenstrom. Serum and urine light chain levels in benign monoclonal gammopathies, multiple myeloma and Waldenstrom's macroglobulinemia. Clin. Exp. Immunol. 3:911-921 (1968).
36. R.P. Roos. B-cell abnormalities in multiple sclerosis. A hypothesis. Arch. Neurol. 42:73-75 (1985).
37. K. Solling. Free light chains of immunoglobulins. Scand. J. Clin. Lab. Invest. 41[Suppl.157]: 1-84 (1981).
38. J. Gordon and J.L. Smith. Free immunoglobulin light chain synthesis by lymphocytes from patients with hypogammaglobulinemia. Clin. Exp. Immunol. 34:288-294 (1978).
39. A.L. Shapiro, M.D. Scharff, J.V. Maizel and J.W. Uhr. Synthesis of excess light chains of gamma globulin by rabbit lymph node cells. Nature. 211:243-245 (1966).
40. H.M. Moutsopoulos, A.D. Steinberg, A.S. Fauci, H.C. Lane and N.H. Papadopoulos. High incidence of free monoclonal lambda light chains in the sera of patients with Sjogren's syndrome. J. Immunol. 130: 2663-2665 (1983).
41. L.C. Burkly, R. Zaugg, H.N. Eisen and H.H. Wortis. Influence of nude and X-linked immune deficiency genes on expression of kappa and lambda light chains. Eur. J. Immunol. 12:1033-1039 (1982).
42. S.T. Ju and M.E. Dorf. Preferential induction of specific lambda isotypic antibodies in mice. J. Immunol. 133:1404-1409 (1984).
43. L.C. Burkly and H.H. Wortis. T cell regulation of light chain expression: Preferential enhancement of Ig production by T cells in the response to DNP. J. Immunol. 135:1577-1581 (1985).
44. N. Geckeler, J. Faversham and M. Cohn. On a regulatory gene controlling the expression of murine lambda light chain. J. Exp. Med. 148:1122-1136 (1978).
45. R.J. Fulton, M. Nahm and J.M. Davie. Monoclonal antibodies to streptococcal group A carbohydrate. II. The $Vk1^{GAC}$ light chain is preferentially associated with serum IgG3. J. Immunol. 131:1326-1331 (1983).
46. H. Kubagawa, M. Mayumi, W. Crist and M. Cooper. Immunoglobulin heavy-chain switching and pre-B leukemias. Nature. 301:340-344 (1983).

47. R.G. Painter, H.J. Sage and C. Tanford. Contributions of heavy and light chains of rabbit immunogl
ding studies on isolated heavy and light chains. Biochem. 11:1327-1337 (1972).
48. G.T. Stevenson. The binding of haptens by the polypeptide chains of rabbit antibody molecules. Biochem. J. 133:827-838 (1973).
49. A.B. Edmundson, K.R. Ely, R.L. Girling, E.E. Abola, M. Schiffer, F.A. Westholdm, M.D. Fausch and H.F. Deutsch. Binding of 2,4-dinitrophenyl compounds and other small molecules to a crystalline lambda-type Bence-Jones dimer. Biochem. 13:3816-3827 (1974).
50. B. Rostrom and H. Link. Oligoclonal immunoglobulins in cerebrospinal fluid in acute cerebrovascular disease. Neurol. 31:590-596 (1981).
51. J.R. Miller, A.M. Burke and C.T. Bever. Occurrence of oligoclonal bands in multiple sclerosis and other CNS diseases. Ann. Neurol. 13:53-58 (1983).
52. J.T. Caroscio, S. Kochwa, H. Sacks, J.A. Cohen and M.D. Yahr. Quantitative CSF IgG measurements in multiple sclerosis and other neurologic diseases. Arch. neurol. 40:409-413 (1983).
53. L.A. Hershey and J.L. Trotter. The use and abuse of the cerebrospinal fluid IgG profile in the adult: A practical evaluation. Ann.Neurol. 8:426-434 (1980).

CEREBROSPINAL FLUID COMPLEMENT COMPONENTS IN MULTIPLE SCLEROSIS

D.A.S. Compston, B.P. Morgan, and
A.K. Campbell

Departments of Neurology and Medical Biochemistry
University of Wales College of Medicine, Heath Park
Cardiff CF4 4XN, U.K.

The physical basis for symptoms, and factors which determine the clinical course in patients with multiple sclerosis (MS) are not well understood. The disease is relapsing during the early stages in 90% of patients, and progressive form onset in the remainder; eventually, up to 80% of patients become disabled to some extent. The major clinical factor determining disability is onset of the progressive phase so that at some stage approximately 60% of patients switch from a relapsing to a progressive course. The development of benign or severe MS may depend more on strategic placement of lesions than on differences in the underlying disease process. The available evidence suggests that the switch to chronic progression depends on the volume of disease in a given part, and occurs when the capacity for synaptic re-organisation, redundancy in affected pathways and other mechanisms of recovery are exhausted.

Despite rapid onset and spontaneous recovery of symptoms expected early in the course, pathologically there is an orderly progression from the perivenous infiltration by inflammatory cells, without myelin breakdown seen in the earliest lesions to myelinolysis, astrocytosis and oligodendrocyte depletion with sparse remyelination observed as plaques evolve. Immunological, imaging and electrophysiological evidence indicates that the disease is more active even in the early stages than the clinical method would suggest. Aetiological factors thought to be involved in the cascade of events leading to myelin damage include environmental events, genetic susceptibility and perturbations in the immune system involving numbers and function of circulating B/T lymphocytes and intrathecal IgG synthesis. Several lines of evidence suggest that the sequence of events may not be the same in all cases and provide evidence for heterogeneity in the pathogenesis of MS. But at some stage the early events must converge and damage myelin through a final common pathway which results in the symptoms and signs by which the disease is defined. Taken together, this indicates that a mechanism of myelin injury is likely to exist which stops short of myelin breakdown. Disease activity, expressed clinically or silent, might then not be due to demyelination at all. Any proposed mechanisms would need to account for rapid onset or recovery of symptoms and be consistent with continuous disease activity despite the intermittent time course of MS. Tissue injury mediated by the complement system fulfills the criteria for a final common pathway of myelin injury occurring in the context of local inflammation, activated non-specifically and capable of causing transient cell damage or alternatively cytolysis depending on threshold events and so providing a conceptual basis for clinicopathological correlations in the central nervous system (CNS) in MS. In formulating this hypothesis, account has been taken of observations specific to MS, and unrelated experimental systems outside the nervous system. The putative mechanisms described are not likely to be the only cause of myelin injury; other cytopathic processes might co-exist and contribute to tissue damage.

The complement cascade involves information of the membrane attack complex (MAC) resulting from the sequential addition of components C5-C9 to C3b, the product of C3 conversion. This latter step itself depends either on activation of the classical pathway by complement-fixing IgG or IgM antibodies often aggregated as immune complexes, or the alternate pathway by polysaccharides. Either can be initiated in other ways and myelin is capable of complement activation by both the classical and alternate pathways (Cyong et al., 1982; Silberberg et al., 1985). The usual consequence of MAC formation on nucleated cells is lysis but under certain conditions a variety of non-lytic and reversible events may occur. There is a large electrochemical gradient of calcium across the cell membrane; damage to a nucleated cell leads initially to a rapid rise in intracellular free calcium and a fall in ATP followed by activation of phospholipases and proteinases together with other changes in the cell and its membrane (Campbell, 1983). These events are all reversible up to a critical threshold point, after which irreversible damage and cell death occur. It has been shown that sub-lytic amounts of the MAC cause a transient rise in intracellular free calcium (Campbell and Luzio, 1981) which in turn, activates metabolic processes within the cell (Hallett et al., 1981; Hallett and Campbell, 1982) and initiates recovery mechanisms (Campbell and Morgan 1985) leading to removal of the potentially lethal MAC by vesiculation and endocytosis (Morgan and Campbell, 1985; Morgan et al., 1986). Inhibitors of the recovery mechanisms have been shown to increase the number of cells reaching the lytic threshold, thereby increasing cell lysis (Edwards et al., 1983; Roberts et al., 1985). T cell mediated cell injury may employ similar mechanisms through the use of cytolysins (Lachmann, 1983, Ward and Lachmann, 1985).

Involvement of complement in disease can be inferred from alterations in concentration of individual components, detection of unstable activation products or from functional tests which involve part of, or the entire, cascade such as the CH50. Despite consumption, the concentration of early components may even rise as a result of local re-synthesis, along with other acute phase proteins. IgG synthesized intrathecally in patients with MS is complement fixing (Ryberg, 1982) and immune complexes can be detected in their CNS (Tachovsky et al., 1976; Coyle et al., 1980). Cerebrospinal fluid concentrations of C2 and C3 are normal and C4 slightly reduced in patients with MS; C3 and C4 activation products are not detectable (Yam et al., 1980; Delasnerie-Laupretre et al., 1982; Jans et al., 1984). The late components are synthesized predominantly in the liver but probably not by cells found in the CNS and have a lower normal concentration. Because of the amplification inherent in the complement cascade, more terminal component molecules are involved in the activation process, leading to significant consumption and measurable changes in their concentration in biological fluids.

Concentrations of the terminal component of complement (C9) have been measured in CSF from patients with MS (Morgan et al., 1984) and isolated demyelinating lesions (Compston et al., 1986a) using an automated 2 site immunoradiometric assay with an absolute sensitivity of 10 ng/ml and working range of 50-2000 ng/ml (Morgan et al., 1983) and are shown in Fig.1. The concentration of any protein detected in CSF will be influenced by plasma concentration, and changes in blood-brain barrier permeability will result in over-estimation of IgG synthesis or under-estimation of complement consumption if CSF concentrations alone are used for assessment. This potential source of error can in part be corrected by calculating an index derived from the ratios of complement components to albumin in plasma and cerebrospinal fluid, analogous to the IgG index (Lefvert and Link, 1985).

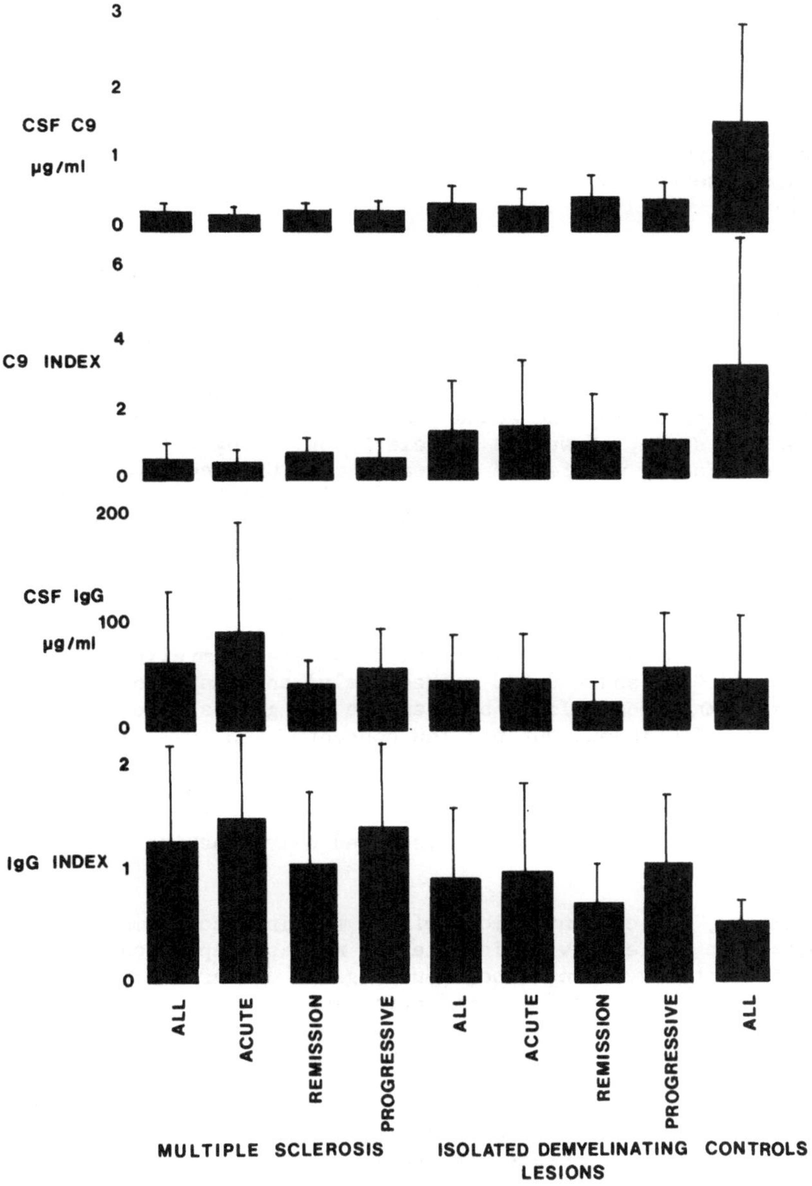

Fig.1. Cerebrospinal fluid concentrations (± standard deviation) of C9 and IgG together with C9 and IgG indices in patients with multiple sclerosis and isolated demyelinating lesions depending on disease activity, compared with controls; for numbers, see text.

Fifty one patients with MS of whom 48 had clinically definite disease were studied; C9, IgG and albumin were measured in CSF and plasma in 14 patients during relapse. These measurements were made during remission in 19 patients and during the progressive phase in 18. C9 and IgG idices were then derived and compared with results in 73 patients without MS including 33 who were considered to be neurologically normal. CSF C9 concentration was lower in all MS patients than controls ($p < 0.00001$); this reduction was seen in acute or progressive phases of the disease and during remission ($p < 0.00001$ for each comparison). This accounted for the lower C9 index observed in MS patients than controls ($p < 0.00001$), which was also present in acute or progressive cases and those in remission ($p < 0.00001$ for each comparison). Other variables from which the C9 index was derived, did not differ between cases and controls. Others have since confirmed this reduction in CSF C9 in MS patients (Sanders et al., 1985). Conversely, mean CSF IgG concentration was higher in all MS patients than controls ($p < 0.0001$); this increase was seen in patients with acute and progressive MS ($P < 0.003$ and < 0.0008) but not those in remission. Mean IgG index was higher in all MS patients than controls ($p < 0.00001$); the increase was observed during acute or progressive phases and in remission ($p < 0.001$).

Having demonstrated reciprocal alterations in C9 and IgG indices in patients with MS which do not depend on disease activity at the time of sampling, 40 patients with isolated demyelinating episodes affecting the optic nerve (6) brain stem (7) or spinal cord (27) were then investigated. More than one site was affected in 2 patients; episodes affecting the spinal cord followed an identified infection in 4 patients. Nineteen individuals were studied during the acute phase, 5 in remission and 16 during the progressive stage, of whom 8 had electrophysiological abnormalities present in clinically unaffected pathways. CSF C9 concentration was lower in all patients with isolated demyelinating lesions than controls ($p < 0.00001$); this reduction was seen in individuals with acute, progressive or stable isolated lesions ($p < 0.003$) for each comparison. C9 index was lower in patients with isolated demyelinating lesions than controls ($p < 0.00001$). The reduction was observed in acute or progressive cases and those in remission ($p < 001$, .001 and .02 respectively). C9 concentration and C9 index were higher in patients with isolated demyelinating lesions than in MS ($p < 0.05$ and < 0.003 respectively) and there were significant differences in many comparisons between the two groups categorised by disease activity. IgG index, but not IgG concentration, was higher in all patients with isolated demyelinating lesions than controls ($p < 0.001$) and this increase was present in individuals with acute and progressive lesions ($p < 0.02$ and < 0.002) but not cases in remission. IgG index was higher in all patients with MS than isolated demyelinating lesions ($p < 0.03$).

In summary, CSF concentrations of the terminal complement component C9 were lower in patients with isolated or multiple episodes of demyelination than in controls having other neurological diseases. The reduced CSF C9 concentration accounted for a reduction in C9 index. The C9 index was lower in MS patients than in cases with isolated demyelinating lesions. C9 indices were abnormal irrespective of disease activity in each group of patients with demyelination.

These findings are consistent with the hypothesis that activation of the complement cascade occurs in the central nervous system in patients with demyelinating disease. The fact that the changes are present even during the first clinically detectable episode suggests that this is not merely a consequence of tissue damage. In order to provide further evidence that the reduction in CSF terminal complement component concentration reflects activation and consumption of C9 in the CNS of patients with demyelination, attempts were then made to localize C9 in fresh frozen white matter from two patients with MS obtained at autopsy compared with tissue removed at craniotomy from 3 patients with other neurological diseases and from one patient without CNS disease (myasthenia gravis) obtained at autopsy, using an immunoperoxidase method (Jasani et al., 1986) which incorporates the same high affinity monoclonal antibody used in the immunoradiometric assay. Perivascular adventitial granular staining of C9 was present in the CNS of both patients with MS, but none of the controls (Fig.2); staining of glial cells and neurones was also observed, but unlike the vascular staining, this may not be disease specific. Staining in MS tissue was most marked in areas within or surrounding moderately recent plaques although some morphologically normal tissue was also affected. C9 was demonstrated in vessels of all sizes including small capillaries. The dense granular staining in blood vessels was almost completely blocked by pre-incubation of monoclonal antibody C9-47 with purified C9 (Compston et al., 1986b). Immunolocalisation of C9 in and around plaques is not necessarily due to MAC formation since antibody C9-47 binds to C9 in both the free and membrane-bound state. However, free C9 is normally present in small quantities in plasma and CSF and the concentration is not increased in either compartment in patients with MS (see above) so that vascular staining is unlikely to be present unless MAC formation had occurred. If C9 is present in association with membrane attack complexes, the possibility exists that these are themselves part of vesicles containing myelin damaged by complement activation and MAC formation, extruded from affected areas as part of a repair process.

Further indirect evidence implicating C9 in the pathogenesis of MS is derived from changes observed during treatment. In a double-blind placebo controlled trial of high-dose intravenous methylprednisolone (Milligan et al., 1986), acute and chronic symptoms improved in actively treated patients and in most the effect was achieved within one week of starting treatment, suggesting that corticosteroids influence rapidly reversible mechanisms of myelin injury. There were simultaneous alterations in CSF cell count, IgG and C9 indices and the percentage of peripheral blood OKT8 positive cells all of which were abnormal at entry; and returned closer to the normal range after active than placebo treatment (Compston et al., 1986c). The most significant effect of methylprednisolone was on the C9 index which increased to 68.7% more than expected on placebo treatment ($p < 0.06$). This finding is consistent with inhibition of intrathecal complement activation. The earliest event after complement injury on cells exposed to the MAC is a rise in intracellular calcium and in the special situation of partially demyelinated axons, this would be expected temporarily to interfere with the propogation of nerve impulses (Bostock and McDonald, 1982). It has recently been demonstrated that conduction in the CNS, reflected by latency of visual evoked potentials, improves in patients with MS during infusion of the calcium channel blocker Verapamil (Gilmore et al., 1985). High-dose intravenous methylprednisolone might achieve similar but less immediate effects by inhibiting complement activation, thereby preventing transient changes in the calcium ion environment of myelinated axons. There is additional evidence to suggest that changes in intracellular calcium might be important in generating both reversible and irreversible myelin injury in demyelinating disease. Vesicular disruption of the myelin membrane has been observed after exposure to a calcium ionophore (Schlaepfer, 1977); the effects are calcium dependent but not necessarily associated with irreversible damage to the myelinating cell (Smith et al., 1985).

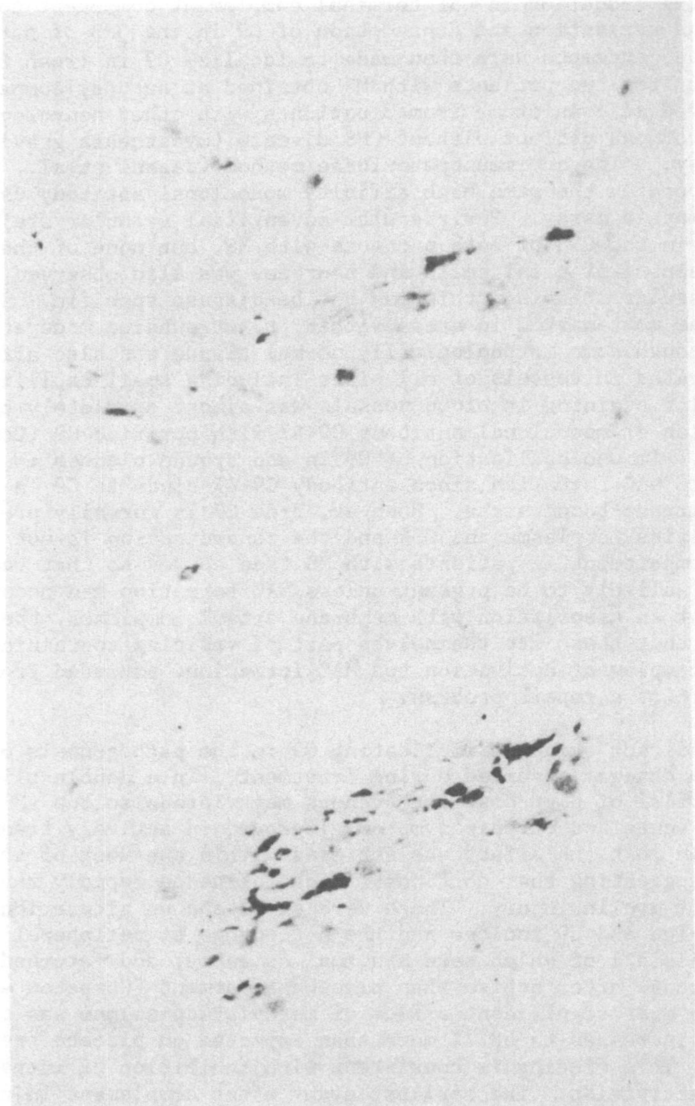

Fig.2. Vascular staining with monoclonal antibody C9-47 in affected white matter from a patient with multiple sclerosis (A) and after preincubation of C9-47 with purified C9 (B).

Although the evidence is consistent with the hypothesis that activation of the complement cascade occurs in the CNS in patients with demyelinating disease, apparently unrelated immunological events undoubtedly occur which may be required for activation of the complement system, independently cytopathic or epiphenomenal. But since myelin itself can activate the complement cascade, through either the alternate or classical pathway, minor degrees of myelin damage could then generate further complement activation irrespective of the cause and thereby amplifying tissue damage. Membrane attack complexes are required for antibody-mediated demyelination of mouse cerebellar explant cultures (Liu et al., 1983) and can themselves, be recovered from rat brain myelin membrane treated with serum complement (Silverman et al., 1984). The area over which these MACs are deposited will be influenced by local availability of C7 since one the C5/6 complex, which is stable and can diffuse away from the activation site without becoming membrane-bound binds C7 the new C5/6 complex is fixed to membrane or rapidly inactivated (Lachmann and Thompson, 1970). The formation of MACs distributed over a wide area, even in response to myelin injury, provides a mechanism for amplifying local tissue damage. However, C9 consumption occurs at times when there is no clinical evidence for demyelination and is not strictly related to the number of sites affected clinically but occurs both in patients with MS and isolated demyelinating lesions. These immunological and clinical findings can be explained by postulating that in demyelination, two types of lesion exist. First there are areas where membrane attack complexes have formed in sufficient concentration irreversibly to damage the membrane causing morphological changes; depending on their anatomical distribution, these lesions, the equivalent of plaques, would produce fixed symptoms or electrophysiological and imaging abnormalities. The second type of lesion would occur in areas where membrane attack complexes have produced a variety of non-lytic effects associated with changes in calcium ion concentrations and resulting either in no symptoms or transient clinical abnormalities with the potential for full recovery. The two types of lesion might co-exist the latter forming a penumbra around plaques and many patients with demyelination do complain of temporary fluctuation in their pre-existing symptoms. Elsewhere, chronic active membrane damage might occur giving rise to no symptoms but nevertheless accounting for persistent immunological and other abnormalities. Non-lytic lesions may considerably outnumber areas of plaque formation in many patients with demyelination, from the earliest clinically identificable stage.

ACKNOWLEDGEMENT

The authors thank Drs. B. Jasani and P. Wilkins for carrying out the histological studies.

REFERENCES

1. H. Bostock and W.I. McDonald. Recovery and function after demyelination. In: Neuronal-glial cell interrelationships. T.A. Sears, ed. Springer-Verlag, Berlin. 287-302 (1982).
2. A.K. Campbell. Intracellular calcium; its universal role as regulator. Chichester: John Wiley and Sons. (1983).
3. A.K. Campbell and J.P. Lucio. Intracellular free calcium as a pathogen in cell damage initiated by the immune system. Experientia. 37: 1110-1112 (1981).
4. A.K. Campbell and B.P. Morgan. Monoclonal antibodies demonstrate protection of polymorphonuclear leycocytes against complement attack. Nature. 317:164-166.
5. D.A.S. Compston, B.P. Morgan, D. Oleesky, R. Fifield and A.K. Campbell. Cerebrospinal fluid C9 in demyelinating disease. Neurology. In press (1986a).
6. D.A.S. Compston, P. Wilkins, G. Cole, B. Jasani and A.K. Campbell. CNS immunolocalisation of C9 in multiple sclerosis. (submitted for publication) (1986b).
7. D.A.S. Compston, N.M. Milligan, P.J. Hughes, J. Gibbs, V. McBroom, B.P. Morgan and A.K. Campbell. A double blind controlled trial of high dose methylprednisolone in patients with multiple sclerosis. 2. Laboratory results. (submitted for publication) (1986c).

8. P.K. Coyle, R.L. Hirsch, P. O'Donnell, B.R. Brooks, S.R. Cohen, R.T. Johnson and J.S. Wolinsky. Cerebrospinal-fluid lymphocyte populations and immune complexes in active multiple sclerosis. Lancet. ii:229-232 (1980).
9. J.C. Cyong, S.S. Witkin, B. Reiger, E. Barbarese, R.A. Good and N.K. Day. Antibody-independent complement activation by myelin via the classical complement pathway. J. Exp. Med. 155:587-598 (1982).
10. N. Delasnerie-Laupretre, C. Suet-Hubert and A. Marcelli-Barge. Cerebrospinal fluid C2 and HLA system in multiple sclerosis. Tissue antigens. 19:79-84 (1982).
11. S.W. Edwards, B.P. Morgan, T.G. Hay, J.P. Luzio and A.K. Campbell. Complement mediated lysis of pigeon erythrocyte ghosts analysed by flow cytometry. Evidence for involvment of a threshold phenomenon. Biochem. J. 206:195-202 (1983).
12. R.L. Gilmore, E.J. Kasarkis and R.G. McAllister. Verapamil-induced changes in central conduction in patients with multiple sclerosis. J.N.N.P. 48:1140-1146 (1985).
13. M.B. Hallett, J.P. Luzio and A.K. Campbell. Stimulation of Ca^{2+} -dependent chemiluminescence in rat polymorphonuclear leucocytes by polystyrene beads and the non-lytic action of complement. Immunology. 44:569-576 (1981).
14. M.B. Hallett and A.K. Campbell. Measurement of changes in cytoplasmic free calcium in fused cell hybrids. Nature. 295:155-157 (1982).
15. H. Jans, A. Heltberg, I. Zeeberg, J. Halkjaer-Kristensen, T. Fog and N.E. Raun. Immune complexes and the complement factors C4 and C3 in cerebrospinal fluid and serum from patients with chronic progressive multiple sclerosis. Acta Neurol. Scand. 69:34-38 (1984).
16. B. Jasani, N.D. Thomas, D.W. Wynford-Thomas and G.R. Newman. Non deleterious inhibition of endogenous peroxidase. Histochemical J. In press (1986).
17. P.J. Lachmann. Are complement lysis and lymphocytotoxicity analogous? Nature. 305:473-474 (1983).
18. P.J. Lachmann and R.A. Thompson. Reactive lysis: the complement-mediated lysis of unsensitised cells. II. The characterization of activated reactor as C56 and the participation of C8 and C9. J. Exp. Med. 131:643-657 (1970).
19. A.K. Lefvert and H. Link. IgG production within the central nervous system: a critical review of proposed formulae. Ann. Neurol. 17:13-20 (1985).
20. W.T. Liu, P. Vanguir and M.L. Shin. Studies on demyelination in vitro: the requirement of membrane attack complex components of the complement system. J. Immunol. 131:778-782 (1983).
21. N.M. Milligan and D.A.S. Compston. A double blind controlled trial of high dose intravenous methylprednisolone in patients with multiple sclerosis: clinical effects. (submitted for publication) (1986).
22. B.P. Morgan, A.K. Campbell, J.P. Luzio and K. Siddle. Immunoradiometric assay for human complement component C9 utilising monoclonal antibodies. Clin. Chim. Acta. 134:85-94 (1983).
23. B.P. Morgan, A.K. Campbell and D.A.S. Compston. Terminal component of complement (C9) in cerebrospinal fluid of patients with multiple sclerosis. Lancet. ii:251-254 (1984).
24. B.P. Morgan and A.K. Campbell. The recovery of human polymorphonuclear leucocytes from sub lytic complement attack is mediated by changes in intracellular free calcium. Biochem. J. 231:205-208 (1985).
25. B.P. Morgan, J.R. Dankert and A.F. Esser. Recovery of human neutrophils from complement attack. Removal of the membrane attack complex by endocytosis and exocytosis. J. Immunol. In press (1986).

26. P.A. Roberts, J. Knight and A.K. Campbell. 2 chloradenosine inhibits complement induced reactive oxygen metabolite production and recovery of human polymorphonuclear leucocytes from complement attack. Biochem. Biophys. Res. Comm. 126:692-697 (1985).
27. B. Ryberg. Antibrain antibodies in multiple sclerosis. J. Neurol. Sci. 54:239-261 (1982).
28. M.E. Sanders, C.L. Koski, D. Robbins, M.L. Shin, E.L. Alexander, M.M. Frank and K.A. Joiner. Detection of activated terminal complement in cerebrospinal fluid. Complement. 2:68 (abs. 196) (1985).
29. W.W. Schlaepfer. Vesicular disruption of myelin stimulated by exposure of nerve to calcium ionophore. Nature. 265:734-736 (1977).
30. D.H. Silberberg, M.C. Manning and A.D. Schreiber. Tissue culture demyelination by normal human serum. Ann. Neurol. 15:575-580 (1984).
31. B.A. Silverman, D.F. Carney, C.A. Johnston, P. Vanguri and M.L. Shin. Isolation of membrane attack complex of complement from myelin membranes treated with serum complement. J. Neurochemistry. 42:1024-1029 (1984).
32. K.J. Smith, S.M. Hall and C.L. Schauf. Vesicular demyelination induced by raised intracellular calcium. J. Neurol. Sci. 71:19-37 (1985).
33. T.G. Tachovsky, R.P. Lisak, A. Koprowski, A.N. Theofilopoulos and F.J. Dixon. Circulating immune complexes in multiple sclerosis and other neurological diseases. Lancet. ii:997-999 (1976).
34. R.H.R. Ward and P.J. Lachmann. Monoclonal antibodies which react with lymphocyte lysed target cells and which cross-react with complement-lysed ghosts. Immunology. 56:179-188 (1985).
35. P. Yam, L.D. Petz, W.W. Tourtellotte and B.I. Ma. Measurement of complement components in cerebrospinal fluid by radioimmunoassay in patients with multiple sclerosis. Clin. Immunol. Immunopathol. 17:492-505 (1980).

INTRATHECAL ANTIVIRAL AND ANTINUCLEIC ACID ANTIBODY SYNTHESIS IN MULTIPLE SCLEROSIS (MS), SUBACUTE SCLEROSING PANENCEPHALITIS (SSPE) AND OTHER NEUROLOGICAL DISEASES (OND)

E. Schuller*, B. Allinquant*, P. Lebon** and J.D. Degos***

* Laboratoire de Neuro Immunologie - INSERM U 134 - Hôpital de la Salpêtrière - 75651 Paris Cedex 13 - France
** Laboratoire de Virologie - INSERM U 43 - Hôpital Saint Vincent de Paul - 75674 Paris Cedex 14 - France
*** Service Neurologie - Hôpital Henri Mondor - 94010 Créteil Cedex - France

The role of common viruses, particularly measles, in the etiology and progression of multiple sclerosis (MS) has remained controversial ever since the original hypothesis of Pierre Marie one century ago. The presence of a high titre of measles antibodies was first reported, 24 years ago, in the CSF of patients with MS (Adams and Imagawa, 1962). Since then, numerous reports have confirmed this observation (Panelius et al., 1971; Castaigne et al., 1973; Norrby et al., 1974; Cremer et al., 1980). The most widely held interpretation of this finding is that the antibodies represent a non-specific immunological reaction with little relationship to the pathophysiology of the disease (Forghani et al., 1978; Arnadottir et al., 1982; Leinikki et al., 1982). Further, the presence of another type of antibody in the CSF of MS patients, that specifically recognizes yeast RNA was described in this laboratory (Schuller et al., 1977). More recently, 2 different antinucleic acid antibodies were found and were shown to be synthesized in the CNS of patients with various neuroimmunological diseases, including MS (Allinquant et al., 1982).

The study reported here, compares the 2 types (antiviral and antinucleic acid) of intrathecal synthesis in MS patients comparatively to a group of SSPE patients and to a third group with other neurological diseases (OND).

PATIENTS AND METHODS

Matched serum and CSF from 3 groups of patients were studied 1) 168 patients with definite MS (McAlpine, 1973), comprising 56 males and 112 females; 2) 31 patients with SSPE; 3) 41 patients with other neurological diseases (OND).

The following analyses were made on the Serum and CSF samples: 1) CSF albumin, calculated from cellulose acetate electrophoresis. 2) Serum and CSF IgG by EID (Schuller and Tömpe, 1974). 3) Titres of anti-measles and anti-rubella antibodies by haemagglutination inhibition assay. 4) Anti RNA (ss-nucleic acid) antibodies in serum and CSF by counter-immuno-electrophoresis as previously described (Schuller et al., 1977).

5) Anti ds-DNA by radio-immunoassay as described (Allinquant et al., 1982) in 83 MS, 7 SSPE and 10 OND.

Neuro-immunological analyses

1- Local CNS IgG synthesis was calculated according to the formula previously described (Schuller and Sagar, 1981).

$$\text{IgG local synthesis (mg/l)} = \text{CSF IgG (mg/l)} - \left[30 + \left(\frac{(\text{CSF albumin} - 240)}{60}(\text{serum IgG g/l})\right)\right]$$

where 30 represents the maximum of normal CSF IgG concentration, 240 mg/l the normal mean CSF albumin concentration and 60 an empirically determined figure for the quantity of IgG transudated from serum to CSF for a transudation coefficient of 0.1% of serum albumin. This formula has been previously applied to a group of 191 cases of MS (15). From this result, one can easily calculate the percentage of local synthesis:

$$\text{\% CSF IgG local} = \frac{\text{IgG local synthesis (mg/l)}}{\text{CSF total IgG (mg/l)}}$$

and by deduction the percentage of IgG of plasmatic origin i.e. % CSF IgG plasmatic.

2- The antibody specific activity in serum (ASS) and CSF (ASCSF) is calculated according to the ratio:

$$\text{ASA} = \frac{\text{1 antibody unit}}{\dfrac{\text{IgG concentration}^{*}\text{ (mg/l)}}{\text{serological titre}^{*}}}$$

* in the fluid studied

ie: reciprocal of the serological titre/total IgG concentration (mg/l).

For convenience, this specific activity is expressed here in units 10^{-3} per mg/l of IgG in serum or CSF.

3- The specific activity of locally synthesized IgG (ASLS) was obtained, using the formula:

$$\text{AS CSF} = (\text{ASS} \times \text{\% CSF IgG plasmatic}) + (\text{ASLS} \times \text{\% CSF IgG local})$$

ie: $$\text{ASLS} = \frac{\text{ASCSF} - (\text{ASS} \times \text{\% IgG plasmatic})}{\text{\% IgG local}}$$

This ASLS is also expressed in units 10^{-3} per mg/l of locally synthesized IgG.

STATISTICAL METHODS

Student's t-test, Chi-squared test and correlation coefficients (r).

RESULTS

Intrathecal IgG synthesis

Local IgG synthesis was present (Table 1) in 145 (86%) of the 168 MS patients, in all SSPE patients and in 18 (44%) patients with OND. In this last group, local IgG synthesis was significantly lower ($p < 0.001$) than in the 2 others. In MS patients, intrathecal production of IgG was significantly lower ($p < 0.001$) than in SSPE.

Table 1. Local synthesis

	in MS (168)	in SSPE (31)	in OND (41)
local IgG synthesis (mean ± SE mg/l)	43.7 ± 3.7** ***	*** 148 ± 35**	*** 16.1 ± 4.9 ***
frequency	86% (145)	100% (31)	44% (18)
local specific antibody synthesis			
frequency			
measles	49% (83)	100% (31)	22% (9)
- only	26% (44)		20% (8)
-+ rubella	23% (39)	ND	2% (1)
rubella	31% (52)	ND	12% (5)
ss-nucleic acid	31% (52)	84% (26)	5% (2)
ds-nucleic acid	7% (6/83)	100% (7/7)	0

Intrathecal specific antibody synthesis

Frequencies of these local syntheses are summarized in Table 1, which indicate the repartition of measles and rubella antibodies in the 96 MS synthesizing such antibodies inside their CNS.

Correlation between viral and anti ss-nucleic acid antibodies in MS

Table 2 indicates the repartition of MS patients in groups defined by absence or presence of viral and/or anti ss-nucleic acid antibodies. As previously observed in another group of MS patients (Schuller et al., 1979), a highly significant ($p < 0.001$) association between these 2 local syntheses can be demonstrated. An other interesting fact is the very significant difference between the means of local IgG synthesis in MS patients with or without local anti ss-nucleic acid antibody synthesis.

Table 2. Local IgG synthesis (mean ± SE mg/l) and local specific antibodies synthesis in 168 MS

	local IgG synthesis
no antibodies (62)	15.1 ± 2.5
viral antibodies only (54)	15.2 ± 2.5***
nucleic antibodies (52)	
- only (10)	72.9 ± 14.7***
-+ viral (42)	93.2 ± 8.2***

Correlations between local (intrathecal) and general anti-measles immunity in MS and SSPE

The means of anti-measles antibody specific activity (ASA) in serum IgG and intrathecal IgG synthesized (calculated from our formula) are given in table 3. Local IgG synthesis means of the 83 MS patients with local anti-measles antibody production and of the 31 SSPE are also indicated. Three types of correlations can be discussed:

a) local antimeasles ASA, which is observed in about half of MS and in all SSPE patients, is always higher than in serum ASA of the same patients. The ratio local ASA/serum ASA is about 6 in SSPE and 9 in MS: a significant ($p < 0.02$) difference can be demonstrated between both in serum, but not in local synthesis (see Table 3).

b) conversely, local IgG synthesis is significantly ($p < 0.001$) higher in SSPE patients than in MS. A negative correlation between local anti-measles ASA and local IgG synthesis was observed in both diseases and was highly significant in MS.

Table 3. Anti measles local and general immunity

	in MS (83)	in SSPE (31)
antibody specific activity (ASA)		
- in serum	11.1 ± 1.0**	28.5 ± 6.7** ($p < 0.02$)
- in local synthesis	97.4 ± 29.7**	180.8 ± 45.7** (NS)
local IgG synthesis (mean ± SE mg/l)	56.1 ± 6.9	148.1 ± 35.5 ($p < 0.001$)
correlations (r)		
ASA serum/ASA LS	0.17 (NS)	0.65 (< 0.001)
ASA LS/local IgG synthesis	-0.36 (<0.001)	-0.20 (NS)

c) no correlation between local and serum anti measles ASA can be established in the 83 MS, contrary to the SSPE group, where such correlation is highly ($p < 0.001$) significant.

Correlations between local (intrathecal) and serum anti ss-nucleic acid ASA in MS and SSPE

The means of anti ss-nucleic acid ASA in serum IgG and intrathecal IgG are given in Table 4. Means of local IgG synthesis in 52 MS patients with local anti ss-nucleic acid antibody production and of the 31 SSPE are also indicated. Three types of correlations can be discussed:

a) local anti ss-nucleic acid ASA, which is observed in about 31% of MS and in 84% of SSPE patients, is lower than serum ASA in MS and higher than serum ASA in SSPE. The ratio local ASA/serum ASA is about 0.7 in MS and 1.5 in SSPE: a significant ($p < 0.05$) difference between local ASA, but not between serum ASA, can be demonstrated in both diseases.

b) no significant difference in the means of local IgG synthesis can be established and no correlation was found between this local IgG synthesis and local anti ss-nucleic acid ASA in both diseases.

c) similarly, no correlation between local and serum anti ss-nucleic acid ASA was observed.

Table 4. Anti ss nucleic acid local and general immunity

	in MS (52)	in SSPE (31)
Antibody specific activity (ASA)		
- in serum	94.7 ± 2.8**	97.1 ± 7.4 (NS)
- in local synthesis	70.2 ± 6.6**	146.4 ± 37.5 (< 0.05)
local IgG synthesis (mean ± SE mg/l)	89.3 ± 7.9	148.1 ± 35.5 (NS)
correlations (r)		
ASA serum/ASA LS	0.05	- 0.06
ASA LS/local IgG synthesis	0.06	- 0.11 (NS)

DISCUSSION

Two important points must be discussed:

The comparison of local immunity in MS and SSPE

Local anti viral antibody synthesis is frequent and very high in MS patients: local measles ASA, for example, is approximately the same in MS and SSPE patients. Conversely, local anti ss-nucleic acid antibody synthesis is frequent and high (compared to serum values), in SSPE, contrary to MS where this synthesis is rare and low, compared to serum values. Moreover, local production of anti ds-DNA antibodies seems constant in

SSPE and extremely rare in MS, as previously reported (Schuller et al., 1985b).

Role of this specific intrathecal antibody synthesis

Local synthesis of viral antibodies in MS patients seems very frequent. The local production of anti-measles antibody has been calculated previously in patients with SSPE (Tourtellotte et al., 1981) and in patients with MS (Albrecht et al., 1983). In the latter study on 23 MS patients, using very sensitive techniques for the detection of viral antibodies, 91% of MS cases demonstrated immune reactivity against one or more viruses; the mean anti-measles antibody titre was significantly greater than in other neurological diseases. As previously published (Schuller et al., 1985a) a longitudinal study has demonstrated stable between anti measles and anti rubella local antibody titres in successive CSF samples of the same MS patients. On the other hand, no correlation was found with any (sex, HLA types) genetic factor, nor with the age of the patients. Our conclusion was in favour of a specific immune response (possibly related to local antigenic stimulation) more than of a "nonsense" intrathecal production.

In the case of anti ss-nucleic acid antibodies, the situation is a little different: their local synthesis is not very different than their serum synthesis in either SSPE or MS. Nevertheless, this local synthesis, as for antiviral antibodies, is not proportional to the amount of local production of IgG or linked to genetic factors.

Whatever, a striking difference exists between MS and SSPE patients concerning anti ss-nucleic acid antibodies, speaking in terms of the frequency and the amount of this local synthesis. This difference contrasts with the great similarity of local anti measles antibody synthesis in both diseases. Finally, these data argue in favour of an intrathecal viral stimulation in MS rather than a non specific response. The apparent defect in anti nucleic acid antibody synthesis could be a contributing factor to this persistance of the virus in the CNS of MS patients.

ACKNOWLEDGEMENTS

This work was supported by grants from INSERM, Association pour la Recherche sur la Sclérose en Plaques and University Paris VI. We thank M. Josien for statistics and presentation of this manuscript.

REFERENCES

1. J.M. Adams and D.T. Imagawa. Measles antibodies in multiple sclerosis. Proc. Soc. Exp. Biol. Med. 111:562-566 (1962).
2. P. Albrecht, W.W. Tourtellotte, J.T. Hicks, S. Hiroshi, E.J. Boone and A.R. Potvin. Intra-blood-brain barrier measles virus antibody synthesis in multiple sclerosis patients. Neurol. (NY). 33:45-50 (1983).
3. B. Allinquant, V. Giraud, M. Piccioti and E. Schuller. Serum and cerebrospinal fluid antibodies to single-stranded and double-stranded nucleic acids in neurological diseases. J. Neuro-Immunol. 3:77-89 (1982).
4. T. Arnadottir, M. Reunanen and A. Salmi. Intrathecal synthesis of virus antibodies in multiple sclerosis patients. Infect and Immunity. 38(2):399-407 (1982).

5. P. Castaigne, F. Cathala, A.F. Chateau, E. Schuller, P. Collomb, R. Baylet, P. Girard and N. Dumas. Les anticorps de rougeole du serum et du LCR. Nouv. Presse Med. 2(14):895-899 (1973).
6. N.E. Cremer, P.J. Kenneth, G. Fein and H. Likosky. Comprehensive viral immunology of multiple sclerosis. II. Analysis of serum and CSF antibodies by standard serologic methods. Arch. Neurol. 37:610-615 (1980).
7. B. Forghani, N.E. Cremer, K.P. Johnson, A.H. Ginsberg and W.H. Likosky. Viral antibodies in cerebrospinal fluid of multiple sclerosis and control patients: comparison between radioimmunoassay and conventional techniques. J. Clin. Microbiol. 7:63-69 (1978).
8. P. Leinikki, I. Shekarchi, M. Livanainen, E. Taskinen, K.V. Holmes, D. Madden and J.L. Sever. Virus antibodies in the cerebrospinal fluid of multiple sclerosis patients detected with ELISA tests. J. Neurol. Sci. 57:249-255 (1982).
9. E. Norrby, H. Link and J.E. Olsson. Measles virus antibodies in multiple sclerosis. Arch. Neurol. 30:285-292 (1974).
10. M. Panelius, A.A. Salmi, P. Halonen and K. Penitinen. Measles antibodies detected with various techniques in sera of patients with multiple sclerosis. Acta Neurol. Scand. 47:315-330 (1971).
11. E. Schuller and L. Tömpe. Electroimmunodiffusion of IgG heavy chains in nanogram quantities with a carboxymethyl-cellulose-agarose gel. Clin. Chim. Acta. 54:131-133 (1974).
12. E. Schuller, B. Allinquant, N. Delasnerie and J. Reboul. Determination of RNA antibodies in serum and CSF by counterimmunoelectrophoresis. J. Immunol. Meth. 14:177 (1977).
13. E. Schuller, P. Lebon, B. Alliquant, N. Moreau, J. Reboul and G. Deloche. Nucleic and viral antibodies in serum and CSF of MS patients. In: "Humoral immunity in neurological diseases". D. Karcher, A. Lowenthal and A.D. Strosberg. Ed Plenum Press. 255-264 (1979).
14. E. Schuller and H.J. Sagar. Local synthesis of CSF immunoglobulins. J. Neurol. Sci. 51:361-370 (1981).
15. E. Schuller and H.J. Sagar. Central nervous system IgG synthesis in multiple sclerosis. Application of a new formula. Acta Neurol. Scand. 67:365-371 (1983).
16. E. Schuller, B. Allinquant, P. Lebon, H. Sagar and A. Govaerts. Measles specific antibody activity in serum and locally synthesized CSF IgG fractions: results in SSPE, MS and other neurological diseases. 2nd International symposium on SSPE, Bergamo (Italy) 22-24 May 1985. To be published by Elsevier (a).
17. E. Schuller, B. Allinquant and C. Mussenger. Anti nucleic acid antibody local synthesis and intrathecal ribonuclease in MS and other neurological diseases. 5th symposium on CSF. Rostock, 6-7 September 1984. In: "Fortschritte der Liquorforschung" Wilheim-Pieck-Universität Rostock. pp.22-30 (1985) (b).
18. W.W. Tourtellotte, B.I. Ma, D.B. Brandes, M.J. Walsh and A.R. Potvin. Quantification of the Novo Central Nervous system IgG measles antibody synthesis in SSPE. Ann. Neurol. 9:551-556 (1981).

CORRELATION OF LYMPHOCYTE PHENOTYPES AND IMMUNE FUNCTION IN MULTIPLE SCLEROSIS (MS)

Jack P. Antel and Avertano Noronha

The University of Chicago, Department of Neurology
Chicago, Illinois

Immune-mediated mechanisms are postulated to contribute to the pathogenesis of multiple sclerosis (MS). The various cellular components mediating and regulating immune reactivity in MS have been evaluated using a wide range of assays which attempt to compare MS patients and controls with regard either to the number of cells belonging to a particular subset as defined by a distinctive cell surface marker or by specific immune functional activities. In many of these studies, no attempts were made to correlate subset enumeration and functional assay parameters. With specific regard to T cell subsets involved in regulating the immune response, one can demonstrate from studies of peripheral blood mononuclear cells (MNCs) that functional derangements occur in suppressor cell activity in MS, which cannot yet be accounted for by a quantitative change in a currently recognized T cell subsets. In this report, we review our data derived from studies of peripheral blood cells supporting this observation and present preliminary data on suppressor activity mediated by T cell lines, an approach which can be applied to T cells derived from the cerebrospinal fluid (CSF) or even brain tissues.

Immune regulatory T cell subsets have been considered in two major categories, namely T helper/inducer and T suppressor cell subsets. These two cell subsets have most commonly been distinguished by the usually mutually exclusive presence of the distinctive cell surface glycoproteins, namely CD4 (T4) and CD8 (T8). The functional immune regulatory properties of these cell subsets were originally defined in assays of T cell dependent B cell secretion of Ig, using pokeweed mitogen (pwm) as a polyclonal activator (1). In this assay system, $T4^+$ cells freshly isolated from peripheral blood and added to cultures of B cells plus accessory cells in the presence of pwm without any prior manipulation will function as inducer/helper cells. $T8^+$ cells in this system, will suppress Ig secretion by the T4-B cell combination, again with no prior activation of the suppressor cell being required. The $T8^+$ cell seems itself, however, to be dependent on interaction with an inducer subset which can be defined on the basis of phenotypic surface markers (Leu 3^+, Leu 8^+) (2). The $T4^+$ and $T8^+$ cell subsets also mediate other functional activities; $T8^+$ cells mediate Class I major histocompatibility (MHC) antigen restricted cytolytic activity whereas $T4^+$ cells are mediators of Class II MHC antigen restricted cytolysis (3).

Suppressor cell function has also been evaluated _in vitro_ using assays in which the putative suppressor-mediating cell subset has been activated with mitogen, usually Concanavalin A (Con A), or antigen, often alloantigen in mixed lymphocyte culture, for some time period (48-96 hours) prior to being added to a population of cells themselves being cultured with a T or B cell activator. In most studies in which this assay has been applied to MS, the activated suppressor cells were exposed to mitomycin C prior to their being added in with responder cells, usually autologous or heterologous MNCs, which in turn are being stimulated with Con A - ie. a predominantly T cell activator (4,5,6). The mitomycin C inhibits further DNA synthesis and proliferation by the suppressor cells, thus permitting one to attribute the subsequently observed ^{3}H-thymidine uptake to the responder cells.

Studies of Con A-activated suppressor cells were initially conducted using unfractionated mononuclear cells (MNCs). Subsequent studies suggested that multiple cell subsets contained within MNCs, including both T and non-T cells, mediated the suppressor activity (7,8). In studies of normal young individuals in which we isolated specific cell subsets contained within the MNC population, either total T cells (ie. E^+ cells that form rosettes with sheep red blood cells), non-T cells (E^- cells), $T8^+$ cells, or $T4^+$ cells and then activated them with Con A, we found that $T8^+$ cells

Table 1. Mean percent suppression mediated by cell subsets isolated from peripheral blood MNCs of normal adults and MS patients with progressive disease

	percent suppression		donor number
	control donors	MS patients	
Unfractionated MNCs	88 ± 1%	32 ± 3%	4
E^+ cells (total T cells)	82 ± 1%	18 ± 2%	4
E^- cells (B cells plus monocytes)	-5 ± 7%		3
$T8^+$ cells**	87 ± 3%	37 ± 4%	4
$T4^+$ cells**	37 ± 2%	28 ± 6%	4

Data indicate mean percent suppression ± standard error of mean (SEM) for the number of donors indicated. For each donor, percent suppression is calculated by the formula:

$$1 - \text{cpm cultures of } \frac{(10^5 \text{ R cells} + 10^5 \text{ S cells} + \text{Con A})}{(10^5 \text{ R cells} + 10^5 \text{ C cells} + \text{Con A})} \times 100\%$$

- S cells = MNCs or subsets thereof which are cultured for 48 hours with Con A and then treated with mitomycin C (50 μg per ml).
- C cells = MNCs or subsets thereof which are maintained in culture for 48 hours without Con A and then treated with mitomycin C.
- ** = $T8^+$ and $T4^+$ cells are cultured with Con A in the presence of 10% accessory cells (ie. E^- cells) in order to obtain cell activation.

were the major mediators of suppression in this assay system (Table 1). Nonactivated mitomycin-treated cells did not significantly effect ^{3}H-thymidine uptake by responder cells.

In the MS patient group, functional abnormalities of immunoregulatory activity mediated by peripheral blood MNCs have been demonstrated in assay systems involving both nonactivated (pwm-induced IgG secretion) and activated (Con A-induced) suppressor cell assays. In evaluating the results of functional assays of immune regulation performed on MS patients, one need consider correlations both with observed quantitative changes in regulatory T cell subsets and with clinical parameters of disease activity. With regard to clinical correlations, we and others have previously demonstrated that Con A-induced suppressor activity mediated by unfractionated MNCs derived from peripheral blood was reduced compared to controls in patients with relapses of MS and was increased during the recovery phase (4-6, 10). The data presented in this report were derived from studies of peripheral blood cells obtained from patients with progressive multiple sclerosis and who were receiving no active immunotherapy. Most of these patients also had cerebrospinal fluid (CSF) analysis performed as part of entry evaluation into a clinical trial with Cyclosporin A.

a. Pokeweed mitogen (pwm)-induced IgG secretion studies

As shown in Fig.1, the levels of IgG secretion by MNCs of progressive MS patients were increased compared to age-matched controls. We found no correlation between the proportion of $T8^+$ or $T4^+$ cells in the MNC population and levels of IgG secretion for either the MS or control groups. Amongst normal young adults, levels of pwm-induced IgG secretion by MNCs varied widely; the levels secreted by a given individual were, however, rather consistent over time (11). In the young adult group, levels of IgG secretion were dependent on T cell regulatory influences, correlating inversely with the functional suppressor capability of the $T8^+$ population (11). In elderly individuals, low IgG secretion values can reflect either decreased B cell response or decline in $T4^+$ helper function but do not correlate with $T8^+$ cell suppressor activity, which declines with age (12, 13). Our studies of MS patients also indicate that their "high" levels of pwm-induced IgG secretion reflect diminished $T8^+$ cell suppressor function (14). The above data were generated using a crossover design experimental paradigm in which the influence of a constant number of $T8^+$ cells isolated by "panning" from MNCs was assessed on heterologous pwm-stimulated cocultures of $T4^+$ cells plus B cells. The levels of suppression observed did vary with the number of $T8^+$ cells added, indicating that cell numbers do need to be considered. Addition of sufficient number of $T8^+$ cells from MS patients could completely suppress IgG secretion, indicating that MS patients do not have a complete lack of functional suppressor cells.

The levels of pwm-induced IgG secretion observed in our group of progressive MS patients were found to be consistently high, as determined by repeated studies on the same individuals performed over a 12-month time period (15) and overall were suggestively higher than those observed in a previously studied group of MS patients with stable disease (16, 17). Note, however, we did not study the stable and progressive patients in a paired manner. Our previous data on stable MS patients did suggest a persistent increase in IgG secretion in the MS population regardless of clinic state. Our newer data suggests that a further superimposed increase may occur in patients in the progressive phase of the disease. We did not find a correlation between levels of pwm-induced IgG secretion in vitro and calculated levels of IgG synthesis within the central nervous system in the progressive MS group.

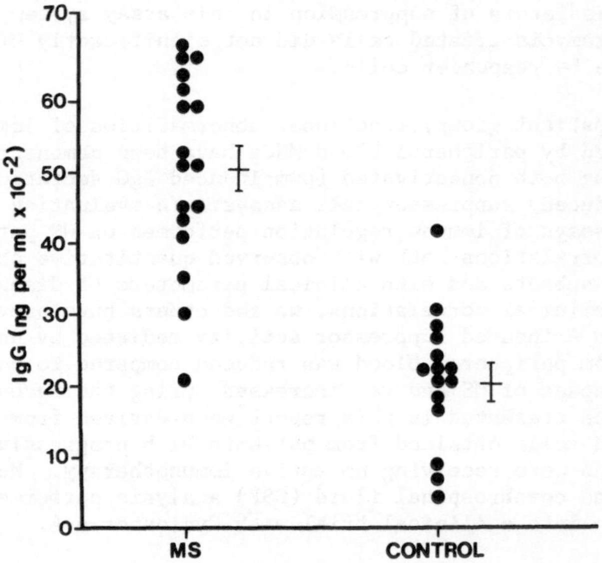

Fig.1. Comparison of levels of pokeweed mitogen-induced IgG secretion by peripheral blood mononuclear cells isolated from progressive MS patients and controls. Data indicate values for individual donors. Mean values ± SEM are given for each group.

The basis for the reduced T8$^+$ cell-mediated suppressor function in "high" secreting normal individuals compared to "low" secretors and for the almost universal finding that progressive MS patients are "high" IgG secretors remains to be defined. Reder et al. (18) demonstrated that in progressive MS patients, the density of T8 antigen expressed per cell was reduced compared to control donors and stable MS patients. One can reduce T8 antigen density on cells by exposing the cells to anti-T8 mAb (OKT8); this results in modulation of the antigen from the cell. We find that reducing T8 antigen density can result in augmented pwm-induced IgG secretion by MNCs from donors who initially were producing less than maximal levels of IgG (Table 2). The observation that T8 antigen density is normal in stable MS patients suggests that the observed reduction in progressive patients is an acquired one. Mechanisms which potentially could account for shifts in T8 antigen density in MS include the effects on lymphocytes of exogenous factors such as anti-lymphocyte antibody, macrophage-released mediators, or myelin or other brain breakdown products, the occurrence of intrinsic changes within the T8 cell, or shifts of particular cell subsets between the systemic circulation and the nervous system. No evidence yet exists for any genetically-determined polymorphisms of the T8 antigen (19).

The T8 cell population mediates cytolytic as well as suppressor activity. Jacobsen et al. (20) have shown that T8 cell-mediated cytolytic activity directed against influenza virus-infected cells is normal in MS. We find that Class I MHC alloantigen-directed cytolysis is preserved in the same group of progressive MS patients who demonstrate exaggerated levels of IgG secretion - ie. reduced suppressor activity (16). This discrepancy in activity between two functions ascribed to the same phenotypic cell subset raises the possibilities that distinct sub-subsets exist within the T8 population or that different inducer mechanisms are involved in suppressor and cytolytic functions.

Table 2. Effect of incubation of MNCs with OKT8 mAb on pwm-induced Ig secretion

Ig Secretion	
No Ab	+ OKT8
1950 ng/ml	3750 ng/ml
2000	2700
2000	3500
2550	3650
825	875
2450	4750
960	3300
1350	3550
1000	4500

MNCs from normal donors were incubated with or without 25 μl of OKT8 monoclonal antibody, diluted 1:10 from reconstituted stock, for 30 minutes on ice and then cultured for 7 days in the presence of pwm.

b. Activated suppressor cell function

In this assay, MNCs or subsets thereof are activated *in vitro*, usually by the mitogen Con A, for 48-96 hours; suppressor activity is determined by assessing the effects of these activated cells on the reactivity of a second cell population. In our specific assay system, we expose Con A-activated cells to mitomycin C and then add these cells to freshly isolated autologous or heterologous MNCs which are cultured with Con A. Non-activated mitomycin-treated cells serve as controls. Suppressor activity is the level of reduction in ^{3}H-thymidine uptake by the responder (R) cells cocultured with activated mitomycin-treated cells compared to uptake by R cells cocultured with control cells, as determined after 72 hours of culture.

In our progressive MS patient group, Con A-induced suppressor activity mediated by unfractionated MNCs was persistently reduced compared to controls (15), permitting one to explore the cellular basis for the observed functional abnormalities. We found no correlation between suppressor activity in this assay and proportion of $T8^+$ or $T4^+$ cells within the MNC population. To determine whether defective Con A-mediated suppression in these patients could be attributed to a specific T cell or non-T cell subset, we compared suppressor activity mediated by total T cells, $T8^+$ cells, and $T4^+$ cells derived from MS patients with similar cell subsets derived from controls donors. We also determined the capacity of accessory cells, either macrophages or E^- cells, from MS patients and controls to support T cell-mediated suppression (9). In order to activate T cells with Con A, one does require a source of accessory cells, and we used either monocytes (plastic adherent cells) or E^- cells. The results of our studies are presented in Tables 1 and 3 and suggest the following:

a. Defective Con A-induced suppressor activity mediated by unfractionated MNCs derived from progressive MS patients is also observed when isolated T cells are used, even when the MS-T cells are cocultured with normal donor accessory cells.

b. Accessory cells from MS patients are capable of supporting high levels of suppressor activity by normal donor T cells.

c. $T8^+$ cells derived from MS patients mediate lower levels of suppression than do equal numbers of $T8^+$ cells derived from control donors.

d. As with our results from the nonactivated suppressor assay (pwm-induced IgG secretion), the functional abnormalities noted in the Con A assay of suppressor function could not be accounted for simply by quantitative changes of currently defined T cell subsets.

Table 3. Mean percent suppression mediated by Con A-activated mitomycin-treated cocultures of T cells and accessory cells derived from MS patients and controls

	accessory cells	
	MS	Control
E^+ cells - MS	-	18 ± 2%
- Control	70 ± 1	82 ± 1
Number studied	2	4

- accessory cells, either plastic-adherent macrophages or E^- cells, are cocultured in a 1:10 proportion with E^+ (T) cells.

The basis for the functional Con A-induced suppressor defects observed in progressive MS patients remain under study. We can show that T cell activators other than Con A can induce suppressor activity; activators which we have examined include OKT3 antibody which acts via the T cell receptor and phorbol myristate acetate (PMA) whose mechanism of T cell activation may bypass the T cell receptor (9). With both reagents, the MS patients again demonstrate lower levels of suppression than do controls. ^{3}H-thymidine uptake by mitogen- or OKT3-activated MNCs or $T8^+$ cell subsets does not differ between MS patients and controls. Addition of interleukin-2 (IL-2) to the cultures, does not augment suppressor levels in the MS population (15).

Whether functional suppressor assays will prove to be either better predictors of disease course or better indicators of response to therapy than will quantitative measures using cell surface markers, will largely depend on development of objective clinical-laboratory methods to document disease course and response to therapeutic agents. We have previously shown that azathioprine (Imuran™) will inhibit pwm-induced IgG secretion by MNCs from MS patients without augmenting Con A-induced suppressor cell activity (17). Cyclosporine A in dosages which markedly inhibit cytolytic activity does not either inhibit IgG secretion or alter Con A-induced suppressor activity (15). The previously noted observation that suppressor function fluctuates in patients with relapsing-remitting form of MS does, however, suggest that the suppressor defect in MS could be amenable to pharmacologic therapy.

The assays outlined above have been conducted on cells freshly isolated from peripheral blood and require considerable cell numbers, far exceeding those that can be derived from cerebrospinal fluid (CSF). Expanded number of T cells or subsets thereof can be derived from the CSF by establishing T cell lines. Santoli et al. (21) have demonstrated that both $T4^+$ and $T8^+$ celllines derived from the CSF maintain their expected helper and suppressor functions respectively. We have generated IL-2 dependent

$T8^+$ cell lines from peripheral blood of MS patients and normal donors and compared their suppressor mediating capabilities with those observed using freshly isolated $T8^+$ cells.

We have used two approaches to generate these $T8^+$ cell lines. In one technique, unfractionated MNCs were initially cultured with OKT3. Beginning on day 4, the cultures were supplemented twice weekly with 50% IL-2, derived from the MLA Gibbon monkey tumor cell line. Feeder cells (autologous or heterologous radiated MNCs) were added after 10-14 days of culture. Cell lines derived from this culture technique were predominantly $T8^+$ and all expressed Tac antigen. These cells, when treated with mitomycin 24-48 hrs after the last IL-2 supplement did not suppress ^{3}H-thymidine uptake by Con A-stimulated fresh responder cells (Table 4), a finding which mimics the lack of suppressor effect of nonactivated freshly isolated cells when exposed to mitomycin.

Table 4. Suppressor activity of $T8^+$ cells maintained as cell lines in culture for > 2 weeks

	$T8^+$ cell lines maintained in 50% IL-2		"panned" $T8^+$ cells maintained with OKT3 and 20% IL-2	
	MS	Control	MS	Control
^{3}H-thymidine uptake in presence of IL-2				
- OKT3	13149 cpm	6951 cpm	2724 cpm	8816 cpm
+ OKT3 (48 hrs)			76630	87721
percent suppression mediated by mitomycin-treated $T8^+$ cells:	-13[(a)]	-13[(a)]	-1[(b)]	-94[(b)]

Data indicate results from individual pairs of MS patients and controls. Suppression is determined by adding 10^5 cells from the $T8^+$ lines, either treated or not treated with mitomycin, to 10^5 Con A-stimulated responder MNCs. (a) cells did not receive OKT3 prior to testing; (b) cells were stimulated with OKT3, 48 hours prior to testing.

In the second method, we initiated the cell cultures with "panning" enriched $T8^+$ cells. The cells were stimulated with OKT3 in the presence of autologous radiated feeders and 20% IL-2. The cells were recultured weekly with fresh feeder cells and OKT3. IL-2 was added biweekly after the first week. As shown in Table 4, the cells were responsive to OKT3 with markedly higher ^{3}H-thymidine uptakes being found compared to those observed with cells exposed only to IL-2, either 20% or 50%. Normal donor $T8^+$ cell lines treated with mitomycin 48 hours after their third exposure OKT3 and added to fresh Con A-stimulated responder cells, induced marked suppression of ^{3}H-thymidine uptake by Con A-stimulated responder cells. OKT3-stimulated, mitomycin-treated $T8^+$ cells from MS patients induced markedly lower levels of suppression (< 10%). These data indicate that the observed functional activated suppressor cell defect noted in MS when freshly isolated cells are used, is maintained for a persistent period in culture. This approach should lend itself both to evaluation of CSF derived suppressor cells and to discerning the basis for the aberrant suppressor findings themselves.

REFERENCES

1. S.F. Schlossman and E.L. Reinherz. Regulation of the immune response. Inducer and suppressor T lymphocyte subsets in human beings. N. Engl. J. Med. 303:370 (1980).
2. P.A. Gatenby, G.S. Kansas, C.Y. Xian, R.L. Evans and E.G. Engleman. Dissection of immunoregulatory subpopulations of T lymphocytes within the helper and suppressor sublineages in man. J. Immunol. 129: 1997 (1982).
3. S.C. Meuer, S.E. Schlossman and E.L. Reinherz. Clonal analysis of human cytotoxic T lymphocytes: $T4^+$ and $T8^+$ effector T cells recognize products of different major histocompatibility complex regions. Proc. Natl. Acad. Sci. (USA). 79:4395 (1982).
4. J.P. Antel, B.G.W. Arnason and M.E. Medof. Suppressor cell function in multiple sclerosis: Correlation with clinical disease activity. Ann. Neurol. 5:338 (1979).
5. R.L. Gonzalez, P.C. Dau and L.E. Spitler. Altered regulation of mitogen responsiveness by suppressor cells in multiple sclerosis. Clin. Exp. Immunol. 36:78 (1978).
6. P.A. Neighbour and B.R. Bloom. Absence of virus-induced lymphocyte suppression and interferon production in multiple sclerosis. Proc. Natl. Acad. Sci. 76:476 (1979).
7. N.K. Damle and S. Gupta. Heterogeneity of Concanavalin A-induced suppressor T cells in man defined with monoclonal antibodies. Clin. Exp. Immunol. 48:581 (1982).
8. H.B. Herscowitz, T. Sakane, A. Steinberg and I. Green. Heterogeneity of human suppressor cells induced by Concanavalin A as determined in simultaneous assays of immune function. J. Immunol. 124:1403 (1980).
9. J.P. Antel, M.B. Bania, A. Reder and N. Cashman. Activated suppressor cell dysfunction in progressive multiple sclerosis. J. Immunol. In press.
10. U. Tjernlund, P. Cesaro, E. Tournier, J.D. Degos, J.F. Bach and M.A. Bach. T cell subsets in multiple sclerosis: A comparative study between cell surface antigens and function. Clin. Immunol. Immunopathol. 32:185 (1984).
11. M. Rosenkoetter, A.T. Reder, J.J.F. Oger and J.P. Antel. T cell regulation of polyclonally-induced immunoglobulin secretion in humans. J. Immunol. 132:1779 (1984).
12. D. Skias, A.T. Reder, M.B. Bania and J.P. Antel. Age-related changes in mechanisms accounting for low levels of polyclonally induced immunoglobulin secretion in humans. Clin. Immunol. Immunopathol. 35: 191 (1985).
13. L.G. Wrabetz, J.P. Antel, J.J.F. Oger, B.G.W. Arnason, J.M. Goust and J.E. Hopper. Age-related changes in in vitro immunoglobulin secretion: comparison of responses to T-dependent and T-independent polyclonal activators. Cell. Immunol. 74:398 (1982).
14. J.P. Antel, M. Rosenkoetter, A. Reder, J.J.F. Oger and B.G.W. Arnason. Multiple sclerosis: Relation of in vitro IgG secretion to T suppressor cell number and function. Neurology. 34:1155 (1984).
15. M.B. Bania, J.P. Antel, A.T. Reder, M.K. Nicholas and B.G.W. Arnason. Suppressor and cytolytic cell function in multiple sclerosis - Effects of cyclosporin A and interleukin-2 (IL-2). Submitted.
16. J.P. Antel, M.K. Nicholas, M.B. Bania, A.T. Reder, B.G.W. Arnason and L. Joseph. Comparison of $T8^+$ cell-mediated suppressor and cytotoxic functions in multiple sclerosis. J. Neuroimmunol. In press.

17. J.J.F. Oger, J.P. Antel, H.H. Kuo and B.G.W. Arnason. Influence of azathioprine (Imuran) on in vitro immune function in multiple sclerosis. Ann. Neurol. 11:177 (1982).
18. A.T. Reder, J.P. Antel, J.J.F. Oger, T.A. McFarland, M. Rosenkoetter and B.G.W. Arnason. Low T8 antigen density on lymphocytes in active multiple sclerosis. Ann. Neurol. 16:242 (1984).
19. V. Sukhatme, S. Singh, C. Stoklosa, J.P. Antel and A.T. Reder. Molecular analysis of the CD8 protein in multiple sclerosis. Submitted.
20. S. Jacobson, M.L. Flerlage and H.F. McFarland. Impaired measles virus-specific cytotoxic T cell responses in multiple sclerosis. J. Exp. Med. 162:839 (1985).
21. D. Santoli, E.C. Defreitas, M. Sandberg-Wollheim, M.K. Francis and H. Koprowski. Phenotypic and functional characterization of T cell clones derived from the cerebrospinal fluid of multiple sclerosis patients. J. Immunol. 132:2386 (1984).

CSF LYMPHOCYTE SUBPOPULATIONS IN MS AND POST-/RABIES/-VACCINATION ENCEPHALOMYELTITIS

Andras Guseo and Bernadett Kalman

Department of Neurology, Central Hospital of Cty. Fejér
Székesfehérvar, Hungary

Lymphocytes and monocytes are the main cytological constituents of the CSF. The cells are blood borne and express the same surface antigen groups, they have the same biological characteristics as those of the peripheral blood. The population of CSF lymphocytes is under continuous fluctuation, even in normal conditions, but somewhat slowlyer than those of the periphery. They undergo local transformation due to local cellular and humoral activities. CSF distribution of T lymphocyte subsets may be expected to bear much closer relation to immunologically active cells within the CNS lesions than peripheral blood lymphocytes, they give better picture of what is happening in the brain, than is given by values in the peripheral blood. Positive correlations have been found between disease activity and number (McAlpine et al., 1955), mitotic activity (Noronha et al., 1980) and responsiveness to MBP (Lisak and Zweiman, 1977), surface phenotypes (Zaffaroni et al., 1985, Antel et al., 1984), abnormal immunological activity (Haffler et al., 1985), T suppressor number and surface antigen density (Antel et al., 1984) and erythrocyte binding capacity in E rosette (Oger et al., 1975, Guseo, 1984).

The advent of monoclonal antibodies specific to various human lymphocyte surface differentiation markers raised hopes that the more exacting phenotypic characterization feasible with technology would allow greater understanding of the immunoregulatory abnormality in MS.

The data available in MS are contributory. One group of investigators don't find any alteration in cell content in MS(Paty et al., 1983, Hauser et al., 1983, Dommasch et al., 1984, Rice et al., 1984, Zabriskie et al., 1985, Albala et al., 1985) and in EAE (Feasly et al., 1984), whereas others described well defined abnormality in cell ratio as well as cell surface characteristics (Noronha et al., 1980, Oger et al., 1982, Cashman et al., 1982, Panitch and Francis 1982, Sandberg-Wollheim 1983, Compston 1983, Hauser et al., 1983, Antel et al., 1984, Bach et al., 1985). The discrepancies noted in these studies raise the fundamental question of whether immune dysfunction plays a primary pathogenic role in multiple sclerosis or whether it merely represents epiphenomena secondary to the disease process.

Methodological problems concerning CSF cell specifications are considerable which explain the fewer number of papers on this subject.

We demonstrate results with an easy and quick method by labelled microbeads using Bio-Rad's Quantigen for helper and suppressor enumeration as well as a similar method developed in our laboratory for the demonstration of optional cell surface antigens among them OKT4, OKT8 and Leu 7.

MATERIAL AND METHODS

120 CSF samples of MS patients in stable condition, with chronic progressive course or with acute exacerbations, have been investigated by the E rosette technique and some of them were investigated parallel by monoclonal antibodies too. In some patients the investigations have been repeated before and after intensive steroid treatment.

3 ml of CSF with normal cell count or 0.5 ml witl lympho-monocytosis pleocytosis should be centrifuged for 5 min. at 500 g. After decantation of CSF 3 drops of Parker 199 (tissue culture medium, Flow Laboratories) should be added.

E-rosettes - as routine method - have been prepared by using the method described by Guseo, 1984. Active (5 minute), avid (the whole surface covered by sheep red blood cells) and late total (24 hour) lymphocytes have been distinguished. Special attention was drown to avid or "giant rosette" lymphocytes (Fig.1a).

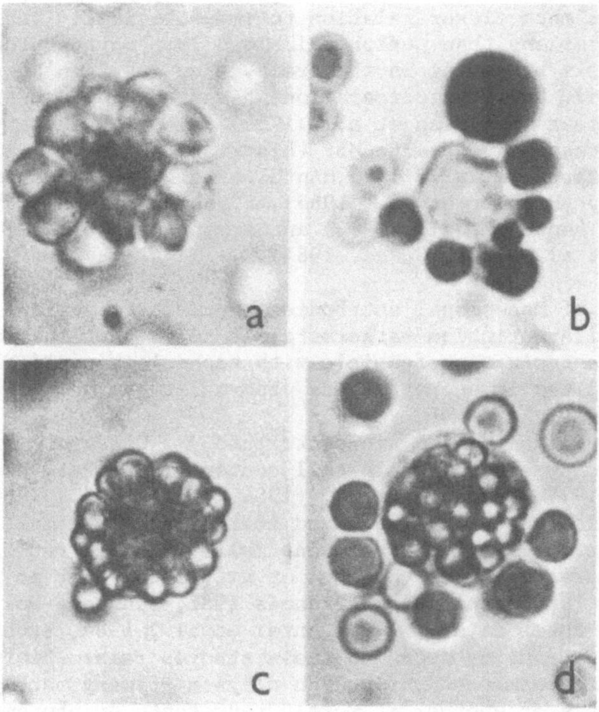

Fig.1. Rosette forming of CSF lymphocytes.
a. Avid E-rosette
b. Bio-Rad OKT8 lymphocyte
c. Own OKT4 avid lymphocyte
d. Own OKT4 and E rosette

50 µl of Immunbead (Quantigen, Bio-Rad) containing suspension should be added to the spined lymphocytes. After 5 min. manual shaking at room temperature, incubate for 5 min. at 36°C and then 60 min. at 4°C. To 10 µl of cell suspension from the apex of the glass tube, add 10 µl of 0.1% toluidine blue solution. Count the labelled and non-labelled lymphocytes in Fuchs-Rosenthal chamber in light microscope binding more than two spheres. OKT4 beads appear as pink, OKT8 as brown spheres (Fig.1b).

Immunbead with OKT4, OKT8 and Leu7 monoclonal antibodies have been prepared using 2.1 um (Estapor Latex PSI 496) unique polyvinyl toluene beads (Rhone-Poulenc, Paris), Guseo 1986 (Fig.1c). Marking of lymphocytes were done similar as described at Quantigen.

Double surface markers have been evaluated using E+OKT4 (Fig.1d), E+OKT8 and E+Leu7 and OKT4+8 markers simultaneously, giving sheep red blood cells (SRBC) and immunbeads at the same time to CSF cell suspensions. Cells with double markers have been evaluated.

RESULTS

Multiple sclerosis

E-rosette: there was no considerable difference in active and total lymphocytes in chronic progressive patients in acute relapse or in remission. The only significant and permanent finding was the decrease of avid cells in acute exacerbations and a slight elevation in chronic progressive disorders (Fig.2). This was found to be a useful marker of disease activity. After a short high dose steroid treatment, a remarkable increase of avid T cells have been observed. A similar tendency was seen after immunosuppressive therapy in MS and non-MS patients too (Guseo 1984).

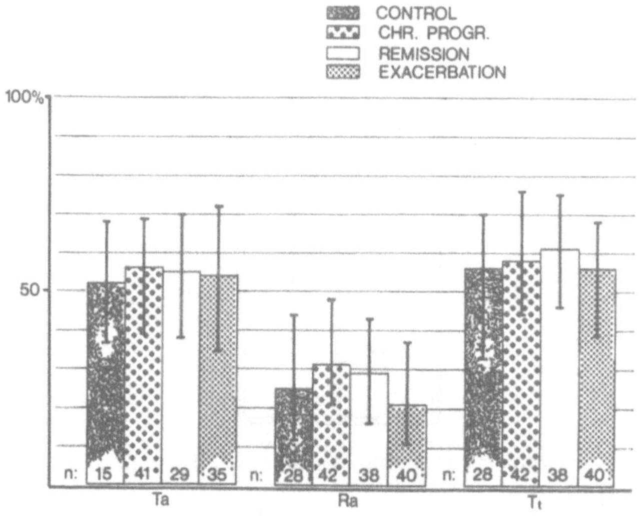

Fig.2. Active (Ta), avid (Ra) and total (Tt) T lymphocytes in MS by the E rosette technique.

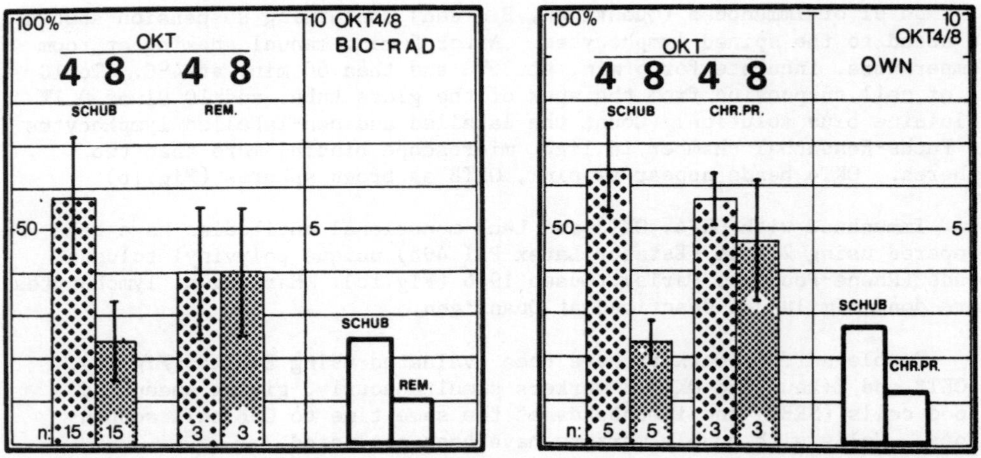

Fig.3. Helper and suppressor cells in the CSF, demonstrated by Bio-Rad and own method in MS.

Monoclonal antibodies: a slight but not significant descrease of suppressor cells has been found in acute relapse in the CSF. In chronic progressive cases the number of suppressor cells was higher and therefore the helper(suppressor ratio fell to 1.0 (Fig.3). After steroid treatment in remission a significant elevation of suppressor cells and fall of helper cells results in a low, nearly normal helper/suppressor ratio.

Comparing the results of both Bio-Rad and own method, the results were concordant (Fig.3).

The number of Leu7 positive cells in chronic progressive cases were higher than those in active phase, but the small number of cases admonish for carefulness (Fig.4).

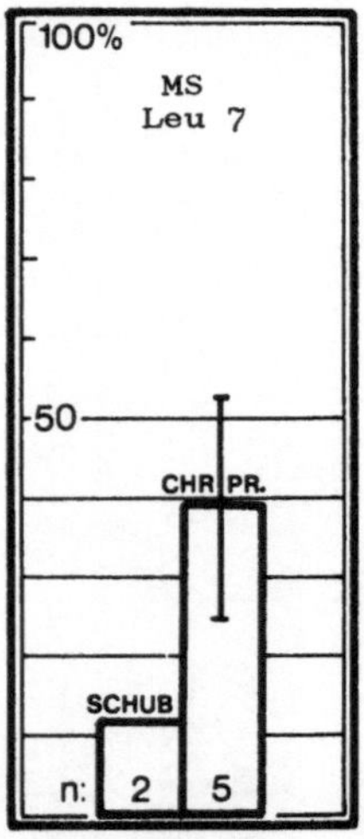

Fig.4. Cytotoxic lymphocyte in MS demonstrated by Leu7 monoclonal antibody coated beads.

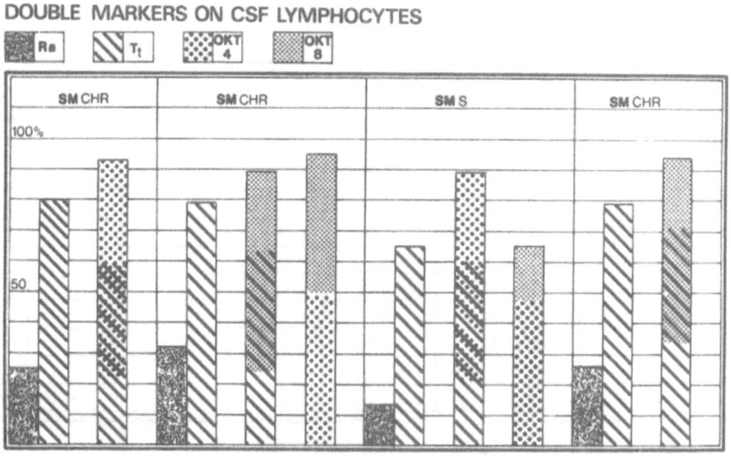

Fig.5. Double markers E+OKT4 and E+OKT8 in MS.

<u>Double markers (E+OKT4, E+OKT8, E+Leu7 and OKT4+8):</u> the aim of this investigation was to find out whether E avid cells belong to the helper or suppressor group. In each investigated case a wide overlap 5-40% of E and monoclonal rosettes as well as 3-5% of OKT4+8 markers have been found on one cell in one acute and three chronic progressive MS cases (Fig.5). In many cases the percentage of Leu7 positive cells was the closest to the number of avid cells. No direct evidence could be drawn to the nature of avid cells by this method.

<u>Post-(rabies)-vaccination encephalomyelitis</u>

<u>Case history:</u> a 34 years old male developed post rabies vaccination encephalomyelitis one day after the 6th consecutive vaccination with the Hempt vaccine. On the 10th day afther the first injection at the clinical admission, fewer, nystagmus, peripheral palsy of the VIIth cranial nerve, right sided hemiparesis and ataxia have been observed. One day later severe paraparesis developed with urinary incontinence. 100 mg Oradexon was started daily after admission completed by plasmapheresis on the next two days and 250 mg Cyclosporin A for 6 days followed by daily 150 mg Azathioprin. CSF was taken at admission and weekly in the acute phase and investigated for cellular and humoral immunological parameters (Fig.6).

A slight elevation of helper T lymphocytes was observed in the CSF during the whole course of the disease. There was a remarkable elevation of avid E-rosettes as well as of total T lymphocytes 10 days after an intensive steroid booster and on the 7th day of Cyclosporin A treatment. From that time a decrease in all cell groups has been observed. The lowest suppressor cell number has been evaluated after Cyclosporin A treatment, which was responsible for a very high helper/suppressor ratio.

The patient was symptom-free 3 months after the start of his clinical signs. His wife and 9 years old daughter were vaccinated at the same time without any clinical complication.

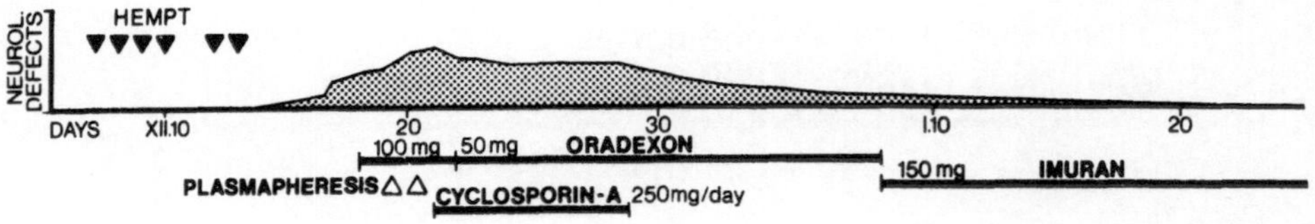

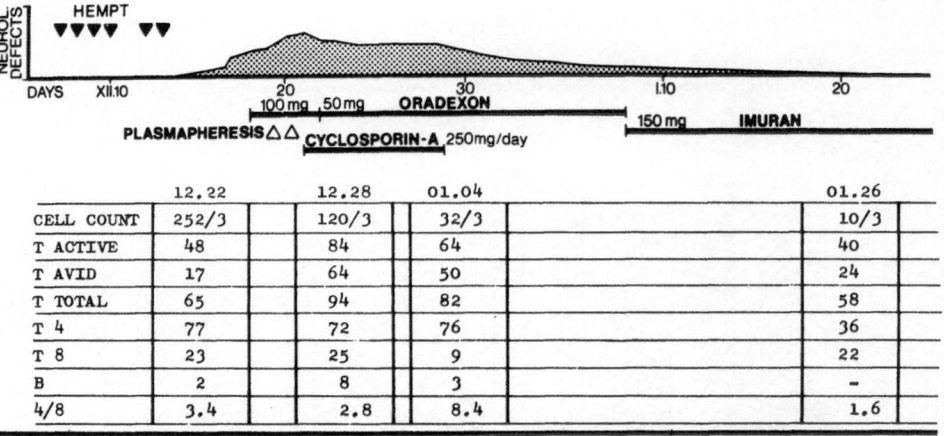

	12.22	12.28	01.04	01.26
CELL COUNT	252/3	120/3	32/3	10/3
T ACTIVE	48	84	64	40
T AVID	17	64	50	24
T TOTAL	65	94	82	58
T 4	77	72	76	36
T 8	23	25	9	22
B	2	8	3	-
4/8	3.4	2.8	8.4	1.6

Fig.6. Post rabies vaccination encephalomyelitis. Clinical course, treatment and CSF cell changes.

DISCUSSION

Immune responses are triggered by cell surface events, therefore in vitro systems which detect receptors on the cell surface, might reveal some specific dynamic aspects of the local immunologic reactions. The nature of avid cells is not yet clear. There are increasing data about the difference of active and avid lymphocytes, Dore-Duffy and Zurier 1979 and Oger et al., 1982 stressed the suppressor nature of avid T lymphocytes, Howard et al., 1984 demonstrated a greater density of SRBC receptors on T suppressor cells than on other T lymphocytes, while Dore-Duffy and Zurier 1979 emphasized their helper nature.

We demonstrated earlier that there is a constant decrease of avid T cells in the CSF in active MS cases and that the low number of avid cells can be normalized by steroid or immunosuppressive treatment, Guseo et al., 1984. All the polyclonal activators were able to induce net increase in total E-receptor content of peripheral blood T lymphocytes after 72 hours culture, whereas beta-endorfin and macrophage synthesized prostaglandin significantly depressed the expression of E-receptor, Oh et al., 1986.

It is well known that in exacerbation among lymphocytes a great number of monocytes reaches the target organ. Their activity and local prostaglandin synthesis may cause the down-regulation of E-receptors on CSF lymphocytes. The induction of new E-receptor antigen is probably responsible for the higher avidity of lymphocytes shortly after steroid treatment.

We have shown a disease activity dependent fluctuation in E avid cells in MS and in a case of monophasic human EAE as well as in benign lymphocytic meningitis (unpublished data), which indicates that E-receptor antigen density may be a functional marker for activated T (suppressor) lymphocytes. It would be interesting to correlate these findings by monoclonal antibodies detecting early and late appearing activation antigens.

The disappearance of T suppressor cells from the periphery, preceeding acute relapse, suggested the segregation of these cells into the target organ. The lower proportion of OKT8^{+} cells in acute exacerbations doesn't support the hypothesis of their actual target homing, which was confirmed by Zaffaroni et al., 1985. Schädlich et al., 1983 didn't find any correlation between OKT8 binding cells in the CSF and the severity of the disease.

Fleischer et al., 1984 demonstrated double OKT4 and 8 markers on the cell surface of clonally expanded CSF lymphocytes. In our investigations helper and suppressor markers have been demonstrated in 3-5% of the lymphocytes. Any lymphocyte subpopulation expresses a number of different surface antigens of a functional significance, which is the result of a continually changing dynamic process. The dynamic variability of the surface molecules emphasizes the careful evaluation of the results.

SUMMARY

A quick and easy light microscopic method was used to demonstrate CSF lymphocyte subpopulations. Decrease of suppressor T lymphocytes in exacerbation and increase in chronic progressive cases have been demonstrated.

By the E rosette, the number of avid T cells decreases in acute exacerbation. This was found to be a useful functional marker.

Fluctuation of CSF lymphocyte subpopulations was noticed in a case of post-(rabies)-vaccination encephalomyelitis during steroid and Cyclosporin A treatment.

REFERENCES

1. M.M. Albala, D. Davignon, L.D. Fast and D.D. Clark. Normal T subsets and lymphocyte activity in multiple sclerosis. Clin. Exp. Immunol. 61:524-547 (1985).
2. J.P. Antel, D.M. Peeples, A.T. Reder and B.G.W. Arnason. Analysis of T regulator cell surface markers and functional properties in multiple sclerosis. J. of Neuroimmunol. 6:93-103 (1984).
3. M.A. Bach, C. Martin, P. Cesaro, J.F. Eizenbaum and J.D. Degos. T cell subsets in multiple sclerosis. A longitudinal study of exacerbating remitting cases. J. of Neuroimmunol. 7:331-343 (1985).
4. N. Cashman, M.A. Bach, C. Martin, J.D. Degos and J.F. Bach. Suppressor/cytotoxic cell perturbations during exacerbations on MS. Neurology. 32:A69 (1982).
5. A. Compston. Lymphocyte subpopulations in patients with multiple sclerosis. 46:105-114 (1983).
6. D. Dommasch, L. Kappos, C. Focke and M. Popp. Longitudinal investigation of T lymphocyte subsets in the peripheral blood of MS patients. Annual report of the Max-Planck-Society Clinical Research Unit for MS. 2:22-23 (1984).
7. P. Dore-Duffy and R.B. Zurier. E-rosette formation in normals and patients with multiple sclerosis: Effect of prostaglandin and aspirin. Clin. Immunol. Immunopathol. 13:261-268 (1979).
8. B. Fleischer, P. Marquardt, S. Poser and H.W. Kreth. Phenotypic markers and functional characteristics of T lymphocyte clones from cerebrospinal fluid in multiple sclerosis. J. of Neuroimmunol. 7: 151-162 (1984).
9. A. Guseo. T lymphocyte subsets in the CSF in various stages of MS. In: "Immunological and clinical aspects of multiple sclerosis". R.E. Gonsette, P. Delmotte, ed. MTP Press Limited, Lancaster. 205-209 (1984).
10. A. Guseo. Rapid determination of CSF lymphocyte subsets by labelled microspheres. J. of Neuroimmunol. In press.

11. D.A. Hafler, M.E. Hemler, L. Christenson, J.M. Williams, H.M. Shapiro, T.B. Strom, J.L. Strominger and H.L. Weiner. Investigations of in vivo activated T cells in multiple sclerosis and inflammatory central nervous system diseases. Clin. Immunol. Immunopathol. 37:163-171 (1985).
12. S.L. Hauser, E.L. Reinherz, C.J. Hoban, S.F. Schlossman and H.L. Weiner. CSF cells in multiple sclerosis: monoclonal antibody analysis and relationship to peripheral blood T cell subsets. Neurology. 33:575-579 (1983).
13. S.L. Hauser, E.L. Reinherz, C.J. Hoban, S.F. Schlossmann and H.L. Weiner. Immunoregulatory T cells and lymphocytotoxic antibodies in active multiple sclerosis. Weekly analysis over a six month period. Ann. Neurol. 13:418-425 (1983).
14. F. Howard, J.A. Ledbetter, J. Wong, C.P. Bieber, E.B. Stinson and L.A. Herzenberg. Human T lymphocyte differentiation marker defined by monoclonal antibodies that block E rosette formation. J. Immunol. 126:2117-2122 (1981).
15. A.B.C. Noronha, D.P. Richman and B.G.W. Arnason. Detection of in vivo stimulated cerebrospinal fluid lymphocytes by flow cytometry in patients with multiple sclerosis. New Engl. J. Med. 303:713-717 (1980).
16. J.F. Oger, B.G.W. Arnason, S.H.W. Ray and J.P. Kistler. A study of B and T cells in multiple sclerosis. Neurology. 25:444-447 (1975).
17. J.F. Oger, J.P. Antel, A. Noronha and B.G.W. Arnason. Changes in T cell subpopulations in the cerebrospinal fluid in multiple sclerosis patients. Neurology. 32, A148 (1982).
18. S.K. Oh, W.L. Farrar and F.W. Ruscetti. Modulation of E-receptor expression on activated T lymphocytes. Clin. Immunol. Immunopathol. 38:55-67 (1986).
19. H.S. Panits and G.S. Francis. T lymphocyte subsets in cerebrospinal fluid in multiple sclerosis. New Engl. J. Med. 307:60-61 (1982).
20. D.W. Paty, L. Kastrukoff, N. Morgano and L. Hiob. Suppressor T-lymphocytes in multiple sclerosis. Analysis of patients with acute relapsing and chronic progressive disease. Ann. Neurol. 14:445-449 (1983).
21. G.P.A. Rice, D. Finney, S.L. Braheny, R.L. Knobler, J.C. Sipe and M.B.A. Oldstone. Disease activity markers in multiple sclerosis. Another look at suppressor cells defined by monoclonal antibodies OKT4, OKT5 and OKT8. J. of Neuroimmunol. 6:75-84 (1984).
22. M. Sandberg-Wollheim. Lymphocyte populations in the cerebrospinal fluid and peripheral blood of patients with multiple sclerosis and optic neuritis. Scand. J. Immunol. 17:575-581 (1983).
23. H.J. Schädlich, Y. Bliersbach, K. Felgenhauer and M. Schieferdecker. OKT8 binding lymphocytes in diseases of the nervous system. J. of Neuroimmunol. 5:289-294 (1983).
24. M. Zaffaroni, D. Caputo, A. Ghezzi and C.L. Cazzullo. T cell subsets in multiple sclerosis: relationships between periheral blood and cerebrospinal fluid. Acta Neurol. Scand. 71:242-248 (1985).

T-CELL MARKERS IN CEREBROSPINAL FLUID OF PATIENTS WITH MULTIPLE SCLEROSIS AND OTHER NEUROLOGICAL DISEASES

E. Tournier-Lasserve[1], N. Cashman[2], E. Roullet[3], O. Lyon-caen[4], J.D. Degos[5] and M.A. Bach

[1] Unité de Pathologie de l'Immunité, Institut Pasteur, Paris
[2] Unité INSERM 25, Hôpital Necker, Paris
[3] Service de Neurologie, Hôpital Saint-Antoine, Paris
[4] Service de Neurologie, Hôpital de la Salpétrière, Paris
[5] Service de Neurologie, Hôpital Henri Mondor, Créteil

INTRODUCTION

Multiple sclerosis (MS) is a demyelinating disease likely resulting from an autoimmune process (1). Indeed, several observations suggest that an immune response develops inside of the central nervous system (CNS) during the active phase of the disease: oligoclonal immunoglobulins are locally produced and secreted into the cerebrospinal fluid (CSF) (2), and plaques of demyelination are infiltrated, especially in perivascular areas, by mononuclear cells comprising mostly T-cells and macrophages (3,4). Neither the target(s) of this immune response nor the respective roles of cellular and humoral immunity are presently known although it has been suggested by reference to the animal models of experimental allergic encephalomyelitis (EAE) that T-cells might play a key role in the pathogenesis of MS as it does in EAE (5). Several authors including ourselves have reported marker and function abnormalities of circulating blood T-cells, generally associated with active phases of the disease (6,9). How relevant are these observations to the analysis of the local autoimmune process remains questionable. Unfortunately however, the direct approach of the events taking place inside of the CNS will be necessarily limited to the histopathological study of a very small number of brains. Cerebrospinal fluid on the other hand is generally thought to give a better image of the CNS than peripheral blood, and is more easily accessible to investigation.

T-cells can be divided into two major subsets according to the expression of the differentiation surface antigens CD4 and CD8 (10,11): these subsets functionnally differ by their ability to recognize nominal antigens either in the context of class II or class I antigens of the major histocompatibility complex (MHC), respectively.

Moreover, in most in vitro assays available, CD4 T-cells behave as helper inducer cells whereas CD8 T-cells exert effector/suppressor activities (10,11). Either subset may show cytotoxic activity depending on whether the target cells express class I and/or class II MHc antigens (10). Upon antigenic or mitogenic activation, T-cell of either subset express a new set of surface molecules such as the receptor for interleukin 2 (IL2), ("Tac" antigen) (12), MHC class II antigens ("DR" antigens), (13,14), and other antigens of so far undefined function (15). Some of these activation antigens are only expressed by cells of the T-cell lineage whereas others, such as DR antigens are present on other cell types such as B-cells or macrophages (14). We have studied the expression of the subset markers CD4 and CD8 on one hand, and of the activation markers Tac and DR on the other hand by CSF cells, in comparison to peripheral blood mononuclear cells (PBMC), in MS patients and patients suffering other neurological diseases (OND).

MATERIAL AND METHODS

Subjects

Studies of CD4 and CD8 T-cell subsets and of T-cell activation markers were performed independently on different groups of MS patients and OND controls. The former study included 40 MS patients (26 relapsing patients, 9 patients in remission and 5 patients with chronic progressive disease) and 15 OND patients, of whom 8 suffered inflammatory diseases of the CNS. The latter study included 14 MS patients (9 relapsing patients, 1 patient in remission, and 4 patients with chronic progressive disease) and 12 OND patients, among whom 10 suffered an inflammatory disease of the CNS.

No patient received either immunosuppressive of corticorsteroïd therapy at the time of study except when otherwise stated. Staff members and blood bank donors served as healthy controls for blood studies.

Cell preparation

Peripheral blood mononuclear cells were obtained by centrifugation of heparinized venous blood over a Ficoll-Hypaque gradient. After 3 washings, PBMC were resuspended in RPMI 1640 (Gibco Laboratories, Grand Island, NY) and supplemented with 5% normal heat-inactivated human serum, at a concentration of 10^6 cells per ml.

Cerebrospinal fluid cells were prepared as already described (16). Briefly 20 ml of CSF were drawn into a polypropylene tube containing 4 ml human serum (to improve cell viability). CSF cells were collected by centrifugation at 400 g during 10 minutes, then washed once in RPMI and finally resuspended in 250 µl RPMI supplemented with 5% normal human serum.

Monoclonal antibodies

The following monoclonal antibodies were used for this study: OKT3 (Ortho Pharmaceuticals, Raritan, New-Jersey, U.S.A.), directed against the CD3 molecule, and IOT1 (Immunotech, Marseille-Lumigny, France) directed against the CD5 molecule served as pan-T-cell markers. Antibodies OKT4

(Ortho) or IOT4 (Immunotech), and OKT8 (Ortho) or IOT8 (Immunotech), were used to detect CD4 and CD8 T-cell subsets respectively. Antibody B.1.49.9 and B8.12.2. (Immunotech) recognized the IL2 receptor ("Tac" antigen) and a monomorphic HLA-DR determinant respectively.

Immunofluorescence assays

Cell fixation of monoclonal antibodies was detected by an indirect immunofluorescence assay using FITC-labelled purified goat anti-mouse IgG antibodies, absorbed on a human IgG immunosorbent as already described (7,16). Reading was performed either visually using a Leitz fluorescence microscope (for the T-cell subset analysis), or by flow-cytometry using a Cytofluograph (Ortho), for studies on T-cell markers of activation.

RESULTS

Distribution of CD4 and CD8 T-cells in blood of MS patients (Table 1)

Patients suffering active MS (relapse or progressive course) displayed, as a group, a T-cell subset imbalance, as compared to OND patients or healthy controls: the mean percentage of CD8+ PBMC was decreased with a correlative increase of the CD4/CD8 ratio. Not all patients however, exhibited such an abnormality, which was most often seen in exacerbating patients shortly before or shortly after the clinical onset of a relapse (2 weeks and one week respectively). MS patients, studied more than a month after the onset of exacerbation, again exhibited high CD4/CD8 ratios, which may result in part from a biased selection of patients suffering prolonged and servere relapse who remained unusually long in the hospital for this reason. MS patients in remission and OND patients showed normal T-cell subset distribution.

CD4 and CD8 cells in CSF of MS patients (Table 2 and Fig.1)

The percentage of CD3 positive cells and the CD4/CD8 ratio among CSF cells from OND patients was higher than that measured among PBMC of the same group or of the group of healthy subjects. The CD4/CD8 ratio in CSF of relapsing MS patients was still higher than that observed in CSF of OND patients, resulting from a significantly lower percentage of CD8+ T-cells in the formers. Again, the most striking abnormalities were seen in patients studied within 2 weeks before or after the clinical onset of relapse. It is noteworthy that many patients studied during the third week of relapse displayed low CD4/CD8 ratios, similar to those observed in patients in remission.

Four patients were investigated more than once. As seen in Fig.1, the highest CD4/CD8 ratio values were always observed at the closest time after the beginning of exacerbation.

Table 1. Changes of blood T-cell subset distribution in active MS

Remission	Relapse					Chronic progression	OND	Healthy controls
	0-14 days before	0-6 days after	7-13 days after	14-20 days after	21-60 days after			
1.7±0.1[a]	3.5±0.6[b]	3.3±0.4	2.2±0.4	1.9±0.3	3.0±0.4	2.8±0.5	2.0±0.2	1.8±0.1
(22)[c]	(7)	(13)	(8)	(8)	(14)	(29)	(15)	(61)

[a] Mean ± SE
[b] Values significantly different from healthy control group are underlined
[c] Number of subjects tested.

Table 2. CSF lymphocyte subsets

% cell reactive with	OND controls	MS remission	MS: exacerbation			MS: chronic progressive form
			2 wks before to 2 wks after	third week	3 wks to 6 mos	
	n=11	n=9	n=11	n=8	n=12	n=5
CD3	89±2	88±2	87±2	90±2	87±2	89±1
CD4	64±3	71±3	69±3	64±3	67±3	65±2
CD8	28±3	23±2	15±1	31±4	20±1	21±1
CD4/CD8 ratio	2.59±0.32	3.17±0.39	4.80±1.28	2.42±0.46	3.63±0.52	3.33±0.30

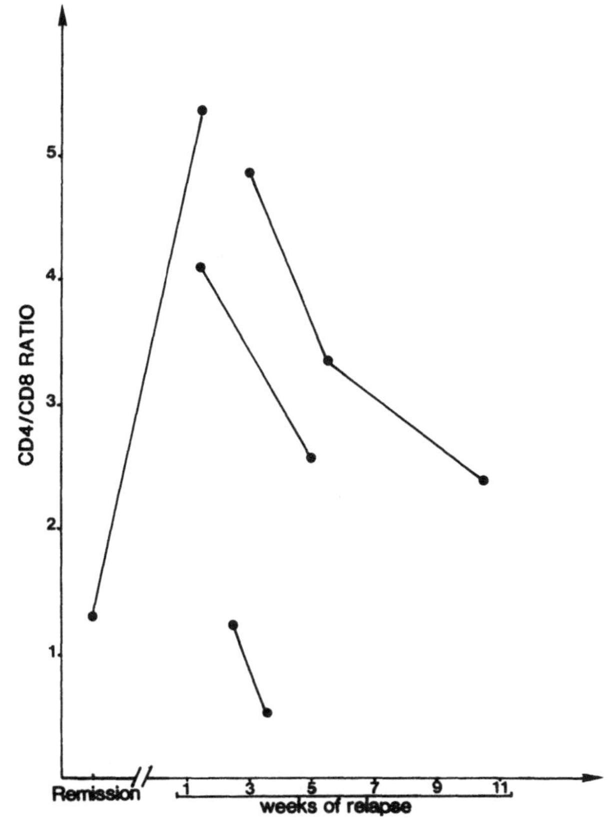

Fig.1. A follow-up of CD4 and CD8 T-cell subsets in CSF of relapsing MS patients.

Expression of Tac and DR antigens by CSF cells of MS and OND patients (Table 3,4,5 and Fig.2)

Low percentages of either Tac$^+$ or DR$^+$ cells were observed among blood lymphocytes of healthy subjects (less than 10% in 97.5% of cases, mean = 3%). Percentages of Tac$^+$ cells among lymphocytes of MS and OND patients were similar to those of healthy subjects. Both patient groups showed a moderate elevation of the percentage of DR$^+$ lymphocytes, which reached statistical significance for OND patients only. A significant increase (by 2 to 3 times) of the percentage of Tac$^+$ and DR$^+$ cells in CSF as compared to blood was noted in MS patients and OND patients without any significant difference between both groups.

Fig.2 shows that high percentages of DR$^+$ CSF cells were observed either shortly after relapse or in chronic progressive forms, whereas high percentages of Tac$^+$ cells were observed in any group of MS patients, including in the patient in remission.

One relapsing MS patient and one patient suffering a Lyme disease were studied more than once. In the MS patients (Table 4), a moderate elevation of Tac+ CSF cells and a more consistent increase of DR+ cells was observed on the first occasion, that is to 2 weeks after the onset of clinical symptoms, prior to any treatment. During the next 3 weeks, while a treatment by ACTH had been started, the percentage of Tac+ cells increased in CSF whereas that of DR+ cells strikingly decreased. The patient suffering a Lyme disease (Table 5) showed at the first study high CSF percentages of Tac+ cells and DR positive cells, which had returned to low values when she was reinvestigated 3 months later, at a time when she was clinically improving but still harboured 70 cells/mm^3 with CSF.

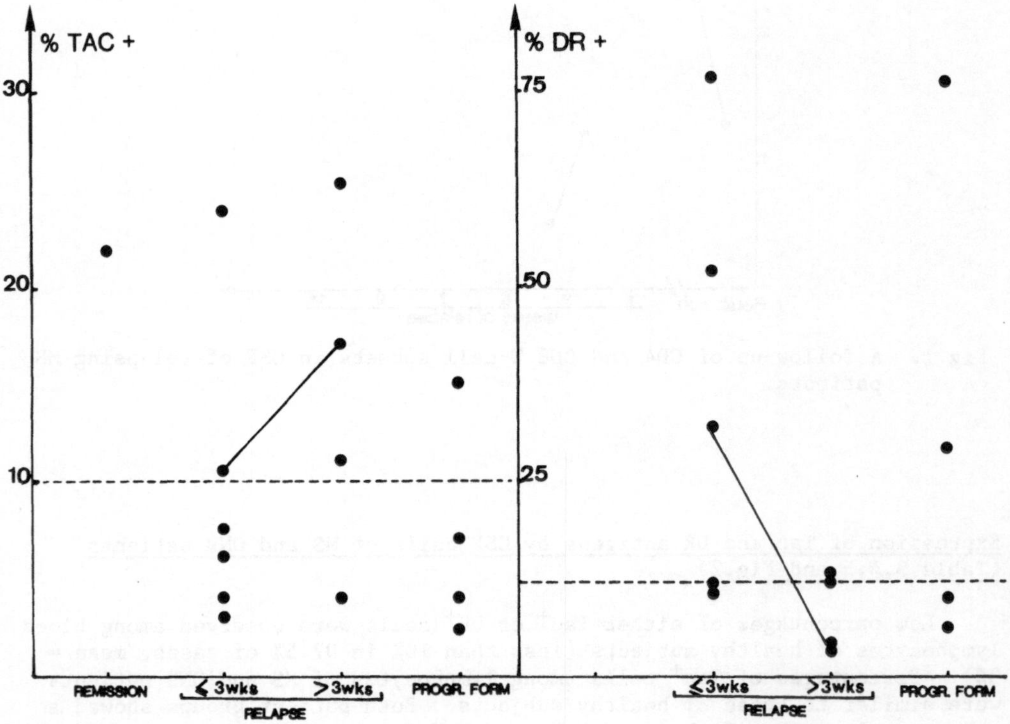

Fig.2. Expression of Tac and DR antigens by CSF cells of MS patients. Dashed lines indicate the 95% confidence upper limit of normal values of either Tac positive or DR positive cells within blood of healty subjects. Values recorded at different times from the same patient are joined by a solid line.

Table 3

SUBJECTS	SOURCE OF CELLS	% T1	% TAC	% DR
MS patients	blood	48±4a 10	4±1 8	8±2 10
	CSF	54±7 11	10±2 14	26±7 13
OND patients	blood	44±3 7	5±2 7	9±2 6
	CSF	57±6 11	15±3 12	32±5 11
subjects	blood	46±5 11	3±1 11	3±1 9

a Mean ± SEM

Table 4. CSF cell kinetic study of one relapsing MS patient

Treatment	Date	Cells/mm^3	% CD5	% Tac	% DR	% CD4	% CD8	CD4/CD8 ratio
None	4/2/85 2-3 weeks post relapse	18	44	10	32	37	30	1.23
ACTH 1mg daily	11/2/85	8	-	15	34	24	47	0.51
ACTH 1 mg every other day	25/2/85	7	46	17	3	-	-	-

Table 5. CSF cell kinetic study of one patient suffering Lyme disease

Date	Cells/mm^3	% CD5	% Tac	% DR	% CD4	% CD8	CD4/CD8 ratio
28/10/84	115	81	15	60	65	75	0.86
10/1/85	70	-	3	2	48	24	2.00

DISCUSSION

We have observed in some active MS patients a relative decrease of the CD8 T-cell proportion, an abnormality which could be detected among PBMC but was more pronounced among the CSF cells (7,8,16). In relapsing patients, this phenomenon appeared to be transient, occurring a few days before or after the clinical onset of exacerbation (8), which likely explains that some groups failed to evidence any T-cell subset abnormality of PBMC in MS patients (17).

The relevance of such a T-cell subset imbalance to the pathophysiology of MS is unclear. CD8 T-cells might migrate massively to the CNS at the time of relapse and thus create a relative deficit of the peripheral CD8 T-cell pool. However our CSF studies do not support this hypothesis, since the early phase of relapse is actually associated to a decrease of the CD8 T-cell percentage. T-cell subset imbalance may also result from the activation and expansion of the pool of CD4 T-cells. Some histopathological studies of MS lesions indicated that CD4 T-cells were predominant within the perivascular infiltrates of plaques and the surrounding white matter (3,4). Conflicting reports of CD8 T-cells being the predominant T-cell type may result from the secondary recruitment and activation of CD8 T-cells (18). A similar biphasic phenomenon has been observed in animal models of EAE: T-cell lines of the "T4" phenotype are the first T-cells observed within the lesions and can transfer the disease to naïve recipients (5,19) whereas "T8" cells may be secundarily observed within the CNS of actively induced EAE (20). In that respect it is worthy to note that activation of either cytotoxic or suppressor function of CD8 T-cells has been shown to require the help of "inducer" CD4 T-cells in all _in vitro_ models of immune response so far studied (10,11).

Changes in the distribution of T-cell subsets in the various body compartment of MS patients likely result from the initial activation of small antigen-reactive T-cell clones (whatever the nature of this antigen) followed by the secondary recruitment, activation and migration of larger T-cell polls. Several studies including the present one indeed demonstrate the presence of activated T-cells within the CNS and the CSF. Thus we found in CSF from MS and OND patients (most of the latter suffering an inflammatory disease) a higher percentage of cells expressing the IL2 receptor (Tac antigen) than in blood, where the percentage of Tac$^+$ cells was not different from that of healthy subjects. We also found an increased percentage of DR positive CSF cells in the same groups of patients but without individual correlation with the percentage of Tac positive cells. DR antigens are normally expressed by resting B-cells and dendritic cells and appear upon activation on T-cells and macrophages (14). We have strong indirect evidence of the presence of DR positive T-cells in CSF in some OND and MS patients in which we simultaneous found elevated percentages of both CD5 positive cells and DR positive cells. Expression of DR antigens and Tac antigen by activated T-cells have been shown to have different kinetics (13,2) which may also explain the lack of correlation between their percentages among CSF cells. Indeed, in the present work, increased percentages of DR positive cells in CSF of relapsing MS patients were recorded at the beginning of the exacerbation period, whereas high numbers of Tac positive cells were observed within the CSF for longer periods, and were even present in one patient in remission. It is interesting to note that no difference could be detected between MS and OND patients in the expression of DR or Tac antigens by CSF T-cells, but it should be reminded that most OND patients actually suffered an inflammatory disease of the central nervous system. Our data are in agreement with those reported by Bellamy et al. (22) who also measured high numbers of Tac positive-cells in the CSF of MS patients (but not in blood) and who demonstrated in addition the presence of Tac positive cells, as well as of IL2 producing cells, within the CNS lesions of MS patients. On the other hand Hafler et al. (23) did not detect any increase of Tac positive cells in the CSF of MS patients with chronic progressive disease but observed both in blood and CSF of these patients high percentages of T-cells expressing another marker of T-cell activation, the Tal antigen (15). Finally, Noronha et al. (24,25), measuring RNA and DNA contents in CSF cells by flow cytometry, also reached the conclusion of the presence of high numbers of activated T cells within CSF of MS patients. Whether these T-cells are locally activated within the CNS, or are triggered at the periphery and then concentrate within the CNS, cannot be concluded from any of these studies and remain a key problem of the pathogenesis of multiple sclerosis.

ACKNOWLEDGEMENTS

The financial support of "Association pour la Recherche sur la sclérose en plaques" (ARSEP) is gratefully acknowledged.

REFERENCES

1. D.E. McFarlin, H. McFarland. Multiple sclerosis. N. Engl. J. Med. 307:1183 (1982).
2. H. Link. Immunoglobulin G and low molecular weight proteins in human cerebrospinal fluid. Chemical and immunological characterization with special reference to multiple sclerosis. Acta. Neurol. Scand. 43 (Suppl.28):11 (1973).
3. H. Nyland, R. Matre, S. Mork, J.R. Bierke and A. Naess. T-lymphocyte subpopulations in multiple sclerosis lesions. N. Engl. J. Med. 307: 1643 (1982).
4. U. Traugott, E.L. Reinherz and C.S. Kaine. Multiple sclerosis: distribution of T-cell subsets within active chronic lesions. Science. 219:308 (1983).
5. C.B. Petinelli and D.E. McFarlin. Adoptive transfer of experimental allergic encephalomyelitis in SJL/J mice after in vitro activation of lymph node cells by myelin basic protein: Requirement for Lyt I +2-T lymphocytes. J. Immunol. 127:1420 (1981).
6. E.L. Reinherz, H.L. Weiner, S.L. Hauser, J.A. Cohen, J.A. Distaso and S.F. Schlossmann. Loss of suppressor T-cells in active multiple sclerosis. Analysis with monoclonal antibodies. N. Engl. J. Med. 303:125 (1980).
7. M.A. Bach, F. Phan Dinh Tuy, E. Tournier, L. Chatenoud, J.F. Bach, C. Martin and J.D. Degos. Deficit of suppressor T cells in active multiple sclerosis. Lancet. 2:1221 (1980).
8. M.A. Bach, C. Martin, P. Cesaro, J.F. Eizenbaum and J.D. Degos. T-cell subsets in multiple sclerosis: A longitudinal study of exacerbating-remitting case. J. Neuroimmunol. 7:331 (1985).
9. A. Compston. Lymphocyte subpopulations in patients with multiple sclerosis. J. Neurol. Neurosurg. Psychiatry. 46:105 (1983).

10. E.L. Reinherz, S.C. Meuer and S.F. Schlossmann. The human T-cells receptor: Analysis with cytotoxic T-cell clones. Immunol. Rev. 74:83 (1983).
11. Y. Thomas, L. Rogozinski and L. Chess. Relationship between human T-cell functional heterogeneity and human T-cell surface molecules. Immunol. Rev. 74:113 (1983).
12. T. Uchiyama, S. Broder and T.A. Waldmann. A monoclonal antibody (anti-Tac) reactive with activated and functionally mature human T-cell. I. Production of anti-Tac monoclonal antibody and distribution of Tac(+) cells. J. Immunol. 126:1393, 7 (1981).
13. G.R. Burmester, B. Jahn, M. Gramatzki, J. Zacher and J.R. Kalden. Activated T-cells in vivo and in vitro: divergence in expression of Tac and Ia antigens in the nonblastoïd small T-cells of inflammation and normal T-cells activated in vitro. J. Immunol. 133:1230 (1984).
14. E.L. Reinherz, P.C. Kung, J.M. Ritz, G. Goldstein and S.F. Schlossmann. Ia determinants on human T-cell subsets defined by monoclonal antibody: activation stimuli required for expression. J. Exp. Med. 150:1472 (1979).
15. D.A. Fox, R.E. Hussey and K.A. Fitzgeral. $Ta_1$1, a novel 105 kd human T-cell activation antigen defined by a monoclonal antibody. J. Immunol. 133:1250 (1984).
16. N. Cashman, C. Martin, J.F. Eizenbaum, J.D. Degos and M.A. Bach. Monoclonal antibody defined immunoregulatory cells in multiple sclerosis cerebrospinal fluid. J. Clin. Invest. 70:387 (1982).
17. G.P.A. Rice, D.F. Finney, S.L. Brahemy, R.L. Knobler, J.C. Sipe and M.B.A. Oldstone. Disease activity markers in multiple sclerosis. Another look at suppressor cells defined by monoclonal antibodies OKT4, OKT5 and OKT8. J. Neuroimmunol. 6:75 (1984).
18. H.L. Weiner, A.K. Bhan and J. Burks. Immunohistochemical analysis of the cellular infiltrate in multiple sclerosis lesions. Neurology (NY). 34: Suppl. 1:112 (1984).
19. S. Sriram, D. Solomon, R.V. Rouse and L. Steinman. Identification of T-cell subsets and B lymphocytes in mouse stain experimental allergic encephalomyelitis lesions. J. Immunol. 129:1649 (1982).
20. W.F. Hickey and W.K. Gonatas. Suppressor T lymphocytes in the spinal cord of Lewis rats recovered from acute experimental allergic encephalomyelitis. Cell. Immunol. 85:284 (1984).
21. A. Yachie, T. Miyawaki, N. Uwadana, S. Ohzeki and N. Taniguchi. Sequential expression of T cell activation (Tac) antigen and Ia determinants on circulating human T cells after immunization with tetanus toxoid. J. Immunol. 131, 731 (1983).
22. A.S. Bellamy, V.L. Calder, M. Feldmann and N. Davison. The distribution of interleukin-2 receptor-bearing lymphocytes in multiple sclerosis: evidence for a key role of activated lymphocytes. Clin. Exp. Immunol. 61:248 (1985).
23. D.A. Hafler, D.A. Fox, M.E. Manning, S.F. Schlossmann, E.L. Reinherz and H.L. Weiner. In vivo activated T lymphocytes in the peripheral blood and cerebrospinal fluid of patients with multiple sclerosis. N. Engl. J. Med. 312:1405 (1985).
24. A.B.C. Noronha, D.P. Richman and B.G.W. Arnason. Detection of in vivo stimulated cerebrospinal-fluid lymphocytes by flow cytometry in patients with multiple sclerosis. N. Engl. J. Med. 303, 713 (1980).
25. A.B.C. Noronha, G.R. Otten, D.P. Richeman and B.G.W. Arnason. Multiple sclerosis: flow cytometry with simultaneous detection of surface antigen and cell cycle phase reveals that activated cells in cerebrospinal fluid are not OKT8-positive. Ann. Neurol. 12, 104 (1982).

THE IDENTIFICATION OF THEOPHYLLINE RESISTANT AND THEOPHILLINE SENSITIVE T CELL BY MONOCLONAL ANTIBODIES AGAINST LEUCOCYTES

Tianbao Wang, Dafei Xu and Zheng Wang

Dept. Pathophysiology, Beijing Institute of Clinical Medicine, Friendship Hospital Beijing, China

Shore et al. showed that T cell, purified by E rosette technique, may be separated by incubation with theophylline into two subsets, one of which lost its ability to form E rosette and was called theophylline sensitive T cell (Tsen), the other one can still form E rosette with SRBC and was called theophylline resistant T cell (Tres). Tres and Tsen have been shown to enhance and to inhibit immune function in vitro as well as in vivo respectively (1). It is worth to investigate the distribution of T4 and T8 antigen on Tres and Tsen using monoclonal antibodies.

MATERIAL AND METHODS

A peripheral mononuclear cell was isolated by the Ficoll-Hapaque fractionating method from normal blood donors. The mononuclear cell was put in a petri dish and incubated at 37°C for 1 hour to remove the adherent cell. A purified lymphocyte was incubated with a fresh prepared sheep red blood cell in the refrigerator overnight to form rosette. The E rosette was isolated by centrifugation and the red blood cell was disrupted by treatment of distilled water. After washing, the E rosette forming cell was incubated with theophylline at 37°C for 1 hour. The cell was washed twice in PBS and incubated again with SRBC at 4°C for two hours. E rosette was separated again and shook with distilled water to disrupt red blood cells. This was Tres. After treatment with theophylline, T cells that did not form rosettes in the supernatant were collected too by another centrifugation. This was Tsen. Both Tres and Tsen were washed and adjusted to a concentration of 5 10^6/ml. To 100 micro 1 of Tres and Tsen cell suspension, 5 micro 1 of monoclonal antibodies were added and incubated in an ice bath for 30 minutes. After washing, cell suspension was incubated with isothiocynate conjugated goat anti mouse $F(ab)_2$ for 30 minutes in an ice bath. After washing, cell suspension was made with glycerol PBS and at least 300 cells were counted under a fluorescence microscope and the percentage of fluorescence positive cells was estimated.

Monoclonal antibodies used in this experiment were gifts kindly sent by Dr. Jose of the Cancer Institute of Australia. It included T44 (corresponds to OKT4), T33 (corresponds to OKT3), Leu2b (corresponds to OKT8), FMC (mab to monocyte and granulocyte), TDR (mab to Ia antigen) and BL14 (mab to B cell line).

RESULTS

The results were shown in Table 1:

Table 1. Identification of Tres and Tsen by some monoclonal antibodies

monoclonal ab	Tres (%)	Tsen (%)	p
T33	76.72 ± 1.60	81.45 ± 4.07	= 0.05
T44	51.87 ± 8.61	17.74 ± 4.93	< 0.001
Leu2b	21.58 ± 6.06	34.83 ± 6.54	< 0.001
FMC	1.83 ± 1.25	1.25 ± 1.36	
TDR	7.77 ± 9.36	4.38 ± 2.88	
BL14	1.50 ± 0.8	2.48 ± 1.97	

It is obviously that Tres is enriched with T4 and Tsen is enriched with T8.

DISCUSSION

T cell subpopulations, especially T helper and T suppressor, are very important in regulating immune function. A variety of techniques have been developed to estimate T helper and T suppressor. The most commonly used, was estimating Fc receptor of IgG and IgM on T cell surface in the past 10 years and it has been gradually replaced by a monoclonal antibody technique. OKT and Leu series of monoclonal antibodies to T subsets were widely used in clinic to evaluate the immune function of patients since 1980 and the phenotypic characteristics defined by OKT and Leu series were considered to be equal to the function of cells. It is increasingly obvious that a monoclonal antibody defined T cell subset is functionally heterogeneic (2). There is a need to look for a technique evaluating T subsets functionally.

Theophylline resistant and theophylline sensitive T cells were shown to enhance and inhibit xenogeneic local GVHR , autologous MLR (1), antigen induced plaque forming cell response and lymphocyte transformation respectively. It is interesting to compare OKT4 and OKT8 defined cells with Tres and Tsen. Divakaran and Wangle found that Tres contained much more OKT4 defined cells, but Tsen contained OKT4 and OKT8 defined cells without a significant difference (3). Birch et al. showed that Tres contained 71.8% OKT4 defined cells and 19.3% OKT8 defined cells, while Tsen contained 23.1% of OKT4 and 53.% of OKT8 defined cells. Our result was consistent with Birch's. It will be interesting to know whether the results in clinical application of Tres and Tsen determination are the same as those using OKT or Leu series monoclonal antibodies.

REFERENCES

1. N.K. Damle and S. Gupta. Scand. J. Immunol. 15:493 (1982).
2. R.E. Balliuex and C.J. Heijnen. Ibid. 74:5 (1983).
3. S. Divakaran and A.G. Wangle. Immunobilo. 165:500 (1983).

REACTIVITY OF CSF CELLS TO NONSPECIFIC STIMULI AND VIRUS ANTIGENS IN VITRO

A. Salmi[1], M. Reunanen[2] and J. Ilonen[3]

[1] Viral Pathogenesis Research Unit, Department of Medical Microbiology and Infectious Diseases
[2] University of Alberta, Canada, Department of Neurology
[3] University of Oulu and National Public Health Institute Oulu, Finland

SUMMARY

We have established short-term in vitro techniques for cultivation of a small number of CSF cells which can be tested for spontaneous proliferation, antigen induced lymphocyte blast transformation or production of immunoglobulins or specific antibodies. The proliferation of lymphocytes was measured by the incorporation of ^{3}H-thymidine and the IgG and antibody production capacity by measuring their amounts in in vitro culture supernatants by enzyme immunoassays. These techniques were used to study the in vitro reactivities of CSF lymphocytes from patients with viral meningitis and multiple sclerosis (MS).

The spontaneous activity of CSF cells was high in acute viral meningitis but it was also elevated in MS patients. When the CSF cells were stimulated with measles, rubella, mumps or herpes simplex antigens, the majority of the MS patients reacted to at least one of these antigens and many had simultaneous reactivity against all. This reactivity varied in samples taken at different times from the same patient but this fluctuation was not clearly connected to the exacerbating- remitting course of the disease.

The in vitro IgG- and antibody production capacity of CSF cells in MS was low. Specific antibodies against different viruses could only occasionally be measured in culture supernatants of CSF cells. The CSF cells from virus meningitis patients produced large amounts of specific antibodies in similar culture conditions.

In conclusion, our results show that in vitro culturing techniques can be used to demonstrate the reactivity of CSF cells against defined antigens. However, these studies have not suggested any specific reactivity or pattern which would explain the etiology of MS.

INTRODUCTION

A large number of immune cells are found in the central nervous system (CNS) of multiple sclerosis (MS) patients. It is likely that some of these cells have an active role in the pathogenesis of MS but unlikely that all of them have a specificity for antigens in the central nervous system. Most cells in the cerebrospinal fluid (CSF) are T cells and only a minority has B- or plasma cell characteristics (Allen et al., 1976, Kam-Hansen et al., 1978). Both of these classes of immune cells are found in the brain compartment itself but the relative number of B cells may be larger in the CNS tissue than in the CSF. Antigen presenting cells needed for immune functions are also found in the CNS. These cells are of hematogenic origin or permanent brain cells with antigen presenting function (Traugott et al., 1983, 1985; Hirsch et al., 1983; Fontana et al., 1984).

As all the necessary components of the immune system reside in the CNS of MS patients, the observed intrathecal immune functions of MS patients (see Walsh and Tourtellotte, 1983) is not unexpected. Revealing the specificities of the CNS immune functions may give important clues about the etiology or pathogenesis of MS. The antibodies produced intrathecally in these patients have been extensively studied in recent years. The bulk of the intrathecally synthesized antibodies seems to represent a random selection of specificities derived from the immunity outside of the CNS (Salmi et al., 1983). Antibodies against myelin components are also synthesized in the CNS of MS patients but their pathogenetic significance is not known.

Immune functions in the CNS of MS patients can not be directly studied but the cells obtained from the CSF specimens of these patients may express at least partially the immune functions occurring in the CNS. The small number of cells in the CSF has hampered studies on the immune functions of MS patients. The development of T- and B-cell cell cloning techniques have opened a way to expand a small number of CSF cells into cell lines or cell clones which can be studied for reactivity in vitro (Ben-Nun et al., 1981, Fleischer et al., 1984, Hafler et al., 1985). Such techniques are very powerful in principle but may also give an incomplete picture of CNS immunity because the properties of the cell lines may not be the same as those of the cells in vivo.

We have developed techniques for directly studying the functions of both the T and B cells from CSF of MS and virus meningitis patients. Although the number of cells in the tests is small, it is possible to demonstrate their spontaneous or antigen-driven proliferative activity as well as measure immunoglobulins and antibodies in the supernatants of in vitro cultivated CSF cells. We summarize here our experience of using these techniques which confirm the presence of immune cells with specificity to more than one virus in the CNS of multiple sclerosis and viral meningitis.

MATERIALS AND METHODS

Patients and specimens

MS patients met the generally accepted diagnostic criteria of definite MS (Schumacher et al., 1965). The exacerbation was defined by deterioration of the patient with new clinical symptoms and signs and the samples representing remission were taken at least three weeks after the onset of ongoing remission. The patients with mumps virus meningitis were hospitalized cases in which the diagnosis was confirmed by serological tests. Neurological control patients represented different neurological conditions without any sign of intrathecal inflammatory diseases.

The CSF samples from patients were transferred to the laboratory immediately after the lumbar puncture, cells pelleted and washed in conical tissue culture tubes, once with HANKS BSS for proliferation assays or twice with medium containing 5% fetal calf serum (FCS) for in vitro antibody synthesis. The cells were finally suspended in RPMI 1640 medium supplemented with bicarbonate, antibiotics and 10% pooled human serum (proliferation assays) or 10% FCS (in vitro antibody synthesis).

Proliferation assays of the mononuclear cells

For the measurement of spontaneous proliferation, 2 x 10^4 CSF cells were incubated immediately after preparation in a test tube for two hours at ±37°C in a 5% CO_2 atmosphere with ^3H-thymidine present at a concentration of 2µCi/ml. The cells were then spun onto microscope slides in a cytocentrifuge. The slides were fixed in Carnoy solution, gelatinized and covered with photographic film (Kodak Autoradiographic Stripping plates AR 10). The exposure time was six days at ±4°C, whereafter the slides were developed and stained with Giemsa stain. The percentage of labelled cells was calculated by counting a minimum of 1000 cells.

Lymphocyte cultures for proliferation assays with viral antigens were prepared similarly in test tubes by adding various viral antigens or VERO cell control antigen to cultures in a final concentration of 2.5 µg/ml (Reunanen, 1983). A total of 2 x 10^4 mononuclear cells suspended in a final volume of 0.4 ml were used in these cultures. ^3H-thymidine was added after six days in culture and after two hours labelling time, the slides were prepared for counting as described above for the spontaneous proliferation assay. When the number of labelled cells in the stimulated cultures was twice that of the control cultures, the tests were considered positive.

In vitro synthesis of immunoglobulins

The tube cultures for in vitro antibody synthesis were incubated with and without pokeweed mitogen (PWM, final concentration 12.5 µg/ml) for 7 days in the same culture condition described for the proliferation assays. One day cultures were harvested for control purposes in some experiments. The volume of CSF cell cultures in conical tubes was 0.4 ml in which a minimum of 5 x 10^4 cells were suspended.

Measurement of in vitro produced IgG and antibodies

The supernatants from CSF cells cultivated in vitro as well as the last washing solutions of the CSF cells were tested for immunoglobulin G (IgG) and specific antibodies by enzyme immunoassays (EIA). The method for IgG measurement has been described earlier (Ilonen et al., 1986). The antibodies to different virus antigens were measured by a modification of antibody-EIA in which plastic microtiter plates were coated with different virus antigens and control antigens (Arnadottir et al., 1982). The antibodies in the sample were bound to this solid phase during one hour incubation at ±37°C. Antibodies to human IgG made in rabbits were then added and the final incubation was with horseradish peroxidase labelled anti-rabbit immunoglobulin antibodies. The results were read as $O.D._{492}$ values in a Multiskan plate reader and were compared to a standard curve with known amounts of different viral antibodies. The criteria for in vitro antibody production were the lack of such antibodies in the control specimen and no reactivity in the assays with control antigen.

RESULTS

Spontaneous activity of CSF cells

As shown in Table 1, cells in CSF obtained from patients with viral meningitis had a high spontaneous activity as measured by ^{3}H-thymidine incorporation in a 2 hour culture immediately after the specimen had been taken (Reunanen et al., 1982). When the same technique was applied to CSF cells from MS patients, it was revealed that they have higher spontaneous stimulation than patients with other neurological diseases (Reunanen, 1982a). Some relapsing-remitting patients had higher spontaneous CSF cell proliferation when in exacerbation than in remission but this was not always true. When the spontaneous proliferation of CSF cells was tested in a long-term follow-up study, it was found that the activity did not correlate with the clinical fluctuations in MS (Reunanen, 1982a).

Table 1. Spontaneous proliferation of CSF cells obtained from MS patients, neurological controls, and mumps meningitis patients. The results are expressed as percent of cells in DNA synthesis immediately after the specimen was taken as measured by uptake of tritiated thymidine.

Patient group	No. of patients	Percentage of cells in DNA synthesis Median	Range
MS, non-relapsing	9	0.45	0 - 1.0
MS, remission	21	0.2	0 - 0.55
MS, exacer-bation	19	0.25	0 - 1.15
Neurological controls	20	0.0	0 - 0.4
Mumps meningitis	6	2.1	0.5 - 4.4

Spontaneous synthesis of immunoglobulins <u>in vitro</u> by CSF cells from mumps meningitis and MS patients were also measured. The cells were washed 2 times, cultured with or without PWM for 7 days and the amount of immunoglobulins in the last washing solution and the culture supernatants were measured in EIA. Table 2 shows that the washing procedure removed most of the immunoglobulins from the specimens but some remnant amounts

Table 2. Production of IgG by CSF cells from MS patients. The amount of immunoglobulins in the final washing solution of the lymphocytes and the lymphocyte supernatants with and without PWM stimulation for 7 days was measured by an enzyme-immunoassay.

Patient	No. of lymphocytes in culture	Amount of immunoglobulin G in supernatant (μg/ml) Wash	No stimul.	PWM stimul.
E.S.	350,000	0.06	19.6	13.0
A.K.	120,000	0.03	0.15	0.26
R.B.	116.000	0.30	0.38	0.60
E.A.	88.000	0.19	0.38	0.31
R.L.	48,000	0.05	0.19	0.13
K.N.	160,000	0.11	0.20	0.20
N.P.	100,000	0.23	0.54	0.60

were occasionally found. IgG was produced without stimulation with PWM by CSF cells from all the patients. Further, the addition of PWM did not increase the spontaneous immunoglobulin production but instead, decreased the amount of IgG found in the culture supernatant in most patients. Taken together, the results show that CSF cells obtained from MS patients are active in vivo and this activity is not correlated with the clinical stage of the patients.

Stimulation of CSF cells with virus antigens

We have tested the CSF cells from mumps meningitis and MS patients for their responsiveness to different viral antigen (Reunanen et al., 1982, 1983). Table 3 summarizes the results of such experiments which show that CSF cells specific for different viral antigens are found both in acute viral meningitis and MS patients. The degree of stimulation of CSF cells from mumps meningitis patients is higher with other than mumps antigen suggesting that tests for the specific T cells are no good indicators of the specificity of the T cells in the brain compartment.

Table 3. Proliferative response of CSF lymphocytes when stimulated in vitro with different virus antigens

Patient group	No. of positive/No of patients tested: Measles	Rubella	Herpes	Mumps
Mumps encephalitis	3/11	2/10	3/11	2/11
Multiple sclerosis	12/20	5/9	7/12	3/5

The CSF cells from 8 MS patients were tested with 3 or 4 of these viral antigens. Three of these patients had CSF cells which responded to at least 3 of these antigens. Such results suggest that CSF cells from MS patients have reactivity against more than one viral antigen. The reactivities of the CSF cells also fluctuate during the clinical course of MS (Reunanen et al., 1983). As there is no clear-cut correlation with exacerbations, the presence of virus-reacting lymphocytes in the CSF of MS patients may not have any etiological or pathogenetic significance.

IgG and antibody production by CSF cells in vitro

We have analysed the viral antibody specificity of immunoglobulins produced in vitro by CSF cells stimulated with PWM from patients with mumps meningitis and multiple sclerosis. CSF cells from all the four pa-

Table 4. In vitro synthesis of IgG and viral antibodies by PWM-stimulated CSF cells from mumps meningitis and multiple sclerosis patients

Patient group	Patients with in vitro IgG synthesis	Patients with in vitro antibody synthesis against: Measles	Rubella	Herpes s.	Adeno	Mumps
Mumps	4/4	2/4	1/4	2/4	0/4	4/4
MS	7/11	4/7	4/7	0/7	1/7	1/7

tients with mumps meningitis studied produced IgG in vitro whereas only 7/11 of CSF cells obtained from MS patients had such synthesis. Supernatants from the cultures contained antibodies which bound to different virus antigens in EIA (Table 4). Although all the meningitis patients had mumps antibodies produced in vitro, small amounts of antibodies to other viruses were simultaneously synthesized. In vitro synthesis of specific antibodies against more than one virus were also observed in some MS patients. Antibodies against measles and rubella viruses were clearly more often found than in antibodies to Herpes simplex or adenoviruses.

DISCUSSION

We have shown that a small number of CSF cells obtained from MS and viral meningitis patients can be used in functional studies in vitro. If proper controls are included in the tests, the results are reliable but the small number of cells limits the tests to a selected few at any time of sampling. Nevertheless, the information obtained may be useful for understanding the pathogenesis of multiple sclerosis.

A significant number of CSF cells from mumps meningitis patients proliferated without any antigenic stimulation whereas spontaneous proliferation of CSF cells from MS patients was observed only slightly more often than in other neurological patients serving as controls. Further, the spontaneous proliferation of CSF cells from the MS patients was not clearly correlated with the clinical exacerbations of the patients. It has also earlier been shown that the CSF cells from MS patients are activated in situ both in exacerbations and in remissions (Sandberg-Wollheim 1974, Dommasch et al., 1977, Reunanen et al., 1978, Noronha et al., 1980). All the available evidence, including the present results, indicate that the immune cells in the central nervous system of MS patients have a spontaneous activity, probably reflecting the CNS inflammation in this disease even during clinically silent remission periods. The spontaneous activity of the CSF cells is also important to take into account when specific reactivities of the CSF cells are studied.

The proliferative response of the CSF cells after antigen stimulation reflects most likely the division of the T cells. We have shown the T cell nature of the proliferating cells only in a few experiments because the small number of cells limits the number of tests (Reunanen, 1982b).It is generally accepted, however, that the proliferative response after antigen stimulation reflects mainly the activity of the T cells, most likely of the helper subtype of cells (Reinherz and Schlossmann, 1980). Our observation that different viral antigens can stimulate CSF cells from MS patients into proliferation suggests that a great variety of T cell specificities may nonspecifically reside in the central nervous system of MS patients at any time. The recruitment of the T cells into the CNS seems to be nonspecific as suggested by the fact that the cellular reactivity is not restricted to the etiological virus in mumps meningitis patients. As nonspecific recruitment of immune cells occurs in all the immunological processes, the presence of different T cell specificities in the inflammation of the CNS, such as infections or demyelinating diseases, is expected. The brain compartment does not seem to be such a privileged area of the body as earlier believed and a small number of T cells can be expected to survey the brain tissue even in healthy individuals. Therefore, the presence of any specificity in the CSF of MS patients can not be taken as proof for their etiological or pathogenic significance.

Immunoglobulins synthesized intrathecally are known to be composed of antibody specificities against a number of different viruses and other antigens (see Walsh & Tourtellotte, 1983). Our results demonstrate that cells from CSF specimens synthesize such specificities also in vitro. It is obvious that only a limited repertoire of B cell can be found in the CSF specimens as the total number of lymphoid cells recovered from an CSF sample rarely exceeds 100,000 and the relative number of B cells is small (Kam-Hansen et al., 1978). Nevertheless, more than one antibody specificity was synthesized in vitro by the CSF cells from MS patients. The antibodies against measles and rubella viruses were more frequently synthesized than those against adeno- and herpes simplex viruses which is in accord with the known frequencies of intrathecally synthesized antibodies in MS patients (Salmi et al., 1983).

It is evident that most of the intrathecally synthesized antibodies in MS patients are not relevant from the disease process point of view. B cells may not enter as easily to a healthy central nervous system as T cells evidently do. When the blood-brain-barrier (BBB) is damaged as in viral meningitis, the barrier is temporarily damaged and the B cells obtain the access to the brain compartment of the body (Hänninen et al., 1980). Our studies on in vitro virus antibody synthesis of the CSF cells from mumps meningitis patients provide a direct proof for this phenomenon. It is also known that B cells can enter the CNS after mechanical trauma and apoplexy. Any such interruption of the BBB may increase the number of B memory cells in the CNS where they seem to be trapped and synthesize immunoglobulins with different but invariable specificities for long period of time in MS patients (Arnadottir et al., 1982, Walsh and Tourtellotte, 1986).

There is now overwhelming evidence that a number of different specificities of T cells and B cells can be found in the CNS of MS patients. As a small number of T cells may be continuously surveying the brain compartment of the body (Hafler & Weiner, 1986), their repertoire may mainly reflect the specificities circulating in the peripheral blood at the time of sampling. On the other hand, memory B cells and plasma cells may rather represent specificities circulating at the time of BBB damage of MS patients. The relatively large number of T cell and B cell specificities in the CNS of MS patients suggests that the intrathecal immune system in these patients represents a random selection of T and B cell specificities circulating in the blood. As a consequence, results of in vitro functional tests directly with the CSF cells or with clones established from CSF cells will by definition mainly reflect this fact. A small number of specificities expressed by these cells may as well be of etiological or pathogenetic significance but such linkage has not yet been demonstrated.

ACKNOWLEDGEMENTS

This work was supported by grants from the Alberta Heritage Foundation for Medical Research, Alberta, Canada and the Sigrid Juselius Foundation, Helsinki, Finland. The authors thank Dr. Garry Lund for his careful review of the manuscript and Ms. Barbara Stringham for her secretarial assistance.

REFERENCES

1. J.C. Allen, W. Sheremata, J.B.R. Cosgrove, K. Osterland and M. Shea. Cerebrospinal fluid T and B lymphocyte kinetics related to exacerbations of multiple sclerosis. Neurology. 26:579 (1976).
2. T. Arnadottir, M. Reunanen and A. Salmi. Intrathecal synthesis of virus antibodies in multiple sclerosis patients. Infect. Immun. 38: 399 (1982).

3. A. Ben-Nun, H. Wekerle and I.R. Cohen. The rapid isolation of clonable antigen-specific T lymphocyte lines capable of mediating autoimmune encephalomyelitis. Eur. J. Immunol. 12:709 (1981).
4. J. Burns, B. Zweiman and R. Lisak. Tetanus toxoid reactive lymphocytes in the cerebrospinal fluid of multiple sclerosis patients. Immunol. Commun. 13:369 (1984).
5. D. Dommasch, W. Grüninger and B. Schultze. Autoradiographic demonstration of proliferating cells in cerebrospinal fluid. J. Neurol. 214:97 (1977).
6. B. Fleischer, P. Marquardt, S. Poser and H.W. Kreth. Phenotypic markers and functional characteristics of T lymphocyte clones from CSF in multiple sclerosis. J. Neuroimmunol. 7:151 (1984).
7. A. Fontana, W. Fierz and H. Wekerle. Astrocytes present myelin basic protein to encephalitogenic T-cell line. Nature. 307:273 (1984).
8. D.A. Hafler, M. Buchsbaum, D. Johnson and H.L. Weiner. Phenotypic and functional analysis of T cells cloned directly from the blood and cerebrospinal fluid of patients with multiple sclerosis. Ann. Neurol. 18:451 (1985).
9. D.A. Hafler and H.L. Weiner. In vivo labelling of peripheral blood T cells using monoclonal antibodies: Rapid trafficking into CSF in progressive multiple sclerosis. Neurology. 36 (Suppl.1):314 (1986).
10. P. Hänninen, P. Arstila, H. Lang, A. Salmi and M. Panelius. Involvement of the central nervous system in acute, uncomplicated measles virus infection. J. Clin. Microbiol. 11:610 (1980).
11. M.R. Hirsch, J. Wietzerbin, M. Pierres and C. Goridis. Expression of Ia antigens by cultured astrocytes treated with gamma-interferon. Neurosci. Lett. 41:199 (1983).
12. J. Ilonen, R. Salonen, T. Hyypiä, K. Lankinen, R. Karttunen and A. Salmi. Immune functions in healthy blood donors with HLA-Dw2 and -Dw3 antigens. Immunobiology. In press. (1986).
13. S. Kam-Hansen, A. Frydén and H. Link. B and T lymphocytes in cerebrospinal fluid and blood in multiple sclerosis, optic neuritis and mumps meningitis. Acta Neurol. Scand. 58:95 (1978).
14. A.B.C. Noronha, D.P. Richman and B.G.W. Arnason. Detection of in vivo stimulated cerebrospinal-fluid lymphocytes by flow cytometry in patients with multiple sclerosis. N. Engl. J. Med. 303:713 (1980).
15. E.L. Reinherz and S.F. Schlossmann. The differentiation and function of human T lymphocytes. Cell. 19:821 (1980).
16. M. Reunanen. Spontaneous proliferation of cerebrospinal fluid mononuclear cells in multiple sclerosis. A longitudinal study. J. Neuroimmunol. 3:275 (1982a).
17. M. Reunanen. Lymphocyte stimulation and viral antibody synthesis in the cerebrospinal fluid of patients with multiple sclerosis. Acta Univ. Oul. D93:1 (1982b).
18. M. Reunanen, J. Ilonen, T. Arnadottir, A. Ahonen and A. Salmi. Mitogen and antigen stimulation of multiple sclerosis cerebrospinal fluid lymphocytes in vitro. J. Neurol. Sci. 58:211 (1983).
19. M.I. Reunanen, J. Ilonen and K. Järvenpää. Proliferating cells in demyelinating states. In: "Myelination and Demyelination", ed. J. Palo. Plenum Press New York and London (1978).
20. M. Reunanen, R. Salonen and A. Salmi. Intrathecal immune responses in mumps meningitis patients. Scand. J. Immunol. 15:419 (1982).
21. A. Salmi, M. Reunanen, J. Ilonen and M. Panelius. Intrathecal antibody synthesis to virus antigens in multiple sclerosis. Clin. Exp. Immunol. 52:241 (1983).
22. M. Sandberg-Wollheim. Immunoglobulin synthesis in vitro by cerebrospinal fluid cells in patients with multiple sclerosis. Scand. J. Immunol. 3:717 (1974).

23. G.A. Schumacher, G. Beebe, R.F. Kibler, L.T. Kurland, J.F. Kurtzke, F. McDowell, B. Nagler, W.A. Sibley, W.W. Tourtellotte and T. Willmon. Problems of experimental trials of therapy in multiple sclerosis. Report by the panel on the evaluation of experimental trials of therapy in multiple sclerosis. Ann. N.Y. Acad. Sci. 122:552 (1965).
24. U. Traugott, E.L. Reinherz and C.S. Raine. Multiple sclerosis: Distribution of T cell subsets within active chronic lesions. Science. 219:308 (1983).
25. U. Traugott, L.C. Scheinberg and C.S. Raine. On the presence of Ia-positive endothelial cells and astrocytes in multiple sclerosis lesions and its relevance to antigen presentation. J. Neuroimmunol. 8:1 (1985).
26. M.J. Walsh and W.W. Tourtellotte. The cerebrospinal fluid in multiple sclerosis. In: "Multiple sclerosis". J.F. Hallpike, C.W. Adams and W.W. Tourtellotte, eds., Williams & Wilkins, Baltimore (1983).
27. M.J. Walsh and W.W. Tourtellotte. Temporal invariance of clonal uniformity of brain and cerebrospinal IgG, IgA and IgM in multiple sclerosis. J. Exp. Med. 163:41 (1986).

ACTIVATED T-CELLS AND ANTIGEN REACTIVITY IN THE CEREBROSPINAL FLUID AND BLOOD OF PATIENTS WITH MULTIPLE SCLEROSIS

David A. Hafler and Howard L. Weiner

From the Center for Neurologic Diseases, Brigham and Women's Hospital and Harvard Medical School, Boston MA 02115

There is increasing evidence that T-cells in tissue compartments outside of the blood/reticuloendothelial systems may represent specific, sequestrated populations of lymphocytes with different immunologic characteristics as compared to the peripheral blood. Evidence for this includes increased numbers of activated lymphocytes in cerebrospinal fluid (CSF) (1) and synovial fluid (2) in localized infections of the central nervous system and articular joints respectively and the finding of increased proportions of antigen specific cytotoxic effector cells in the CSF of subjects with viral meningoencephalitis (3). Thus, studies of activation and specificity of CNS derived T lymphocytes may assist in understanding the pathophysiology of inflammatory diseases such as multiple sclerosis.

In this report, we present data that a marker of T memory cells, Ta_1, is found in increased frequency from CSF lymphocytes obtained from CSF of both multiple sclerosis subjects with other noninflammatory neurologic diseases. This will be discussed in context of direct single cell cloning experiments which do not show an increased frequency of either myelin basic protein (MBP) or proteolipid protein (PLP) reactive cells in the CSF of MS patients studied.

METHODS

Patients

Patients with clinically definite multiple sclerosis were studied during visits to the outpatient Multiple Sclerosis Clinical and Research Unit at the Brigham and Women's Hospital or on the day of admission to the hospital. The control populations consisted of age-matched patients with other neurologic diseases, and age-matched healthy subjects (4).

Patients had received no steroids for one month or immunosuppressive drugs for nine months at the time of blood drawing.

Production of monoclonal antibodies and analysis of lymphocytes

The production and characterization of the monoclonal antibodies anti-T3, anti-T4, anti-T8, anti-$T11_3$, anti-Ta_1 and anti-interleukin-2 receptor have been described previously (4,5).

Cytofluorographic analysis of cell populations was performed by means of indirect immunofluorescence with fluorescein-conjugated goat antimouse IgG (Tago, Burlingame, Calif.) on a flow cytometer using a linear scale. Background fluorescence activity was determined with control ascites fluid obtained from mice immunized with a nonsecreting hybridoma. The percentage of activation antigen-positive T cells was calculated by dividing the number of activation antigen-positive cells by the total number of T3-positive cells. The average percentages of T3-positive mononuclear cells were not statistically different in the different groups. All cytofluorographic analyses were performed by persons with no knowledge of the patient's clinical status or diagnosis.

Preparation and staining of spinal-fluid lymphocytes

Between 3 and 15 ml of cerebrospinal fluid was centrifuged at 400xg for 10 minutes, and the cell pellet was resuspended in 400 of RPMI-1640 (Gibco, Grand Island, N.Y.) supplemented with 10 per cent heat-inactivated human AB serum (Pel Freeze Biologicals, Hawthorne, N.J.). Aliquots of cells were then placed in 96-well microtiter plates and stained, and the percentage of positive cells was scored independently by two observers using a Zeiss fluorescence microscope as previously described (4). From 75 to 100 cells were counted per sample, except as noted.

Isolation of lymphocytes

Human peripheral-blood mononuclear cells were isolated from heparinized venous blood by means of centrifugation on a Ficoll-Hypaque density gradient (Pharmacia Fine Chemicals, Piscataway, N.J.). In certain cases, purified T-cells were prepared from mononuclear cells by rosetting with sheep red cells (M.A. Bioproducts, Walkersville, Md.) using standard procedures (4).

IL-2

T-cell growth factor (IL-2)-conditioned medium was produced by incubating 2.5 x 10^6 lymphocytes/ml (obtained from the Red Cross during apheresis and cryopreserved before use) with 0.5 x 10^6 LAZ 156 cells/ml (obtained from Dr. Herbert Lazarus, Dana-Farber Cancer Institute, Boston, MA), 5 μg/ml of PHA-P (Wellcone Research Laboratories, Beckenham, England), and 3 ng/ml of phorbol myristate acetate (Sigma, St. Louis, MO) in tissue culture medium containing 1% heat-activated human AB serum for 48 hours at 37°C in a 7.5% CO_2 environment. Conditioned IL-2 medium was obtained by separating the cells by centrifugation followed by filtration through a Millex 0.22-mm filter (Milliport Corpóration, Bedford, MA). No further purification to remove the lectin was performed.

Limiting dilution cloning

CSF or blood lymphocytes were diluted in tissue culture medium containing 1 x 10^6/ml irradiated (5,000 rads) autologous mononuclear cells and PHA-P at a final concentration of 0.5 μg/ml in V-bottom 96-well plates (Flow Laboratories, McLean, VA) in a 100-μl volume. At 48 hours, 100 μl of 20% IL2 was added to each well. Plates were fed every 4 days and sample wells were counted to monitor cell growth. Between days 10 and 14 each V-bottom well was transferred to a round-bottom 96-well plate with 1 x 10^5 irradiated autologous feeder cells per well. Growth-positive wells, which were ascertained by microscopic analysis, were split, followed 3 to 4 days later by transfer into 24-well plates. Clones were subsequently fed every 3 to 4 days with 10% IL-2 and complete medium. Irradiated autologous "feeder" cells were added every 2 weeks. After 4 weeks there were enough cells to perform analysis and phenotyping.

T-cell separation of Ta_1 subpopulations

T-lymphocytes were incubated for 30' at 4°C with a 1:125 dilution of anti-Ta_1, then resuspended at a concentration of 10 x 10^6 cells/ml in media consisting of PBS with 2% human AB serum (Pe Freez, Rodgers, AK), 100 units/ml penicillin, and 100 g/ml of streptomycin (Gobco, Grand Island, NY); 3 cc of the cell suspension was placed on the rabbit anti-mouse coated petri plate, and after two hours of incubation at 4°C, non-adherent cells were harvested by gently rinsing the dish with 10 cc aliquots of ice-cold media. These cells consisted of the Ta_1 depleted population used in subsequent experiments. Plates were then incubated at 37°C for 30' to allow lightly adherent cells to lift off the plate surface; these were removed by rinsing the plates and then discarded. Strongly adherent cells were then harvested by vigorous pipetting, followed by scraping and consisted of the Ta_1 enriched population.

Proliferation assays

The proliferative response of T-cell clones against white matter antigens and MBP was assayed by incubating 40,000 T-cells in a 96-well round-bottom plates in 100 µl of tissue culture medium with 3,000 autologous adherent antigen presenting cells (APC) irradiated with 5,000 rads. After 48 hours, cells were pulsed with 2 µCi of ^{3}H-thymidine and harvested 18 hours later on an automated cell harvester. Delta counts per minute were calculated by subtracting proliferation of T-cells alone from counts obtained in the presence of APC or APC an antigen. As a positive control, each clone was incubated separately with 20% IL-2.

RESULTS

The percentage of cells bearing the T-cell differentiation marker Ta_1 in patients with multiple sclerosis, healthy controls, and patients with other neurologic diseases were measured. Two standard deviations from the mean percentage of Ta_1+ cells from normal controls was used as an upper limit of normal (14.3%). As seen in Fig.1, twenty of thirty five patients with progressive multiple sclerosis were abnormal, as compared with four of eighteen patients with stable or improving multiple sclerosis, one of seventeen patients with other neurologic diseases, and one of fourteen normal controls ($p<0.0002$, Fisher's exact test). The number of patients with increased Ta_1+ cells was comparable in both the stable and improving groups (Fig.1).

To determine whether the Ta_1 activation antigen was preferentially expressed on T4+ or T8+ cells, isolated T4 or T8 populations from selected patients were analysed. Representative fluorescent histograms from a single patient (Fig.2) demonstrated the presence of Ta_1+ cells in both major functional T-cell subsets.

The cerebrospinal fluid was examined in 20 patients with multiple sclerosis, and 19 patients with other neurologic diseases, including 6 determinations on five patients with acute inflammatory central nervous system diseases who had a pleocytosis (greater than five cells per cubic millimeter). Staining was performed on all samples of spinal fluid, although in four patients with other neurologic disease and less than one cell per cubic millimeter in the spinal fluid, only 20 lymphocytes could be counted because of the small volumes of spinal fluid obtained. Staining was performed with anti-T3, anti-Ta_1, and anti-interleukin-2-receptor monoclonal antibodies. Table 2 shows the average cell counts of patients with multiple sclerosis and patients with other neurologic diseases with and with out pleocytosis. As previously reported (4), the majority of cells in the spinal fluid were T-cells and there was no significant difference in the percentage of mononuclear cells positive for the T3 antigen in any of the different groups. The mean percentage of Ta_1+ T-cells (± SEM) in spinal fluid in patients with progressive multiple sclerosis was 42 ± 3%. In contrast, patients with acute inflammatory central nervous system diseases (greater than five cells per cubic millimeter) had 9.6 ± 1.8% Ta_1+ cells. In patients with noninflammatory neurologic diseases (less than two cells per cubic millimeter), the mean percentage of Ta_1+ T-cells (39 ± 5.4%) were similar to that in patients with multiple sclerosis, although the total number of lymphocytes was low 0.7 ± 0.16 cells per cubic millimeter (Fig.3). In the spinal fluid of three patients with stable multiple sclerosis, the percentage of Ta_1+ cells ranged from 36 to 54%.

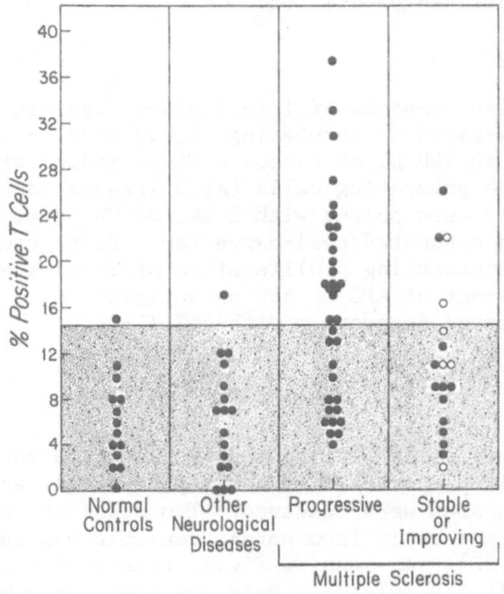

Fig.1. Percentage of Ta_1-positive T-cells in the peripheral blood of patients and controls. Open circles represent patients who were recovering from an attack thad had occurred in the prior eight weeks The stippled area shows 2 S.D. from the mean percentage of Ta_1-positive T-cells for control subjects (P<0.0002, Fisher's exact test). (4)

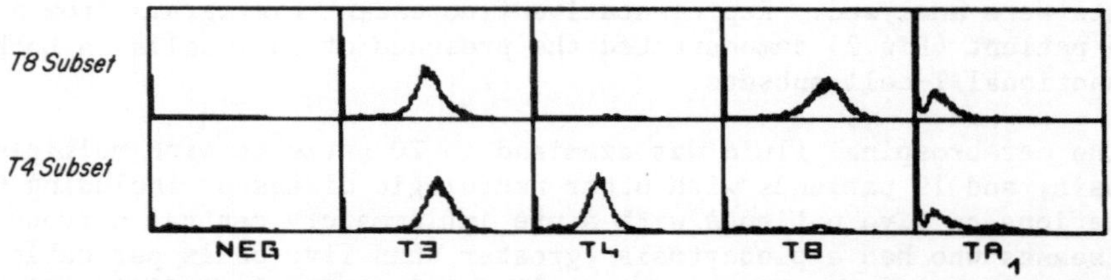

Fig.2. Ta_1-positive lymphocytes in both T4 and T8 subsets from a patient with multiple sclerosis. Subsets were prepared by complement-mediated lysis of the reciprocal populations and stained with anti-T3, anti-T4, anti-T8, anti Ta_1, and control ascites. Cytofluorographic analysis using a log scale was then performed. The T8 subset shows staining with anti-T3, anti-T8, and anti-Ta_1, and no staining with anti-T4; the reciprocal T4 subset also shows staining with anti-Ta_1. (4)

Table 1. Peripheral-blood T-cell activation antigens in patients with multiple sclerosis (MS), patients with other neurologic diseases, and controls

Category	No. of Subjects	Mean Age (Range)	Sex Distribution	% Reactivity with Monoclonal Antibodies[a]		
				Anti-Ta_1	Anti-$T11_3$	Anti-IL-2 Receptor
Progressive MS	35	42 (17-65)	17M, 18F	16±1[b]	6±1	< 1
Stable or improving MS	18	34 (18-52)	7M, 11F	11±2[c]	7±2	< 1
Other neurologic diseases	17	40 (14-65)	8M, 9F	6±1[d]	5±1	< 1
Normal controls	14	42 (19-65)	7M, 7F	6±1	4±1	< 1

[a] Results are expressed as mean percentages ± S.E.M. The percentage of reactive cells was calculated by dividing the percentage of activation antigen-positive cells by the percentage of T3-positive cells in peripheral blood. IL denotes interleukin.

[b] $p<0.001$ as compared with patients with other neurologic diseases or controls (two-tailed t-test).

[c] $p<0.05$ as compared with patients with progressive MS (two-tailed t-test) or normal controls (two-tailed t-test).

[d] $p<0.02$ as compared with patients with stable or improving MS (two-tailed t-test).

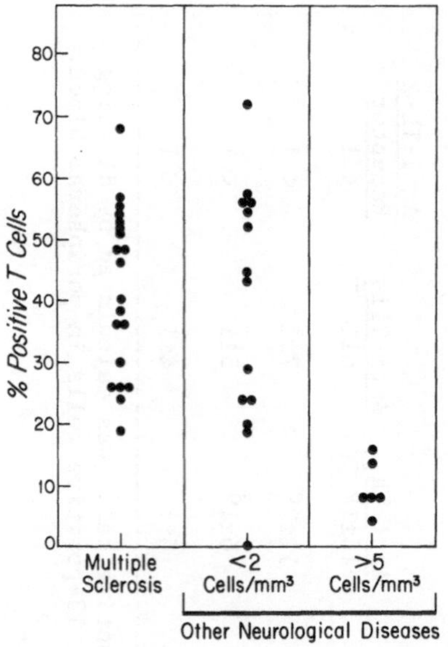

Fig.3. Percentage of cerebrospinal fluid T-cells reactive with anti-Ta_1 monoclonal antibody in patients with multiple sclerosis and patiens with other neurologic diseases. Patients with other neurologic diseases were divided into sub-groups with inflammation (>5 cells per cubic millimeter) and without inflammation (<2 cells per cubic millimeter) ($p<0.0001$, Fisher's exact test). (4)

To determine whether there was a correlation between the percentage of Ta_1+ cells in the peripheral blood and spinal fluid of the patients studied, linear regression analysis was performed. In patients with other neurologic diseases that were studied, there was a positive correlation between the percentage of Ta_1+ cells in the peripheral blood and in the spinal fluid ($R=0.54$, $p < 0.05$). This correlation was also present when patients with other neurologic diseases and either less than 2 or greater than 5 cells per cubic millimeter were analysed separately ($R=0.52$ for both cases) (Fig.4). This correlation was not seen in patients with multiple sclerosis in whom there tended to be an negative correlation between the proportion of Ta_1+ cells in blood and spinal fluid ($R=0.28$), although it was not statistically significant ($p > 0.2$) (Fig.4). There was minimal staining of spinal fluid lymphocytes with the monoclonal antibody that recognized the interleukin-2 receptor in patients with multiple sclerosis (0.6%), and in patients with noninflammatory neurologic diseases (0%). In the group with inflammatory neurologic diseases, however, 9.8% of the lymphocytes bore the interleukin-2 receptor. (Table 2) ($p < 0.01$, two-tailed t-test).

As previously mentioned, the Ta_1 antigen is present on T-cell lines and clones irrespective of cell cycle. Because of the increased proportions of Ta_1 positive cells found in MS blood and the sequestration of Ta_1 positive cells in CSF as compared to peripheral blood of MS subjects as well as normal subjects, Ta_1 was further investigated. T-lymphocytes obtained from normal human subjects were separated into Ta_1+ and Ta_1- subpopulations and their functions studied. Whereas Ta_1+ cells constitute 10-15% of E-rosette positive lymphocyte population, most, if not all of the anamnestic response to the recall antigens tetanus toxoid and mumps, resided in the Ta_1+ population (Fig.5). Increased proliferation was not due simply to increased inducer cell function within the Ta_1+ subpopulation (data not shown). Thus, the Ta_1 antigen appears to be a marker for pre-

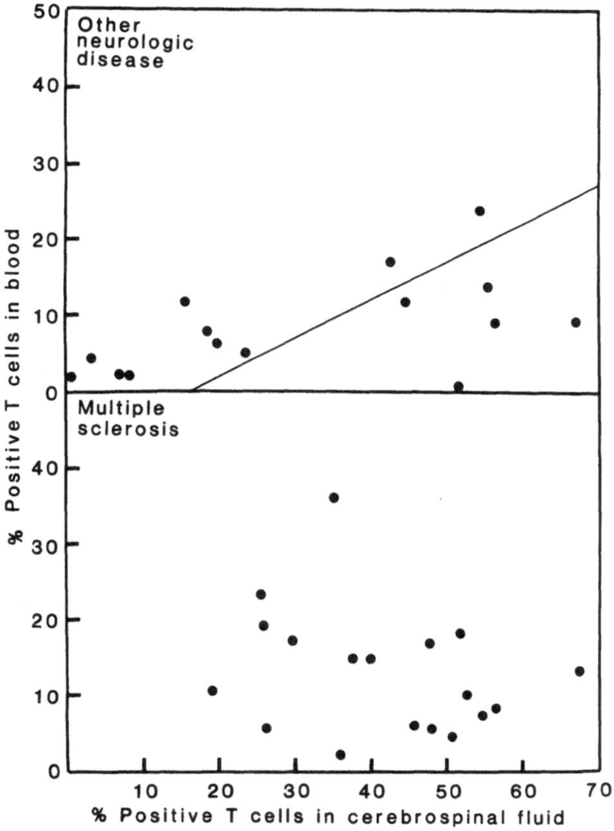

Fig.4. Correlation of the percentage of Ta_1+ cells in blood and cerebrospinal fluid. Correlation between blood and CSF in subjects with other neurological diseases ($R=0.54$, $p<0.05$) and multiple sclerosis ($R=0.28$, $p>0.2$).

viously activated T-cells in peripheral blood, and this subpopulation may include T-memory cells.

In order to determine if there was an increased frequency of white matter, myelin basic protein or proteolipid protein reactive T-cells in the CSF or peripheral blood of MS patients, mononuclear cells were directly cloned and plated prior to other in vitro manipulation, then stimulated with PHA and IL-2. Slightly less than half (1/2.1 and 1/2.6, respectively) of the cells plated grew. Two hundred and thirty five clones were generated from the cerebrospinal fluid, and one hundred and twenty six clones from the peripheral blood from six patients with progressive multiple sclerosis. Nineteen additional clones were generated from the cerebrospinal fluid of a patient herpes zoster meningoencephalitis. As can be seen in Table 3, none of the clones derived from either the blood or the CSF proliferated to myelin basic protein or proteolipid protein. Clones were also tested for reactivity against a crude white matter homogenate and again no proliferation was observed. Clones were also established from a patient with post viral encephalomyelitis. Four of nine (44%) T4 clones from the CSF, and one our of thirteen (9%) cloned from the peripheral blood reacted to myelin basic protein, but at low levels. None of the T8 clones demonstrated any reactivity to myelin basic protein, and none of the clones proliferated to proteolipid protein (Table 3).

Table 2. Activation antigens on cerebrospinal fluid (CSF) T-cells from patients with progressive multiple sclerosis (MS) and patients with other neurologic diseases without and with pleocytosis (> 5 lymphocytes per cubic millimeter).

Category	No. of subjects	CSF lymphocyte count[a]	Reactivity with monoclonal antibodies[b]		
			Anti-T3	Anti-Ta_1	Anti-IL-2 receptor
Progressive MS	20	3.9±1.6	88±2.4	42±3.0[c]	0.6±0.3
Other neurologic diseases					
> 5 cells/mm^3	6	36±13	85±3.0	9.6±1.8	9.8±4.4[d]
< 2 cells/mm^3	14	0.7±0.16	82±4.4	39±5.4[e]	0

[a] Per cubic millimeter. Values are means ± S.E.M.

[b] Results are expressed as mean percentage ± S.E.M. The percentage of activation antigen-reactive T-cells was calculated by dividing the percentage of activation antigen-positive cells by the percentage of T3-positive cells. IL denotes interleukin.

[c] $p < 0.001$ as compared with patients with other neurologic diseases and pleocytosis (two-tailed t-test).

[d] $p < 0.01$ as compared with patients with MS or other neurologic diseases without pleocytosis (two-tailed t-test).

[e] $p < 0.01$ as compared with patients with other neurologic diseases and pleocytosis (two-tailed t-test).

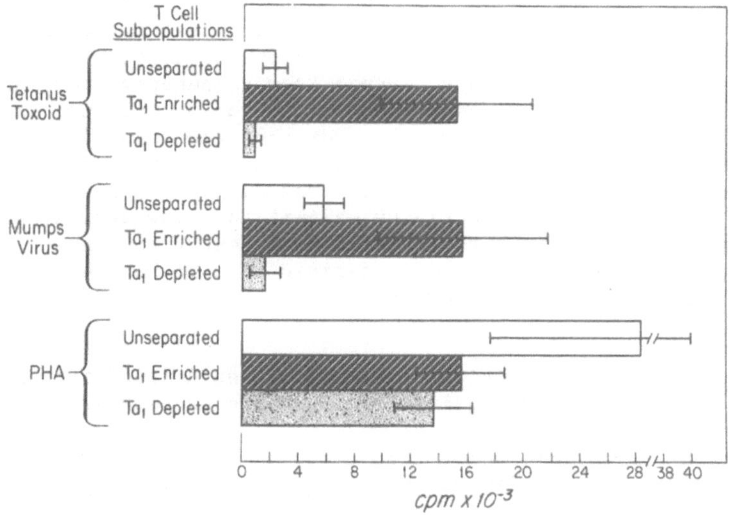

Fig.5. Average proliferative responses (±SEM) of unseparated T-cells, Ta_1 enriched, and Ta_1 depleted populations after plate adherence separation to tetanus toxoid, mumps virus, and PHA separate experiments ar shown (see methods section). Unseparated vs. Ta_1 enriched and Ta_1 depleted vs. Ta_1 enriched proliferative responses were significantly different ($p<0.05$, paired two tailed t test). (16)

Table 3. Antigen proliferation of T-cell clones derived from brain parenchyma CSF and blood against myelin basic protein and proteolipid protein

T-cell origin	Myelin basic protein	Proteolipid protein
Multiple sclerosis CSF	0/235	0/132
Multiple sclerosis brain	0/57	0/57
Multiple sclerosis blood	0/126	0/78
Post viral encephalomyelitis		
T4 CSF	4/9 (44%)	0/9
T8 CSF	0/10 (0%)	0/10
T4 Blood	1/13 (8%)	0/13
T8 Blood	0/5 (0%)	0/5
Herpes zoster encephalitis	0/7	ND

The antigen specificity of clones generated from the cerebrospinal fluid of the patient with herpes zoster meningoencephalitis were also tested against the herpes zoster virus. Five of nineteen clones proliferated to herpes zoster, and all of these were T4+T8- (data not shown). One T4+T8+ clone was also derived from the CSF, and this clone did not proliferate to herpes zoster. None of the clones proliferated to myelin basic protein or to mumps virus (Table 3).

In order to begin to assess whether antigen reactive cells may be found in the plaque of patients with multiple sclerosis, T-cells were directly cloned from two plaques derived from an autopsy specimen of an MS patient (13). Forty six clones were derived from one plaque, and eleven clones were derived from another. In addition, fourteen clones were generated from the peripheral blood. Again, none of the clones proliferated to either myelin basic protein or proteolipid protein (Table 4). Thus, myelin basic protein reactivity, albeit to a low degree, was seen only in the CSF and blood of the subject with post viral encephalomyelitis, but not in any of the specimens derived from either multiple sclerosis blood, cerebrospinal fluid or brain.

Table 4. Antigen proliferation of T-cell clones derived from multiple sclerosis plaque against myelin basic protein and proteolipid protein

T-cell origin	Myelin basic protein	Proteolipid protein
Plaque # 1	0/11	0/11
Plaque # 2	0/46	0/46
Blood	0/14	0/14

DISCUSSION

The Ta_1+ antigen appears to be a marker for previously activated T-cells and this subpopulation may include T memory cells (5). Ta_1 is not linked to cell cycle growth, as opposed to IL-2 and transferrin receptors which are growth factor receptors. Thus, once Ta_1 appears on the T-cell surface after activation, it remains on the T-cell surface, as opposed to IL-2 and transferrin receptors which disappear after T-cell activation (6,7). In the peripheral blood, patients with progressive multiple sclerosis had an increased expression of the differentiation antigen Ta_1, as compared to patients with inactive multiple sclerosis and patients with other neurologic diseases and healthy controls. This was in contrast to the expression of the activation antigens $T11_3$ and interleukin-2-receptor which were not increased in patients with multiple sclerosis (4).

Interestingly, Ta_1+ cells were found in the cerebrospinal fluid of both multiple sclerosis and other neurologic disease patients. The proportion of Ta_1+ cells in patients with inflammatory neurologic diseases in the CSF was lower than in patients with other neurologic disease or with multiple sclerosis. This may have been due to the presence of cytotoxic effector cells or NK cells that were Ta_1 negative. The high proportion of Ta_1+ cells in the cerebrospinal fluid of subjects, many of whom were essentially normal subjects, was of interest. It has been postulated that activated T-cells preferentially cross the blood brain barrier. Thus, one might expect that a marker of post differentiated T-cells or "memory" cells could be found in a higher proportion of CSF T-cells, which was consistent with our observation. These findings also suggest that CSF T-lymphocytes exhibit different characteristics than peripheral blood lymphocytes.

There were very few T-cells bearing the IL-2 receptor in MS CSF, and no IL-2 receptor positive cells seen in non-inflammatory CSF. In patients with acute inflammation such as meningitis and encephalitis, there were increases in IL-2 receptor positive cells. It is of note that a number of investigators have found IL-2 receptor positive cells in active plaques of patients with multiple sclerosis (8,9). This may suggest that the CSF compartment does not entirely reflect central nervous system processes. An alternative possibility is that either macrophages, astrocytes, or another antigen presenting cells are continually inducing IL-2 receptor expression in the brain but not CSF. It is also likely that whereas continuous stimulation may be occurring in the active plaques, once the T lymphocyte enters the CSF no further stimulation occurs. In this regard, we have recently used anti-T11 monoclonal antibodies which bind to the T-cell surface without T-cell lysis and do not cross into the CSF in an attempt to measure the traffic of T-cells from the blood into the CSF. These experiments have suggested there is very rapid movement of T-cells from the blood to the CSF (10). It may be possible to use a similar approach to measure the trafficking of activated cells in patients with multiple sclerosis.

Frequency analysis in delayed type hypersensitivity reactions have suggested that the frequency of antigen reactive cells is low in the spleen and lymph node after antigenic challenge (11,12). It has, therefore, been generally thought that the frequency of antigen reactive cells in the CSF would also be low. However, Kreth and his co-workers have found that in viral infections with known antigens, such as mumps, there is sequestration of antigen specific cytotoxic effector cells in the cerebrospinal fluid (3). We have also found a high degree of antigen reactivity in the CSF of a patient with herpes zoster meningoencephalitis. However, using the same methodology of direct single cell clonal analysis, we and others have failed to demonstrate myelin basic protein or proteolipid reactivity in the CSF or in the brain plaque themselves of patients with multiple sclerosis (13-15). It should be noted that high frequencies of CSF antigen reactive cells have been observed only with acute viral infections and not chronic inflammatory processes. It is possible that high frequencies of antigen reactive clones might only be found during initial phases of disease induction, and with time the high frequency of antigen reactivity may be lost and replaced by a chronic nonspecific inflammatory reaction. We are presently investigating T-cell receptor gene rearrangements to look for frequent T-cell clonotypes in brain, CSF, or blood of patients with multiple sclerosis.

ACKNOWLEDGEMENTS

We would like to thank Ms. Deborah Benjamin for her expert technical assistance and Ms. Marianne Berry for her excellent help with preparation of the manuscript.

REFERENCES

1. A.B.C. Noronha, D.P. Richman and B.G.W. Arnason. Detection of in vivo stimulated cerebrospinal-fluid lymphocytes by flow cytometry in patients with multiple sclerosis. N. Eng. J. Med. 303:713-7 (1980).
2. R.I. Fox, S. Fong, N. Sabharwal, S.A. Carstens, P.C. Kung and J.H. Vaughan. Synovial fluid lymphocytes differ from peripheral blood lymphocytes in patients with rheumatoid arthritis. J. Immunol. 128:351-4 (1982).
3. B. Fleischer and H.W. Kreth. Clonal analysis of HLA-restricted virus specific cytotoxic T lymphocytes from cerebrospinal fluid in mumps meningitis. J. Immunol. 130:2187-2190 (1983).

4. D.A. Hafler, D.A. Fox, M.E. Manning, S.F. Schlossmann, E.L. Reinherz and H.L. Weiner. In vivo activated T lymphocytes in the peripheral blood and cerebrospinal fluid of patients with multiple sclerosis. NEJM. 312:1405-1411 (1985).
5. D.A. Fox, R.E. Hussey and K.A. Fitzgerald. Ta_1, a novel 105 kd human T-cell activation antigen defined by a monoclonal antibody. J. Immunol. 133:1250-6 (1984).
6. I.S. Trowbridge and M.B. Omary. Human cell surface glycoprotein related to cell proliferation is the receptor for transferrin. Proc. Natl. Acad. Sci. USA. 87:3039-43 (1981).
7. D.A. Cantrell and K.A. Smith. Transient expression of interleukin 2 receptors: consequences for T-cell growth. J. Exp. Med. 158:1895-1911 (1983).
8. A.S. Bellamy, V.L. Calder, M. Feldmann and A.N. Davison. The distribution of interleukin 2 receptor bearing lymphocytes in multiple sclerosis: evidence for a key role of activated lymphocytes. Clin. Exp. Immunol. 61:248-256 (1985).
9. F.M. Hofman, R.I. von Hanwehr, C.A. Dinarello, S.B. Mizel, D. Hinton and J.E. Merrill. Immunoregulatory molecules and IL-2 receptors identified in multiple sclerosis brain. J. Immunol. 136:3239-3248 (1986).
10. D.A. Hafler and H.L. Weiner. In vivo labelling of peripheral blood T-cells using monoclonal antibodies: rapid trafficking into CSF in progressive multiple sclerosis. Neurology (Abst.). 36:314 (1986).
11. R.G. Miller, H-S Teh and R.A. Phillips. Quantitative studies of the activation of cytotoxic lymphocyte precursor cells. Immunol. Rev. 35:38 (1977).
12. R.J. Fallis, M.L. Powers and H.L. Weiner. Adoptively transferred chronic EAE: changes in CNS T-cell phenotypes and frequency of MBP reactive T-cells following relapse. Ann. Neurol. (Abst). In press.
13. D.A. Hafler, M. Buchsbaum, D. Johnson and H. Weiner. Phenotypic and functional analysis of T-cells cloned directly from the blood and cerebrospinal fluid of patients with multiple sclerosis. Ann. Neurol. 18:451-458 (1985).
14. B. Fleischer, P. Marquardt, S. Poser and H.W. Kreth. Phenotypic markers and functional characteristics of T lymphocyte clones from cerebrospinal fluid in multiple sclerosis. J. Neuroimmunol. 7:151-162 (1984).
15. D.A. Hafler, A.D. Duby, D. Benjamin, J. Seidman and H.L. Weiner. Analysis of T-cell receptor beta chain gene rearrangements in T-cells cloned directly from active MS plaques. Neurology. 36:314 (1986).
16. D.A. Hafler. Antigen reactive memory T-cells are defined by Ta_1. J. Immunol. In press (1986).

CELL MEDIATED HYPERSENSITIVITY TO MYELIN ANTIGENS IN CEREBROSPINAL FLUID AND BLOOD IN MULTIPLE SCLEROSIS AND SUBACUTE SCLEROSING PANENCEPHALITIS

Anna Czlonkowska, Margarita Vainiene, Zenon Rzepecki,
Maciej Poltorak, Bozena Iwinska and Janina Korlak

Psychoneurological Institute, Sobieskiego 1/9 02 957
Warsaw, Poland

INTRODUCTION

In the present work, we compared cell-mediated hypersensitivity to myelin basic protein (MBP), cerebroside, ganglioside and encephalitogenic peptide in multiple sclerosis (MS) and subacute sclerosis panencephalitis (SSPE). Both these diseases are characterized by widespread damage of the nerve tissue but differ in the pathogenesis. In MS, autoimmunization is supposed to play an important role and viral infection initiating that process has so far not been proved (1). In SSPE, virus infection is commonly accepted as an initiating factor and autoimmune phenomena are secondary (2, 3).

MATERIALS

For each of the studied antigen different group of MS, SSPE other neurological disease patients (OND) and healthy controls were used.

MS patients were diagnosed according to the criteria of Rose (4). SSPE diagnosis was established on the basis of clinical and psychological examination, the presence of periodic complex in electroencephalography and the detection of rising measles antibodies in CSF and PB. Patients were in the second or third stage of the disease defined according to the criteria of Jabbour (5).

OND - group consisted with patients with noninflammatory neurological diseases as epilepsy, ischialgia, transient cerebral ischemia, extrapyramidal diseases, alcoholic polyneuropathy, myelosis funicularis and mental retardation.

Persons referred to as the healthy control group displayed neurose, reactive psychoses or psychopathies and revealed no abnormalities upon neurological examination.

METHODS

Study of lymphocyte sensitization

Antigen-active rosette forming cells assay (Ag-ARFC) was applied. The method of Falsburg and Edelman (6) was used with some modifications introduced by Offner et al. (7) and Czlonkowska et al. (8).

The results are given as the percentage of active rosette forming cells (ARFC) and the percentage of ARFC after stimulation with antigen (Ag-ARFC). From these values the antigen sensitization index (Ag-SI), i.e. Ag-ARFC: ARFC ratio was calculated. The subject was regarded as positively reacting with the antigen when the Ag-SI was in excess of 1,15 (in the case of MBP, in the presence of at least one concentration of protein).

Antigens. MBP was prepared from the rabbit spinal cord by the method of Deibler et al. (9). The protein was dissolved in saline and 20 or 40 ng in 10 µl were added to 0,1 ml of lymphocyte culture. Purified cerebroside (type IV) and ganglioside (type III) of bovine brain were obtained from Sigma. Cerebroside was first dissolved in ethanol but final dilution was done in saline. Ganglioside was dissolved only in saline. One concentration of lipids, 5 pg in 10 µl was added to 0,1 ml of lymphocytes culture. Human allergic encephalitogenic peptide (Phe-Ser-Trp-Gly-Ala-Glu-Gly-Gln-Arg) was obtained from Interchem, Munich. Peptide was dissolved in saline and working solution contained 10 ng in 10 µl.

Study of lymphocyte subsets

Immunoperoxidase slide assay. We used the method of Morich et al. (10). Peripheral blood (PB) lymphocytes were separated on a ficoll/hypaque gradient, washed, and then cytocentrifuged smear was prepared. Cerebrospinal fluid (CSF) cells cytocentrifuged sediment was done without washing. Cells were fixed in 0,01% glutaraldehyde for 10 min at 4°C, or in acetons for 10 min at -20°C.

As primary antibodies, we used hybridoma supernatants containing monoclonal immunoglobulin (kindly provided by Dr. P. Beverly, University College, London) : 1.UCHT 1 (staining nearly all T cells, OKT3-like antibody), 2.UCHT 4 (staining suppressor/cytotoxic cell, OKT8-like antibody). To detect helper/inducer cells, we used the OKT4 antibody (Ortho).

To identify the cells which bound the monoclonal antibodies, we used a rabbit anti-mouse IgG, swine anti-rabbit IgG, rabbit peroxidase antiperoxidase complex (Dako) and, as a substrate, 0,06% diaminibenzidina (Sigma). Cells were counterstained with 1% toluidine blue.

The slides were viewed by light microscopy. Positive cells exhibited a dark brown ring or sometimes spots, patches or caps. The percentage of positive cells was determined by counting 100 cells in CSF and 200 in PB on each slide.

For statistical analysis, Willcoxon U test and the chi^2 test were used.

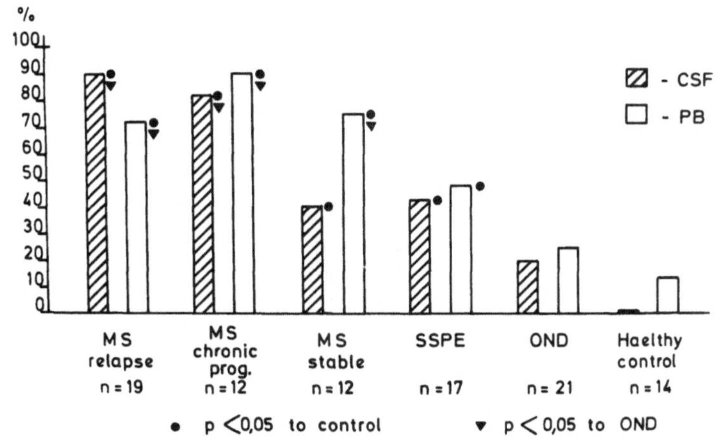

Fig.1. Percentage of subjects showing sensitization to MBP.

RESULTS

Stimulation of ARFC by MBP

(Fig.1) The incidence of reactivity to MBP is highest in MS patients being in active stage of the disease. 80-90% of MS patients have positive reaction both in CSF and PB. In the stable stage, reactivity is lower in CSF than in PB. About 50% of patients with SSPE respond to MBP in CSF and blood. There is no difference in frequency as compared to the OND group. In the healthy control group, nobody has a positive reaction in CSF, but a few persons to MBP in PB.

Stimulation of ARFC by glycolipids

(Fig.2 and 3). The percentage of persons reacting with galactocerebroside is highest in the active MS group (80-100%) as well in CSF as in PB. However, more than 30% of the patients of the SSPE and OND group

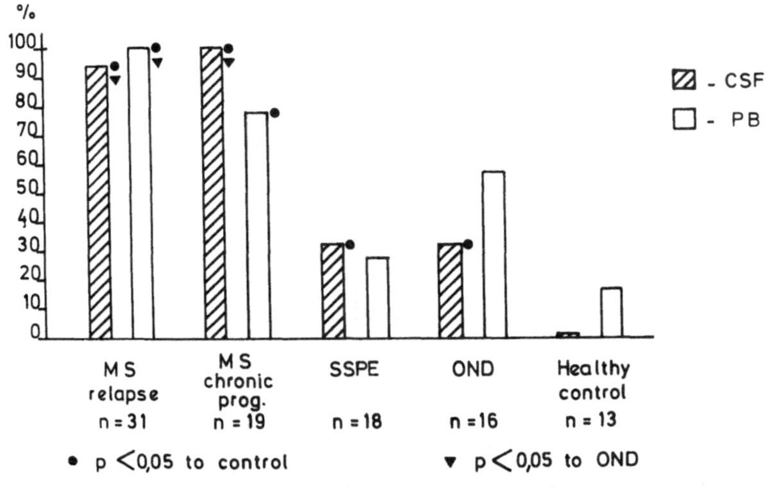

Fig.2. Percentage of subjects showing sensitization to galactocerebroside.

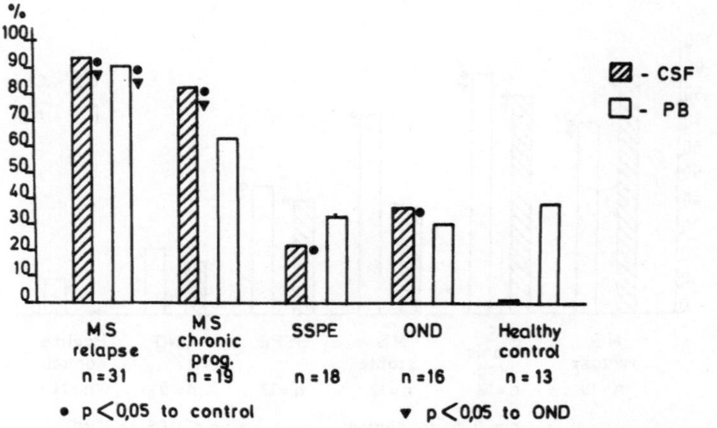

Fig.3. Percentage of subjects showing sensitization to ganglioside.

react positively with galactocerebroside in CSF and PB. In the healthy control group, nobody answers positively on CSF, but on PB, 15% have positive reaction. With ganglioside, similarly as with galactocerebroside, the highest incidence of reactivity is noticed in the active MS group. The reaction is also positive in about one third of the patients with SSPE and OND, as well in CSF as in PB. Nobody from the healthy control group reacted positively on CSF, but nearly 50% had positive reaction on PB.

Stimulation of ARFC by encephalitogenic peptide

(Fig.4). Encephalitogenic peptide is less immunogenic than MBP and glycolipids. In MS the frequency of sensitization in CSF and PB is only 30% and in SSPE it is even lower. Nobody from the group of noninflammatory OND reacted with the peptide.

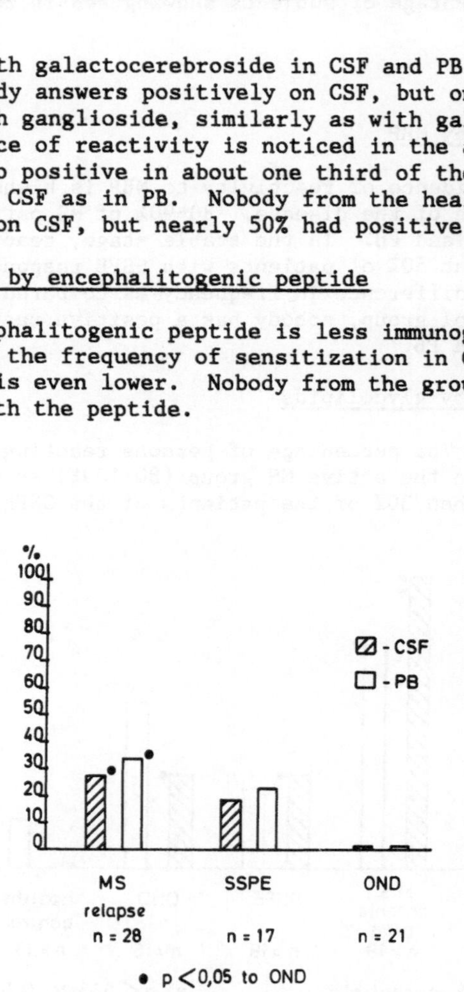

Fig.4. Percentage of subjects showing sensitization to encephalitogenic peptide.

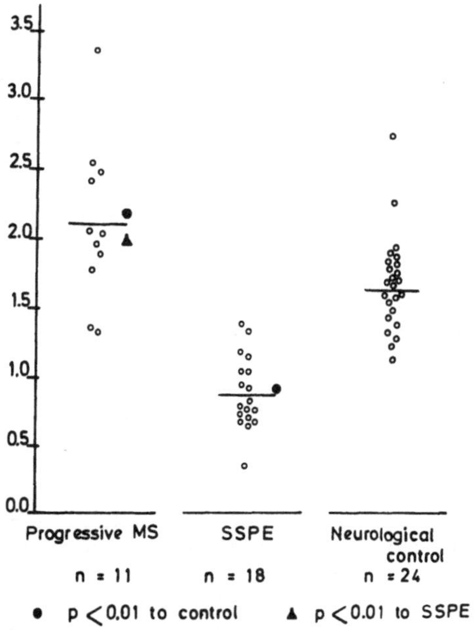

Fig.5. T_h/T_s ratio in CSF

Subpopulation of T cells

(Fig.5 and 6). In MS the T_h/T_s ratio is, as well in CSF as in PB, higher than in SSPE and control. In SSPE the T_h/T_s ratio is lower than in control and MS.

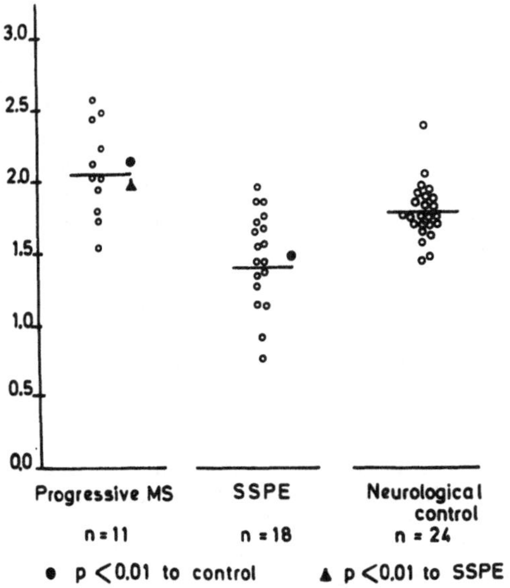

Fig.6. T_h/T_s ratio in blood.

DISCUSSION

The presence of myelin components as MBP (11, 12) or lipids (13, 14) was demonstrated in the CSF and PB in various neurological diseases. It is supposed that damage of the nerve tissue and release of own antigens may be factors facilitating autoimmunization (1, 15).

The reactivity of PB and CSF lymphocytes to brain antigens is still controversial. Because of the immunogenic and potentially encephalitogenic properties of MBP, a lot of attention has been focused on the immune response to MBP in human pathology, but the results obtained in different laboratories, are not consistent (16, 17, 18).

For our study of sensitization to brain antigens, we have used antigen stimulated ARFC assay. The Ag-ARFC test is regarded as an in vitro method, showing the existence of in vivo cell mediated hypersensitivity to studied antigen (6, 19).

To the study of cell mediated immunity to MBP, Ag-ARFC was used first by Hashim et al. (20) in experimental allergic encephalitis. Later, others, using Ag-ARFC, have found a high incidence of reactivity of PB lymphocytes to MBP in MS (7, 21, 22, 23). Offner et al. (7, 21) did not notice any difference in sensitization according to the intensity of disease process, but Ilyas and Davison (22) found a higher incidence in the active stage of MS. In our study, higher reactivity to MBP in PB was observed in relapse and in chronic progressive stage. The reactivity of PB lymphocytes with MBP was not MS specific and a similar phenomenon, however to a smaller degree, was also observed in OND.

Studies with the use of the CSF were done only sporadically (24, 25). Lisak et al. (25) using the lymphocyte transformation test, showed reactivity of CSF cells to MBP of MS patients being in relapse or in a chronic progressive stage and of patients with an active demyelinative disease other than MS.

The problem of a delayed type of hypersensitivity to lipid components of myelin was not so extensively studied as that to MBP. Certain authorities maintain that these haptens are unable to initiate cell-mediated immunity (26, 27). However, Nagai et al. (28) injecting ganglioside into experimental animals, were able to demonstrate blastoid cell transformation in vitro upon culturing of lymphocytes with myelin-containing ganglioside antigen. Recently, Offner et al. (29) demonstrated, in vivo and in vitro, in Lewis rats delayed type of hypersensitivity to ganglioside after immunization with the spinal cord and CFA.

In our work, like Offner and Konat (30) and Ilyas and Davison (22) found, most of MS patients react positively with ganglioside and cerebroside. However, we don't confirm that this phenomenon is highly specific for MS as it is observed in OND only sporadically. We have found that about 50% of the patients with noninflammatory OND are sensitized to cerebroside, and more than 30% to ganglioside. We also observed that some persons without any damage to nerve tissue, have in PB lymphocytes reacting with glycolipids. Similarly as in the case of MBP, we did not find sensitization to glycolipids in the CSF of the healthy control group. However, most CSF of MS patients and 30-40% of persons with OND, showed reactivity with MBP and glycolipids.

Frick (31) has studied in MS, sensitization to human encephalitogenic peptide, using a cell mediated cytotoxicity test, and observed the response only in MS patients. In our study we also found lack of reactivity in cases of noninflammatory neurological diseases, but a reaction was present in the SSPE group, although it was less frequent than among the MS patients.

Humoral immune responses to MBP in SSPE have been studied previously in several laboratories (2, 32), but the problem of cellular immunity is less known. In our work, we found that lymphocyte sensitization to MBP, glycolipids and encephalitogenic peptide in SSPE, is much lower than in MS.

Johnson et al. (33) have found that 8 of 17 patients with measles encephalitis demonstrated lymphocyte proliferative responses to MBP, but only 6 of 40 patients with measles without encephalitis. In our study, reactivity with MBP was observed in about 50% of SSPE patients. 20-30% SSPE patients reacted with glycolipids and encephalogenic peptide. The reactivity to the studied antigens in SSPE was not greater than in the OND group.

When comparing lymphocytic reactivity to MBP and glycolipids in PB and CSF, we can suggest that the active sensitization to myelin components in the CSF is caused by breakdown of tolerance to the own antigens, released during the course of the disease. Sporadically observed sensitization in PB, in healthy control, can be caused by cross reactivity with environmental factors.

It is interesting why the incidence of cell mediated hypersensitivity to brain antigens is higher in MS than in SSPE. Antibodies to MBP are synthesized in SSPE to a similar degree as in the active stage of MS (2). If we presume that sensitization to brain antigen is a secondary phenomenon to brain damage, we should expect greater reactivity in SSPE. In fact, reactivity in SSPE was not different, than in other noninflammatory neurological diseases. In our OND group, damage to the brain tissue was less pronounced as in SSPE.

It was found by us, similarly like by others (34, 35), that a low proportion of T suppressor cells in MS can be a factor enhancing autoimmunity. Contrary, in SSPE we noticed a lower T_h/T_s ratio. Measles virus infection of lymphocytes (36) and constant antigenic stimulation in SSPE may cause alterations of immunoregulation. Although humoral immunity is well preserved or even exaggerated, cell mediated immunity can be to some extent suppressed, as was observed in a previous study of a non-specific immunity in SSPE (38).

REFERENCES

1. B.H. Waksman. The pathogenetic significance of cross reactions in autoimmune disease of the nervous system. Immunology Today. 5:346 (1984).
2. J. Ruutiainen, T. Arnadottir, G. Molnar, A. Salmi and H. Frey. Myelin basic protein antibodies in the serum of CSF of multiple sclerosis and subacute sclerosing panencephalitis. Acta Neurol. Scand. 64:196 (1981).
3. H.H. Budka, Lassmann and Th. Popow-Kraupp. Measles virus antigen in panencephalitis. Acta Neuropathol. 56:52 (1982).
4. A.S. Rose, G.W. Ellison, L.W. Myers and W.W. Tourtellotte. Criteria for the clinical diagnosis of multiple sclerosis. Neurology. 26:20 (1976).
5. J.T. Jabbour, J.H. Garcia, H. Lemmi, J. Regland, D.A. Duenas and J.L. Sever. Subacute sclerosing panencephalitis; a multidisciplinary study of eight cases. J. Amer. Med. 207:2248 (1969).

6. J.P. Felsburg and R. Edelman. The active E rosette test, a sensitive in vitro correlate for human delayed-type hypersensitivity. J. Immunol. 118:62 (1972).
7. H. Offner, G. Konat, N.E. Raun and J. Clausen. E rosette forming lymphocytes in multiple sclerosis patients. Basic protein stimulation of rosette-forming cells. Acta Neurol. Scand. 57:380 (1978).
8. A. Czlonkowska, M. Poltorak, W. Cendrowski and J. Korlak. Sensitization of cerebrospinal fluid and peripheral blood lymphocytes to myelin basic protein in multiple sclerosis. Acta Neurol. Scand. 66:121 (1982).
9. G.E. Deibler, E. Martenson and M.W. Kiese. Large scale preparation of myelin protein from central nervous tissue of several mammalian species. Preparat. Biochem. 2:139 (1972).
10. F.J. Morich, F. Momburg, G. Moldenhauer, K.U. Hartmann and K.J. Bross. Immunoperoxidase slide assay (IPSA) a new screening method for hybridoma supernatants directed against cell surface antigens compared to other binding assays. Immunobiol. 164:192 (1983).
11. S.R. Cohen, B.R. Brooks, B. Jubelt, R.M. Herndon and G.M. McKhann. Myelin basic protein in cerebrospinal fluid. In: J.H. Wood (ed.) Neurobiology of cerebrospinal fluid. Vol.1. Plenum Press, New York. (1980).
12. C. Jacque, A. Delassalle, G. Rancurel, M. Raoul, B. Lesourd and J.C. Legrand. Myelin basic protein in CSF and blood. Arch. Neurol. 39:557 (1982).
13. W.W. Tourtellotte and A.F. Haerer. Lipids in cerebrospinal fluid. Part 12. In multiple sclerosis and retrobular neuritis. Arch. Neurol. 20:605 (1969).
14. Y. Nagai, J.J. Kanfer and W.W. Tourtellotte. Preliminary observations of gangliosides of normal and multiple sclerosis cerebrospinal fluid. Neurology. 23:945 (1973).
15. P.Y. Paterson, E.D. Day, C.C. Whitaker. Neuroimmunological diseases: Effector cell responses and immunoregulatory mechanisms. Immunological Rev. 55:89 (1981).
16. R.A.C. Hughes, I.A. Gregson and R.A. Metcalfe. Multiple sclerosis-lymphocyte transformation with multiple sclerosis and normal brain myelin basic protein and subcellular fractions. Acta Neurol. Scand. 65:161 (1982).
17. V. Wicher, W. Olszewski and F. Milgrom. Age-related reactivity of lymphocytes from multiple sclerosis patients to myelin basic protein. Int. Arch. Allergy Appl. Immun. 66:136 (1981).
18. C.J.J. Brinkman, W.M. Nillesen, O.R. Hommes, K.J.B. Lamers, B.E.J. de Pauw and P. Delmotte. Cell-mediated immunity in multiple sclerosis as determined by sensitivity of different lymphocyte populations to
19. J. Wybran and E. Dupont. The active E rosette: an early marker for T cell activation. Ann. Immunol. Inst. Pasteur. 133D:211 (1982).
20. G.A. Hashim, D.H. Lee and J.C. Pierce. Antigen-stimulated rosette formation by T lymphocytes in experimental allergic encephalomyelitis. Neurochemical Res. 2:99 (1977).
21. H. Offner, C. Rostogi, G. Konat and J. Clausen. Stimulation of active E-rosette forming lymphocytes by myelin basic protein and specific antigens from multiple sclerosis brains. J. Neurol. Sci. 42:349 (1979).
22. A.A. Ilyas and A.N. Davison. Cellular hypersensitivity to gangliosides and myelin basic protein in multiple sclerosis. J. Neurol. Sci. 59:85 (1983).
23. G.A. Hashim and M. Brewen. Myelin basic protein-responsive blood T lymphocytes in patients with multiple sclerosis. J. Neurosc. Res. 13:349 (1985).

24. R.P. Lisak and B. Zweiman. In vitro cell mediated immunity of cerebrospinal fluid lymphocytes to myelin basic protein in primary demyelinating disease. N. Engl. J. Med. 297:850 (1977).
25. R.P. Lisak, B. Zweiman and J. Whitaker. Spinal fluid basic protein immunoreactive material and spinal fluid lymphocyte reactivity to basic protein. Neurology. 31:180 (1981).
26. B. Niedieck. On the glycolipid hapten of myelin. Prog. Allergy. 18:353 (1975).
27. S. Leibowitz. Glycolipid haptens in disease of the nervous system. In: A. Boese (ed.) Search for the cause of multiple sclerosis and other chronic diseases of the central nervous system. Verlag Chemie, Weinheim. pp. 117:126 (1980).
28. Y. Nagai, T. Momoi, T. Saito, M. Mitsuzawa and S. Ontani. Ganglioside syndrome, a new autoimmune neurological disorder experimentally induced with brain ganglioside. Neurosc. Lett. 2:107 (1976).
29. H. Offner, B.A. Standage, D.R. Burger and A.A. Vandenbark. Delayed type hypersensitivity to gangliosides in the Lewis rat. J. Neuroimmunol. 9:147 (1985).
30. H. Offner and G. Konat. Stimulation of active E-rosette forming lymphocytes from multiple sclerosis patients by gangliosides and cerebrosides. J. Neurol. Sci. 46:101 (1980).
31. E. Frick. Cell-mediated cytotoxicity by peripheral blood lymphocytes against basic protein of myelin, encephalitogenic peptide, cerebrosides and gangliosides in multiple sclerosis. J. Neurol. Sci. 57:55 (1982).
32. H.S. Panith, P. Swoveland and K.P. Johnson. Antibodies to measles virus react with myelin basic protein. Neurology. 29:548 (1979).
33. T.R. Johnson, D.E. Griffin, R.L. Hirsch, J.S. Wolinsky, S. Roedenbeck, I.L. De Soriano and A. Vaisberg. Measles encephalomyelitis - clinical and immunologic studies. N. Engl. J. Med. 310:137 (1984).
34. E.L. Reinherz, H.L. Weiner, S.L. Hauser, J.A. Cohen, J.A. Distaso and S.F. Schlossman. Loss of suppressor T cells in active multiple sclerosis - Analysis with monoclonal antibodies. N. Engl. J. Med. 303:125 (1980).
35. M.A. Bach, C. Martin, P. Cesaro, J.F. Eizenbaum and J.D. Degos. T cell subsets in multiple sclerosis. J. Neuroimmunol. 7:331 (1985).
36. J.G. Fournier, M. Tardieu, P. Lebon, O. Robain, G. Pensot, S. Rozenblatt and M. Bouteille. Detection of measles virus RNA in lymphocytes from peripheral blood and brain perivascular infiltrates of patients with subacute sclerosing panencephalitis. N. Engl. J. Med. 313:910 (1985).
37. P. Arneborn and G. Biberfeld. T-lymphocyte subpopulations in relation to immunosuppression in measles and varicella. Infection Immunity. 39:29 (1983).
38. M. Vainiene, A. Czlonkowska and J. Korlak. Subacute sclerosing panencephalitis: influence of the clinical course and treatment with isoprinosine on non-specific cell-mediated and humoral immunity. Acta Neurol. Scand. 67:275 (1983).

SPECIFICITY OF CLONES AND T CELL LINES FROM CEREBROSPINAL FLUID IN VIRAL MENINGOENCEPHALITIS AND MULTIPLE SCLEROSIS

H.W. Kreth, P. Marquardt and R. Martin

Children's Hospital, University of Würzburg
D-8700 Würzburg, FRG

INTRODUCTION

It is now recognized that MS is a T cell-mediated disease initiated at the time around puberty in genetically susceptible individuals. The disease is frequently accompanied by a moderate pleocytosis. The majority of the CSF exudate cells are T cells of the $OKT4^+$ phenotype.

Since MS is a localized inflammatory disorder, the impression has always been that immunological studies should concentrate on CSF lymphocytes. However, until recently, CSF cells have been too difficult to study by conventional immunological methods because of their small numbers.

The advance of modern tissue culture techniques has led to a revolution in clinical immunology. With the use of Interleukin-2 (IL-2) as T cell growth factor, it is now possible to expand and propagate very small quantities of T cells and analyse their functions and specificities at the single cell level.

This technique has already been applied to MS, and CSF T cell lines and clones have been established and tested for reactivity against viral and neural antigens in different laboratories (1,2,3,4). The data and their relevance to the pathogenesis of MS are extremely difficult to interpret. There is an urgent need for background information on the composition of T cell specificities in chronic inflammatory CNS disorders with well-defined etiologies.

In this study, we will therefore first present data on the antigen specificities of CSF T cells in acute and chronic viral infections. Subsequently, we will try to relate these observations to those found in patients with MS.

EXPERIMENTAL PROTOCOL

In these experiments, in vivo activated CSF T cells were always directly expanded without any prior in vitro restimulation. We may therefore assume that no selection for certain subpopulations or certain specificities should have occurred before the cloning procedure. Details can be found elsewhere (5). In short: Freshly isolated or frozen and thawed

CSF cells are seeded at limiting dilution into histoplates in the presence of irradiated feeder cells (50 Gy) and a crude preparation of TCGF containing submitogenic concentrations of PHA.

The cloning efficiencies ranged from 4-10%. Before functional testing, T cell colonies were always propagated in mitogen-free TCGF (Lymphocult-T-LF, Biotest, Frankfurt, FRG).

Since not all expanded T cell populations are monoclonal in the strict sense of the word, the term "T cell colony" (TCC) will be used.

LOCAL T CELL RESPONSE IN MUMPS MENINGITIS

We initially developed the method described above by using CSF T cells derived from a child with mumps meningitis (5). In this study, recruitment of T cells into the CNS was highly antigen-specific. Furthermore, bulk cultures of CSF cells and CSF T cell clones revealed almost identical patterns of reactivity as far as restriction elements and antigen specificities were concerned. This was an important observation suggesting that the information obtained from cloned T cell populations is in fact reliable.

A similar high enrichment of antigen-specific T cells has also been found in measles encephalitis (6).

To demonstrate what the incidence of specifically sensitized T cells is like in mumps meningitis, we will briefly describe one of our recent experiments. In this case, CSF cells were derived from a 7-year-old boy who presented with severe headaches, vomiting and nuchal rigidity 2 days after onset of parotitis. Cells were seeded at 1 cell and 3 cells per well. Out of a total of 190 T cell colonies a sample of 51 was selected at random and used for phenotypic analysis and functional studies. As shown in Fig.1. there is a predominance of $OKT8^{+}$ T cell colonies displaying strong cytotoxicity against mumps virus-infected autologous B lymphoblastoid cell lines. The lytic activity of $OKT4^{+}$ TCCs was usually much less. Only 3 $OKT4^{+}$ TCCs reacted against mumps virus in the presence of autologous presenter cells in a 3-day lymphoproliferative assay. The results are presented in Table 1.

It should be noted that TCC 41 has a remarkable specificity, in as far as it reacted not only to mumps and sendai virus but also upon exposure to cardiolipin (diphosphatidylglycerol). Evidently, this T cell colony is specific for phospholipid! The reactivity towards mumps and sendai viruses can be explained by the fact that both are enveloped viruses that mature by budding from host cell membranes.

It might be speculated that induction of phospholipid- and/or glycolipid-specific T cells is a frequent event during infections with enveloped viruses. This might have important implications for the pathogenesis of chronic demyelinating disorders (7).

Table 1. Proliferative response of CSF T cell colonies derived from a patient with mumps meningitis (L.A.)

Colony		cpm[^{3}H]-TdR Uptake in the presence of autologous presenter cells and:						
No		Medium	Mumps	Sendai	Cerebrosides	Cardiolipin	MPB	PHA
13	(T8$^+$)	1560*)	1465	1700	1385	77	1400	3820
30	(T4$^+$)	498	<u>3095</u>	253	511	50	420	9595
41	(T4$^+$)	447	<u>1185</u>	<u>1127</u>	295	<u>3537</u>	336	2260
58	(T8$^+$)	109	166	105	67	57	106	5525
60	(T4$^+$)	344	<u>3675</u>	293	278	75	254	7556
63	(T8$^+$)	920	1085	910	1050	154	240	6850

*) Means of triplicate cultures.

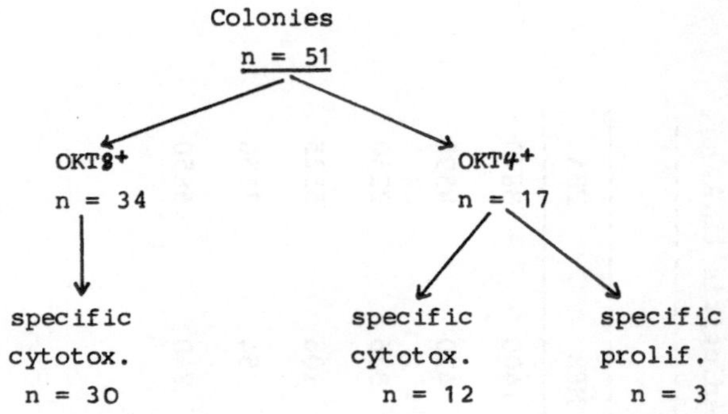

Fig.1. Functional analysis of T cell colonies derived from CSF of a patient with mumps meningitis (L.A. *12/11/78).

CSF T CELL SPECIFICITIES IN PROGRESSIVE RUBELLA PANENCEPHALITIS (PRP).

A completely different pattern was found in a patient with chronic rubella panencephalitis. This patient, a 15-year-old girl, had experienced uncomplicated rubella at the age of 8 years. Three years later, she presented with intellectual deterioration, choreiform movements and grand-mal seizures. A diagnosis of chronic rubella panencephalitis was made because of typical laboratory findings in serum and CSF (8). Now, 5 years after initial diagnosis, the patient is still alive with her CSF still showing a persistent lymphoid pleocytosis and marked oligoclonal bands specific for rubella virus.

In this case, a total of 336 clones and oligoclonal T cell lines were established in 2 independent cloning experiments. Surface marker analysis revealed that the majority of TCCs had the OKT4$^+$ phenotype. As summarized in Fig.2. all T cell populations were tested in proliferative assays against rubella virus and autoantigens. About 75% of TCCs were also assayed for cytotoxicity against rubella virus-infected autologous and allogeneic PHA-blasts. Compared with the findings in mumps meningitis, there are striking differences. First of all, the antigen specificity of CSF T

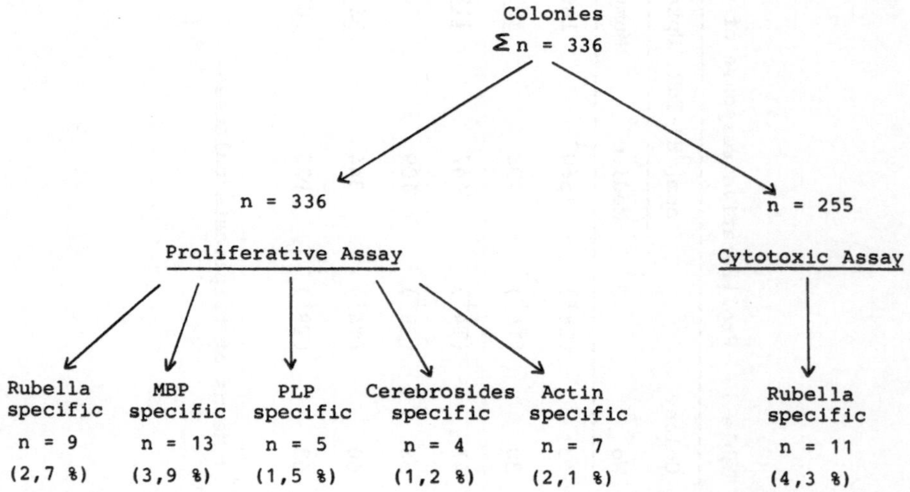

Fig.2. Functional analysis of T cell colonies derived from CSF of a patient with progressive rubella panencephalitis.

Table 2. Antigen-specific proliferative response of CSF T cell colonies from a patient with progressive rubella panencephalitis

Colony		cmp[^{3}H]-TdR Uptake in the presence of autologous presenter cells and:					
No		Medium	Rubella Virus	MBP	PLP	Cerebrosides	PHA
277/B	($T4^+$)	145*)	<u>3 365</u>	136	335	295	54 070
212	($T4^+$)	113	<u>14 620</u>	330	395	277	50 190
135	($T4^+$)	196	90	<u>1 033</u>	67	63	7 204
265	($T4^+$)	96	450	<u>1 685</u>	n.d.	n.d.	12 595
314	($T4^+$)	318	70	156	<u>1 570</u>	268	12 815
349	($T4^+$)	50	77	45	<u>2 148</u>	70	5 210
108	($T4^+$)	125	70	110	265	<u>860</u>	10 385
358	($T4^+$)	54	170	95	628	<u>3 200</u>	930

*) Means of triplicate cultures.

cells in PRP is low. What is most exciting, however, is the emergence of colonies specific for brain autoantigens such as myelin basic protein (MBP), cerebrosides and proteolipidprotein (PLP). On quantitative terms, autoreactive colonies almost seen to outweigh virus-specific TCCs. A representative sample of rubella- and autoantigen-specific TCCs are shown in Table 2. In more recent experiments, these colonies have been restimulated by antigen in the presence of irradiated autologous presenter cells without losing their antigen specificity.

FUNCTIONAL CHARACTERISTICS OF CSF T CELLS IN MULTIPLE SCLEROSIS

There is now good evidence for the presence of a rather high fraction of *in vivo* activated T cells in cerebrospinal fluid of patients with MS (9,10). The cells can easily be expanded *in vitro* into growing colonies by using the direct expansion protocol. As already published by us (2), the majority of colonies express OKT4 antigens, and about 50% of them are capable of exerting lectin-dependent cytotoxicity.

We have tested several hundred clones and oligoclonal T cell lines from several patients for specific reactivity, either cytotoxic or proliferative, against a panel of viral (measles, mumps, parainfluenza type 3, rubella, EBV) and nonviral antigens (myelin basic protein, glycolipids).

As far as viral antigens are concerned no specific reactivity was observed with the exception of a single $OKT8^+$ clone that was capable of killing autologous but not allogeneic mumps virus-infected target cells (2). However, the significance of this observation, in particular, whether this clone has any causal relationship to the patient's disease, is not clear. With regard to autoantigens (MBP, cerebrosides, gangliosides), we will present one of our more recent experiments. In this case, the patient was a 23-year-old male with clinically definite MS. CSF cells were taken during an exacerbation of his disease. As summarized in Fig.3, one out of 91 colonies responded vigorously to cerebrosides, 3 reacted moderately to myelin basic protein and 19 displayed a mild degree of proliferation upon exposure to gangliosides. The pattern of reactivity for representative T cell colonies is shown in Table 3.

Table 3. Proliferative response to autoantigens in the presence of autologous presenter cells of representative T cell colonies derived from a patient with MS

Colony		cpm[^{3}H]- TdR incorporated in response to				
No		Medium	MBP	Cerebrosides	Gangliosides	PHA
2	($T4^+$)	75	76	50	<u>495</u>	1215
7	($T4^+$)	260	<u>815</u>	220	375	1550
12	($T4^+$)	70	155	128	<u>436</u>	1520
19	($T4^+$)	220	<u>650</u>	330	295	1170
29	($T4^+$)	132	75	55	<u>445</u>	2290
33	($T4^+$)	106	210	<u>13325</u>	360	2365
79	($T4^+$)	185	<u>460</u>	216	220	10180

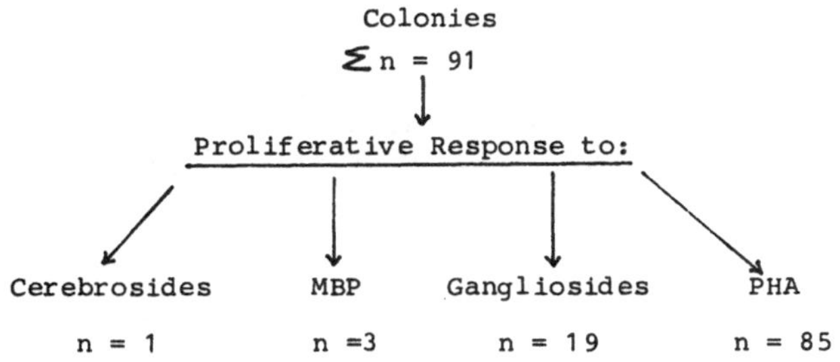

Fig.3. Functional analysis of T cell colonies derived from a patient with MS.

The reason for the mild degree of proliferation upon exposure to MBP and gangliosides is not known at present.

SUMMARY AND CONCLUSIONS

The findings reported above can be summarized as follows: the incidence of specifically antigen-reactive T cells in CSF is very high during the acute phase of viral infections of the CNS. This observation which was originally made in mumps meningitis and measles encephalitis (5,6) has more recently also been confirmed for varicella cerebellitis. The results also agree with those from animal studies (11). Furthermore, $OKT8^+$ cytotoxic T cells are the prevailing cell type.

In progressive rubella panencephalitis (PRP), a disease of several years' duration, virus-specific T cells can still be found. However, the incidence is rather low (around 5%). These cells might easily be missed if too small a sample of CSF clones or T cell lines is functionally analysed. It is conceivable that with longer duration of the disease the fraction of rubella-specific T cells among CSF exudate cells might be further diminished.

Another characteristic of this chronic inflammatory CNS disorder is that the majority of T cells belong to the $OKT4^+$ subpopulation. Obviously, $OKT4^+$ T cells, whether cytotoxic or noncytotoxic, are not able to eradicate rubella virus from the CNS.

The most important observation, however, is that virus infections of the CNS give rise to autoreactive T cell populations. This is most striking in chronic rubella panencephalitis. The extent to which these T cells contribute to the overall immunopathology of the disease, is not known.

What is the relevance of these findings for MS? First of all, if MS is triggered by a virus, and even if the virus persists in the CNS, the incidence of specifically reactive T cells in such a protracted disease of long duration may be extremely low (e.g. < 1/1000). Thus, it is certainly not reasonable to test hundreds and hundreds of clones against a large panel of viral antigens in order to identify the originally triggering pathogen.

Cloning of CSF T cells, however, might help us to identify the relevant brain antigens if virus-induced autoimmunization is indeed one of the major pathomechanisms in MS.

REFERENCES

1. J.R. Richert, D.E. McFarlin, J.W. Rose, H.F. McFarland and J.I. Greenstein. Expansion of antigen-specific T cells from cerebrospinal fluid of patients with multiple sclerosis. J. Neuroimmunol. 5:317 (1983).
2. B. Fleischer, P. Marquardt, S. Poser and H.W. Kreth. Phenotypic markers and functional characteristics of T lymphocyte clones from cerebrospinal fluid in multiple sclerosis. J. Neuroimmunol. 7:151 (1984).
3. R.B. Clark, P. Dore-Duffy, J.O. Donaldson, M. Kathryn Pollard and S.P. Muirhead. Generation of phenotypic helper (inducer and suppressor) cytotoxic T-cell lines from cerebrospinal fluid in multiple sclerosis. Cell. Immunol. 84:409 (1984).
4. D. Santoli, E.C. Defreitas, M. Sandberg-Wollheim, M.K. Francis and H. Koprowski. Phenotypic and functional characterization of T cell clones derived from the cerebrospinal fluid of multiple sclerosis patients. J. Immunol. 132:2386 (1984).
5. B. Fleischer and H.W. Kreth. Clonal analysis of HLA-restricted virus-specific cytotoxic T lymphocytes from cerebrospinal fluid in mumps meningitis. J. Immunol. 130:2187 (1983).
6. B. Fleischer and H.W. Kreth. Clonal expansion and functional analysis of virus-specific T lymphocytes from cerebrospinal fluid in measles encephalitis. Human Immunol. 7:239 (1983).
7. H.E. Webb and J.K. Fazakerley. Can viral envelope glycolipids produce autoimmunity, with reference to the CNS and multiple sclerosis? Neuropathology and applied neurobiology. 10:1 (1983).
8. J.S. Wolinsky, B.O. Berg and C.J. Maitland. Progressive rubella panencephalitis. Arch. Neurol. 33:772 (1976).
9. A.B.C. Noronha, D.P. Richman and B.G.W. Arnason. Detection of in vivo stimulated cerebrospinal fluid lymphocytes by flow cytometry in patients with multiple sclerosis. N. Engl. J. Med. 303:713 (1980).
10. D.A. Hafler, D.A. Fox, M.E. Manning, S.F. Schlossman, E.L. Reinherz and H.L. Weiner. In vivo activated T lymphocytes in the peripheral blood and cerebrospinal fluid of patients with multiple sclerosis. N. Engl. J. Med. 312:1405 (1985).
11. J.L. Hurwitz, R. Korngold and P.C. Doherty. Specific and nonspecific T-cell recruitment in viral meningitis: possible implications for autoimmunity. Cell. Immunol. 76:397 (1983).

ACTIVATION OF AN ENCEPHALITOGENIC T LYMPHOCYTE LINE WITH A CELL FREE SUPERNATANT CONTAINING BASIC PROTEIN AND I-REGION GENE PRODUCTS

Arthur A. Vandenbark[1,2,3], Peter Teal[1] and Halina Offner[1,3]

[1]Neuroimmunology Research Laboratory, VA Medical Center Portland, OR
[2]Department of Microbiology and Immunology, Oregon Health Sciences University, Portland, OR
[3]Department of Neurology, Oregon Health Sciences University, Portland, OR

BACKGROUND

Antigen specific T lymphocyte activation requires the recognition of antigen in the context of Class I or Class II major histocompatibility complex (MHC) gene products (1). Class I or Class II MHC restriction has been associated with the two major subsets of T lymphocytes (2). Antigen presentation with Class II (Ia) MHC products takes place on the surface of accessory cells (APC) such as macrophages, dendritic cells, or Langerhans cells which usually express Ia (3), or on other cell types such as endothelial cells (4) or astrocytes (5) in which Ia expression can be induced by gamma interferon (gamma-IFN). The I region genes which code for the Ia molecules also function to regulate the immune response, influencing the magnitude and nature of the responses to various antigenic determinants (6-9)/ The determinants which are recognized by T cells appear to be the product of unique interactions between processed antigen fragments and the available Class II MHC molecules on the surface of the accessory cells (10-12). Of relevance to this article, the T cell activation signal apparently needs not to remain associated with the antigen presenting cell, and may be shed into the surrounding medium (13-17).

In animals developing experimental autoimmune encephalomyelitis (EAE), immune response to myelin basic protein (BP) is also restricted by Class II MHC molecules. In the Lewis rat, the dominant epitope(s) of guinea pig or rat myelin basic protein encompasses the region surrounding residue 79 (18). Immunization of Lewis rats with whole GP-BP and subsequent selection of T cells lines using the complete BP molecule results in a T cell response restricted to the 68-88 amino acid fragment, in spite of the antigenic capabilities of other regions of GP-BP (19). The immunodominance of the epitope(s) surrounding residue 79 is probably related to the potent encephalitogenic and delayed type hypersensitivity (DTH) inducing capabilities associated with this region. Furthermore, T lymphocyte lines from Lewis and Brown Norway rat strains, which differ in their RT-1 haplotypes, recognized distinct determinants on guinea pig myelin basic protein (19). However, F_1 (Lewis x BN) T cell lines could recognize either the Lewis or the BN determinant depending on which APC type was used to select the line (20), suggesting that Ia molecules on the APC might influence which determinant on GP-BP is immunodominant.

In this article, we will evaluate the activation signal which stimulates GP-BP reactive T lymphocytes to proliferate and to transfer both delayed type hypersensitivity reactions - measured by ear swelling - and clinical signs of EAE. The experimental approach included: a) defining the role of accessory cells in antigen presentation, b) determining if the activation signal could be produced and shed as a cell free supernatant from accessory cells, c) evaluating the role of activated T cell products on the production of the stimulation signals, and d) determining the specificity and Ia restriction of the activation signal.

EXPERIMENTAL RESULTS

Antigen specific activation of T cell lines is strain restricted

To determine if antigen specific T cell lines were MHC restricted, GP-BP and PPD specific lines from either Lewis or Brown Norway rats were stimulated with GP-BP or PPD presented by either syngeneic or allogeneic thymocytes. As is shown in Table 1, each line responded best when stimulated with syngeneic APC and relevant antigen. Allogenic APC were unable to present the relevant antigen, but could induce responsiveness to Con A (Table 1). These data indicate clearly that specific activation of the T cell lines required that the immunizing antigen are present in combination with syngeneic accessory cell signals.

Table 1. Antigen specific activation of rat T cell lines is strain restricted.

Responder T cell line	Source of APC	Proliferation response[a] (CPM x 10^{-3} ^{3}H-Tdy Uptake) Control	Con A	GP-BP	PPD
LE/BP	LE TX	3 ± 1	232 ± 10	265 ± 17	2 ± 1
	BN TX	1 ± 1	166 ± 7	3 ± 1	0 ± 0
BN/BP	LE TX	3 ± 1	196 ± 9	3 ± 1	1 ± 0
	BN TX	2 ± 1	166 ± 2	123 ± 13	1 ± 0
LE/PPD	LE TX	7 ± 2	226 ± 16	8 ± 2	269 ± 15
	BN TX	8 ± 1	190 ± 11	8 ± 1	28 ± 5
BN/PPD	LE TX	1 ± 0	178 ± 8	1 ± 0	1 ± 0
	BN TX	2 ± 1	199 ± 10	2 ± 1	166 ± 6

[a] Each value represents mean ± standard deviation of lymphocyte proliferation in triplicate wells containing 2 x 10^4 T cells and 2 x 10^6 irradiated thymic APC plus medium, Con A, or antigen, and incubated for 72 hr, the last 18 hr in the presence of 0.5 μCi ^{3}H-Tdy.

Production of processed antigen

Additional experiments were designed to determine if the T cell activation required direct cell-cell contact with APC, or if a cell free signal released by the APC into the culture medium could stimulate the T cells. APC populations (irradiated thymocytes, TX) were pulsed for 24 hrs with relevant or irrelevant antigens, and culture supernatants were collected after spinning out the cells at 400 x g. The supernatant was added back to resting BP-1 cells for 2-3 days incubation, and the proliferation response was measured by ^{3}H-Tdy uptake. As is shown in Table 2, response was observed only when the cells were stimulated with supernatants produced by syngeneic APC pulsed with the relevant antigen for each line. No stimulatory effect on resting BP-reactive T cells was observed when supernatants from TX were combined with native GP-BP (data not shown), suggesting that the stimulatory signal contained a processed form of GP-BP. Henceforth, supernatants which stimulated the T cell lines will be referred to as processed antigen (e.g. pGP-BP), although these supernatants undoubtedly contained native or unprocessed antigen as well. These data indicate that a cell free form of processed antigen was produced and released by antigen-pulsed APC. This cell free activation factor was relatively inefficient as a T cell stimulant, inducing less than 10% of the response observed in the presence of APC. However, the cell free supernatant showed the same MHC restriction pattern (Table 2) as was observed with APC present (Table 1).

Table 2. Response of T cell lines to supernatants of antigen-pulsed APC[a]

Responder T cell line	Source of APC	Proliferation Response (CPM x 10^{-3} ^{3}H-Tdy Uptake) to Supernatants from APC pulsed with: Medium	GP-BP	PPD
LE/BP	LE TX	0.3 ± 0.2	6.6 ± 1.1	0.4 ± 0.2
	BN TX	0.5 ± 0.2	0.6 ± 0.3	0.3 ± 0.1
BN/BP	LE TX	1.5 ± 0.4	1.2 ± 0.2	0.7 ± 0.2
	BN TX	1.5 ± 0.7	8.5 ± 0.5	1.3 ± 0.6
LE/PPD	LE TX	0.3 ± 0.2	0.8 ± 0.6	27.0 ± 2.0
	BN TX	0.7 ± 0.5	0.3 ± 0.3	0.7 ± 0.3

[a] 60 x 10^{6} thymic accessory cells (APC) were pulsed for 24 hrs with medium, 25 µg GP-BP, or 25 µg PPD in 1 ml. The cells were sedimented by centrifugation at 400 x g for 10 min, and 100 µl supernatant were added to triplicate wells containing 2 x 10^{4} resting T cells. The cells were incubated for 72 hr, the last 18 hr with 0.5 µCi ^{3}H-tdy. Values represent mean ± standard deviation.

Activated T lymphocytes enhance production of processed antigen

The greatly enhanced response of the T cell lines in the presence of APC suggested that T cell activation might contribute to the production of processed antigen. To test this possibility, supernatants were collected after 6 hrs incubation from the usual stimulation mixture of APC (TX), T

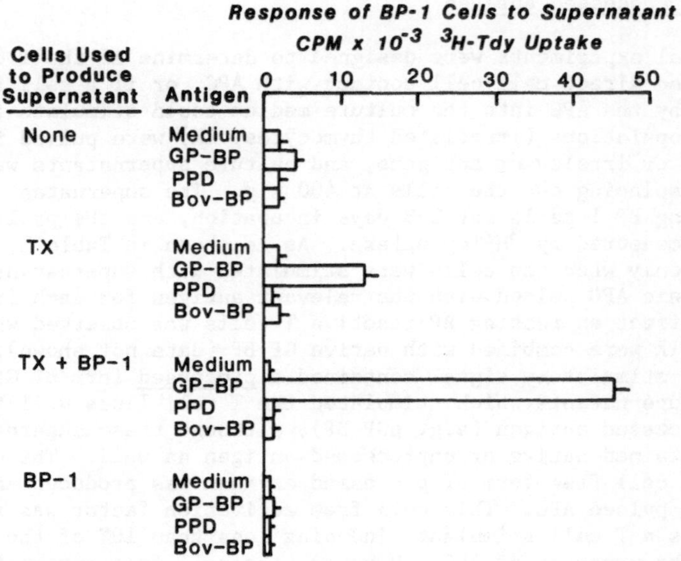

Fig.1. Stimulation of GP-BP specific T lymphocytes with cell free supernatants. Supernatants were produced and collected after 4 hours using the cell and antigen mixtures shown in the figure. These supernatants were added to triplicate microtiter wells containing 2 X 10^4 resting BP-1 T lymphocytes and the cultures incubated for 3 days, the last 18 hours with ^{3}H-Tdy. The cells were collected on glass fiber filters and counted by standard liquid scintillation techniques.

lymphocytes, and antigen, and added to resting T cells of the same specificity. As is shown in Fig.1, the combination of BP-1 cells (from Lewis rats) plus Lewis TX plus GP-BP was far more efficient than TX plus antigen alone at producing the stimulatory signal. BP-1 cells plus GP-BP, or medium plus GP-BP or any cell combination without GP-BP could not produce the stimulatory supernatant factor.

Further preliminary experiments were carried out to optimize the production of the supernatant factor and established the following: 1) The best ratio of TX:T cell ranged from 25:1 to 40:1. 2) Supernatant activity was dependent on the concentration of APC used. 3) Optimal supernatant activity reached a plateau between 10 and 25 µg/ml antigen. Based on these observations, processed antigen was produced for subsequent experiments using 1.5 x 10^6 resting BP-1 cells plus 60 x 10^6 TX plus 10-25 µg antigen per ml of stimulation medium.

To evaluate the kinetics of pGP-BP production, stimulated culture supernatants were collected and tested at various times after the addition of GP-BP. The production of GP-BP was detectable at 30 min, reached optimal levels by 4-6 hrs, and decreased substantially by 24 hrs. The pGP-BP produced by either the BP-1 line plus TX or the GP-BP reactive D9 clone (kindly provided by Dr. Irun Cohen of the Weizmann Institute, Israel) plus TX could stimulate both BP-1 and D9 cells (data not shown), suggesting that the pGP-BP activity was not limited to the T cell line used in the pGP-BP production.

pGP-BP activity is I-A and epitope restricted

As was shown in Table 1 above, stimulation of BP reactive T cells required presentation of BP by histocompatible APC. To determine if Class II MHC determinants were involved in the activation of the BP-1 line, we utilized monoclonal antibodies against the I-A and I-E MHC products (OX-6 and OX-17 respectively, kindly donated by Dr. Steven Brostoff of the Medical University of South Carolina) to inhibit stimulation by APC or pGP-BP. As is shown in Fig.2, addition of anti-I-A but non anti-I-E antibodies inhibited stimulation of the BP-1 cells by both TX and by pGP-BP. Addition of both OX-6 and OX-17 resulted in the same degree of inhibition as OX-6 alone. As we showed previously (22), the effect of OX-6 is directed at the APC population rather than the activated T cells.

The data presented in Fig.1. indicated that only processed GP-BP, but not processed Bov-BP or PPD could stimulate the BP-1 T cell line which was selected against GP-BP and which is known to respond to epitope(s) near amino acid residue 79 within the 68-84 peptide fragment of GP-BP. To evaluate further the epitope specificity of the BP-1 activation signal, we used two monoclonal antibodies to GP-BP (kindly donated by Dr. Robert Fritz of Emory University) to attempt to inhibit the pGP-BP activity. These antibodies have been characterized previously for their reactivity to GP-BP (23). Antibody 15-32 binds the N terminal region of the 43-88 peptide, and 22-17 binds the C terminal region of the 68-88 peptide. Neither antibody alone nor both antibodies together inhibited the activa-

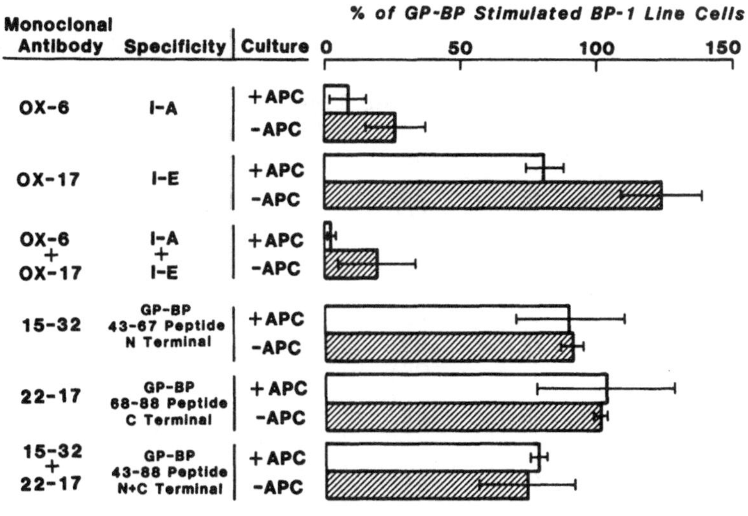

Fig.2. Effects of monoclonal antibodies on the activation of BP-1 cells by TX plus GP-BP (+APC), or by pGP-BP (-APC). Triplicate microtiter cultures containing 2 X 10^4 BP-1 cells, 2 X 10^6 TX and 2 μg GP-BP (+ APC), or 2 X 10^4 BP-1 cells (100 μl) plus 100 μl pGP-BP (-APC), were incubated with 2 μg of various antibodies or without antibody for a total of 3 days, the last 18 hr with ^{3}H-Tdy, and were harvested and counted by liquid scintillation procedures. All values were derived from pooled data from 3 separate and complete experiments. Numbers represent % of uninhibited control cultures, which were 145 ± 24 X 1063 CPM (+APC) and 119 ±32 X 10-3 CPM (-APC).

tion of BP-1 cells by TX or by pGP-BP (Fig.2) at concentrations as high as 10 μg/ml, suggesting that the epitope recognized by the T cell line was neither blocked nor conformationally disturbed by interaction of GP-BP with the antibodies.

Contribution of antigen specific and nonspecific factors in supernatants

Although the data presented above suggested that both specific antigen and Ia molecules were required for proliferation of BP-1 cells, it seemed plausible that other nonspecific, mitogenic factors, released during the 4-6 hr incubation of BP-1 cells with TX and GP-BP, might contribute to the response of resting BP-1 cells. To evaluate antigen nonspecific effects, PPD or OVA specific T lymphocyte lines were activated with TX and their homologous antigen for 4 hrs, and the supernatants from these cultures were added to resting homologous T cells or to resting BP-1 cells. As is shown in Table 3, supernatants from the activated PPD specific line produced strong activation (135 ± 8 CPM x 10^{-3}) of resting PPD T cells. The same supernatant produced low but detectable stimulation (5 ± 0 versus 1 ± 0 CPM x 10^{-3} background) when added to resting BP-1 cells. Addition of GP-BP during the PPD-specific activation of the PPD T cell line produced a supernatant which stimulated resting BP-1 cells to a degree comparable with supernatant produced by APC plus activated BP-1 cells (37 ± 2 versus 40 ± 2 CPM x 10^{-3}, Table 3). In this example, the antigen specific signal thus contributed about 90% of the stimulation, the remainder coming from antigen nonspecific products of T cell activation.

Table 3. Effects of supernatants from antigen activated T cell lines on Lewis GP-BP reactive T cells[a]

Supernatant production			Proliferation response: CPM x 10^{-3} ^{3}H-Tdy uptake		
TX + T cell line	Antigen	Responder line	No Inhibitor	+ OX-6	+OX-17
BP-1	GP-BP	BP-1	40 ± 2	4 ± 0	44 ± 2
PPD	PPD	PPD	135 ± 8		
	PPD	BP-1	5 ± 0	4 ± 0	6 ± 0
	PPD + GP-BP	BP-1	37 ± 2	5 ± 0	44 ± 0
OVA	OVA	OVA	33 ± 3		
	OVA	BP-1	2 ± 0	1 ± 1	1 ± 0
	OVA + GP-BP	BP-1	30 ± 3	1 ± 1	33 ± 4

[a] Supernatants were produced by incubating 60 x 10^6 irradiated thymocytes with 1.5 x 10^6 T lymphocytes and antigen (GP-BP, 10 μg/ml; PPD and OVA, 25 μg/ml) for 4 hr. Supernatants were collected, centrifuged at 400 x g for 10 min, and 100 μl were added to 2 x 10^4 responder T lymphocytes in 100 μl stimulation medium in microtiter wells. Anti-I-A (OX-6) or anti-I-E (OX-17) monoclonal antibodies were also added to some wells (2 μg/well). The cultures were incubated for 72 hr, the last 18 hr with 0.5 μCi ^{3}H-Tdy, before harvesting and counting. Values include mean ± standard deviation of triplicate cultures, and are representative of 4 such experiments.

The PGP-BP signal produced by either PPD activated PPD specific T cells or GP-BP activated BP-1 T cells was inhibitable with OX-6 but not OX-17 antibodies to the level of the nonspecific stimulation (4000 CPM), further implicating the need for I-A but not I-E gene products in the antigen specific activation signal (Table 3). However, treatment of the antigen nonspecific component of the activation signal with OX-6 did not inhibit T cell response, suggesting lack of Ia restriction. When OVA specific T cells were used to produce supernatants, a similar pattern of responsiveness was observed as described using the PPD T cell line (Table 3). Evaluation of 9 such experiments indicated that the nonspecific component contributed from 3 to 40% of the total stimulatory activity found in the supernatants.

A similar protocol was used to evaluate antigen specific and nonspecific stimulation of supernatants produced by allogeneic APC in the presence of activated T cells. As is shown in Table 4, antigen specific T cell lines responded best to supernatants containing homologous antigen produced by syngeneic APC in the presence of syngeneic activated T cells. Supernatants produced by allogeneic APC in the presence of activated T cells often contained significant nonspecific effects (e.g. supernatant from Lewis APC plus Lewis PPD specific T cells plus PPD induced 30,000 CPM versus a background of 5,000 CPM when added to BN BP reactive T cells), but the addition of homologous antigen (BP in this case) produced little additional antigen specific effect (4,000 additional CPM in the above example). These results indicate clearly that the predominant component of the cell free supernatant effect was antigen specific and strain restricted. However, the antigen nonspecific effects were often significant, but were not strain restricted.

Table 4. Effects of activated T cell products on supernatant activity[a]

Responder T cell line	APC source	Proliferation response ($CPM \times 10^{-3}$ ^{3}H-Tdy uptake) to supernatants from APC pulsed with: Medium	Activated T cell Products	Activated T cell Products + Antigen
LE/BP	LE TX	2 ± 1	20 ± 1	115 ± 7
	BN TX	1 ± 1	2 ± 1	9 ± 4
BN/BP	LE TX	5 ± 2	30 ± 3	34 ± 4
	BN TX	4 ± 1	28 ± 3	72 ± 5
LE/PPD	LE TX	8 ± 4	8 ± 2	117 ± 15
	BN TX	2 ± 0	21 ± 2	37 ± 5

[a] Supernatants were produced by incubating 60×10^6 irradiated thymocytes (APC) with 1.5×10^6 T lymphocytes and antigen (GP-BP and/or PPD, 25 µg/ml) for 4 hr. Supernatants were collected, centrifuged at 400 x g for 10 min, and 100 µl were added to 2×10^4 responder T lymphocytes in 100 µl stimulation medium in microtiter wells. The cultures were incubated for 72 hr, the last 18 hr with 0.5 µCi ^{3}H-Tdy, before harvesting and counting. Values include mean ± standard deviation of triplicate cultures, and are representative of 4 such experiments.

Separation and reconstitution of pGP-BP activity

In previous experiments, supernatants of activated T cell cultures were obtained by sedimenting the cells at 400 x g for 10 min. This process removed the cells, but could not remove macromolecular complexes, shed cell membranes, or microsomal components from the preparation. To evaluate further the contribution of these components to pGP-BP activity, supernatants produced by centrifugation at 400 x g were ultracentrifuged at 100,000 x g before testing on resting BP-1 or OVA T cells. As is shown in Table 5, the pGP-BP stimulated BP-1 (42 ± 4 CPM x 10^{-3}) but not OVA T cells (5 ± 1). Some of the proliferation activity was retained in the supernatant after ultracentrifugation (10 ± 2) but this activity still required the presence of I-A molecules, since activity could be reduced by OX-6 but not OX-17. Even less activity after ultracentrifugation was associated with the pellet (4 ± 1). Reassociation of the ultracentrifuged pellet or supernatant with native BP produced activity roughly equivalent to the supernatant alone. However, vigorous mixing of the pellet and ultrasupernatant resulted in reconstitution of most of the starting prolife-

Table 5. Processed GP-BP activity does not sediment at 100,000 x g

Processed GP-BP	T lymphocyte response		
	Proliferation (CPM x 10^{-3})		Clinical EAE
Supernatant treatment	BP-1 line	OVA line	BP-1 line
1. 400 x g	42 ± 4	5 ± 1	2.0 (2/2)
2. 100,000 x g, 4 hr			
Supernatant	10 ± 2	3 ± 1	
+ OX-6	3 ± 0	2 ± 0	
+ OX-17	11 ± 1	3 ± 0	
+ GP-BP	10 ± 3	3 ± 0	
Pellet	1 ± 1	ND	
Pellet + Supernatant	32 ± 3	ND	2.0 (2/2)
Fitrate, 0.45 microns	3 ± 2	ND	
3. No supernatant	1 ± 0	1 ± 0	0.0 (0.6)
4. GP-BP or OVA alone	2 ± 1	2 ± 1	0.0 (0/4)

Processed GP-BP was prepared by incubating 600 x 10^6 irradiated thymocytes with 25 x 10^6 BP-1 T cells plus 100 µg GP-BP in a total of 10 ml medium for 4 hr at 37C. After centrifugation at 400 x g to remove cells, the supernatant was ultracentrifuged further at 100,000 x g for 4 hr to remove membrane fragments. The supernatant obtained after ultracentrifugation was filtered through an 0.45 u membrane to remove any remaining residue. The membrane pellet was collected separately and recombined with medium, native GP-BP or utracentrifuged supernatant. Various fractions were tested for their ability to induce GP-BP specific proliferation of BP-1 cells, as well as to activate BP-1 cells to transfer clinical EAE (a score of 2.0 = hind leg weakness and limp tail).

ration (32 ± 3) and encephalitogenic activity (Table 5). Filtration of the ultracentrifuged supernatant reduced the proliferative activity of pGP-BP to the same level as the ultracentrifuged pellet or to the level observed in the ultrasupernatant that was OX-6 treated.

Activation of encephalitogenic and DTH-inducing activities with pGP-BP

To evaluate the encephalitogenic and DTH inducing properties of pGP-BP activated T lymphocytes, BP-1 or D-9 T cells were incubated with pGP-BP for 24 hours before passive transfer into native rats. As is shown in Table 6, pGP-BP activated T cells transferred both clinical EAE and DTH reactions in a cell dose dependent manner. The activity was greater in supernatants collected after 6 hours than after 24 hours. Although pGP-BP appeared to represent an adequate signal for T cell activation, its encephalitogenic and DTH inducing activities per cell were less than for APC activated BP-1 cells (Table 6). In four direct comparisons, the pGP-BP induced about half as much BP-1 proliferation (48 ± 9%) as activation in the presence of APC plus GP-BP.

Table 6. Transfer of EAE and DTH with Processed GP-BP activated line cells

Activation[a]	Dose of T cells Transferred	Maximum signs EAE[b]	DTH (mm x 10^{-2} ear swelling)[c]
6 hr sup.	5 x 10^6	4.0 (2/2)	Not done
	3 x 10^6	1.4 (4/4)	25 ± 7
	1 x 10^6	0.9 (3/4)	23 ± 9
24 hr sup.	3 x 10^6	0.8 (3/4)	22 ± 2
	1 x 10^6	0.4 (2/4)	21 ± 8
TX + GP-BP	3 x 10^6	3.5 (2/2)	33 ± 4
	1 x 10^6	2.5 (2/2)	37 ± 7
None	3 x 10^6	0.0 (0/3)	5 ± 2

[a] Active supernatant was produced by incubating 10 μg GP-BP with 2.5 x 10^6 BP-1 T cells and 60 x 10^6 irradiated thymocytes (TX) in 1 ml medium for 6 hrs at 37C. The cells were pelleted by centrifugation (400 x g) and 4 ml supernatant was added to 5 x 10^6 resting BP-1 or D-9 T cells. The cells were harvested after 24 hrs and injected i.p. into recipient rats. Alternatively, 3 x 10^6 T cells were activated with GP-BP presented by 100 x 10^6 TX in 10 ml stimulation medium for 3 days prior to transfer.

[b] Clinical EAE was scored as: 0 = no signs; 1 = flaccid tail, incontinence; 2 = hind leg weakness; 3 = paralysis; 4 = death.

[c] Ear thickness was measured with a pressure sensitive micrometer prior to intradermal injection of 20 μg GP-BP in 0.1 ml. Ear thickness was measured after 24 and 48 hrs and swelling determined by subtracting pretest values. Values represent mean 24 hr measurement ± standard deviation for each group.

CONCLUSIONS

The data presented above describe for the first time the production and properties of a cell free form of BP which can induce a GP-BP specific T effector lymphocyte line to proliferate and to transfer clinical EAE and DTH reactions. The activation signal was produced optimally during the accessory cell-dependent activation of T lymphocytes and contained the relevant epitope of GP-BP for the T lymphocytes as well as functional I-A but not I-E region gene product(s). Since the active supernatant had increased stimulatory activity for stimulatory activity for T cells relative to native GP-BP, it appears to have been potentiated by exposure to the APC. Thus we refer to the active supernatant as processed GP-BP (pGP-BP). The cell free pGP-BP produced activation comparable to APC, and confirms previous observations which indicated that both antigen and MHC products are required for specific T cell response to antigen (1-2). However, an association between antigen and Ia similar to that shown recently by Babbitt et al. (12) remains to be demonstrated.

The activation of the BP-1 T cell line by GP-BP appears to have several features in common with results described earlier by Puri and Lonai (12), Erb and Feldmann (13), and Friedman et al. (17). These reports suggested that accessory cells could produce a cell free factor (Ia containing antigen complex, IAC, genetically related factor, GRF, and processed avidin, PA, respectively) containing antigen and syngeneic Ia that bound and activated T helper cells. Furthermore, the IAC activity was enhanced by the presence of an antigen nonspecific macrophage product. Our results extend and refine these observations using a T cell line which recognized a defined region of GP-BP (19) in combination withI-A gene products from Lewis rat accessory cells (22), as well as T cell lines of other specificities from both Lewis and BN rats.

Although relatively small amounts of processed antigen could be produced by pulsing APC for 24 hr with antigen (Table 2), its activity reflected the same antigen specific and strain restricted properties observed when T cells were stimulated with APC plus antigen (Table 1). Much greater stimulatory activity could be recovered if a different antigen specific T lymphocyte line plus its homologous antigen was also included with the APC and relevant antigen to be processed (Fig.1, Tables 3 and 4). This additional antigen processing activity clearly resulted from T cell activation, possibly by release of gamma-IFN which is known to enhance Ia expression and antigen processing by APC (4-5). However, products from syngeneic or allogeneic activated T cells alone (without the relevant antigen to be processed) produced variable levels of nonspecific stimulation (3-40%) on resting T cells. Treatment of the supernatant with anti I-A but not anti I-E specific monoclonal antibodies inhibited T cell activation to the level of the antigen nonspecific stimulation (Fig.2 and Tables 3 and 5), but had no further inhibitory effect on the nonspecific factors. The relative contribution of specific and nonspecific factors are presented schematically in Fig.3.

Further experiments suggested that most of the pGP-BP was present in complexed form, since, after centrifugation, most of the pGP-BP activity was lost from both the supernatant fraction and from the sedimented microsomal fraction (Table 5). Activity in the residual ultrasupernatant fraction appeared to be due partly to antigen nonspecific, Ia restricted stimulation, since activation could be reduced further by treatment with anti I-A antibody. It is likely that the ultrasupernatant activity was due to a combination of nonspecific factors from activated lymphocytes and nonsedimentable pGP-BP, rather than soluble BP/I-A complexes, since filtration of this supernatant through 0.22μ pores reduced activity to the background (Table 5). However, similar to the report of Friedman et al. (17), the

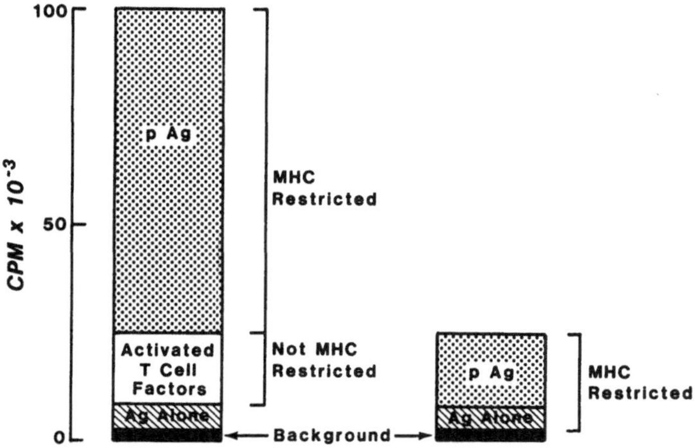

Fig.3. Schematic showing composition of the stimulatory supernatants produced by APC pulsed with antigen, and APC pulsed with antigen in the presence of activated T cell products.

reconstituted pellet and ultrasupernatant fractions reacquired nearly full activity.

The cell free supernatant containing the processed form of GP-BP (pGP-BP) possessed the same biological activities associated with the APC mediated activation of line cells. Incubation of GP-BP specific BP-1 line or D-9 clone cells with thymic APC plus GP-BP but not other antigens, resulted in rapid proliferation, and activation leading to clinical EAE and DTH reactions in recipient Lewis rats. Incubation of BP-1 or D-9 T cells with pGP-BP induced all the same activities, although less activity was observed on a per cell basis. Proliferation induced by pGP-BP was approximately half that observed when TX plus native GP-BP was used, and EAE and DTH inducing activities were also decreased (Table 6). Indeed, significant stimulatory activity for BP-1 cells remained associated with the GP-BP pulsed APC after the supernatant activity was removed (data not shown). It thus appears that the cell free pGP-BP represents only a portion of the total activation signal produced by the APC.

Our results suggest that in the presence of APC, basic protein can be released into the surrounding environment as a cell free factor that can trigger and amplify the BP-1 T cell activation. A proposed sequence of events presented in Fig.4. might include: 1) A small amount of GP-BP may be processed rapidly by residual Ia positive APC to trigger a few nearby T cells. 2) The activation of these T cells may cause the release of gamma-IFN (or similar factors) which 3) induces the APC to produce increased levels of processed BP which are shed with Ia positive membrane fragments to 4) form T cell activation complexes which amplify the activation of the T cell population. This effect may be of physiologic importance in the induction and recruitment of blood-borne encephalitogenic T lymphocytes by brain capillary endothelial cells (24-25), or by microglial cells or astrocytes (5) which are attracted to areas of local inflammation within the brain parenchyma. Additionally, since amplification of BP processing by APC can be enhanced by products of any activated T cell, the response of inflammatory T cells within the CNS to nonencephalitogenic CNS components or non CNS antigens (eg. persistant viruses) could facilitate processing of endogenous BP, and could result in 'bystander activation ' of encephalitogenic T cells.

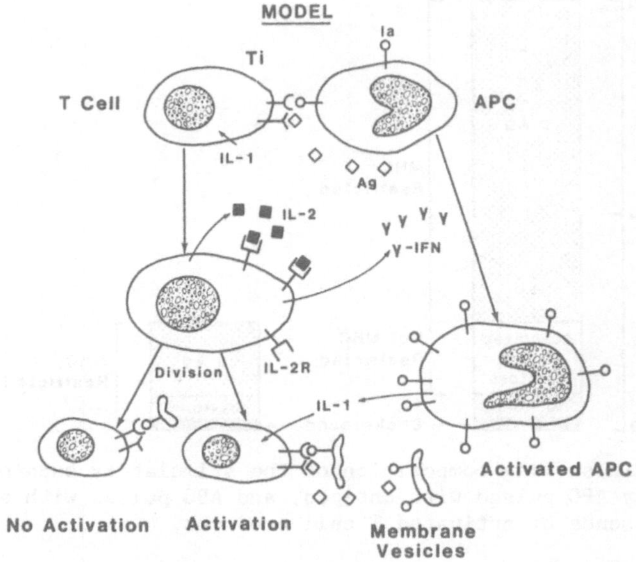

Fig.4. Model of suggested interactions between T lymphocytes and APC.

ACKNOWLEDGEMENTS

This project was supported in part by the Veterans Administration, USA, by BRSG RR05412 Award by the Biomedical Research Support Grant Program, Division of Research Resources, National Institutes of Health, by the American Cancer Society, Oregon Division, and by FIDIA of Italy.

REFERENCES

1. K. Haskins, J. Kappler and P. Marrack. The major histocompatibility complex-restricted antigen receptor on T cells. Ann. Rev. Immunol. 2:51 (1984).
2. S.C. Meuer, O. Acuto, T. Hercend, S.F. Schlossman and E.L. Reinherz. The human T-cell receptor. Ann. Rev. Immunol. 2:23 (1984).
3. H.M. Grey and R. Chestnut. Antigen processing and presentation to T cells. Immunol. Today. 6:101 (1985).
4. J.S. Pober, A. Gimbrone, R. Cotran, C. Reiss, S.J. Burakoff, W. Fierz and K.A. Ault. Ia expression by vascular endothelium is induced by activated T cells and by human gamma-interferon. J. Exp. Med. 158:1339 (1983).
5. W. Fierz, B. Endler, K. Reske, H. Wekerle and A. Fontana. Astrocytes as antigen-presenting cells. I. Induction of Ia antigen expression on astrocytes by T cells via immune interferon and its effect on antigen presentation. J. Immunol. 134:3785 (1985).
6. B. Benacerraf and R.V. Germain. The immune response genes of the major histocompatibility complex. Immunol. Rev. 38:70 (1978).
7. E.R. Unanue. Antigen-presenting function of the macrophage. Ann. Rev. Immunol. 2:395 (1984).
8. S. Howie and W.H. McBride. Cellular interactions in thymus dependent antibody responses. Immunol. Today. 3:273 (1982).
9. H.O. McDevitt. Speculations on how Ia antigens (Ir genes) influence the specificity of the immune response. Annales D'Immunologie. 135:227 (1984).

10. I.R. Cohen and J. Talmon. H-2 genetic control of the response of T lymphocytes to insulins. Priming of nonresponder mice by forbidden variants of specific antigenic determinants. Eur. J. Immunol. 10: 284 (1980).
11. A.S. Rosenthal. Determinant selection and macrophage function. Immunol. Today. 3:33 (1982).
12. B.P. Babbit, P.M. Allen, G. Matsueda, E. Haber and E.R. Unanue. Binding of immunogenic peptides to Ia histocompatibility molecules. Nature. 317:359 (1985).
13. P. Erb and M. Feldmann. The role of macrophages in the generation of T helper cells. III. Influence of macrophage-derived factors in helper cell induction. Eur. J. Immunol. 5:759 (1975).
14. J. Puri and P. Lonai. Mechanism of antigen binding by T cells. H-2(I-A)-restricted binding of antigen plus Ia by helper cells. Eur. J. Immunol. 10:273 (1980).
15. A. Friedman and I.R. Cohen. Molecular events in the processing of avidin by antigen-presenting cells (APC). I. The immune response of T lymphocytes to avidin is regulated by H-2-linked Ir genes. Immunogenetics. 18:267 (1983).
16. A. Friedman, R. Zerubavel, C. Gitler and I.R. Cohen. Molecular events in the processing of avidin by antigen-presenting cells (APC). II. Identical processing by APC of H-2 highand low-responder mouse strains. Immunogenetics. 18:277 (1983).
17. A. Friedman, R. Zerubavel, C. Gitler and I.R. Cohen. Molecular events in the processing of avidin by antigen-presenting cells (APC). III. Activation of T-lymphocyte lines and H-2 restriction are mediated by processed avidin associated with I-region gene products. Immunogenetics. 18:291 (1983).
18. C-H.J. Chou, F.C-H. Chou, T.J. Kowalski, R. Shapira and R.F. Kibler. The major site of guinea-pig myelin basic protein encephalitogenic in Lewis rats. J. Neurochem. 28:115 (1977).
19. A.A. Vandenbark, H. Offner, T. Reshef, R. Fritz, C-H.J. Chou and I.R. Cohen.. Specificity of T lymphocyte lines for peptides of myelin basic protein. J. Immunol. 135:229 (1985).
20. E. Beraud, T. Reshef, A.A. Vandenbark, H. Offner, R. Fritz, C-h.J. Chou, D. Bernard and I.R. Cohen. Experimental autoimmune encephalomyelitis mediated by T lymphocyte lines: Genotype of antigen presenting cells influences immunodominant epitope of basic protein. J. Immunol. 136:511 (1986).
21. A.A. Vandenbark, T. Gill and H. Offner. A myelin basic protein specific T lymphocyte line which mediates experimental autoimmune encephalomyelitis. J. Immunol. 135:223 (1985).
22. H. Offner, S.W. Brostoff and A.A. Vandenbark. Antibodies against I-A and I-E determinants inhibit the activation and function of encephalitogenic T lymphocyte lines. Cellular Immunol. In press. (1986).
23. R.B. Fritz and C-H.J. Chou. Epitopes of peptide 43-88 of guinea pig myelin basic protein. Localization with monoclonal antibodies. J. Immunol. 130:2180 (1983).
24. D.R. Burger and R.M. Vetto. Vascular endothelium as a major participant in T lymphocyte immunity. Cellular Immunol. 70:357 (1982).
25. A.A. Vandenbark. Critical immunologic events in multiple sclerosis: overview and summary. Res. Monographs in Immunology. 7:257 (1984).

LYMPHOCYTE CLONES FROM THE SPINAL FLUID OF PATIENTS WITH MULTIPLE SCLEROSIS AND CONTROLS

Gary Birnbaum, Linda Kotilinek and Sandra Aubitz

Department of Neurology
University of Minnesota, School of Medicine, Box 92
Minneapolis, Minnesota 55455

INTRODUCTION

Large numbers of lymphocytes are present in both the brains and spinal fluids of patients with multiple sclerosis (MS). The antigen(s) responsible for drawing these immunocompetent cells into the central nervous system (CNS) is not known. Neither is the role these cells play in the CNS demyelination found in MS patients. Many attempts have been made to identify the specificities of both the antibodies and lymphocytes in brains and spinal fluids of MS patients. Results have been variable. Some laboratories have identified antibodies reactive with a variety of viral (1,2) and brain (3,4) antigens. Cells have also been obtained from MS CSF that react with myelin basic protein (5) and viral antigens (6). It is not clear whether these lymphocyte responses are primary to the disease or secondary to a nonspecific recruitment of lymphocytes into the central nervous system.

In a previous publication (7) we reported that large numbers of lymphocytes from the spinal fluids of MS patients responded to autologous and/or allogeneic antigens. In addition, we were able to demonstrate that the patterns of these responses were relatively restricted suggesting that many of the lymphocytes present in MS CSF may have been drawn there and clonally expanded as a result of a specific immune reaction rather than a nonspecific recruitment secondary to the release of lymphokines. We attempted to determine whether lymphocytes reactive to allogeneic and autologous antigens also crossreacted with a variety of viral and central nervous system antigens such as measles virus, myelin basic protein and galactocerebroside. While some clones were found which did respond to galactocerebroside and tetanus toxoid, the numbers were very small and no particular patterns of response could be detected (unpublished observations).

Since there appears to be a genetic predisposition for MS, we hypothesized that development of the disease may be related to a particular pattern of immune response to an environmental antigen. Should this be the case, similarities in antigen receptor idiotype on T-lymphocytes in MS CSF may be demonstrable. Similarities in anti-acetylcholine receptor antibody idiotypes in patients with myasthenia gravis (8) and anti-DNA idiotypes in lupus erythematosis (9) lent support to our hypothesis.

Many of the lymphocytes present in MS CSF are activated (10,11). These in vivo activated cells may be particularly relevant in terms of the demyelinating process and possibly the pathogenesis of the disease. The following paper describes our preliminary efforts to isolate and clone in vivo activated lymphocytes from the CSF of MS patients in controls and to identify whether the antigen receptor idiotypes on these cells are similar among MS patients.

To do this, we established cultures of lymphocytes from MS and control CSF in the presence of delectinated Interleukin-2 (IL-2). Since only activated lymphocytes have receptors for IL-2, only such cells would respond to this lymphokine. After one week of culture, blast cells were isolated and cloned and used as antigens to stimulate autologous peripheral T-cells. Responding peripheral T-cells were cloned and assayed for their reactivity, both to the original clone used for stimulation and to other clones obtained from the same CSF or different CSFs. The patterns of responses of these T-cell activated clones were measured.

METHODS AND PROCEDURES

Cerebrospinal fluid

Fresh spinal fluid was obtained from MS patients and controls undergoing lumbar puncture for therapeutic or diagnostic purposes. With the patient's permission, approximately five to seven cc of CSF was obtained. CSF having more than 50 x 10^3 RBCs or a ratio of RBC: WBC of more than 2:1 were discarded. Spinal fluid was centrifuged at 50XG for ten minutes at room temperature. Pelleted cells, varying in number from 10,000 to 1.5 million were aliquoted into individual round bottom wells of a 96-well tissue culture plate with no more than 50,000 cells/well. Culture medium consisted of RPMI 1640 (Gibco, Grand Island, NY) with 15 per cent pooled human serum antibodies and an optimal concentration of delectinated IL-2 (Cellular Products Inc., Buffalo, NY). Cultures were incubated at 37°C in 95 per cent air and 5 per cent CO_2. Cultures were re-fed with fresh IL-2 on day 3-4 of culture.

Enrichment of activated cells and preparation of clones

After seven days of culture, cells were harvested and washed three times in medium. Blast cells were isolated using a discontinuous Percoll gradient as described previously (7). Blast cells accumulating at the 50 and 55 per cent Percoll interfaces were pooled, washed, counted and aliquoted into 64-well Terasaki histocompatibility-typing plates at a concentration of one-half cell per well. Feeder cells (7.5 x 10^3/well) consisting of irradiated 2.5 x 10^3 autologous peripheral blood lymphocytes and 5 x 10^3 pooled normal allogeneic Epstein-Barr virus (EBV) transformed B-cells were used. Nondelectinated interleukin-2 was added at this point to promote cell growth. Details of our technique have been previously described (7). Briefly, after 10 to 14 days wells, containing large numbers of clone cells, were harvested and placed into flat-bottom 96-well plates and cultured with additional feeder cells and interleukin-2. When clones had filled these wells, cells were transferred to larger wells in 24-well flat-bottom plates. Feeder cells and interleukin-2 were again added. After one to two weeks, those clones which showed greatest proliferation were harvested, washed and used as antigens in our T-T culture system.

Preparation of T-anti-T-cell clones

The technique of Lamb and Feldmann was used (12). Autologous peripheral blood lymphocytes were harvested on a discontinuous Ficoll. Hypaque gradient (7). Lymphocytes were cultured for five days with clones of T-cells obtained from activated cells in autologous CSF. Responding blast cells were enriched on Percoll gradients as described above, cloned, and expanded as above. These "T-anti-T" clones were used in our antigen specificity assays.

Antigen specificity assays

"T-anti-T" clones were washed and placed into round bottom 96-well tissue culture plates at a concentration of 10^4 cells/well. Clones were stimulated with either the original stimulating CSF clone or clones obtained from both autologous and allogeneic CSF at a responder: stimulator ratio of 1:1. 2.5 x 10^3 irradiated autologous PBL/well acted as antigen presenting cells. Patterns of response were investigated. In addition, T-anti-T clones were stimulated with a pool of EB virus transformed B-cells from normal and MS individuals as well as with lymphocytes obtained from autologous peripheral blood. After 48 hours cultures were pulsed with tritiated thymidine and the amount of thymidine incorporation was determined using standard liquid scintillation counting techniques.

RESULTS

Cloning of in vivo activated cells

Cells were obtained from 46 CSF, consisting of 26 CSF from MS patients and 20 patients with other neurologic diseases (OND). Cell numbers in 7 cc CSF varied from 2 x 10^3 to 72 x 10^4. Following treatment with delectinated IL-2 and subsequent cloning, clones were obtained from 19 CSF (10 MS CSF and 9 OND CSF). Numbers of clones obtained did not correlate with absolute numbers of cells in the CSF but rather with the acuteness of the inflammatory CNS process. These data support our hypothesis that predominantly in vivo activated cells appear to be responsive to delectinated IL-2 and thus present as blast cells after culture with this lymphokine. There was great variability in the growth rates of clones. Only those demonstrating the greatest proliferative potential were used in our T-anti-T assays.

Growth of T-anti-T clones

When peripheral blood lymphocytes from MS and control individuals were stimulated with autologous T-cell clones from spinal fuid, good proliferative responses were observed and responsive cells could be cloned. Again, great variability in growth rates of clones was noted. However, even actively proliferating clones eventually died after two or three months of continuous culture. This occurred in the face of repeated antigenic stimulation and IL-2 administration. Occasionally clones could be "rescued" by "subcloning". This consisted of placing 5,000 clone cells into a flat-bottom well of a 96-well tissue culture plate and restimulating that restricted number of cells with the original antigen stimulating clone. A new burst of proliferation was observed and cells could be expanded further for variable periods of time (an additional two to three months).

Patterns of T-anti-T responses

Two hundred sixteen T-anti-T clones from eight patients (7 MS and 1 OND) were assayed for their responsiveness to the original stimulating spinal fluid clone as well as to other autologous spinal fluid clones and allogeneic spinal fluid clones. In addition, responsiveness to pools of EB virus transformed allogeneic cells and autologous non-T-cells were de-

Table 1. "Public" response of T cell reactive T cell clones

CSF #	Stimulator	CPM of responding clone 1-31'-5	1-31'-10
1(OND)	1-31	1171	1351
	1-29	80	165
	1- 9	158	207
	3-13	427	440
	38	1654	5380
	5	217	826
	-	85	160
	IL-2	14779	21840
	MS Pool	100	182
	N Pool	1244	2823

CSF #	Stimulator	2-18'-1
2(MS)	2-18	1275
	2-11	114
	3-2	633
	3-6	1150
	3-13	2593
	3-38	226
	4- 8	129
	4-11	216
	4-15	271
	5-13	199
	5-20	1096
	6- 4	301
	6- 9	291
	7- 7	200
	7-16	206
	8- 2	113
	8- 5	348
	8-10	253
	Autol.PBL	98
	-	63
	MS Pool	1812
	N Pool	2235
	N LCL	479
	IL-2	3779
	0.1% PHA	420

Legend: Peripheral blood lymphocytes were cultured with clones derived from in vivo activated T-cells in autologous CSF. Responding cells were cloned and these T-anti-T cell clones were assayed for their proliferative responses to the original stimulating clone and to panels of clones from autologous and allogeneic CSF. Results are expressed as the geometric mean of the counts per minute.

termined. Results of four representative clones are shown in Tables 1 and 2. Several patterns were noted. Many T-anti-T clones did not respond to the originally stimulating clone or to any of the other autologous and allogeneic clones. Other clones responded to all stimulating clones and to allogeneic pooled cells. Other clones responded to the original stimulating clones and to selected clones from both autologous and allogeneic CSF (Table 1). Most of these clones also responded to a pool of EBV transformed cells and/or autologous non-T-cells from peripheral blood. We have called these clones specific for a "public" antigen. Least common, but definite in their patterns of reactivity, were clones that responded to the original stimulating clone and to particular other clones from autologous and allogeneic CSF but not to pooled allogeneic cells or to autologous non-T-cells (Table 2). Such clones may be responding to a T-cell receptor idiotype and thus may be responding to a "private" antigen.

Table 2. "Private" responses of T cell reactive T cell clones

CSF #	Stimulator	CPM of responding clone 2-6'-4	2-6'-5	2-18'-9
2(MS)	2- 6	1630	1197	ND
	2-18	ND+	ND	1356
	2- 1	179	197	ND
	2-11	167	158	151
	3- 2	473	365	333
	3- 6*	575	658	600
	3-13	3070	1373	1925
	3-38	368	225	299
	4- 8	402	278	191
	4-11	252	227	197
	4-15	205	153	189
	5-13	212	150	173
	5-20*	530	537	499
	6- 4	202	222	195
	6- 9	205	195	145
	7- 7	193	220	173
	7-16	253	225	153
	7-17	260	187	175
	8- 2	210	177	173
	8- 5	193	168	186
	8-10	243	207	191
		157	145	134
	MS Pool	202	138	133
	N Pool	672	385	222
	NLCL	750	347	292
	IL-2	5513	3355	3374
	0.1% PHA	663	763	401
	-	205	153	142

+ ND - Not done
* Background CPM = 500
Legend: Our procedure is identical to that described in Table 1.

DISCUSSION

Our results must be considered preliminary but we have been successful in growing and cloning in vivo activated T-lymphocytes from the spinal fluids of MS and control individuals. We have succesfully used these clones as antigens in an autologous T-anti-T-cell culture system in the hope of obtaining T-cell clones that respond to the antigen specific receptors on in vivo activated autologous CSF T-cells. If successful, we may be able to determine whether the patterns of idiotypes on spinal fluid T-cells from MS patients are similar and whether they could serve as a genetic marker, a diagnostic test and/or a means of determining the role of these in vivo activated cells in the development of disease.

Large numbers of our T-anti-T clones responded to autologous antigens. To decrease the number of such reactive cells and to enrich for T-cells responding to idiotype, we are in the process of adapting the technique of Zoschke and Bach (13) for selective killing of autologously activated cells using bromodeoxyuridine (BuDR). Preliminary results suggest that this technique is effective in reducing numbers of autologously reactive cells and in increasing our yield of clone specific T-cells.

REFERENCES

1. B. Rostrom, H. Link, M.A. Laurenzi, S. Kam-Hansen, E. Norby and B. Wahren. "Viral antibody activity of oligoclonal and polyclonal immunoglobulins synthesized within the central nervous system in multiple sclerosis". Annals of Neurology. 9:569-574 (1981).
2. T. Arnadottir, M. Reunanen, O. Meurman, A. Salmi, M. Panelius and P. Halonen. "Measles and rubella virus antibodies in patients with multiple sclerosis. A longitudinal study of serum and CSF specimens by radio-immuno-assay." Archives of Neurology. 36:261-265 (1979).
3. M.K. Gorny, Z. Wroblewska, D. Pleasure, S.L. Miller, A. Wajgt and H. Koprowski. "CSF antibodies to myelin basic protein and oligodendrocytes in multiple sclerosis and other neurological diseases." Acta Neurologica Scandinavica. 67:338-347 (1983).
4. C-H. Jen Chou, FC-H Chou, W.W. Tourtellotte and R.F. Kibler. "Devic's syndrome: antibody to glial fibrillary acidic protein in cerebrospinal fluid". Neurology. 34:86-88 (1984).
5. R.P. Lisak and B. Zweiman. "In vitro cell mediated immunity of cerebrospinal fluid lymphocytes to myelin basic protein in primary demyelinating diseases." New England Journal of Medicine. 297:850-853 (1977).
6. M. Reunanen, A. Salmi, J. Ilonen and E. Herva. "Proliferation of multiple sclerosis cerebrospinal fluid lymphocytes after stimulation with measles virus antigens." Acta Neurologica Scandinavica. 62: 293-299 (1980).
7. G. Birnbaum, L. Kotilinek, M. Schwartz and M. Sternad. "Spinal fluid lymphocytes responsive to autologous and allogeneic cells in multiple sclerosis and controlled individuals." Journal of Clinical Investigation. 74:1307-1317 (1984).
8. A. Vincent. "Idiotype restriction in myasthenia gravis antibodies." Nature. 290:293-294 (1981).
9. N.I. Abdou, H. Wall, H.B. Lindsley, J.F. Halsey and T. Suzuki. "Network theory in autoimmunity. In vitro suppression of serum anti DNA antibody binding to DNA by anti-idiotypic antibody in systemic lupus erythematosis." Journal of Clinical Investigation. 67:1297-1304 (1981).

10. A.B.C. Noronha, D.P. Richman and B.G.W. Arnason. "Detection of in vivo stimulated cerebrospinal fluid lymphocytes by flow cytometry in patients with multiple sclerosis." New England Journal of Medicine. 303:713-717 (1980).
11. D.A. Hafler, D.A. Fox, M.E. Manning, S.F. Schlossman, E.L. Reinherz and H.L. Weiner. "In vivo activated T-lymphocytes in the peripheral blood and cerebrospinal fluid of patients with multiple sclerosis." New England Journal of Medicine. 312:1405-1411 (1985).
12. J.R. Lamb and M. Feldmann. "A human suppressor T-cell clone which recognizes an autologous helper T-cell clone." Nature. 300:456-458 (1982).
13. D.C. Zoschke and F.H. Bach. "Specificity of antigen recognition by human lymphocytes in vitro." Science. 170:1404-1406 (1970).

IL-2 RECEPTOR EXPRESSION ON T CELL LINES DERIVED FROM PERIPHERAL BLOOD AND CEREBROSPINAL FLUID OF MULTIPLE SCLEROSIS PATIENTS

Elaine C. Defreitas+, M. Sandberg-Wolheim* and Hilary Koprowski+

+ The Wistar Institute, Philadelphia, PA 19104
* Department of Neurology, University of Lund, Lund, Sweden

INTRODUCTION

Receptors for interleukin 2 (IL-2) on T cells appear after activation of these cells by mitogen (1) or antigen (2). Studies on the regulation of the IL-2 receptor (IL-2R) were made possible by the development of a receptor-ligand binding assay (3) and a monoclonal antibody (mAb) against an epitope on the human IL-2 molecule (4). This mAb, called anti-Tac, detects both high and low affinity receptors for IL-2 (5). Expression of high affinity receptors was found to correlate with T cell proliferation (6). Expression of both types of receptors decayed with time and was independent of receptor-saturating concentrations of IL-2 (6).

Since multiple sclerosis (MS) is a disease characterized by central nervous system (CNS) immune abnormalities (7), and alterations in T cell subpopulations during the disease process (8), we examined T cell lines and clones from cerebrospinal fluid (CSF) and peripheral blood (PB) for IL-2R expression. This report documents that IL-2R on T cells from MS patients are not downregulated at the same rate as are those on T cells from normal individuals.

MATERIALS AND METHODS

Patients

PB and CSF samples were obtained from 4 patients with MS as determined by the criteria of McDonald and Halliday (9) and also from normal donors. All samples were obtained with full, informed consent. All donors used had been immunized previously for medical reasons with tetanus toxoid (TT) and Bacillus Calmette-Guerin (BCG).

Establishment of T-cell lines and clones

Antigen and mitogen-activated T cell lines were established from PB and CSF of normal donors and MS patients as follows (10): PBMC were purified on Lymphoprep(Nyegaard, Olso, Norway) by density centrifugation. Cells were suspended in RPMI 1640, 10% normal heat-inactivated human AB serum, 2 mM glutamine and penicillin-streptomycin (thereafter known as growth media), to 4 x 10^6/ml. Parallel cultures received phytohemagglutinin-purified (PHA-P; 1 μg/ml: Burroughs Wellcome, England), TT (10 μg/ml: Connaught Labs, Willowdale, Ontario), or purified protein derivative (PPD) of BCG (20 μg/ml: Connaught Labs, Willowdale, Ontario). After 7 days at 37°C, nonadherent cells were washed and resuspended to 10^5/ml in growth media with 50 ng/ml recombinant (r) IL-2 (courtesy of Dr. J. Besemer, Sandoz Ltd., Vienna, Austria). When cultures reached densities of 10^6/ml, cells were resuspended to 10^5/ml in complete growth media plus r IL-2. Every 2 wk, T cell lines were restimulated by addition of antigen or mitogen and 10^6 PBMC irradiated with 8000 rads from a 157 Cesium source [thereafter known as accessory cells (AC)]. Mitogen-stimulated T cell lines were stimulated with AC from a single allogeneic donor; antigen-stimulated T cell lines were stimulated with AC from the autologous donor.

Each CSF-derived T cell line was prepared from a single spinal tap by immediate centrifugation of CSF and washing of CSF-derived cells. All CSF cells were stimulated with antigen or mitogen in the presence of 4 x 10^6 autologous or allogeneic AC, respectively. CSF T cell lines were expanded as PB-derived lines. After 6 wk in culture, all antigen-stimulated lines were $T3^+$, Leu 3^+, Leu 2^-. Mitogen-activated lines were $T3^+$, Leu 3^+ and Leu 2^+.

IL-2 receptor expression

T cell lines and clones were evaluated for IL-2R expression using anti-Tac mAb (4), courtesy of Dr. Warner Greene, NCI, Bethesda, MD. Briefly, 10^6 cells were incubated with a 10^{-4} dilution of anti-Tac purified ascites for 60 min at 4°C. After washing, an optimal dilution of FITC-conjugated F(ab)'2 goat anti-mouse IgG (Cappel Labs, Cochranville, PA) was added for 30 min at 4°C. After washing, cells were analyzed for fluorescence by flow cytometry on the Ortho System 50 cytofluorgraph. Controls were cells treated with normal mouse serum and the second antibody.

IL-2 dependent proliferation

Proliferation of T cell lines and clones to rIL-2 was evaluated by seeding 2 x 10^4 viable cells in triplicate microtiter wells in 100 μl growth media. Varying concentrations of rIL-2 in 20 μl volumes were added. After varying times, cultures were pulsed with 10 μCi/ml ^{3}H-thymidine (Td) for 18 hr and harvested for liquid scintillation counting. In certain experiments (Fig.3), the pulse period was 5 hr.

RESULTS

Kinetics of expression of IL-2 R on antigen-specific T cell lines from PB of MS patients and normal donors

T cell lines specific for tetanus toxoid and purified protein derivative of BCG were generated from PB cells of two normal donors and two MS patients by repeated stimulation with antigen and autologous AC. Each line was >97% $T3^+$, Leu 3^+. To determine the kinetics of IL-2 R expression after activation with antigen, T cell lines were "rested" in the absence of exogenous IL-2 for 3 days. After stimulation with antigen and fresh autologous AC, the expression of IL-2R was measured using the mAb anti-Tac.

The appearance of Tac-positive cells on lines from normal donors increased after stimulation and reached a maximum by day 3 (Fig.1A). Supplementation of media with saturating concentrations of IL-2 on day 4 resulted in expansion of Tac-positive T cells which reached a maximum on day 7. Thereafter, percentage of IL-2R-positive cells steadily declined despite continuous supplementation with r IL-2 (Fig.1A).

Leu 3^+ cell lines from two MS patients generated against identical antigens, showed a markedly different pattern. Before antigen activation, all MS lines contained significantly more Tac-positive cells than did those from normals (Fig.1B). After activation, the maximal percentage of IL-2-positive cells was achieved within 2 days. After IL-2 addition, the preparations of Tac-positive cells increased within 2 days. Continuous supplementation with IL-2 resulted in cell populations which continued to express IL-2R for more than 22 days after antigenic stimulation. Tac-expression and proliferation in r IL-2 by MS Leu3^+ cells did not continue indefinitely; by day 40, most T cells became IL-2R negative and stopped dividing.

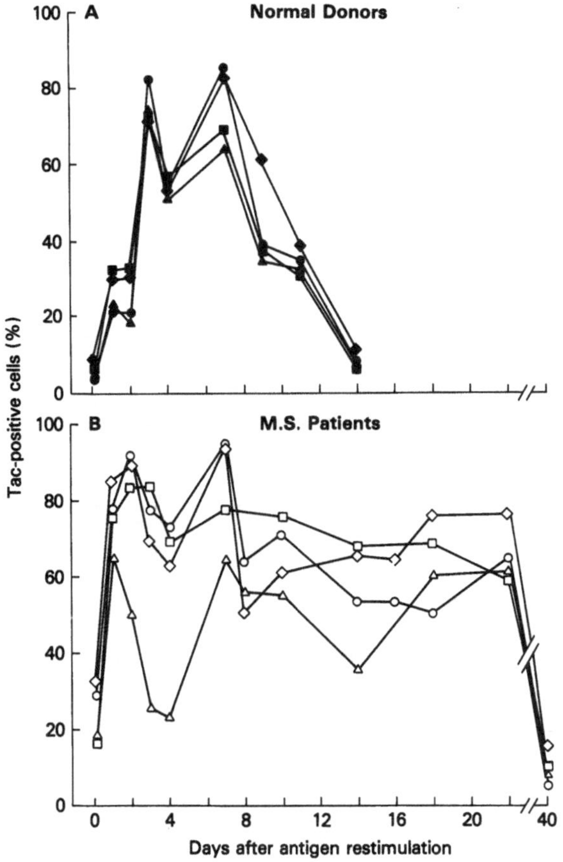

Fig.1. IL-2 receptor expression on T cell lines derived from PB and CSF of MS patients.

Kinetics of expression of IL-2R on mitogen- and antigen-activated T cells from CSF of MS patients and normal donors

Since IL-2R expression on normal PB-derived T cells has been shown to be regulated by macrophages/monocytes or their products (11), similar experiments were performed on MS CSF T cells polyclonally activated with mitogen (PHA-P) and a single allogeneic source of AC.

A representative experiment is shown in Fig.2. Leu 3^+ antigen-activated T cells from CSF of two MS patients and Leu2^+ and Leu 3^+ mitogen-activated CSF T cells from four MS patients were stimulated on day zero either with antigen and autologous AC or PHA-P and allogeneic AC. Tac expression was markedly elevated on all lines until day 22. As with PB-derived lines, all MS CSF-derived lines replicated in r IL-2 for more than 3 weeks (data not shown). Replication of cells and IL-2R expression slowly diminished and ceased by day 40-50 (data not shown). In contrast, mitogen-activated CSF T cell lines from 3 normal donors expressed Tac (and grew in r IL-2) for only 11-14 days.

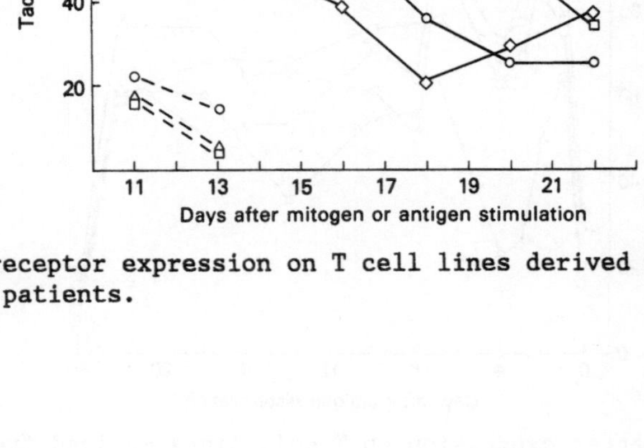

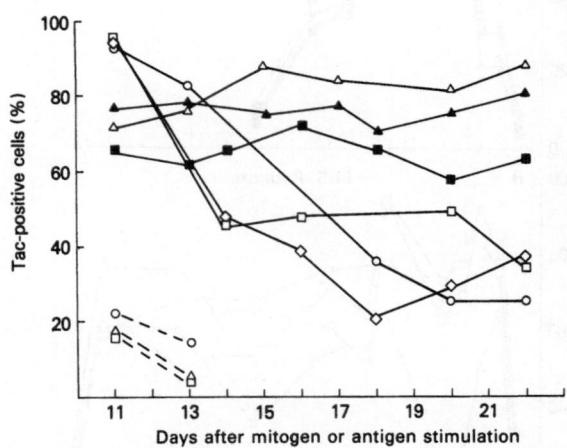

Fig.2. IL-2 receptor expression on T cell lines derived from PB and CSF of MS patients.

Decrease of IL-2R expression and proliferation by PB-derived T cells after IL-2 withdrawal

To maintain cycling T cells in vitro, cultures must be supplemented with free IL-2. Depletion of IL-2 from the extracellular space results in cessation of DNA synthesis and IL-2R negative cells which are at G_0 in their cycle (6). We wished to compare this process in MS and normal T cell lines.

Seven days after antigenic stimulation, when all lines were maximally Tac-positive, cells were extensively washed and placed in IL-2-free media. Fig.3. shows the Tac expression and proliferative response of T cell lines from both groups. Initially, all lines were highly Tac-positive and in active DNA synthesis. By day one, more than half of the normal T cells in all four lines from normal subjects became Tac-negative and proliferation was markedly decreased (Fig.3A). By day 3, all normal lines were IL-2R negative and had ceased synthesizing DNA.

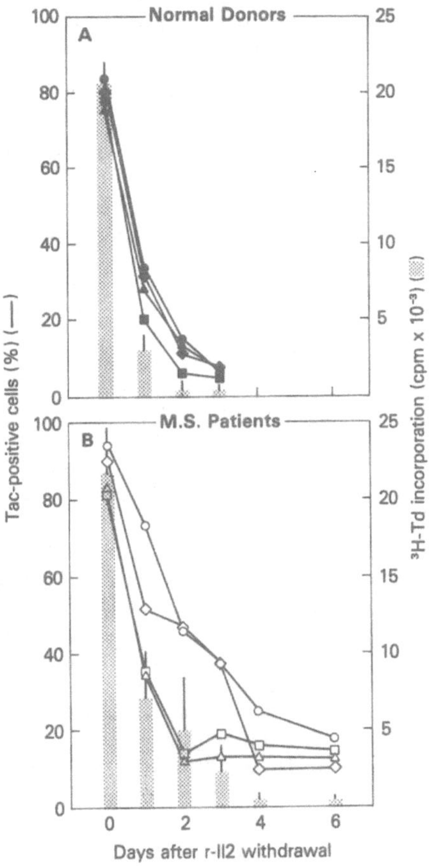

Fig.3. IL-2 receptor expression on T cell lines from PB and CSF of MS patients.

Fig.3B illustrates the different pattern seen with MS T cell lines. Although the proportion of Tac-positive cells also decreases in the absence of IL-2, this occurs more slowly with MS T cell lines than with normal. As late as day 6, when normal cells are Tac-negative and noncycling, Tac-positive cells can be detected in all four lines from MS. The mean proliferative responses of MS lines are significantly higher compared to normals up to day 4 after IL-2 removal indicating the prolonged presence of cells in DNA synthesis.

Comparison of the proliferative response to IL-2 of MS and normal CSF-derived T cell lines

Since the proliferation of IL-2R-positive T cells in known to depend on the number of high affinity IL-2R as well as the concentration of IL-2, we compared the responses of MS and normal T cells at varying concentrations of IL-2.

Table 1 shows the results of one such experiment. As shown, CSF T cells from MS patients were more responsive to limiting concentrations of r IL-2 than T cells from normals, suggesting that either a greater proportion of MS CSF T cells were expressing high affinity IL-2 receptors or that, compared to normals, these cells had a greater number of high affinity receptors per cell.

Table 1. Proliferative response to r IL-2 of MS and normal CSF T cell lines

CSF T cell lines[a]	r IL-2 (ng/ml)[b]		
	50	10	1
Normal 1	9310	2872	1210
2	8717	2244	986
MS # 01-12	20691	18474	5449
# 13-10	26318	19796	4959
# 20-1	26268	18999	5001

[a] All CSF T cell lines were stimulated with PHA-P (1) μg/ml and AC from a single allogeneic donor. After 3 days, all cultures were supplemented with r IL-2 (50 ng/ml) and grown for an additional 8 days.

[b] To determine response to varying concentrations of r IL-2, T cells were washed, seeded in microtiter at 2×10^4 per well and given r IL-2 at the concentrations listed. After two days, all wells were pulsed with ^{3}H-Td for 18 hr and harvested. Results expressed are the mean ^{3}H-Td (cpm) of triplicate samples. SEM was less than 10% of the mean.

Recent experiments directly comparing the average number of IL-2R expressed by MS and normal CSF-derived T cells have been performed in collaboration with Dr. Warner Greene at the NIH. These experiments show that on day 14 post-stimulation normal CSF T cell lines express less than 300 total receptors per cell while MS CSF T cells express between, 20,000 to 50,000 total receptors per cell. Approximately 10% of these receptors are of high affinity. Dot blot analysis using the cDNA probe for the IL-2R showed active mRNA transcription of this gene in MS CSF T cells but none in normal (data not shown).

DISCUSSION

The results presented here, demonstrate differences in the expression of IL-2R and responsiveness to IL-2 by T cells from MS patients and normal individuals.

PB-derived, antigen-induced, $Leu3^{+}$ T cells from MS patients developed maximal IL-2R expression within two days of stimulation and more importantly, did not downregulate their Tac expression until after day 22 in r IL-2. There was a marked heterogeneity in the proportion of Tac-positive cells among the lines tested; however, all lines became IL-2 R-negative by day 40-45 after initial activation. Tac-positivity of these MS cell lines was concordant with continued DNA synthesis and growth suggesting that at least a proportion of these cells express high affinity IL-2R known to be responsible for the proliferative effects of IL-2.

The IL-2R expression by Leu 3^{+} antigen-induced T cell lines from PB of normal donors reported here, is in full accord with the results of others (1, 2, 12). IL-2R expression in all studies reached a maximum within 4 days after mitogenic or antigenic stimulation and decreased thereafter despite the presence of saturating IL-2 concentrations. By day 11-13, normal T cell lines and clones had become IL-2R negative. In all reports, the IL-2-dependent proliferative response paralelled the expression of IL-2R. These data indicate a physiological basis for the empirical observations that most antigen-induced T cell lines and clones require periodic restimulation with antigen and AC.

Since most immune abnormalities in this disease are found within the CNS, we also examined T cells derived from CSF. The delayed downregulation of IL-2R compared to normal CSF T cell lines was also observed. These data suggest that once activated by specific antigen _in vivo_, CSF T cells in MS patients would remain viable and perhaps functional for inordinately long periods of time especially if IL-2 were available _in situ._ If so, one might predict that freshly isolated CSF T cells would express IL-2R. Reports from other laboratories on this subject, however, have been conflicting (13, 14).

Removal of IL-2 from a cycling normal T cell population has been shown to decrease the number of S phase cells within 24 hr (6). Within 3-4 days, these cells had accumulated in G_0, ceased active DNA synthesis, and were Tac-negative. In this report, normal T cell lines deprived of Il-2 behaved similarly. MS T cells, however, continued to synthesize DNA and expressed IL-2R for a longer period of time. This effect may be attributed to an increased number of high affinity IL-2R on cells complexed to ligand, resulting in continuous membrane signaling for replication in the absence of exogenous IL-2. Alternatively, MS T cell lines may be constitutively producing IL-2 which maintains cycling, Tac-positive cell populations.

To approach the question of increased numbers of high affinity IL-2R on MS cells, the proliferative response to varying IL-2 concentrations was measured. The markedly lower concentrations of r IL-2 necessary to induce DNA synthesis in MS CSF T cells compared to normal and the higher proportion of proliferating MS CSF T cells at the same IL-2 concentration suggested that MS cells display a greater average density of high affinity IL-2R. The latter possibility is currently being evaluated by direct measurements of IL-2R affinity.

The mechanism responsible for our observations is unknown. Recent studies have indicated that monocytes (11) and interleukin 1 (15), play a critical though as yet undefined role in the induction of high affinity

IL-2R on human T cells. Since all antigen-specific T cell lines were activated with antigen and autologous (i.e., MS) AC, it was possible that the MS monocytes played a unique contributory role in the altered IL-2R expression of MS T cell lines. However, MS T cell lines stimulated with mitogen and normal allogeneic AC showed a similar pattern of Tac prolongation. Therefore, delayed downregulation of Tac on MS T cells could not be attributed to MS monocytes or their products. Another, as yet unexplored possibility is that T cell lines from MS patients are autoreactive and are experiencing constant antigenic stimulation with self-MHC antigens which upregulates the Tac molecule. The ability of soluble T cell products to achieve this effect has been reported by Teshigaware et al. (16) who described a soluble factor produced by human-T cell leukemia virus (HTLV) I-infected T cells which upregulates Tac on a Tac-negative leukemic cell line.

Another possibility is that the expression of IL-2R on MS T cells is under different transcriptional regulation. For example, HTLV I infection of normal human T cells results in constitutive prolonged expression of IL-2R which appears to be the direct effect of a viral protein encoded by the tat gene of HTLV I (17). This protein upregulates transcription of the mRNA for IL-2R. Our recent report (18) suggests the involvement of a virus in MS similar but not identical to HTLV I. The role of this putative virus or any of its gene products has yet to be determined.

ACKNOWLEDGEMENTS

We thank Dr. J. Besemer (Sandoz Ltd., Vienna, Austria) for the r IL-2 and Dr. Warner Greene (NIH, Bethesda, MD) for the anti-Tac mAb. Excellent technical assistance was provided by Ms. Kathy Schonely and Margaret Boufal. We appreciate the efforts of Mr. Jeffrey Faust with the flow cytometry and Ms. Marie Lennon for preparation of the manuscript. This work was supported by Grant AI-19987 from the NIH and B84-19X-06265-03B from the Swedish Medical Research Council.

REFERENCES

1. D. Cantrell and K.A. Smith. J. Exp. Med. 158:1895-1911 (1983).
2. A. Reske-Kunz, D. Steldern, E. Rude, H. Osawa and T. Diamantstein. J. Immunol. 133:1356-1361 (1984).
3. R.J. Robb, A. Munck and K.A. Smith. J. Exp. Med. 154:1455-1474 (1982).
4. T. Uchiyama, S. Broder and T.A. Waldmann. J. Immunol. 126:1393-1397 (1981).
5. R.J. Robb, W. Greene and C.M. Rusk. J. Exp. Med. 160:1126-1146 (1984).
6. D. Cantrell and K.A. Smith. Science. 224:1312-1316 (1984).
7. M. Sandberg-Wollheim. Scand. J. Immunol. 17:575-581 (1981).
8. N. Cashman, C. Martin, J. Eizenbaum, J. Degos and M. Bach. J. Clin. Invest. 70:387-392 (1982).
9. W.E. McDonald and A.M. Halliday. Br. Med. Bull. 33:4-9 (1977).
10. E.C. Defreitas, B. Dietzschold and H. Koprowski. Proc. Natl. Acad. Sci. USA. 82:3425-3429 (1985).
11. H. Wagasugi, J. Bertoglio, T. Tursz and D. Fradelizi. J. Immunol. 135:321-327 (1985).
12. D. Kaplan, V. Braciale and T. Braciale. J. Immunol. 133:1966-1969 (1984).
13. A. Bellamy, V. Calder, M. Feldmann and A. Davison. Clin. Exp. Immunol. 61:248-256 (1985).

14. D. Hafler, D. Fox, M. Manning, S. Schlossman, E. Reinherz and H. Weiner. N. Engl. J. Med. 312:1405-1411 (1985).
15. J. Kaye, S. Gillis, S. Mizel, E. Shevach, T. Malek, C. Dinarello, L. Lachman and C. Janeway. J. Immunol. 133:1339-1345 (1984).
16. K. Teshigaware, M. Maeda, K. Nishino, T. Nikaido, T. Uchiyama, M. Tsudo, Y. Wano and J. Yodoi. J. Mol. Cell. Immunol. 2:17-26 (1985).
17. M. Kronke, W. Leonard, J. Depper and W. Greene. Science. 228:1215-1217 (1985).
18. H. Koprowski, E.C. Defreitas, M.E. Harper, M. Sandberg-Wollheim, W. Sheremata, M. Robert-Guroff, C. Saxinger, F. Wong-Staal, M. Feinberg and R.C. Gallo. Nature. 318:154-160 (1985).

FINE ANALYSIS OF CYTOLYTIC AND NATURAL KILLER T LYMPHOCYTES IN THE CEREBROSPINAL FLUID OF MULTIPLE SCLEROSIS AND OTHER NEUROLOGICAL DISEASES PATIENTS

Wim E.J. Weber [1], Wim A. Buurman [2], Marc M.P.P. Vandermeeren[1], Rob H.J. Medaer [3] and Jef C.M. Raus [1]

[1] Department of Immunology, Dr. L. Willemsinstituut, University Campus, Diepenbeek, Belgium
[2] Department of Surgery, Academic Hospital Maastricht, University Limburg, Maastricht, The Netherlands
[3] The Multiple Sclerosis and Rehabilitation Clinic, Overpelt, Belgium

INTRODUCTION

Numerous immune abnormalities have been reported in multiple sclerosis (MS) patients. These include elevated immunoglobulin levels in the cerebrospinal fluid (CSF) (1-3), decrease in CD8+ lymphocytes in the peripheral blood (4-6), infiltration of T lymphocytes in the typical brain lesions (7-10), T cells reactive against myelin basic protein in peripheral blood and CSF (11-14), and the presence of activated T lymphocytes in peripheral blood and CSF (15-18). Although the significance of these abnormalities remains unclear, they suggest that T cells play a role in the pathogenesis of the disease (3,19-21).

The central nervous system (CNS) compartment is normally isolated from the periphery. To study local immune responses within the CNS, it is therefore essential to use CSF lymphocytes, since these cells may bear a much closer relation to active cells in the lesions. As the cell number obtained by a single lumbar puncture is usually very low, several investigators have expanded CSF T cells into lines and clones with the use of Interleukin 2 (IL-2) (30). Lines and clones from cells stimulated in vitro, in bulk cultures, however, do not necessarily reflect the original T cell population, due to possible selection by the in vitro culture. To overcome this problem, we have developed a sensitive T lymphocyte microculture system, utilizing a mitogenic anti-CD3 (formerly called T3, ref.33) monoclonal antibody and exogenous IL-2, that allows clonal expansion of essentially all human T lymphocytes into populations suitable for functional assays. This procedure enabled us to measure precursor frequencies of cytolytic and natural killer T lymphocytes in human lymphoïd cell populations, starting from very low cell numbers (34).

In the present investigation, we have used this system to quantitate directly the frequencies of cytotoxic and natural killer T lymphocyte-precursors in the cerebrospinal fluid of 12 MS patients and 11 patients with other neurological diseases (OND). It will be shown that in patients with CNS disorders of inflammatory nature, the relative number of T cells with cytolytic and/or natural killer potential in the CSF, is increased, and that a substantial number of these cells is of the CD4+ phenotype.

MATERIALS AND METHODS

Patient samples

Patient samples were obtained from the inpatient and outpatient units of the MS and Rehabilitation Clinic, Overpelt, Belgium. Diagnosis of definite MS was reached according to recently formulated criteria (35). The patients were not receiving any within several weeks prior to study. CSF (10-15 ml) was obtained by lumbar puncture performed for diagnostic purposes. The sample was centrifuged immediately at 200 g for 5 minutes. The supernatant fluid was taken off and used for normal routine diagnostic procedures and the cells were resuspended in 0.5 ml of fetal calf serum (FCS). Lumbar punctures were never performed for research purposes. Of some patients blood samples were drawn at the same time. For these samples informed consent was obtained after a full explanation of the procedure.

Isolation of cells

Peripheral blood mononuclear cells (PBMC) of fresh heparinised blood were isolated by centrifugation over Ficoll-Paque density gradient (Pharmacia Fine Chemicals, Uppsala, Sweden). PBMC, used as feeders, were obtained from normal healthy plasma donors through the Belgian Red Cross Blood Transfusion Service. The cells were frozen in a microprocessor-controlled biofreezer (Cryoson MIC 15, Midden-Beemster, The Netherlands), subsequently stored in the liquid nitrogen and thawed when needed. These feeders were heavily irradiated (10,000 rad from a 60Co source), before use. CSF cells were isolated by centrifugation, resuspended in 0.5 ml FCS and stored at 20°C until they were plated. Plating of cells was always carried out within 12 hrs. after the lumbar puncture, unless stated otherwise.

Culture conditions

Culture medium was RPMI 1640 (GIBCO Europe, Ghent, Belgium), supplemented with penicillin, streptomycin, L-glutamin, sodium pyruvate, nonessential aminoacids, 10 mM HEPES buffer and 10% heat-inactivated FCS. Limiting dilution cultures were performed as described (34). Briefly, viable PBMC or CSF cells were seeded in limiting numbers (from 0.25 to 10 cells/well) in round-bottom microtiterplates (Greiner, Nürtingen, FRG), containing 10^5 irradiated feeder cells and a predetermined optimal concentration of anti-CD3 monoclonal antibody WT32 (1/1, 250 dilution of ascites), which was a kind gift of Dr. Capel, Nijmegen, The Netherlands (36, 37). Cells were cultured at 37°C in a humidified atmosphere containing 5% CO2. After 48 hrs. 0.5% recombinant Interleukin-2 (rIL-2) was added (recombinant IL-2, Janssen Chimica, Beerse, Belgium). Cultures were refed at weekly intervals with 10^5 irradiated feeders and rIL-2. Microwells were inspected daily for proliferation through an inverted microscope between days 10-18.

Cytotoxicity assays

At day 18 of culture, all microcultures containing growing cells were split into two aliquots. One aliquot was kept in continuous culture with the use of IL-2 and the other one was used to test for cytolytic activity. Half of this aliquot was screened for lectin-dependent cytotoxicity and the other half for natural killer (NK) activity, as described (34).

Briefly, five thousand target cells (K 562 or P 815) were labelled with 51 Chromium (Na2Cr304, Radiochemical Centre, Amersham, U.K.) using a standard protocol and incubated for 4 hrs. with the effector cells in a final volume of 200 µl in round-bottom microwells. In the assay for lectin-dependent killing 0.2 µg phytohemagglutinin (PHA-M, Difco Laboratories, Detroit, MI) was added to each microwell. After incubation, supernatant was harvested using supernatant collection cartridges (Skatron, Oslo, Norway) and 51Cr-release was measured in a gamma counter. Maximum release was determined in wells containing target cells and a detergent; spontaneous release by incubating the targets with RPMI medium. In all experiments maximal release exceeded spontaneous release by more than seven times. Effectors were arbitrarily defined positive for lytic activity when 51Cr-release exceeded mean spontaneous release by more than 3 S.D.

<u>Phenotypic analysis</u>

Phenotyping of the cultured cells was performed by indirect immunofluorescence using anti-CD4 and anti-CD8 monoclonal antibodies (anti-leu 2 and anti-leu 3, Becton Dickinson, Erembodegem, Belgium) through a fluorescence microscope. 10^5 cells were divided into three microwells of a Terasaki microtest-tray (U-bottom nr. 860173, Greiner, Nürtingen, FRG), washed twice with phosphate buffered saline (PBS) + 2% FCS + 0.01% NaN3, and incubated for 30 min. at 4°C with anti-leu 2 and anti-leu 3, and with control non-relevant monoclonal antibody, diluted 1/10 in PBS + 2% FCS + 0.01% NaN3. After two washes, fluorescein-conjugated goat anti-mouse IgG antibody (Becton-Dickinson, Erembodegem, Belgium) was added at an appropriate dilution, and incubated for another 30 min. at 4°C, followed by three washes. Pellets were resuspended in 25 µl glycerol-glycine buffer and transferred to a flat-bottom Terasaki microtray (Nr. 726180, Greiner, Nürtingen, FRG) and were then read through an inverted fluorescence microscope. Background staining, obtained after incubation with a non-relevant monoclonal antibody, followed by the incubation with the fluorescein-conjugated second antibody, was negligible in all experiments.

Determination of the percentage of T lymphocytes in the mononuclear cells, derived from CSF or purified from peripheral blood, was done by indirect immunofluorescence using anti-CD3 monoclonal antibody (Anti-leu 4, Becton-Dickinson, Erembodegem, Belgium) and fluorescein-conjugated goat anti-mouse IgG on a FACS 420 (Becton-Dickinson, Erembodegem, Belgium) as previously described (34).

<u>Frequency analysis statistics</u>

Minimal estimates of precursor frequency were obtained by using the maximal likelihood method from the Poisson distribution relationship of the number of cells plated per culture and the percentage of non-responding (negative for proliferation or cytolytic activity) cultures, as described by Strijbosch et al. (Manuscript submitted).

RESULTS

<u>Frequency of proliferating T cells in CSF and peripheral blood</u>

Frequency of T cells, proliferating under the described culture conditions, was assessed in the CSF of 12 MS patients and 11 patients with other neurological diseases (OND). Viable cells were seeded at 0.25, 0.5, 1.0, 2.0 and 10 cells per microwell (50 microwells for each dilution), and screened daily for proliferation between days 10-18. In a typical experiment, with CSF cells from an MS patient suffering an exacerbation, proliferation was observed in 13/50 (26%), 19/50 (36%), 26/50 (52%), 41/50

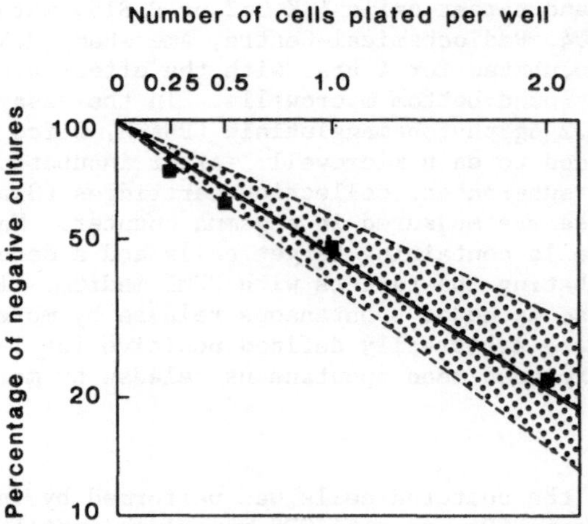

Fig.1. Limiting dilution analysis of proliferating T cells in the CSF of patient nr. 1 (MS patient suffering an exacerbation), under the culture conditions described in Materials and Methods. Each point is based on 50 microcultures. The regression line was fitted to the data by maximum likelihood method. The shaded area represents the 95% confidence interval.

(82%) and 50/50 (100%) of the microcultures established with 0.25, 0.5, 1.0, 2.0 and 10 cells per well, respectively. The numbers of cells in the proliferating cultures ranged from 5-20 x 10^4 per well at day 18 of culture. Calculated by maximum likelihood method, frequency of proliferating cells was 0.75 or 1 cell in 1.33 plated cells (Fig.1). It appeared to be important, however, to plate the cells shortly after drawing of the CSF. In a control experiment, CSF cells of patient 1 were plated 30 hrs. after lumbar puncture, which resulted in a frequency of proliferating T cells of 0.32. Other experiments also demonstrated that cloning efficiencies decreased rapidly, when cells were not plated within 12 hrs. of eased rapidly, when cells were not plated within 12 hrs. of puncture (data not shown). The percentage of T lymphocytes in the original population, as measured by FACS analysis, was 71%. This demonstrates that virtually all T cells in this CSF sample had given rise to a clonal progeny.

Tables 1 and 2 summarize frequencies of proliferating T cells in the CSF of MS and OND patients. Of five patients in each group these frequencies were also determined in the peripheral blood. It can be seen that in most cases the frequency of proliferating T cells was essentially equal to the percentage of T cells in the starting population.

<u>Precursor frequency of T cells with cytolytic and natural killer potential in CSF and peripheral blood of MS and OND patients</u>

Frequencies of cytolytic T lymphocyte-precursors (CTL-p, i.e. a cell that can give rise to a measurable cytolytic T lymphocyte clone) and natural killer-precursors (NK-p, i.e. a cell that can give rise to a progeny expressing natural killer function) in CSF and peripheral blood of MS and OND patients was measured by screening all the proliferating T cell microcultures (established from either CSF or blood as described) at day 18 of culture. Microcultures were screened for lectin-dependent lysis and natural killing in a 51 Chromium-release assay. Lectin-dependent lysis was assessed with murine mastocytoma P815 target cells in the presence of PHA, to detect all T cells with a lytic machinery, regardless of specificity. NK function was screened using human erythroleukemic K562 cells as tar-

Table 1. Frequencies of proliferating T lymphocytes derived from CSF and peripheral blood of MS patients

Patient nr.	Diagnosis	Cell origin	Cells/mm^3	% T cells[c]	Fraction of proliferating T cells T cells (95% interval)
1[d]	MS-ex[a]	CSF	2	71	0.75 (0.54 - 0.94)
2	MS-ex	CSF	3	85	0.81 (0.66 - 0.96)
3	MS-ex	CSF	3	79	0.81 (0.63 - 1.01)
4	MS-ex	CSF	2	52	0.42 (0.25 - 0.59)
5	MS-ex	CSF	2	70	0.73 (0.53 - 0.93)
6	MS-ex	CSF	3	62	0.54 (0.49 - 0.59)
7	MS-ex	CSF	5	65	0.62 (0.41 - 0.83)
		Periph.blood		56	0.53 (0.34 - 0.71)
8	MS-ex	CSF	1	76	0.74 (0.65 - 0.85)
		Periph.blood		61	0.58 (0.37 - 0.79)
9	MS-chron[b]	CSF	2	76	0.78 (0.68 - 0.83)
10	MS-chron	CSF	3	75	0.74 (0.53 - 0.95)
		Periph.blood		82	0.81 (0.77 - 0.85)
11	MS-chron	CSF	3	100	0.99 (0.61 - 1.01)
		Periph.blood		66	0.62 (0.55 - 0.72)
12	MS-chron	CSF	2	70	0.71 (0.65 - 0.95)
		Periph.blood		67	0.70 (0.51 - 0.95)

[a] MS-ex: MS patient suffering an exacerbation

[b] MS-chron: patient with chronic progressive MS

[c] The percentage of T cells in the original population was determined by FACS analysis as described in materials and methods

[d] Data from Fig.1.

Table 2. Frequencies of proliferating T lymphocytes derived from CSF or peripheral blood of OND patients

Patient nr.	Diagnosis	Cell origin	Cells/mm^3	% T cells[b]	Fraction of proliferating T cells (95% interval)
13	Heredo-ataxia	CSF	1	60	0.51 (0.36 - 0.64)
		Periph.blood		73	0.75 (0.66 - 0.86)
14	Syringomyelia	CSF	1	76	0.74 (0.56 - 0.91)
15	Neurosis	CSF	1	58	0.39 (0.30 - 0.48)
16	Lumbar disc	CSF	1	62	0.61 (0.44 - 0.82)
		Periph.blood		63	0.64 (0.61 - 0.74)
17	Vertigo	CSF	1	59	0.41 (0.29 - 0.54)
		Periph.blood		61	0.46 (0.41 - 0.50)
18	Schizophrenia	CSF	1	76	0.75 (0.53 - 1.01)
19	S.S.P.E.[a]	CSF	10	80	0.39 (0.25 - 0.53)
20	Acoustic neurinoma	CSF	10	78	0.83 (0.72 - 0.94)
		Periph.blood		62	0.63 (0.59 - 0.72)
21	Encephalitis	CSF	40	100	0.97 (0.89 - 1.04)
		Periph.blood		59	0.63 (0.39 - 0.86)
22	Guillain-Barré	CSF	6	66	0.61 (0.56 - 0.75)
23	Encephalitis	CSF	20	80	0.76 (0.69 - 0.91)

[a] Subacute sclerosing panencephalitis

[b] The percentage of T cells in the original population was determined by FACS analysis as described in Materials and Methods

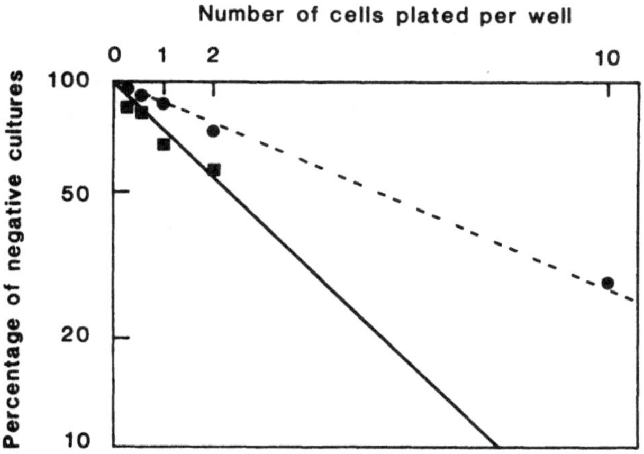

Fig.2. Frequency analysis of CSF cells (derived from patient nr.1), developing into cytolytic and natural killer effector populations. After 18 days of culture, as described in Materials and Methods, each proliferating CSF T lymphocyte microculture was tested for cytolytis of P815 targets in the presence of PHA (■) and for natural killer activity against K562 cells (●). Each point is based on 50 microcultures. The regression lines were fitted to the data by maximum likelihood method.

gets. The frequency of CTL-p in the CSF of patient 1 was 0.29 (95% confidence interval 0.16 - 0.34) and frequency of NK-p was 0.13 (95% confidence interval 0.07 - 0.18) (Fig.2). The frequency of proliferating T lymphocytes in this CSF was 0.75. It could therefore be calculated that 38% and 17% of all the proliferating microcultures expressed CTL and NK potential, respectively. Relative numbers of microcultures with CTL and with NK function as percentages of the total of proliferating T lymphocyte microcultures, established from CSF or peripheral blood, are given in Tables 3 and 4. It appeared that all T cell populations, capable of NK function, were also capable of lysing P815 targets in the presence of PHA.

CTL-p frequency in the CSF of the MS patients ranged from 33 - 93%. These frequencies in the peripheral blood, of the patients tested, were lower than in the CSF (patient nrs. 7,10,11,12). In the CSF of patients with OND CTL-p frequency ranged from 27-100%. When the MS patients studied were classified into two groups, namely those suffering an exacerbation and those suffering a chronic progressive form, and when the OND patients group was split into a subgroup with inflammatory CNS diseases and a subgroup with non-inflammatory diseases, differences in percentages of CTL-p between the patient groups became apparent (Fig.3).

NK-p frequency in the CSF of the MS patients ranged from 17 - 79%, in the non-inflammatory OND group from 13 - 32%, and in the inflammatory OND group from 9 - 82%. NK-p frequencies generally showed a similar pattern as the CTL-p frequencies, although differences were less pronounced.

Table 3. Fractions of proliferating T cells with cytolytic and natural killer potential, in the MS patients

Patient nr.	Cell origin	Fractions (in %) of T cell microcultures lysing P 815 + PHA[a]	K 562[b]
1[c]	CSF	38	17
2	CSF	58	29
3	CSF	58	17
4	CSF	57	19
5	CSF	63	52
6	CSF	93	79
7	CSF	87	40
	Periph.blood	29	8
8	CSF	77	33
9	CSF	33	10
10	CSF	82	55
	Periph.blood	47	25
11	CSF	85	25
	Periph.blood	56	22
12	CSF	68	21
	Periph.blood	63	21

[a] Effectors lysing P 815 targets in the presence of PHA were arbitrarily defined as cytolytic

[b] Natural killer activity was screened using K 562 target cells

[c] Data from Fig.2.

Table 4. Fractions of proliferating T lymphocytes with cytolytic and natural killer potential in CSF and peripheral blood of OND patients

Patient nr.	Cell origin	Fractions (in %) of T cell microcultures lysing P 815 + PHA[a]	K 562[b]
13	CSF	45	21
	Periph.blood	45	18
14	CSF	40	23
15	CSF	36	13
16	CSF	44	32
17	CSF	75	15
	Periph.blood	45	19
18	CSF	27	15
19	CSF	71	28
20	CSF	100	82
	Periph.blood	63	37
21	CSF	70	48
	Periph.blood	52	36
22	CSF	71	9
23	CSF	63	29

[a] Effectors lysing P 815 in the presence of PHA were defined cytolytic

[b] Natural killer function was screened with K 562 cells.

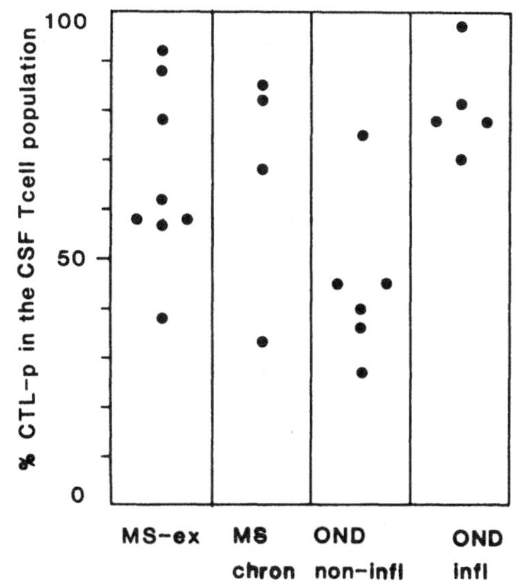

Fig.3. Percentages of CTL-p in the CSF T cell population, derived from MS-patients suffering an exacerbation (MC-ex), suffering a chronic progressive form (MS-chron), and from patients with OND of non-inflammatory character (OND non-infl) and with OND of inflammatory nature (OND infl). Differences in CSF CTL-p frequencies between OND-infl and OND-non-infl patients groups reached statistical significance ($p < 0.05$ by Wilcoxon ranksum test).

Table 5. Fractions of cytolytic and natural killer effectors in CSF T lymphocyte subsets

Patient	Diagnosis	CD4+[a]		CD8+[a]	
nr.		CTL (%)[b]	NK (%)[c]	CTL (%)[b]	NK (%)[c]
2	MS-ex	23	6	100	100
3	MS-ex	25	10	100	100
4	MS-ex	20	20	95	25
5	MS-ex	52	50	86	57
8	MS-ex	52	16	100	71
11	MS-chron	83	28	-	-
18	OND non-infl	5	-	100	63
21	OND infl	82	45	-	-
22	OND infl	57	-	100	33
23	OND infl	50	21	100	46

[a] Expanded CSF T cell microcultures (established with 0.25 and 0.5 cell/well) were phenotyped and tested functionally as described in Materials and Methods. Per patient a minimum of 30 CSF T cell clones was tested.

[b] Cytolysis was tested with P 815 targets in the presence of PHA.

[c] Natural killer function was tested with K 562 targets.

Relation of cytolytic and natural killer activity with the CD4+ and CD8+ phenotype of T cell microcultures expanded from the CSF of MS and OND patients

The proliferating CSF T cell populations, which were likely to be of monoclonal nature, since they were established by plating 0.25 and 0.5 CSF cell/microwell, were analysed for expression of the CD4 or the CD8 surface molecule. Per patient a minimum of 30 clones was analysed. Generally, per patient 1 or 2 clones were found to be CD4+ and CD8+; these were left out for calculation of percentages. Table 5 gives the relative numbers of clones with CTL and with NK potential as percentages of the total number of CD4+ and CD8+ CSF clones. Almost all CD8+ CSF clones expressed cytolytic potential, as did a substantial percentage of the CD4+ CSF clones.

DISCUSSION

Although numerous abnormalities in the humoral immune response of MS patients have been reported (1-3), recent investigations indicate that T lymphocyte-mediated processes may play a central role in the actual brain lesion formation. Abnormalities in T cell subsets in peripheral blood and CSF (4-6), and increases of activated T lymphocytes in the peripheral blood and the CSF were demonstrated (15-18). Moreover, the presence of lymphocytes in the 'plaque' areas of the MS brain could be demonstrated (7-10). For a full appreciation of the role, which these cells play in the pathogenesis of MS, it is important to study the functional properties of T cells present in the brain compartment. As the number of T cells obtained by a single lumbar puncture is usually too low for direct functional assays, these cells have been expanded into long-term lines and clones with the use of IL-2 (22-32). Bulk cultures of T cells, expanded with Il-2, however, do not necessarily reflect the actual composition of the original cell population. To overcome this problem, we have developed a sensitive T lymphocyte microculture system, with the mitogenic anti-CD3 monoclonal antibody WT32 as polyclonal T cell activator, irradiated feeder cells, and exogenous IL-2 (34), that allows virtually all human T cells to expand clonally into populations of a size suitable for functional assays. In the present study, using this system, we have quantitated precursor frequencies of T cells with proliferative potential, with cytolytic potential, and with natural killer potential, in the CSF and peripheral blood of 12 MS and OND patients.

Frequency analysis of T cells with proliferative potential demonstrated clearly that, under the appropriate culture conditions, virtually all CSF and peripheral blood T lymphocytes expand into a clonal progeny of 5-20 x 10^4 cells in 14-18 days of culture. Moreover, this microculture system allowed us to show that MS and OND patients do not differ in regard of proliferative capacity of T cells in the CSF or the peripheral blood. This contrasts with previous studies, reporting a reduced proliferative capacity of both CSF (38) and peripheral blood (13,39) T lymphocytes, derived from MS patients.

The microculture system has been used to quantitate directly the precursor frequency of T cells with cytolytic and with natural killer potential in the CSF and peripheral blood of MS and OND patients. Frequency analysis of CTL-p was done in a lectin-dependent lysis assay to detect all T cells, capable of cytolysis, regardless of specificity. It was found that 37 - 93% of all T cells derived from the CSF of MS patients developed into a measurable cytolytic T lymphocyte clone. Frequency of CTL-p in the CSF of patients with inflammatory OND was higher than those in the patients with non-inflammatory OND ($p < 0.05$ by Wilcoxon ranksum test). CTL-p frequencies in the CSF of the MS patients and the patients with inflammatory OND were increased to those in their peripheral blood, although these differences did not reach statistical significance.

Natural killer function was screened using K 562 target cells. It appeared that 17 - 93% of T lymphocytes in the CSF of MS patients gave rise to a population expressing NK function. In the MS group and the inflammatory OND group NK-p frequencies were increased compared to those in the peripheral blood. Although the differences between the MS patients and the inflammatory OND patient groups on the one hand and the non-inflammatory OND group on the other hand did not reach statistical significance, they do suggest that in central nervous system disorders with an inflammatory character (including MS), the relative number of T cells with cytolytic and/or natural killer potential in the brain compartment are increased compared to the peripheral blood compartment. Hafler et al. (30), establishing T lymphocyte clones from the CSF of 6 MS patients, with a microculture system involving PHA, found CTL-p frequencies in the CSF to be generally equal to those in the blood. The lower cloning efficiency and the use of other target cells in the lectin-dependent lysis assay may be responsible for the difference between these data and the data presented here. In our experiments we detected NK-precursors in the CSF, that could be expanded and functionally tested. This accords with previously published data by Santoli et al. (28), although others failed to detect natural killer cell-precursors in the CSF of MS patients (23, 30).

Almost all CD8+ CSF clones, whether derived from MS or OND patients, were capable of lectin-dependent cytolysis. This observation is in agreement with results previously published by us and others, demonstrating that essentially all peripheral blood CD8+ lymphocytes (from normal healthy volunteers) can give rise, under appropriate culture conditions, to a clonal progeny expressing lectin-dependent cytotoxicity (34, 40,41). Our data are in accordance with results of Fleischer et al. (23), Santoli et al. (28) and Hafler et al. (30), showing that essentially all CD8+ T clones and lines, derived from the CSF from MS patients, are capable of cytolytic activity.

A significant proportion of CD4+ T lymphocyte clone obtained from the CSF appeared to have cytolytic potential, as reported (23, 30). In the experimental animal model for multiple sclerosis it has recently been shown that rat myelin basic protein (MBP)-specific T lymphocyte lines, capable of mediating experimental auto-immune encephalomyelitis, are cytolytic T cells with a helper phenotype (42,43). A similar observation was made for human myelin basic protein (MBP)-specific T cell clones and also for human T lymphocyte clones cytotoxic for measles virus-infected cells. Anti-MBP and anti-measles T cell clones, which are both hypothesized to play a role in MS, are of the CD4+, phenotype and are capable of cytolytic function (44, 45) (W. Weber, manuscript submitted). It is so far unknown whether CD4+ cytolytic T lymphocytes play a special role in the cellular immune response.

In conclusion, employing the high efficiency T lymphocyte microculture system, were were able to demonstrate that the relative numbers of T cells with cytolytic and with natural killer potential in the CSF of patients with inflammatory CNS diseases are increased, compared to numbers in the CSF of patients with non-inflammatory CNS disorders. In MS patients, these increases were less pronounced. However, in all the MS patients studied, relative numbers of T cells with cytolytic and with natural killer potential were increased in the CSF, compared to peripheral blood. In addition, it appeared that in the CSF of all patients studied, a surprising high number of T cells with cytolytic potential was of the CD4+ phenotype.

ACKNOWLEDGEMENTS

We would like to thank Dr. J. Raps and co-workers (Dept. Radiotherapy, Virga Jesse Hospital, Hasselt , for irradiating the cells, the Belgian Cross Blood Transfusion Service, Hasselt, for human buffy coat cells, Dr. H. Heyligen and Mrs. D. Peeters for FACS analysis, and Dr. P. Capel for his kind gift of monoclonal antibody WT32.

REFERENCES

1. A.I. Levinson, M. Sandberg-Wollheim and R.P. Lisak. Analysis of B-cell activation of cerebrospinal fluid lymphocytes in multiple sclerosis. Neurology. 33:1305-10 (1983).
2. R.P. Roos. B-cell activation in multiple sclerosis. Arch. Neurol. 42:73-5 (1985).
3. D.E. McFarlin and H. McFarland. Multiple sclerosis. N. Engl. J. Med. 307:1183-8 (1982).
4. E.L. Reinherz, H.L. Weiner, S.L. Hauser. Loss of suppressor T cells in active multiple sclerosis. Analysis with monoclonal antibodies. N. Engl. J. Med. 303:125-29 (1980).
5. M. Sandberg-Wollheim. Lymphocyte populations in the cerebrospinal fluid and peripheral blood of patients with multiple sclerosis and optic neuritis. Sca. J. Immunol. 17:575-81 (1983).
6. D. Rukavina, J. Sepcic, M. Doric, P. Ledic, L. Zaputovic and P. Eberhardt. Lymphocyte subpopulations in the blood and cerebrospinal fluid of multiple sclerosis patients in active disease. Acta Neurol. Sca. 69:182-5 (1984).
7. U. Traugott, E.L. Reinherz and C.S. Raine. Multiple sclerosis: distribution of T cell subsets within active chronic lesions. Science. 218:308-10 (1983).
8. U. Traugott, E.L. Reinherz and C.S. Raine. Multiple sclerosis. Distribution of T cells, T cell subsets and Ia-positive macrophages in lesions of different ages. J. Neuroimmunol. 4:201-21 (1983).
9. H.W. Kreth, R. Dunker, H. Rodt and R. Meyermann. Immunohistochemical identification of T lymphocytes in the central nervous system of patients and subacute sclerosing panencephalitis. J. Neuroimmunol. 2: 177-83 (1982).
10. S.L. Hauser, A.K. Bhan and F.H. Gilles. Immunohistochemical staining of human brain with monoclonal antibodies that identify lymphocytes, monocytes and the Ia antigen. J. Neuroimmunol. 6:197-205 (1983).
11. A. Czlonkowska, M. Poltorak, W. Cendrowski and J. Korlak. Sensitization of cerebrospinal fluid and peripheral blood lymphocytes to myelin basic protein in multiple sclerosis. Acta Neurol. Sca. 66:121-7 (1982).
12. R.P. Lisak and B. Zweiman. In vitro cell-mediated immunity of cerebrospinal fluid lymphocytes to myelin basic protein in primary demyelinating diseases. N. Engl. J. Med. 297:850-3 (1977).
13. H. Offner, J. Amnitzboll, T. Clausen, T. Fog, K. Hyllested and E. Einstein. Immune responses of lymphocytes with multiple sclerosis to phytohaemagglutinin, basic protein of myelin, and measles antigen. Acta Neurol. Sca. 50:373-81 (1974).
14. W. Sheremata, J.B.R. Cosgrove and E.H. Eylar. Multiple sclerosis and cell-mediated hypersensitivity against myelin A1 protein.
15. J. Golaz, A. Steck and L. Moretta. Activated T lymphocytes in patients with multiple sclerosis. Neurology. 33:1371-3 (1983).
16. D.A. Hafler, D.A. Fox, M.E. Manning, S.F. Schlossman, E.L. Reinherz and H.L. Weiner. In vivo activated T lymphocytes in the peripheral blood and cerebrospinal fluid of patients with multiple sclerosis. N. Engl. J. Med. 312:1405-12 (1985).

17. A.B.C. Noronha, D.P. Richman and B.G.W. Arnason. Detection of in vivo stimulated cerebrospinal fluid lymphocytes by flow cytometry in patients with multiple sclerosis. N. Engl. J. Med. 303:713-17 (1980).
18. D.A. Hafler, M.E. Hemler and L. Christenson. Investigation of in vivo activated T cells in multiple sclerosis and inflammatory central nervous system diseases. Clin. Immunol. Immunopathol. 37:163-71 (1985).
19. M.V. Livanainen. The significance of abnormal immune responses in patients with multiple sclerosis. J. Neuroimmunol. 1:141-72 (1981).
20. B.H. Waksman. Mechanisms in multiple sclerosis. Nature. 318:104-5 (1985).
21. R.P. Lisak. Multiple sclerosis: evidence for immunopathogenesis. Neurology. 30(2):99-105 (1980).
22. B. Fleischer and H.W. Kreth. Clonal analysis of HLA-restricted virus-specific cytotoxic T lymphocytes from the cerebrospinal fluid in mumps meningitis. J. Immunol. 130:2187-90 (1983).
23. B. Fleischer, P. Marquardt, S. Poser and H.W. Kreth. Phenotypic markers and functional characteristics of T lymphocyte clones from cerebrospinal fluid of patients with multiple sclerosis. J. Neuroimmunol. 7:151-62 (1984).
24. R.B. Clark, E.G. Lingenheld, J.O. Donaldson and M.K. Pollard. Compartmentalized immune responses: antigen-specificity of cerebrospinal fluid T-cell lines maintained in the absence of antigen. Clin. Immunol. Immunopathol. 36:176-86 (1985).
25. G. Birnbaum, L. Kotilinek, M. Schwartz and M. Sternad. Spinal fluid lymphocytes responsive to autologous and allogeneic cells in multiple sclerosis and control individuals. J. Clin. Invest. 74:1307-17 (1984).
26. B. Fleischer and U. Bogdahn. Growth of antigen specific, HLA restricted T lymphocyte clones from cerebrospinal fluid. Clin. Exp. Immunol. 52:38-44 (1983).
27. J. Burns, B. Zweiman and R. Lisak. Tetanus toxoid reactive T lymphocytes in the cerebrospinal fluid of multiple sclerosis patients. Immunol. Commun. 13(4):361-9 (1984).
28. D. Santoli, E.C. Defreitas, M. Sandberg-Wollheim, M.K. Francis and H. Koprowski. Phenotypic and functional characterization of T cell clones derived from the cerebrospinal fluid of multiple sclerosis patients. J. Immunol. 132:2386-92 (1984).
29. B. FLeischer and H.W. Kreth. Clonal expansion and functional analysis of virus-specific T lymphocytes from cerebrospinal fluid in measles encephalitis. Hum. Immunol. 7:239-48 (1983).
30. D.A. Hafler, M. Buchsbaum, D. Johnson and H.L. Weiner. Phenotypic and functional analysis of T cells cloned directly from the blood and cerebrospinal fluid of patients with multiple sclerosis. Ann. Neurol. 18:451-8 (1985).
31. J.B. Burns, B. Zweiman and R.P. Lisak. Long term growth in vitro of human cerebrospinal fluid T lymphocytes. J. Clin. Immunol. 1:195-200 (1981).
32. J.R. Richert, D.E. McFarlin and J.W. Rose. Expansion of antigen-specific T cells from cerebrospinal fluid of patients with multiple sclerosis. J. Neuroimmunol. 5:317-24 (1983).
33. IUIS-WHO Nomenclature Subcommittee. Announcement. J. Immunol. 134:659 (1985).
34. W.E.J. Weber, W.A. Buurman, M.M.P.P. Vandermeeren and J.C.M. Raus. Activation through CD3 molecule leads to clonal expansion of all human peripheral blood T lymphocytes: functional analysis of clonally expanded cells. J. Immunol. 135:2337-42 (1985).
35. C.M. Poser, D.W. Paty and W.I. Scheinberg. New diagnostic criteria for multiple sclerosis: guidelines for research protocols. Ann. Neurol. 13:227-31 (1983).

36. J. Van Wauwe, J.R. de Mey and J.G. Goossens. OKT3: a monoclonal anti-human T lymphocyte antibody with potent mitogenic properties. J. Immunol. 124:2708-11 (1980).
37. W.J.M. Tax, H.W. Willems, P.P.M. Reekers, P.J.A. Capel and R.A.P. Koene. Polymorphism in mitogenic effect of IgG1 monoclonal antibodies against T3 antigen of human T cells. Nature. 304:445-7 (1983).
38. S. Kam-Hansen, H. Link, A. Fryden and E. Möller. Reduced in vitro response of CSF lymphocytes to mitogen stimulation in multiple sclerosis. Scand. J. Immunol. 161-9 (1979).
39. J.P. Antel, M. Weinreich and B.G.W. Arnason. Mitogen responsiveness and suppressor cell function - influence of age and disease activity. Neurology. 28:999-1003 (1974).
40. A. Moretta, G. Pantaleo, L. Moretta, J.C. Cerottini and M.C. Mingari. Direct demonstration of the clonogenic potential of every human peripheral blood T lymphocyte. J. Exp. Med. 157:743-54 (1983).
41. A. Moretta, G. Pantaleo, L. Moretta, M.C. Mingari and J.C. Cerottini. Quantitative assessment of the pool size and subset distribution of cytolytic T lymphocytes within resting or alloactivated peripheral blood T cell populations. J. Exp. Med. 158:571-85 (1983).
42. A. Ben-Nun, H. Wekerle and I.R. Cohen. The rapid isolation of clonable antigen-specific T lymphocyte lines capable of mediating autoimmune encephalomyelitis. Eur. J. Immunol. 11:195-9 (1981).
43. D. Sun and H. Wekerle. Ia-restricted encephalitogenic T lymphocytes mediating EAE lyse auto-antigen presenting astrocytes. Nature. 320: 70-2 (1986).
44. S. Jacobson, J.R. Richert, W.E. Biddison, A. Satinsky, R.J. Hartzmann and H.F. McFarland. Measles virus-specific human cytotoxic T cell clones are restricted by class II HLA antigens. J. Immunol. 133: 754-7 (1984).
45. J. Burns, A. Rosenzweig, B. Zweiman and R.P. Lisak. Isolation of myelin basic protein-reactive T cell lines from normal human blood. Cell. Immunol. 81:435-40 (1983).

T CELLS IN THE CSF OF MS PATIENTS: ANALYSIS OF OLIGOCLONALITY WITH THE USE OF A T-CELL RECEPTOR cDNA PROBE

Francien T.M. Rotteveel and Cornelis J. Lucas

Central Laboratory of the Netherlands, Red Cross Blood Transfusion Service and Laboratory for Experimental and Clinical Immunology, University of Amsterdam, P.O. Box 9190, 1006 AD, Amsterdam, The Netherlands

ABSTRACT

Characterization of T cells present in the cerebrospinal fluid (CSF) of patients with multiple sclerosis (MS) may contribute to an understanding of the putative immunopathologic role of these cells. To analyse the diversity of T cells in the CSF of MS patients, 30 cloned T-cell lines from each of two MS patients were surveyed for their patterns of T-cell receptor (TCR) ß-chain gene rearrangements.

DNA from the (CSF-derived) T-cell clones was digested with a number of restriction endonucleases. The gene rearrangement patterns were analysed with a T-cell receptor ß-chain-specific cDNA probe. Southern blot analysis of the DNA of these T-cell clones indicated that all clones have rearrangements in the TCR ß-chain genes. So far, no indications were obtained for identical rearrangement patterns in multiple clones from a single patient.

These results suggested that if there is an oligoclonal population of T cells, it represents a relatively minor fraction of the total number of T cells in the CSF of MS patients.

INTRODUCTION

Multiple sclerosis (MS) is characterized by demyelinated areas in the white matter of the central nervous system (CNS). These plaques are associated with a perivascular infiltrate of mononuclear cells, predominantly T lymphocytes and macrophages (Traugott et al., 1983). MS may be an autoimmune disease that results from or is associated with a persistent viral infections of the central nervous system (McFarland and McFarlin, 1979). In spite of increasing evidence for involvement of the immune system, the etiology of MS is still unknown. Findings regarding the cerebrospinal fluid (CSF) strongly support the notion that lymphocytes contribute to the pathogenesis. The CSF of MS patients contains IgG of restricted heterogeneity, most of which is synthesized within the CNS (Tourtellotte et al., 1984) and which is mainly IgG1. Moreover, pleocytosis of lymphoid cells in the CSF is regularly observed. Another argument for involvement of an immune response is the association of MS with the MHC-class II antigen

HLA-DR2. A disease-MHC association implies a role for T lymphocytes in the disease. It is assumed that cells in the CSF reflect, at least in part, the cells participating in processes in the CNS.

Several laboratories have tried to characterize lymphocytes that can be isolated from the CSF of MS patients. With regard to T-cell subset analysis, the available data are not consistent. A trend towards a relative decrease of T8-positive cells in the CSF of patients with active MS, as compared to stable MS patients, has been reported (Panitch et al., 1982; Sandberg-Wollheim et al., 1983; Cashman et al., 1982; Hommes and Brinkman, 1984). However, Hauser et al., (1983) could not detect abnormalities in the distribution of T-cell subsets in active MS.

Many of the CSF T cells appear to be activated. Noronha et al., (1980) reported a relative increase in the percentage of cells in the G1- and S-phase. It was reported that in MS patients an increased number of IL-2 receptor (Tac)-positive cells occurs in the CSF as compared to PBL (Bellamy et al., 1985; Bach et al., this volume). On the other hand, Hafler et al., (1985) could not detect differences in the number of Tac-positive lymphocytes in the CSF from MS patients. These authors reported an increase in CSF T lymphocytes bearing the T-cell-specific activation antigen, Ta1.

It has not been established whether the observed expansion of the T-cell population in the CSF reflects proliferation of specific T cells. It might be expected that the limited heterogeneity of the IgG is paralelled by a similar oligoclonality of participating T cells. If this is the case, identification of predominantly occurring T cells, likely to be involved in the immunopathologic process, is extremely useful for the study of the specificity and function of these cells.

A method to analyse heterogeneity of T cells is the recently developed technique of analysis of T-cell receptor (TCR) genes. The T-cell receptor for antigens has been identified as a heterodimer composed of disulfide-linked alpha- and ß-chain glycoproteins. The organization of the ß-chain gene complex has been well characterized (Toyonaga et al., 1985). Analysis reveals that, in striking similarity to the immunoglobulin genes, the gene segments are organized into clusters containing variable (V), diversity (D), joining (J) and constant (C) region genes (Hedrick et al., 1984; Siu et al., 1985). The human ß-gene complex contains two nearly identical C genes (C-ß-1 and C-ß-2), each with its own J-ß cluster and a single D-ß-gene segment (Sims et al., 1984). Rearrangements of these gene segments, resulting in VDJ joining, are required for expression of a functional, specific T-cell receptor.

In this study, we have analysed the heterogeneity of T cells in the CSF of MS patients through detection of T-cell receptor ß-chain gene rearrangements, using a specific cDNA probe. Both polyclonally activated cultures of 10^4 CSF cells from 5 MS patients as well as 30 clones of CSF T cells from two chronic progressive MS patients were analysed.

MATERIALS AND METHODS

Cloning of lymphocytes from CSF

Lymphocytes from CSF were collected by centrifugation and stored frozen in liquid nitrogen. To clone T lymphocytes, CSF cells were seeded at an average of 1 cell/well in the presence of 10^4 irradiated autologous PBL in IL-2-containing conditioned medium with 1% phytohemagglutinin (PHA). The IL-2-containing medium was partially replaced every 3 to 4 days.

Every 7 to 10 days, irradiated, autologous PBL was added as feeder cells in the presence of 1% PHA.

DNA extraction and Southern blot analysis

DNA was prepared after cell lysis and proteinase-K digestion, by phenol extraction and ethanol precipitation. The high molecular-weight DNA was digested with the restriction endonucleases Bam H1, Hind III or Eco RI (Boehringer). A lymphoblastoid B-cell line or amnion cells served as a source of genomic DNA containing a TCR ß-germline configuration. The digested DNA was subjected to electrophoresis and, after denaturation and neutralization, transferred to nitrocellulose filters by Southern blotting (1975). Phage lambda-DNA digested with Hind III was used as molecular-weight marker. Hybridization was carried out with a nick-translated, ^{32}P-labelled DNA probe for 18 h at 42°C (Maniatis et al., 1982). The TCR ß-cDNA clone 4D1, used as a probe in these studies, was prepared and described by Jones et al., (1985). Professor Strominger kindly provided the cDNA clone via Dr. C.J.M. Melief.

DNA fragments hybridizing to the probe were detected by autoradiography.

RESULTS

T cells from the CSF of 2 MS patients were clonally expanded in the presence of Il-2 (Rotteveel et al., 1985). Both the MS patiens were in a chronic progressive state and their CSF contained oligoclonal IgG. The clones were obtained by direct limiting dilution of thawed samples of CSF cells. The advantage of this method to analyse CSF cells is that any predominantly occurring T cells are directly available for further study. As another advantage, various cells cannot overgrow each other. The configuration of the TCR ß-chain gene locus in 30 T-cell clones from the CSF of 2 MS patients was studied by Southern blot analysis.

In their germ-line form, the gene segments encoding the two C-ß genes were present on a single Bam-H1 DNA fragment (24 kb), on two Eco RI DNA fragments (4 and 11 kb) and on three Hind-III DNA fragments. (3.5, 6.5 and 8 kb) as shown in Fig.1. The 4-kb Eco RI fragment is not altered by any V, D,J rearrangement, but the C-ß-1-containing Eco RI fragment (11 kb in germ-line form) is altered in size by most rearrangements affecting V, D_1, J_1 and is eliminated by rearrangements between V, D_2, J_2.

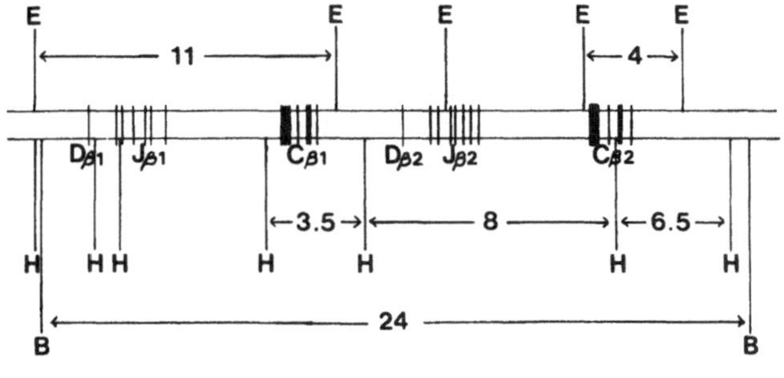

Fig.1. Restriction-enzyme map of the human TCR ß-chain locus (Toyonaga et al., 1985). Restriction enzymes : E, Eco RI; H, Hind III; B, Bam H1. DNA fragments hybridizing with the Cß probe are depicted. The lenght is given in kilo bases (kb).

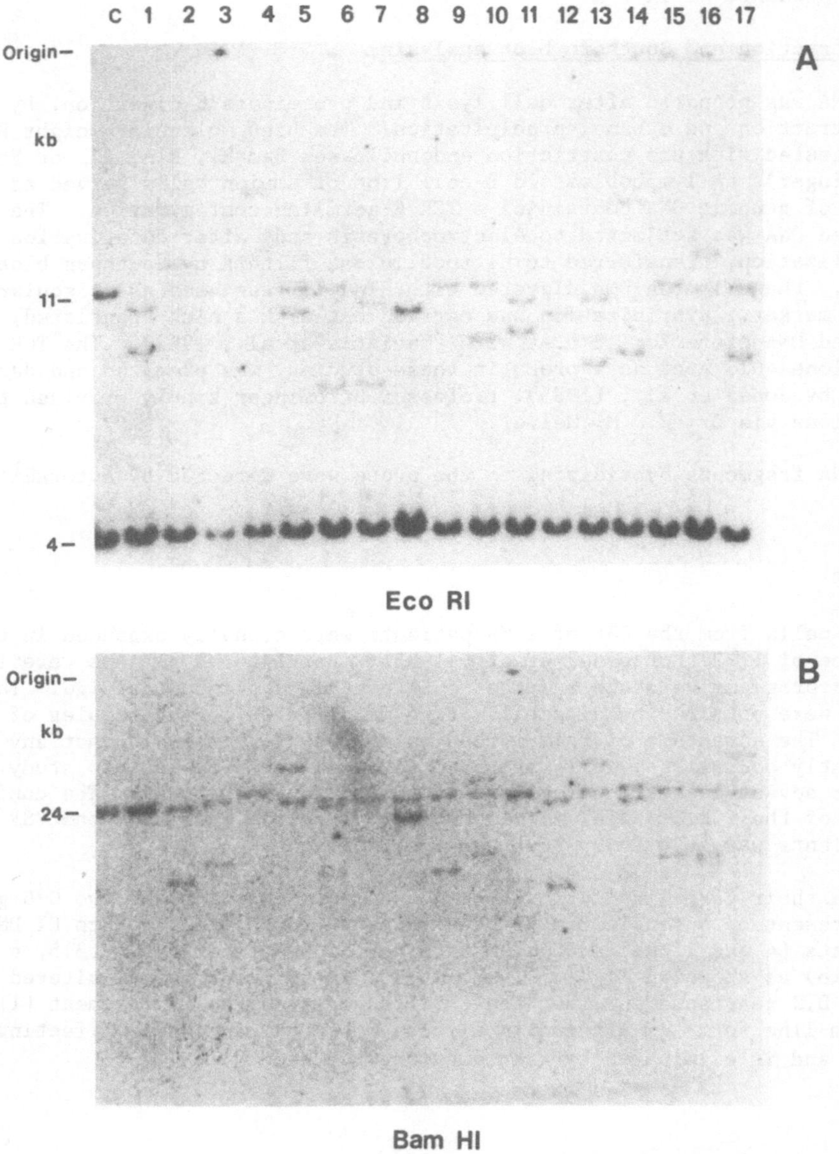

Fig.2. Southern blot analysis of the TCR ß-chain gene rearrangements from CSF-derived T-cell clones of one MS patient. DNAs were digested with Eco RI or Bam H1 and examined by hybridization with the use of a TCR ß-chain cDNA probe. A, Eco RI; B, Bam H1. Lane 1, amnion cells (germ-line configuration); lanes 2-18, CSF T-cell clones.

Analysis of the CSF T-cell clones showed that all T-cell clones had rearrangements of C-ß-1 and/or C-ß-2 genes. After Eco RI digestion, mostly two bands were observed in addition to the 4-kb band, demonstrating rearrangement of TCR genes, see e.g. lanes 3 and 4 of Fig.2A. This finding most likely reflects the occurrence of rearrangements probably being abortive.

Examination of the rearrangement patterns indicate that among the 30 T-cell clones from the CSF of both of the 2 MS patients, no sets of clones with the same rearrangements could be detected. At least on one occasion, the DNA-band patterns in the Southern blots of two clones appeared identical when two different DNA digests were analysed, but proved different when the DNA was digested with a third restriction enzyme. Identification of predominantly occurring T cells in the CSF (perhaps involved in the immunopathology of MS) is thus not yet possible.

DNA from polyclonally stimulated CSF bulk cultures, derived from 5 MS patients, did not show any bands above the background smear, as expected for a polyclonal T-cell population. Minden et al., (1985) have shown that DNA from a monoclonal population of T cells is already detectable in a mixture with fibroblast DNA if their DNA comprises 5% of the total DNA. Therefore, the results of the bulk cultures also indicate that a predominant occurrence of a certain TCR ß-chain gene rearrangement within the CSF T cells probably is unlikely to exist.

DISCUSSION

Demyelination in the CNS of patients with multiple sclerosis is probably the result of an inflammatory, immunologically specific response. It is likely that a limited number of relevant epitopes of brain antigens are recognized by participating T cells. This could result in proliferation of epitope-specific lymphocytes within the CNS lesions. Therefore, the T-cell response within the CNS in MS patients might be oligoclonal. The immunoglobulins in the CNS are oligoclonal and their subclass suggests T-cell dependency. This also could imply that a limited number of T-cell specificities is involved in the intrathecal immune response.

Pleocytosis of the CSF in an inflammatory disease of the brain (Sindbis virus infection) is a result of leakage of mononuclear cells from the meninges into the CSF (Moench and Griffin, 1984). In addition, it has been shown that in the case of mumps meningitis and measles encephalitis the cells present in the CSF are predominantly virus-specific (Fleischer and Kreth, 1983a, 1983b). Therefore, in the case of MS, we assume that at least a fraction of the cells in the CSF are involved in the immunopathology of MS.

To study the oligoclonality of T cells, we have analysed T-cell receptor gene rearrangements of T-cell clones from CSF. The clones were obtained by direct limiting dilution of CSF cells in the presence of a polyclonal activator and IL-2. In this way, cloned, specific cells are directly available for further study. In a, so far, limited, study we have not yet obtained evidence for an appreciable oligoclonality of CSF T cells. From each of two CSF samples available, 30 T-cell clones were obtained. All clones are different from each other based on the observation that all show unique rearrangements of the T-cell receptor ß-chain genes.

At this point, it is still impossible to estimate the extent to which T cells in the CSF might be oligoclonal; therefore, we cannot yet identify the cells likely to be involved in the inflammatory process. The data suggest that if there is an oligoclonal population of T cells, it represents a relatively minor fraction of the total T cells in CSF of MS patients. This is in agreement with the results of other experiments in which T-cell receptor gene rearrangements in polyclonally activated cultures of 10 000 CSF mononuclear cells were analysed.

The presence in the CSF of the T cells which are involved in the CNS immunopathology might be related to disease activity. It is not unlikely that the frequency of these T cells is increased during early phases of an exacerbation when pleocytosis is often highest.

Another method to identify the T cells relevant in the inflammatory process within the CNS of MS patients might be to elute and clone cells from brain-biopsy material.

ACKNOWLEDGEMENT

We gratefully thank Dr. van Walbeek and Professor Koetsier for providing us with CSF and blood samples from MS patients. Wies Vasmel has helped tremendously in the initial phases of this study. We acknowledge inspiring discussions with Erik Braakman and thank Wim Zeijlemaker for critically reading the manuscript.

This study was financially supported by the Foundation for Medical Research FUNGO, which is subsidized by the Netherlands Organization for the Advancement of Pure Research (ZWO) (grant no. 13-40-05).

REFERENCES

1. A.S. Bellamy, V.L. Calder, M. Feldmann and A.N. Davison. The distribution of interleukin-2 receptor bearing lymphocytes in multiple sclerosis: evidence for a key role of activated lymphocytes. Clin. Exp. Immunol. 61:248 (1985).
2. N. Cashman, C. Martin, J.F. Eizenbaum, J.D. Degos and M.A. Bach. Monoclonal antibody-defined immunoregulatory cells in multiple sclerosis cerebrospinal fluid. J. Clin. Invest. 70:387 (1982).
3. B. Fleischer and H.W. Kreth. Clonal analysis of HLA-restricted virus-specific cytotoxic T lymphocytes from cerebrospinal fluid in mumps meningitis. J. Immunol. 130:2187 (1983a).
4. B. Fleischer and H.W. Kreth. Clonal expansion and functional analysis of virus-specific T lymphocytes from cerebrospinal fluid in measles encephalitis. Human Immunol. 7:239 (1983b).
5. D.A. Hafler, D.A. Fox, M.E. Manning, S.F. Schlossman, E.L. Reinherz and H.L. Weiner. In-vivo activated T lymphocytes in the peripheral blood and cerebrospinal fluid of patients with multiple sclerosis. New. Engl. J. Med. 312:1405 (1985).
6. S.L. Hauser, E.L. Reinherz, C.J. Hoban, S.F. Schlossman and H.L. Weiner. CSF cells in multiple sclerosis: monoclonal antibody analysis and relationship to peripheral blood T-cell subsets. Neurology. 33:575 (1983).
7. S.M. Hedrick, E.A. Nielsen, J. Kavaler, D. Cohen and M.M. Davis. Sequence relationships between putative T-cell receptor polypeptides and immunoglobulins. Nature. 308:153 (1984).
8. O.R. Hommes and C.J.J. Brinkman. T-cell subsets in spinal fluid of multiple sclerosis patients. J. Neuroimmunol. 6:123 (1984).
9. N. Jones, J. Leiden, D. Dialynas, J. Fraser, M. Clabby, T. Kishimoto, J.L. Strominger, D. Andrews, W. Lane and J. Woody. Partial primary structure of the alpha and ß chains of human tumor T-cell receptors. Science. 227:311 (1985).
10. T. Maniatis, E. Fritsch and J. Sambrook. Molecular cloning: a laboratory manual. In: Cold Spring Harbor Laboratory, Cold Spring Harbor, N.Y. (1982).
11. H.F. McFarland and D.E. McFarlin. Cellular immune response to measles, mumps and vaccinia viruses in multiple sclerosis. Ann. Neurol. 6:101 (1979).

12. M.D. Minden, B. Toyonaga, K. Ha, Y. Yanagi, B. Chin, E. Gelfand and T. Mak. Somatic rearrangement of T-cell antigen receptor gene in human T-cell malignancies. Proc. Natl. Acad. Sci. USA. 82:1224 (1985).
13. T.R. Moench and D.E. Griffin. Immunocytochemical identification and quantitation of the mononuclear cells in the cerebrospinal fluid, meninges and brain during acute viral meningoencephalitis. J. Exp. Med. 159:77 (1984).
14. A.B.C. Noronha, D.P. Richman and B.G.W. Arnason. Detection of in-vivo stimulated cerebrospinal fluid lymphocytes by flow cytometry in patients with multiple sclerosis. New Engl. J. Med. 303:713 (1980).
15. H.S. Panitch and G.S. Francis. T-lymphocyte subsets in cerebrospinal fluid in multiple sclerosis. New Engl. J. Med. 307:560 (1982).
16. F. Rotteveel, E. Braakman and C.J. Lucas. Towards cloning of lymphoid cells from cerebrospinal fluid. In: Multiple Sclerosis Research in Europe, O.R. Hommes, ed. Lancaster, MTP Press, pp 167-174 (1985).
17. M. Sandberg-Wollheim. Lymphocyte populations in the cerebrospinal fluid and peripheral blood of patients with multiple sclerosis and optic neuritis. Scand. J. Immunol. 17:575 (1983).
18. J.E. Sims, A. Tunnacliffe, W.J. Smith and T.H. Rabbits. Complexity of human T-cell antigen receptor ß-chain constant- and variable-region genes. Nature. 312:541 (1984).
19. G. Siu, S.P. Clark, Y. Yoshikai, M. Malissen, Y. Yanagi, E. Strauss, T.W. Mak and L. Hood. The human T-cell antigen receptor is encoded by variable, diversity and joining gene segments that rearrange to generate a complete V-gene. Cell. 37:393 (1985).
20. E.M. Southern. Detection of specific sequences among DNA fragments separated by gel electrophoresis. J. Mol. Biol. 98:503 (1975).
21. W.W. Tourtellotte, M.J. Walsh, R.W. Baumhefner, S.M. Staugaitis and P. Shapshak. The current status of multiple sclerosis intra-blood-brain-barrier IgG synthesis. In: Multiple Sclerosis: Experimental and Clinical Aspects, L. Scheinberg and C.S. Raine, eds., New York. (1984).
22. B. Toyonaga, Y. Yoshikai, V. Vadasz, B. Chin and T.W. Mak. Organisation and sequences of the diversity, joining and constant region genes of the human T-cell receptor ß-chain. Proc. Natl. Acad. Sci. USA. 82:8624 (1985).
23. U. Traugott, E.L. Reinherz and C.S. Raine. Multiple sclerosis: distribution of T-cell subsets within active chronic lesions. Science. 219:308 (1983).

MOUSE HEPATITIS VIRUS-INDUCED DEMYELINATION: AN EXPERIMENTAL ANIMAL MODEL SYSTEM OF AUTOIMMUNE SENSITIZATION OF THE CENTRAL NERVOUS SYSTEM

M.J.M. Koolen* and C.J. Lucas

*Scripps Clinic and Research Foundation, La Jolla, CA and Central Laboratory of The Netherlands, Red Cross Blood Transfusion Service and Laboratory for Experimental and Clinical Immunology of the University of Amsterdam, Amsterdam, The Netherlands

INTRODUCTION

It is well established that viruses are etiologically related to chronic progressive central nervous system (CNS) disease. Viral infections can also result in other neurological diseases which, besides meningitis and encephalitis, include syndromes like Guillain-Barré syndrome and Reye's syndrome. Many of the virus-induced illnesses meant here represent uncommon complications of primary infections with often common viruses. Other diseases can result from activation of latent or silent viruses. Subacute sclerosing panencephalitis (SSPE) is a progressive degenerative disorder caused by persistent infection of neurons by measles virus (Ter Meulen and Hall, 1978; Johnson, 1982). SSPE is a rare, late complication of childhood measles, and the time span between the initial attack and the onset of SSPE may be a decade or longer. So far, details of the host-virus interactions leading to SSPE are largely unknown. Experiments designed to demonstrate measles virus-specific T cells in the cerebral spinal fluid (CSF) of SSPE patients have thus far remained unsuccessful (Lucas et al., unpublished data).

These and other observations could imply that viruses and virus-like infectious agents indeed play an important role in several progressive demyelinating diseases in humans. Although no clear causal relationships have been established so far, it has been speculated that a virus might be involved in the etiology of multiple sclerosis (MS) (Johnson, 1975). Epidemiological studies of its geographic distribution have shown regions of high and low prevalence. Emigration data indicate that the disease is acquired in childhood from an environmental factor, probably an infectious agent (Kurtzke, 1983; Dean et al., 1971; Alter et al., 1978). Epidemiologic association of MS occurrence with outbreaks of both measles and the related canine distemper viruses implicated these agents, but definitive etiology has not been established (Stroop and Baringer, 1982; Ter Meulen and Hall, 1978). Norrby and coworkers (1978) as well as other groups demonstrated measles virus specificity of the oligoclonal IgG in the CSF. However, despite the use of a multidisciplinary approach to establish causal relationships between viruses and human demyelinating disease, a putative MS virus has so far not been found.

Little is known about immune responses to viruses within the CNS. Only very small numbers, if any, of immunocompetent cells are normally found in the CNS. There is no organized lymphoid tissue in the brain (Medawar, 1948). Also only few, if any, phagocytic cells are found in the CNS. Thus, an invading virus will not be immediately processed. One can envisage that after virus invasion of the CNS time elapses before lymphocytes are recruited and inflammatory reactions are started. Clearance of a virus might thus be delayed giving the virus a head-start.

It is important to realize, however, that the immune response may play a dual role in viral infections. It functions as a host defence mechanism, but it also is an important factor in tissue destruction and disease expression. These two sides might be in delicate balance as is illustrated by the effects of anti-lymphocyte serum on the outcome of Herpes Simplex infection in mice. Administration of the immunosuppressive serum prior to invasion of the CNS increases the incidence of death. Administration of the anti-lymphocyte serum after CNS invasion diminishes the illness and prolongs survival (Nahmias et al., 1969). Thus, T lymphocytes can contribute to the severity of a virus-induced CNS disease. On the other hand, a meningitis is the price which has to be paid for clearing a virus from the CNS.

MOUSE HEPATITIS VIRUS-INDUCED DEMYELINATION

Faced with the questions summarized above, many investigators focused their research on animal model systems of CNS disease to define precisely the factor(s) which determine the course of CNS infection and destruction (Koolen and Buchmeier, 1986). Studies performed in these animal model systems have revealed that completely unrelated viruses, such as paramyxo-,corona-, rhabdo-, arbo-, retro-, herpes-, picorna-viruses and several others are able to cause a demyelinating infection in the CNS. Therefore, these animal model systems allow us to study in detail the function of specific macromolecular components and genes of viruses and their interaction with the host leading to the ultimate production of the disease. Insight into the molecular basis of viral CNS pathogenesis and the role of host factors, such as genetic background and immune response, might finally unravel this complex. It has to be kept in mind, however, that most of the models involve intracerebral infection routes and that thus the studied disease is investigator-mediated.

The interactions of virus- and host-specific factors, studied in probably one of the best-characterized animal model systems, e.g. mouse hepatitis virus-induced demyelinating disease in the CNS of mice and rats, will be reviewed here.

Mouse hepatitis virus (MHV) strain JHM (MHV-4) and strain A-59 (MHV-A59) are members of the coronaviridae, a group of viruses which also includes a number of human cold viruses (Tyrrell et al., 1968; Siddell et al., 1983). In susceptible non-immune mice, the neurotropic strain MHV-4 causes a fatal encephalitis accompanied by demyelination whereas, under similar conditions, infection with the neurohepatotropic strain A-59 is followed by an acute hepatitis as well (Koolen et al., 1983). Demyelination following infection with wild-type virus is a direct effect of virus infection of the oligodendrocyte. This demyelination usually remains unnoticed because of wide-spread destruction of CNS neurons. Resistance of mice to this lethal disease is controlled by a single autosomal gene on chromosome 7, which is expressed at the level of neurons and macrophages (Knobler et al., 1981). Infrequent survivors of the acute encephalomyelitis undergo chronic demyelination (Lampert et al., 1973; Weiner, 1973; Lavi et al., 1984). Using temperature-sensitive (ts) mutants and spontaneously arising variants of MHV, a high incidence of chronic demyelination can be induced in susceptible mice. Demyelinating disease induced with a specific ts-mutant of MHV-4, designated ts-8, is characterized by selective destruction of oligodendrocytes (Haspel et al., 1978). This pathological finding is called primary demyelination.

Similar evidence of a shift from acute fatal to subacute demyelinating disease has been reported for MHV-4 variants and the mutant ts-342 of MHV A-59. Buchmeier and coworkers (personal communication) as well as others (Fleming et al., 1986) have attempted to define the factor(s) which determine neurotropism and limit the spread of infection in vivo in the CNS. Using monoclonal antibodies (MAb) of defined specificity in a passive transfer model to define viral proteins, it was shown that MAb against two topographically distinct sites on the E2-peplomer glycoproteins of MHV-4 are able to block development of fatal encephalitis following immune-complex (IC) infection with wild-type virus leading to selective destruction of oligodendrocytes. Specific variants of MHV-4, selected by growing wild-type virus in the presence of the individual MAb, no longer caused acute fatal encephalitis but, instead, induced chronic demyelinating disease (Koolen and Buchmeier, 1986).

Unlike ts-8, ts-mutant ts-342 of MHV-A59, however, shows no specific cell tropism in vivo as well as in primary brain tissue-culture cells in vitro. Both wild-type MHV-A59 and ts-342 are able to infect both astrocytes and oligodendrocytes although not all cells are infected. In addition, Lavi et al., 1984, have shown that the demyelinating disease present in mice, which survive the initial acute encephalitis/hepatitis with wild-type MHV-A59, can proceed in the absence of detectable infectious virus and/or viral antigens. These observations, confirmed by our own observations, suggest that a cytolytic infection of oligodendrocytes is unlikely to be the cause by which MHV-A59 induces demyelination.

Recently, we were able to define the difference in pathogenic properties of wild-type virus and ts-342 at the molecular level by studying the replication of both viruses in primary mouse brain astrocytes in vitro. In contrast to wild-type virus, ts-342 shows an abortive infection in astrocytes, which is not observed in normal tissue-culture cells. Revertants of ts-342 regained the properties of wild-type virus indicating that the ts-mutation of ts-342, together with host-specific factor(s), are responsible for a reduced synthesis of the viral envelope proteins E1 and E2. Replication of ts-342 in vivo is restricted to the brain (Koolen et al., submitted for publication). Revertant viruses have in-vivo pathogenic properties similar to wild-type MHV-A59, which suggests that the point mutation that led to the ts-phenotype is responsible for reduced neuropathogenicity of the mutant (Van Berlo et al., 1986). These findings suggest that mutant virus can cause and abortive infection in astrocytes in vivo.

In addition, these findings suggest that molecular changes in viral surface proteins modify the outcome of virus-host interactions which is expressed in an altered neurological disease. In addition, the interesting paradox, that virus-induced pathology persists in the absence of demonstrable infectious virus, suggests that other mechanisms are involved in the ongoing disease. Based on the observation that completely unrelated viruses can function as an initial trigger of similar demyelinating diseases, might imply autoimmune sensitization as a general mechanism. It is not unlikely that stimulation of specific cell-mediated immune response against viral antigens and/or host components of myelin, such as myelin-basic protein (MBP), are triggered early in the infectious process and contribute to the chronic demyelinating disease. This might be related to molecular mimicry. Alternatively, virus may persist in limited cell populations, such as the basal ganglia (Fishman et al., 1985) and astrocytes

(Van Berlo et al., 1986) and continually re-initiate the demyelinating process at the primary level during episodes of unresponsiveness of the immune system.

In recent studies with the mutant ts-342, we have observed significant levels of proliferation, measured as ^{3}H-thymidine incorporation, when lymphocytes from virus-infected mice were cultured in the presence of either viral antigen or MBP. The responder cells were shown to be T lymphocytes and depletion of the L_3T_4 population in vivo reduced the proliferative response from MBP to baseline levels, while proliferative responses to viral antigen were still present. These results suggest that different subsets of T lymphocytes are involved in the ts-342-induced demyelinating disease.

Recently, we have shown (Koolen et al., submitted for publication) that athymic nude mice infected intracerebrally with the ts-342 mutant succumb to a fatal hepatitis, but these animals also developed a demyelinating disease. These observations suggest that cellular immune factors are involved in protecting mice against lethal infection, and that initiation of demyelination can occur independently of a cellular immune response. Further studies are now in progress to characterize these responses and the mechanism of demyelination at the cellular level. In addition, we will try to clone the responsible cells.

A POSSIBLE ROLE OF ASTROCYTES IN VIRUS-INDUCED DEMYELINATION

The speculation that mutant virus causes an abortive infection in astrocytes in vivo could also provide a mechanism for the escape of the virus from the surveillance of the immune system.

Recent studies have shown that astrocytes become activated after exposure to either mouse hepatitis virus in vitro or to lymphokines released as part of the systemic reaction to virus (Neta et al., 1981; Wong et al., 1984; Massa et al., 1986). Activated astrocytes share with macrophages the property of presenting antigen together with the class-II MHC antigen Ia (Fontana et al., 1984; Cammer et al., 1978). Zurbriggen and coworkers (1986) showed recently that canine oligodendrocytes in vitro can be damaged by toxic factors as a result of infection of astrocytes with canine distemper virus. Therefore, these properties of astrocytes might enable them to participate directly in the immune response to brain antigens and thereby support brain damage following an initial viral infection. We have not yet studied the expression of Ia determinants on brain cells after infection with the MHV-ts-342 virus.

Traugott and coworkers as well as others have reported that Ia antigens were also expressed on astrocytes and endothelial cells in multiple sclerosis lesions. Furthermore, it was demonstrated that cells at the edge of the MS lesion expressed the interleukin-2 (IL-2) receptor and also exhibited positive staining with antibodies to IL-1, IL-2 and prostaglandin E (J.E. Merrill, this volume). This suggests that astrocytes are participating in an active immune event leading to the formation of the MS lesion.

Although the etiological agent of MS has still to be identified, viruses are generally considered likely candidates (McFarlin and McFarland, 1982). To study MS, the idea of a 'hit-and-run' effect or of persistence of an abortive infection is certainly disconcerting from a virologist's point of view. It implies that, by the time clinical MS appears, the causative agent may have disappeared or escapes detection.

Clearly, the similarities in pathological events of a MS lesion and experimental virus-induced demyelination of the CNS in animals indicate that animal model systems are at the moment the most rewarding systems to elucidate the mechanism of demyelination at the cellular level. Future studies have to be focused on the interaction of virus- and host-specific neuronal cells as well as on the contribution of these cells in generating a local immune response. This information can then be applied in a systematic attempt to interpret multiple sclerosis.

ACKNOWLEDGEMENTS

We thank Jim Johnston and Jetty Gerritsen for the preparation of this manuscript.

M.J.M. Koolen is the recipient of a long-term fellowship from EMBO (grant no. ALTF 287-1984).

REFERENCES

1. M. Alter, E. Kahana and R. Loewenson. Migration and risk of multiple sclerosis. Neurology (Minneap.) 28:1089 (1978).
2. W. Cammer, B.R. Bloom, W.I. Norton and S. Gordon. Degradation of basic protein in myelin by neutral proteinases secreted by stimulated macrophages: A possible mechanism of inflammatory demyelination. Proc. Acad. Sci. USA. 75:1554 (1978).
3. G. Dean and J.F. Kurtzke. On the risk of multiple sclerosis according to age at immigration to South Africa. Brit. Med. J. 3:725 (1971).
4. P. Fishman, J. Gass, P. Swoveland, E. Lavi, M. Highkin and S. Weiss. Infection of the basal ganglia by a murine coronavirus. Science. 229:877 (1985).
5. J.O. Fleming, M.D. Trousdale, F.A.K. El-Zaatari, S.A. Stohlman and L.P. Weiner. Pathogenicity of antigenic variants of murine coronavirus JHM selected with monoclonal antibodies. J. Virol. In press. (1986).
6. A. Fontana, W. Fierz and H. Wekerle. Astrocytes present myelin basic protein to encephalitogenic T-cell lines. Nature. 307:273 (1984).
7. M.V. Haspel, P.W. Lampert and M.B.A. Oldstone. Temperature-sensitive mutants of mouse hepatitis virus produce a high incidence of demyelination. Proc. Natl. Acad. Sci. USA. 75:4033 (1978).
8. R.T. Johnson. Viral infections of the nervous system. Raven Press, New York. (1982).
9. R.T. Johnson. The possible viral etiology of multiple sclerosis. In: Advances in neurology, vol.13, pp.1-46, W.J. Friedlander, ed. Academic Press, New York. (1975).
10. R.L. Knobler, M.V. Haspel and M.B.A. Oldstone. Mouse hepatitis virus type-4 (JHM strain)-induced fatal central nervous system disease. I. Genetic control and the murine neuron as the susceptible site of disease. J. Exp. Med. 153:832 (1981).
11. M.J.M. Koolen and M. Buchmeier. Experimental models of virus attenuation and demyelinating disease. Microbiol. Sci. 3:68 (1986).
12. M.J.M. Koolen, A. Osterhaus, G. van Steenis, M. Horzinek and B.A.M. van der Zeijst. Temperature-sensitive mutants of mouse hepatitis virus strain A59: Isolation, characterization and neuropathogenic properties. Virology. 125:393 (1983).
13. J.F. Kurtzke. Some epidemiological trends in multiple sclerosis. TINS 6:75 (1983).
14. P.W. Lampert, J.K. Sims and A.J. Kniazeff. Mechanism of demyelination in JHM virus encephalomyelitis. Electron microscopic studies. Acta Neuropathol. (Berlin). 24:76 (1973).

15. E. Lavi, D.H. Gilden, Z. Wroblewska, L.B. Rorke and S.R. Weiss. Experimental demyelination produced by the A59 strain of mouse hepatitis virus. Neurology. 34:587 (1984).
16. P.T. Massa, R. Dorries and V. ter Meulen. Viral particles induce Ia antigen expression on astrocytes. Nature. 320:543 (1986).
17. P.B. Medawar. The fate of skin homografts transplanted to brain, to subcutaneous tissue and to the anterior chamber of the eye. Brit. J. Exp. Pathol. 29:58 (1948).
18. D.E. McFarlin and H.F. McFarland. Multiple sclerosis. New Engl. J. Med. 307:1183 (first part); New Engl. J. Med. 307:1246 (second part). (1982).
19. A.J. Nahmias, M.S. Hirsch, J.M. Kramer and F.A. Murphy. Effect of antithymocyte serum on herpes virus hominis (type 2) infection in adult mice. Proc. Soc. Exp. Biol. Med. 132:696 (1969).
20. R. Neta, S.B. Salvin and M. Sabaawi. Mechanisms in the in-vivo release of lymphokines. I. Comparative kinetics in the release of six lymphokines in inbred strains of mice. Cell. Immunol. 64:203 (1981).
21. E. Norrby. Viral antibodies in multiple sclerosis. Progr. Med. Virol. 24:1 (1978).
22. W.G. Stroop and J.R. Baringer. Persistent, slow and latent viral infections. Progr. Med. Virol. 28:1 (1982).
23. S.G. Siddell, R. Anderson, D. Cavanagh, K. Fujiwara, H.D. Klenk, M.R. Mac-Naughton, M. Pensaert, S.A. Stohlman, L. Sturman and B.A.M. van der Zeijst. Coronaviridae. Intervirology. 20:181 (1983).
24. V. ter Meulen and W.M. Hall. Slow virus infections of the nervous system: virological, immunological and pathogenic considerations. J. Gen. Virol. 41:1 (1978).
25. D.A. Tyrrell, J.D. Almeida, D.M. Berry, C.H. Cunningham, D. Hamre, M.S. Hofstad, L. Malluci and K. McIntosh. Coronaviruses. Nature. 220:650 (1968).
26. M.F. van Berlo, G. Wolswijk, J. Calafat, M.J.M. Koolen, M.C. Horzinek and B.A.M. van der Zeijst. Restricted replication of mouse hepatitis virus A59 in primary mouse brain astrocytes correlates with reduced pathogenicity. J. Virol. 58:426 (1986).
27. L.P. Weiner. Pathogenesis of demyelination induced by a mouse hepatitis virus (JHM virus). Arch. Neurol. 28:293 (1973).
28. G.H.W. Wong, P.F. Bartlett, I. Clark-Lewis, F. Battye and J.W. Schrader. Inducible expression of H-2 and Ia antigens on brain cells. Nature. 310:688 (1984).
29. A. Zubriggen, M. Vandevelde and M. Dumas. Secondary degeneration of oligodendrocytes in canine distemper virus infection in vitro. Lab. Invest. 54:424 (1986).

CHARACTERISTICS OF THE CSF INFLAMMATORY EXUDATE IN MURINE LYMPHOCYTIC CHORIOMENINGITIS

Peter C. Doherty, Jane E. Allan, Jane E. Dixon, Zsuzsanna Tabi and Rhodri Ceredig

Department of Experimental Pathology, The John Curtin School of Medical Research, Canberra ACT 2601, Australia

Mice that are injected intracerebrally (i.c.) with lymphocytic choriomeningitis virus (LCMV) develop an acute, fatal neurological disease within 6 to 8 days. This is the best model that we have available for the experimental analysis of T cell-mediated immunopathology in a virus infection (1, 2). There are a variety of reasons why this is so. The virus itself is relatively non-lytic, and is maintained in nature as an inapparent infection of mice that is acquired <u>in utero</u> (3). The disease process that occurs in adult animals requires that the T cell compartment be intact: congenitally athymic nu/nu mice, or mice depleted of T cells by a variety of procedures, remain asymptomatic and become carriers of virus following i.c. injection with LCMV. Fatal neurological disease can be induced in adult mice, that have been infected with LCMV and then immunosuppressed with cyclophosphamide, by the adoptive transfer of virus-immune spleen populations: the effectors that are involved in triggering the inflammatory process are Thy 1^+, and must share at least one class I major histocompatibility complex (MHC) allele with the virus-infected recipients. Class I MHC-related immune response (Ir) gene effects modulate the severity of the disease process, and the rapidity with which immunopathology develops (4).

The participation of class I MHC-restricted T cells is essential for the development of both symptoms and meningitis, which occur in the absence of any major damage mediated by the virus itself in contrast to other more lytic infections (3, 6, 7). As a consequence, the extravasated cells that are present in cerebrospinal fluid (CSF) have presumably localized there as a direct result of the interaction between virus-immune T cells and virus-infected target cells in the central nervous system (CNS). The LCMV model thus provides an almost unique opportunity to study the nature of an inflammatory process induced by virus-immune T cells. This account concentrates on the characteristics of the mononuclear cells that can be recovered from the CSF inflammatory exudate.

EXPERIMENTAL MODELS

The findings that are related here depend on the use of two experimental systems. In the <u>direct</u> model, mice are injected i.c. with 1,000 LD50 of the neurotropic Armstrong (Arm) E350 LCMV. Samples of CSF are taken from the cisterna magna (7) for analysis at intervals thereafter. The indirect model utilizes a passive transfer system: mice are injected i.c. with 1,000 LD50 of Arm LCMV, immunosuppressed 4 or 5 days later with 200 mg/kg of cyclophosphamide (cy), and, on the following day, given immune spleen cells from donors that were primed 8 days previously with the viscerotropic WE3 LCMV (8). The recipient mice develop severe choriomeningitis at 3 or 4 days after cell transfer, depending on the strain of mouse used and the dose of cells given. For instance C57Bl/6J mice, which generate a potent cytotoxic T lymphocyte (CTL) response, show evidence of severe inflammation (and may die) at 72 hours after the intravenous (i.v.) inoculation of 2.0×10^7 immune spleen cells, whereas CBA/H mice (which are much weaker CTL responders (9)) take 96 hours to develop a disease of comparable magnitude (10). The onset of severe inflammatory process is paralleled by the generation of potent cytotoxic T lymphocyte (CTL) effectors in the spleen and CSF of the recipients: these CTL are, at least on day 3 or day 4 after cell transfer, essentially of donor origin.

The nature of the clinical disease also depends on the dose of virus given to the recipients. If this is low, and the immune spleen cells are transferred within 2 days of injection of virus into the recipients, the mice may survive following the development of severe, transient choriomeningitis (11, 12). This has been interpreted as indicating that mice may recover after cell-mediated elimination of virus-infected cells from the choroid plexus, ependyma and meninges, provided that not too many host cells are infected by the time that CTL invasion occurs.

The other point worth noting is that in the indirect model the function of the adoptively-transferred immune spleen cells may be subject to hybrid resistance (Hr) effects (10). This is a complex, and ill-understood, phenomenon (13) which has been discussed in greater detail elsewhere (10). The consequence of Hr is, for instance, that the function of C57Bl/6J (but not CBA/H) immune spleen cells may be largely suppressed in (CBA x C57Bl/6J) F1 recipients. The possible role of Hr should be kept in mind when assessing findings from any T cell transfer system which uses F1 recipients.

CELLULAR CONSTITUENTS OF THE INFLAMMATORY EXUDATE

Our experiments have concentrated on the involvement of natural killer cells, monocyte/macrophages and T cells. All of which would seem to have the potential for mediating immunopathology.

(A) Natural killer cells

Natural killer (NK) cells are present in spleen from about day 3 after inoculation with LCMV, and can also be found in blood (14, 15). Not surprisingly, when CSF is taken from C57Bl/6J mice injected i.c. with virus 6 days previously, evidence of potent NK activity is found in the inflammatory exudate (Expts. 1 and 2, YAC-1 targets, Table 1). As mice are starting to die by day 6 (16), the obvious question is whether or not the NK effectors are contributing to the development of symptoms. Attempts at resolving this by using NK-deficient beige (bg/bg) mice (17), or by treatment with antibody to the asialo GM_1 ganglioside (anti $ASGM_1$) (18), did not generate particularly clear results. The bg/bg mice died of LCM at the same time as their phenotypically normal bg/+ littermates, and there was no consistent difference in the severity of meningitis. Use of the anti-$ASGM_1$ antibody in this direct model for inducing LCM did not have any reproducible effect (16).

Table 1. Cytotoxic activity of cells from lymphoid tissue from lymphoid tissue and CSF

		% specific ^{51}Cr release[c]	
		YAC-1	MC57G-LCMV
Direct model[a]	spleen	46	23
Expt.1	lymph node	21	31
(50:1)	CSF	42	26
Expt.2	spleen	29	0
(50:1)	lymph need	36	28
	CSF	71	28
Indirect model[b]	spleen	15	43
(30:1)	lymph node	12	28
	CSF	8	41

[a] C57Bl/6J mice were incubated i.c. with 1,000 LD50 of Arm LCMV 6 days previously.

[b] C57Bl/6J mice were injected i.c. with LCMV, immunosuppressed 5d later by treatment with 200 mg/kg of Cy, and given d8 LCMV-immune spleen cells on the following day. Samples of CSF were taken after a further 72h.

[c] Lysis of YAC-1 targets is a measure of NK activity, while CTL killing is detected on the MHC-compatible MC57G-LCMV target.

Treatment of the cy-suppressed, recipient mice with anti-$ASGM_1$ was also tried in the indirect, adoptive transfer model (19). The anti-$ASGM_1$ was found both to reduce the level of meningeal inflammatory process, and to eliminate completely all evidence of CTL activity from the spleens of the recipients. T cells are known to be $ASGM_1$ positive and, in these immunosuppressed recipients, anti-$ASGM_1$ can apparently remove the donor CTL, though this does not seem to occur in immunologically intact mice. Cyclophosphamide treatment reduces NK activity (10, 20) and thus, perhaps, the number of cells in lymphoid tissue that will competitively bind anti-$ASGM_1$.

The question of the need, or otherwise, for NK effectors to contribute to the development of fatal LCM was, however, resolvedby the adoptive transfer approach (19). No evidence of NK activity was found in spleen or CSF of Cy-suppressed, virus-infected recipients dying at 72 to 96 hours after the inoculation of immune spleen cells (Expt.3, YAC-1 targets, Table 1). It thus seems likely that the final cause of clinical LCM is not NK-mediated cytotoxic damage.

(B) Monocyte/macrophage

The presence and distribution of monocyte/macrophages in the CSF, meninges, choroid plexus and ependyma has been approached using two different types of immunohistochemical techniques. Brains from clinically-affected mice were perfused with periodate-lysine-paraformaldehyde (21), embedded in RAL paraffin wax and sections were then stained with the F4/80 monoclonal antibody (mAb), which is considered to be specific for cells of the monocyte/macrophage series (22), and with mAb to class II MHC glycoprotein (Ia). Histochemical analyses were made following staining with a peroxidase-labelled second antibody. The other approach was to stain isolated CSF cells with mAbs to the Pgp-1 (phagocyte glycoprotein) marker (23) and, following incubation with fluorescinated anti-Ig, analyse the cell populations by flow microfluorimetry (FMF) using a FACS 440 (Becton Dickinson). The advantage of Pgp-1 is that there are two different alleles in the readily available mouse strains (23), thus enabling the relative contributions of the donor and recipient to be assessed in the adoptive transfer model. The disadvantage is that, as discussed in the later, section on T cells, the marker is not found solely on cells of the monocyte/macrophage series (23).

The results of a typical histological analysis are shown in Table 2. In the experiment presented here approximately 22% of the inflammatory cells involved in the choriomeningitis were found to be $F4/80^+$ in mice with symptoms following direct i.c. injection of virus, while 45% were $F4/80^+$ in the disease induced by adoptive transfer (line 1, Table 2). It is interesting that many fewer cells were Ia^+ in the latter case: this may be a result of the treatment with Cy 96 hours previously. Cells classed as monocytes (crescent shaped nucleus) were often Ia^-, while all macrophages that obviously contained ingested material were Ia^+. The other intriguing point that has emerged from this study is that, though gamma interferon (which is secreted by many T cells (24)) has been shown to induce Ia^+ expression on vascular elements (25) there was littele evidence of Ia^+ blood vessels in these clinically-affected mice.

Table 2. Distribution of $F4/80^+$ and Ia^+ cells in CSF inflammatory exudates of mice with clinical LCM

		Direct model[a]		Indirect model[b]	
		$F4/80^{+}$[c]	Ia^+	$F4/80^+$	Ia^+
% of total inflammatory cells		22	12	45	9
% of F4/80 and Ia cells in different categories	monocytes	13	5	13	3
	macrophages	73	78	70	73
	tissue macrophages	15	17	16	27

[a] C57Bl/6J mice dying at 7 days after i.c. injection of LCMV.

[b] C57Bl/6J mice with symptoms at 72h after the adoptive transfer of syngeneic immune spleen cells.

[c] Both monoclonal antibodies are IgG_{2b}:F4/80[22] is specific for cells of the monocyte/macrophage series, while the anti-Ia (M5/114.15.2, TIB120, American type culture collection) binds to common determinants expressed on molecules encoded at both I-A and I-E.

More than 50% of the inflammatory cells that were isolated from CSF of mice showing symptoms of LCM were Pgp1$^+$ (lines 1 and 2, Table 3). An adoptive transfer experiment (line 3, Table 3) indicated that the larger cells in this Pgp1$^+$ population were predominantly of recipient origin. There was also a set of generally smaller, donor-derived Pgp1$^+$ cells which is discussed later in the section on T cells. The most likely explanation is that the majority of the larger Pgp1$^+$ cells belong to the monocyte/macrophage series, though they could also represent a proportion of other cell types of haemopoietic origin. However, there are very few polymorphonuclear leucocytes present in the LCM inflammatory exudate.

Table 3. The Pgp-1 phenotype of large, freshly isolated CSF cells from mice with clinical LCM

Mouse strains	% of CSF positive[c]	
	Pgp-1.1	Pgp-1.2
C57Bl/6J (B6)[a]	0	56
BALB/c.H-2^b [a]	53	0
B6 BALB/c.H-2^b [b]	45	0

[a] Mice sampled at 6 days after i.c. inoculation with virus.

[b] CSF taken at 96h after i.v. inoculation of 1.0 x 10^7 B6 immune spleen cells into Cy-suppressed, virus-infected, BALB/c.H-2^b recipients.

[c] Cells stained by indirect immunofluorescence with alpha-Pgp-1.1 mAb RAM or alpha-Pgp-1.2 mAb C71 and analysed by FMF; values represent % positively stained above controls stained with the inappropriate alpha-Pgp-1 mAb.

It is thus clear that there are many monocyte/macrophages involved in the LCM inflammatory process, whether induced by direct inoculation of virus or by adoptive transfer of immune spleen cells. This has not, to date, helped us to determine the role, or otherwise, of these cells in the induction of clinical LCM (26). The resolution of this question may rest with the experiment of Baenziger and colleagues (27), which demonstrated that cloned CTL can induce fatal LCM following i.c. inoculation into lethally-irradiated, virus-infected recipients.

(C) T cells

We showed many years back that the inflammatory process in murine LCM contains virus-immune CTL (28): this has now been confirmed for both the direct and the indirect models (MC57G-LCM targets, Table 1) (16). Furthermore, the disease is only induced by class I MHC-restricted effectors (5), and the inflammatory process is triggered by T cells that are Lyt2$^+$ L3T4- (manuscript in preparation). Recent experiments have concentrated on using FMF to analyse the phenotype of the T cells in the CSF. The findings for the direct and indirect (adoptive transfer) models are somewhat different.

C,i Direct model

It has proved quite difficult to demonstrate that there are significant (above background due to staining by the second antibody) numbers of T cells present in CSF taken from clinically affected mice that were injected i.c. with LCMV 6 days previously. Also, limiting dilution analysis has, to date, indicated that only about 1:1,000 of the LCM inflammatory exudate cells can be clonally expanded in vitro to give LCMV-specific CTL: this compares with 1:80 to 1:160 for a comparable inflammatory process induced by vaccinia virus (29). Even so, a frequency of 1:1,000 would mean that the CSF of a clinically affected mouse contains 50 to 100 LCMV-specific CTL[2], which may well be sufficient to cause dysfunction. It is also possible that our findings are an underestimate of the number of LCMV-immune T cells in the CNS, perhaps because many of the specifically reactive lymphocytes are intimately associated with virus-infected cells in the ependyma, choroid plexus and meninges, and are not free-floating in the CSF. This is one of the next questions that we have to address.

A significant number of T cells can, however, be shown to be present in CSF by criteria other than CTL-mediated lysis. The inflammatory cells from clinically-affected mice were incubated in vitro for 5 days in the presence of phorbol ester (PMA), calcium ionophore and interleukin-2 (IL-2), a procedure which is known to expand T cell populations (30). The cells surviving at 5 days were then assessed by FMF and shown to be 95% $Thy1^+$ (Table 4). The dominant population was $Lyt2^+$, and many of the lymphocytes expressed IL-2 receptors (31). An intriguing finding is that the majority of these T cells are apparently $Pgp1^+$ (Table 4) as described for T cells activated by Concanavalin A, though most of the Pgp^+ cells found in freshly recovered CSF are larger in size and are probably monocyte/macrophages (Table 3). The next experiments will be concerned with analysing the virus specificity of the in vitro-expanded T cells, using the limited dilution approach.

Table 4. The surface phenotype of CSF cells cultured for 5 days in the presence of PMA, Ionomycin and IL-2[a]

Monoclonal antibody	Surface positive	% cells positive[b] by FMF
AT83	Thy 1.2	95
53.6.7	Lyt-2	78
GK1.5	L3T4	10
RAM	Pgp-1.1	85
PC61	IL-2R	65

[a] CSF cells were cultured at 5 x 10^5/ml with PMA 3ng/ml, Ionomycin 500 ng/ml and IL-2 40U/ml.

[b] Cells were stained by indirect immunofluorescence and analysed by flow microfluormetry (FMF); values represent % positively stained above controls stained with the second step reagent alone.

C, ii Indirect model

The situation with the adoptive transfer model is much more in accord with expectations from the results of CTL assays (16). There is a substantial population of activated T cells in the CSF as shown by the presence of $Thy1^+$ $Lyt2^+$ cells which are $Pgp1^+$ (donor phenotype; Table 5). A proportion of larger cells were also bearing the recipient Pgp1 phenotype. These $Thy1^+$ cells are presumably equivalent to the activated T cells that were expanded in vitro from the day 6 CSF cells (direct model). The fact that T cells are $Pgp\text{-}1^+$ in CSF emphasizes their "activated" status. The obvious question raised is why the findings for FMF of freshly-isolated CSF from the direct and indirect models are divergent. The one, major difference which we are aware of between the models is that CSF from mice injected i.c. with virus 6 days previously contains potent NK effectors, while we could not find any evidence of NK activity in virus-infected, cy-suppressed recipients that had developed immunopathology as a consequence of the adoptive transfer of immune cells (16). Perhaps the NK cells simply dilute the number of T cells present in CSF in the direct model.

Table 5. Surface phenotype of freshly-isolated CSF cells from BALB/c $H\text{-}2^b$ (Pgp-1.1) recipients given immune B6 (Pgp1.2) immune spleen cells 6 days previously

Surface[a] marker	% of CSF[b] positive
Pgp1.1	36
Pgp1.2	43
Thy1	57
Lyt2	51
L3T4	11

[a] As described in Table 4.

[b] The Pgp1.1 cells were generally larger, though there is some overlap.

SUMMARY

The CSF inflammatory process in murine LCM is triggered by $Thy1^+$ $Lyt2^+$, $L3T4^-$, class I MHC-restricted T cells, and is modulated by class I MHC Ir gene effects. Lymphocytes that are lytic for class I MHC compatible, virus-infected target cells are present in the inflammatory exudate. However, from flow microfluorimetric (FMF) analysis of freshly-isolated CSF populations, it has proved surprisingly difficult to demonstrate that many T cells have localized to the site of virus-induced inflammatory process in mice that were injected i.c. with virus 6 days previously and are clinically affected. Limiting dilution analysis indicates that as few as 1:1,000 of these CSF cells may by LCMV-specific CTL precursors. Even so, a significant population of T cells can be expanded from the CSF by incubation in vitro with phorbol ester, calcium ionophore and Il-2. The majority of these T cells are $Lyt2^+$, but their specificity profiles have not yet been determined. This may prove a useful, general method for recovering small numbers of T cells from sites of pathology. In contrast, the

CSF of virus-infected, cyclophosphamide-suppressed mice that have developed LCM as a consequence of the adoptive transfer of immune spleen cells does contain a substantial component of Thy1$^+$, Lyt2$^+$ cells that can be demonstrated by FMF of freshly-isolated inflammatory exudate.

Another difference between the inflammatory process caused by direct inoculation of LCMV and that resulting from the adoptive transfer of immune spleen cells is that there are potent NK effectors in the former, but not in the latter, case. Apparently NK-mediated cytotoxicity is not essential for the development of neurological symptoms. Large numbers of macrophages are also present in the inflammatory site and are, from adoptive transfer protocols, considered to be predominantly of recipient origin. However, it is not clear whether macrophages play any role in the induction of neurological symptoms.

ACKNOWLEDGEMENTS

We thank Diana Hartley for capable technical assistance.

REFERENCES

1. P.C. Doherty and R.M. Zinkernagel. T cell-mediated immunopathology in viral infections. Transplant. Rev. 19:89 (1974).
2. J.E. Allan, J.E. Dixon and P.C. Doherty. Nature of the inflammatory process in the central nervous system of mice infected with lympho cytic choriomeningitis virus. Curr. Top. Microbiol. Immunol. In press (1986).
3. M.J. Buchmeier, R.M. Welsh, F.J. Dutko and M.B.A. Oldstone. The virology and immunobiology of lymphocytic choriomeningitis virus infection. Adv. Immunol. 30:275 (1980).
4. J.E. Allan and P.C. Doherty. Consequences of a single Ir-gene defect for the pathogenesis of lymphocytic choriomeningitis. Immunogenetics. 21:581 (1985).
5. P.C. Doherty, M.B.C. Dunlop, C.R. Parish and R.M. Zinkernagel. Inflammatory process in murine lymphocytic choriomeningitis is maximal in H-2K or H-2D compatible interactions. J. Immunol. 117:187 (1976).
6. P.C. Doherty and W. Gerhard. Breakdown of the blood-cerebrospinal fluid barrier to immunoglobulin in mice injected intracerebrally with a neurotropic influenza A virus. J. Neuroimmunol. 1:227 (1981).
7. P.C. Doherty and R. Korngold. Characteristics of poxvirus-induced meningitis: virus-specific and non-specific cytotoxic effectors in the inflammatory exudate. Scand. J. Immunol. 18:1 (1983).
8. J.E. Allan and P.C. Doherty. Consequences of cyclophosphamide treatment in murine lymphocytic choriomeningitis: evidence for cytotoxic T cell replication in vivo. Scand. J. Immunol. 22:367 (1985).
9. D. Moskophidis and F. Lehmann-Grube. The immune response of the mouse to lymphocytic choriomeningitis virus III. Differences in numbers of cytotoxic T lymphocytes in spleens of mice of different strains. Cell. Immunol. 77:279 (1983).
10. P.C. Doherty and J.E. Allan. Hybrid resistance modulates the inflammatory process induced by lymphocytic choriomeningitis virus-immune T cells. Immunology. 57:515 (1986).
11. A.R. Thomsen, M. Volkert and O. Marker. The timing of the immune response in relation to virus growth determines the outcome of LCM infection. Acta Path. Microbiol. Scand. Sect. C. 87:47 (1979).

12. J.E. Allan and P.C. Doherty. Immune T cells can protect or induce fatal neurological disease in murine lymphocytic choriomeningitis. Cell. Immunol. 90:401 (1985).
13. E.A. Clarke and R.C. Harmon. Genetic control of natural cytotoxicity and hybrid resistance. Adv. Cancer Res. 31:227 (1980).
14. R.M. Welsh and R.M. Zinkernagel. Heterospecific cytotoxic cell activity induced during the first three days of acute lymphocytic choriomeningitis infection in mice. Nature. 268:646 (1977).
15. L. Stitz, A. Althage, H. Hengartner and R.M. Zinkernagel. Natural killer cells vs cytotoxic T cells in the peripheral blood of virus-infected mice. J. Immunol. 134:598 (1985).
16. J.E. Allan and P.C. Doherty. Natural killer cells contribute to inflammation but do not appear to be essential for the induction of clinical lymphocytic choriomeningitis. Scand. J. Immunol. In press. (1986).
17. R.M. Welsh and R.W. Kiessling. Natural killer cell response to lymphocytic choriomeningitis virus in beige mice. Scand. J. Immunol. 11:363 (1980).
18. H. Yong, G. Yogeswaran, J.F. Bukowski and R.M. Welsh. Expression of asialo GM_1 and other antigens and glycolipids on natural killer cells and spleen leukocytes in virus-infected mice. Nat. Immun. Cell Growth Regul. 4:21 (1985).
19. P.C. Doherty and J.E. Allan. In vivo treatment with antibody to the asialo GM_1 ganglioside inhibits both the adoptive transfer of inflammatory process in murine lymphocytic choriomeningitis and the generation of anti-viral cytotoxic T lymphocytes in cyclophosphamide-suppressed recipients. Manuscript submitted for publication.
20. N. Hanna and I.J. Fidler. Role of natural killer cells in the destruction of circulating tumor emboli. J. Natl. Cancer Inst. 65:801 (1980).
21. I.W. McLean and P.K. Nakane. Periodate-lysine paraformaldehyde fixative. A new fixative for immunoelectron microscopy. J. Histochem. Cytochem. 22:1077 (1974).
22. J.M. Austyn and S. Gordon. A monoclonal antibody directed specifically against the mouse macrophage. Eur. J. Immunol. 10:805 (1981).
23. I.S. Trowbridge, J. Lesley, R. Hyman and J. Trotter. Biochemical characterization and cellular distribution of a polymorphic, murine cell-surface glycoprotein expressed on lymphoid tissues. Immunogenetics. 15:299 (1982).
24. P.M. Taylor and B.A. Askonas. Diversity in the biological properties of anti-influenza cytotoxic T cell clones. Eur. J. Immunol. 13:707 (1983).
25. J.S. Pober, T. Collins, M.A. Grimbrone Jr., R.S. Cotran, J.D. Gitlin, W. Fierz, C. Clayberger, A.M. Kirensky, S.J. Burakoff and C.S. Reiss. Lymphocytes recognize human vascular dermal fibroblast Ia antigens induced by recombinant immune interferon. Nature. 305:726 (1983).
26. A.R. Thomsen and M. Volkert. Studies on the role of mononuclear phagocytes in resistance to acute lymphocytic choriomeningitis virus infection. Scand. J. Immunol. 18:271 (1983).
27. J. Baenziger, H. Hengartner, R.M. Zinkernagel and G.A. Cole. Induction or prevention of immunopathological disease by cloned cytotoxic T cell lines specific for lymphocytic choriomeningitis virus. Eur. J. Immunol. In press (1986).
28. R.M. Zinkernagel and P.C. Doherty. Cytotoxic thymus-derived lymphocytes in cerebrospinal fluid of mice with lymphocytic choriomeningitis. J. Exp. Med. 138:1266 (1973).
29. J.L. Hurwitz, R. Korngold and P.C. Doherty. Specific and non-specific T-cell recruitment in viral meningitis:possible implications for autoimmunity. Cell. Immunol. 76:397 (1983).

30. A. Truneh, F. Albert, P. Goldstein and A.M. Schmitt-Verhulst. Early steps of lymphocytic activation by-passed by calcium ionophores and phorbol ester acting in synergy. Nature. 313:318 (1985).
31. R. Ceredig, J.W. Lowenthal, M. Nabholz and H.R. MacDonald. Expression of interleukin-2 receptors as a differentiation marker on intrathymic stem cells. Nature. 314:98 (1985).

IDENTIFICATION OF THE INFLAMMATORY CELLS IN THE CENTRAL NERVOUS SYSTEM DURING ACUTE VIRAL ENCEPHALITIS

Diane E. Griffin, Thomas R. Moench, Jay L. Hess and Richard T. Johnson

Departments of Medicine and Neurology
The John Hopkins University of Medicine, Baltimore
Maryland 21205

INTRODUCTION

The inflammatory response to viral infections of the central nervous system (CNS) is characteristically composed of mononuclear cells. The full development of this response is an immunologically specific event that is dependent on the presence sensitized T lymphocytes (1-4) and CNS mast cells (5,6). We have used a murine model of acute, non-fatal meningoencephalitis caused by Sindbis virus to study the inflammatory cells appearing in all compartments of the CNS during infection and recovery from infection.

Sindbis virus is alphavirus closely related to Western and Eastern equine encephalitis viruses. This virus replicates rapidly and pantropically in neuronal, ependymal and glial cells of the brains of intracerebrally-inoculated mice. Virus is cleared from the CNS within 7-8 days after infection and mice recover uneventfully (7). Thus, studies of such mice can be used to clarify and dissect various components of the immune response to defined foreign antigens within the CNS.

TIME COURSE OF THE INFLAMMATORY RESPONSE

A mononuclear inflammatory response is reproducibly elicited in the cerebrospinal fluid (CSF), the meninges and the brains of Sindbis virus-infected mice. All of these inflammatory reactions begin tree days after infection co-incident with the development of cellular and humoral virus-specific immunity (1,8). Although both perivascular cuffing and the CSF pleocytosis appear at the same time, the time course of subsequent cellular infiltration differs in the brain and CSF (Fig.1) (9). CSF cells reach their maximum numbers rapidly, 4-5 days after infection, while maximal parenchymal inflammation does not occur until 6-10 days after infection. These observations suggested that the types of mononuclear cells appearing in these two important CNS compartments might be different.

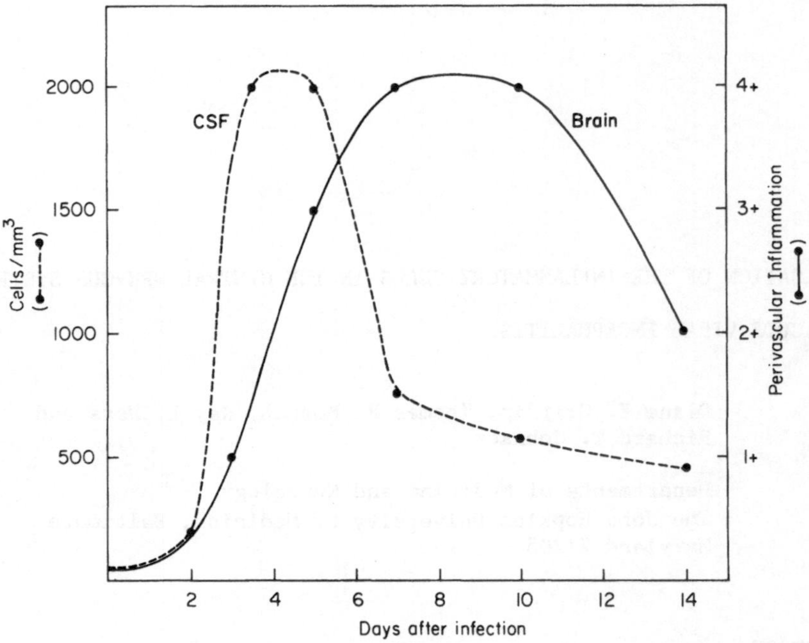

Fig.1. Time course of the development of the mononuclear inflammatory response in the cerebrospinal fluid (CSF) and brains of mice inoculated intracerebrally with Sindbis virus (9,10).

CHARACTERIZATION OF THE MONONUCLEAR CELLS

Immunocytochemical analysis of the types of mononuclear cells was performed using the avidin-biotin peroxidase method (9) and monoclonal antibodies specific for T helper/inducer cells (Lyt-1), T cytotoxic/suppressor cells (Lyt-2), B cells (RA32C2) and monocyte/macrophages (F4/80). Cells in the parenchymal perivascular cuffs are composed of T cells, B cells, monocytes and a variable number of unidentified cells (Fig.2). In the earliest phase only T cells are identifiable. B cells and monocytes gradually become more abundant with time and become the predominant cells during the recovery phase of the infection. T helper/inducer ($T_{H/I}$) cells increase with time while the percentage of T cytotoxic/suppressor ($T_{c/s}$) cells remains the same. This results in $T_{H/I}$ to $T_{c/s}$ ratios ranging from 2:1 (d3-5) to 5:1 (d10) at various phases of the response (Fig.3). It is postulated that T helper/inducer cells provide the immunologic specificity for the inflammatory response and are therefore among the earliest cells from the peripheral blood to arrive at the site of virus replication. Upon antigenic stimulation these lymphocytes produce a variety of lymphokines including chemotactic factors for monocytes and probably for B cells (12,13). The delayed appearance of macrophages and B cells in the perivascular cuffs suggest that these cells are recruited to the local area of virus replication secondarily by the earlier appearing virus-sensitized T lymphocytes. The cellular composition of parenchymal inflammation is similar to that of a classic delayed type hypersensitivity response (14).

The cells in the CSF are more homogeneous than those in perivascular cuffs. They are T cells and unidentified cells early (d3-5) shifting to essentially all T cells later (d7-10) (Fig.2). Only very small numbers (<2%) of B cells and monocytes are present at any time. Appearance of antiviral antibody in the CSF correlates not with the presence of B cells or any other type of cell in the CSF but rather with the appearance of B cells in the brain parenchyma (Fig.4) suggesting that B cells are differentiating and producing IgG and IgA locally in the brain parenchyma which then appears in the CSF. T cells of the helper/inducer phenotype are always more numerous than T cells of the cytotoxic/suppressor phenotype with ratios varying from 1.4:1 (d3-7) to 3:1 (d10-14) (Fig.3). It is not clear why these T cells do not recruit monocytes and B cells into the CSF as well as the brain parenchyma. This may be a manifestation of the major histocompatibility complex (MHC) region-restricted interaction of T lymphocytes with virus-infected cells or tissues (16-20). The MHC restriction implies that antigen-specific T cells, in order to lyse infected cells (19), or be stimulated to lymphokine production (17,18), must recognize not only a specific viral antigen, but viral antigen on infected cells. Cell-associated virus for T cell recognition is found in the brain parenchyma, but primarily cell-free virus is found in the CSF. Monocytes and B cells may therefore be recruited into the brain parenchyma but not into the CSF.

Despite using markers for T cells, B cell and macrophages, the major subclasses of immune cells, not all of the mononuclear cells present could be identified. Since most of the unidentified cells are present at the earliest time points in the inflammatory response it was postulated that some of these cells may be natural killer (NK) cells which tend to be induced early in viral infections (9). Assays for NK cell activity in the CSF using the YAC-1 target cell showed that NK activity was much higher in the CSF than in the blood or spleens of the same animals on d3, was slightly elevated on d5 and essentially equal to blood on d7 (Fig.5) indicating that NK cells are induced by viral infection and are present in high concentration in the CNS during encephalitis. These data suggest that many of the CSF cells unidentifiable by immunocytochemical staining may be NK cells (21).

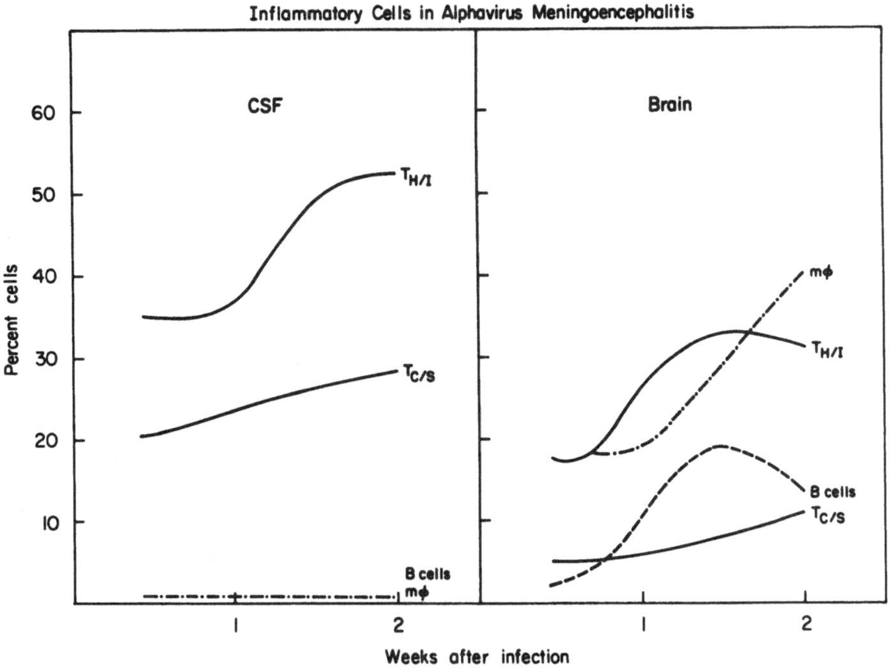

Fig.2. Types of mononuclear cells found in the cerebrospinal fluid (CSF) and brain perivascular cuffs of mice inoculated intracerebrally with Sindbis virus (9,11).

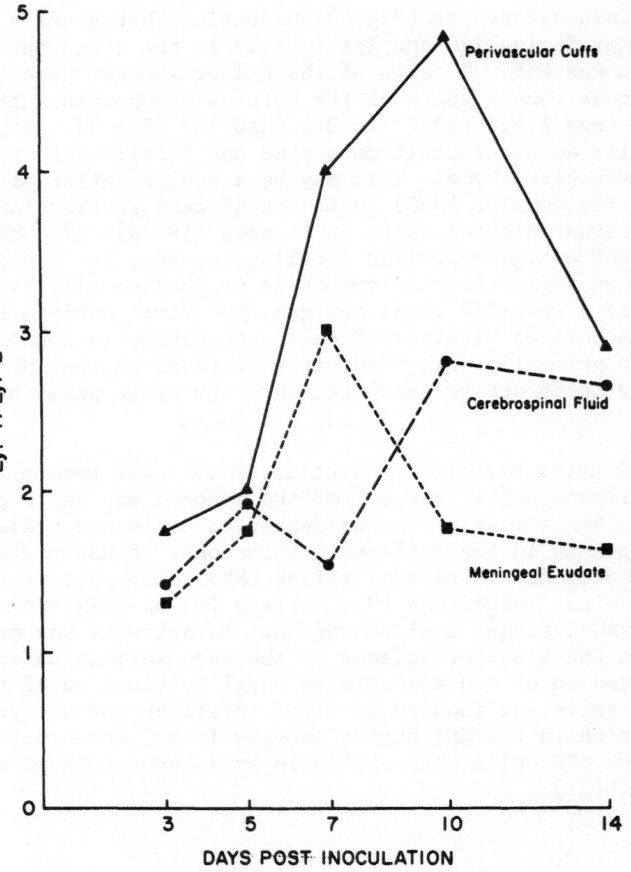

Fig.3. Ratios of cells with the helper/inducer phenotype (Lyt 1) to T cells with the cytotoxic/suppressor phenotype (Lyt 2) in different central nervous system compartments of mice inoculated intracerebrally with Sindbis virus (9).

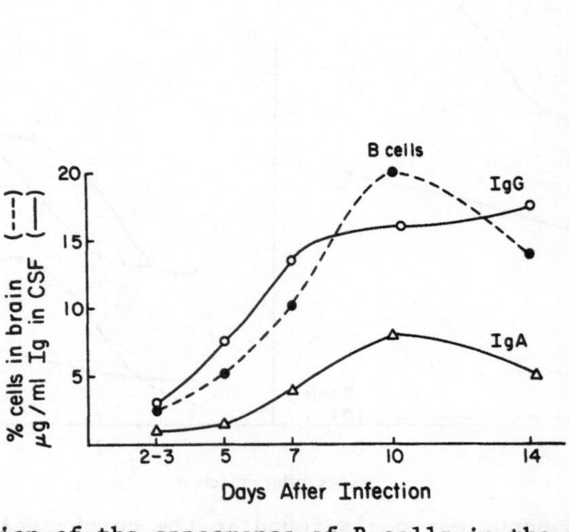

Fig.4. Correlation of the appearance of B cells in the perivascular cuffs of the brain and IgG and IgA in the cerebrospinal fluid (9,15).

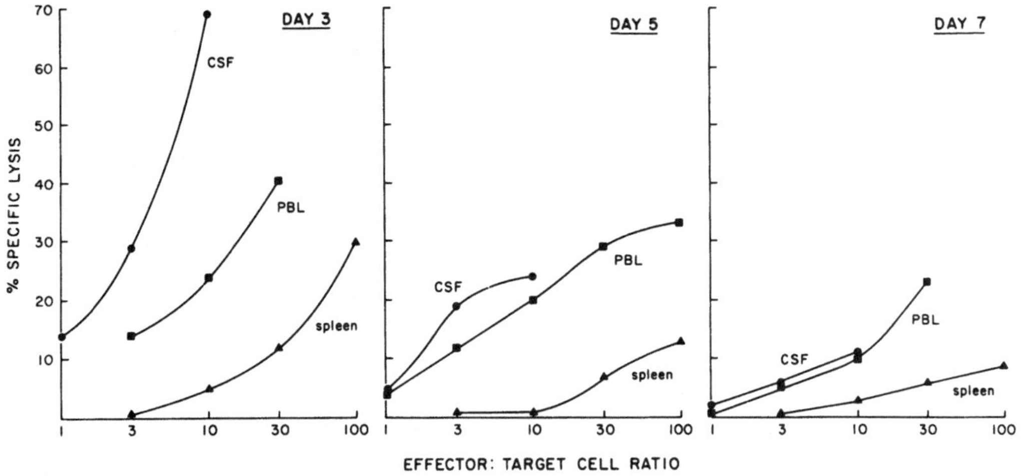

Fig.5. Natural killer cell activity in the spleen, peripheral blood (PBL) and cerebrospinal fluid (CSF) of mice inoculated intracerebrally with Sindbis virus (21).

STUDIES IN MAN

Studies similar to those done in mice have been done on patients with Japanese encephalitis, an acute flavivirus infection with a mortality of 25%. The data from these studies show that the inflammatory response in man to acute viral encephalitis is very similar to that in mice (22,23) (Table 1). During Japanese encephalitis CSF has a higher proportion of T cells and a lower proportion of B cells and macrophages than the perivascular cuffs in the brain parenchyma or the peripheral blood. The proportion of T cells in the CNS which are of the T_4 (helper/inducer) phenotype is increased, compared to blood. In addition, brain and CSF have 15 to 50% unidentified cells suggesting the possible presence of NK cells as a part of the local response to response to viral encephalitis.

Table 1. Mononuclear cells in the Brains, CSF and Blood of patients with Japanese encephalitis (22,23)

Source	Cells (%) T	T4	T_8	B	Mo	% ID	T_4/T_8
Brain	36	-	6	11	17	63	-
CSF	69	48	15	7	7	84	4.2
Blood	44	29	15	26	18	90	2.2

SUMMARY

During acute viral encephalitis, significant differences in the composition of the inflammatory response in the CSF and parenchymal compartments of the CNS are present. The inflammatory infiltrate in CSF reaches a peak and resolves before that of the parenchyma. Few macrophages and B cells are found in the CSF, whereas these cells are prominent components of the parenchymal infiltrate, especially at later time points. Among the T cells present, the representation of the helper/inducer and cytotoxic/ suppressor phenotypes is different in CSF and brain parenchyma, but the helper/inducer phenotype is always most abundant. These studies demonstrate that CSF may not reflect either functionally or phenotypically the composition of inflammatory cells present at the parenchymal site of CNS pathology. Furthermore, these data suggest that the "normal" response to acute viral infection of the CNS is an influx of mononuclear cells which are T cells primarily of the helper/inducer phenotype in the CSF and T cells accompanied by B cells and macrophages in the brain parenchyma.

ACKNOWLEDGEMENTS

This work was supported in part by a grant from the National Multiple Sclerosis Society and by grants NS 18596, NS 07000 and NS 21916 from the National Institutes of Health.

REFERENCES

1. H.F. McFarland, D.E. Griffin and R.T. Johnson. Specificity of the inflammatory response in viral encephalitis. I.Adoptive immunization of immunosuppressed mice infected with Sindbis virus. J. Exp. Med. 136:216-226 (1972).
2. P.C. Doherty and R.M. Zinkernagel. T-cell-mediated immunopathology in viral infections. Transplant. Rev. 19:89-120 (1974).
3. R.V. Blanden. T cell response to viral and bacterial infection. Transplant. Rev. 19:56-88 (1974).
4. M.L. Berger. Immunologic requirements for the adoptive transfer of ectromelia virus meningitis. J. Neuropath. Exp. Neurol. 41:18-33 (1982).
5. F. Mokhtarian and D.E. Griffin. Role of mast cells in virus-induced CNS inflammation in the mouse. Cell. Immunol. 86:491-500 (1984).
6. D.E. Griffin and Q. Mendoza. Identification of the mononuclear cells in the brains of mast-cell deficient (W/W^V) and normal mice during Sindbis-virus induced encephalitis. Cell. Immunol. 97:454-459 (1986).
7. R.T. Johnson, H.F. McFarland and S.E. Levy. Age-dependent resistance to viral encephalitis: Studies of infections due to Sindbis virus in mice. J. Infect. Dis. 125:257-162 (1972).
8. D.E. Griffin. Role of the immune response in age-dependent resistance of mice to encephalitis due to Sindbis virus. J. Infect. Dis. 133: 456-464 (1976).
9. T.R. Moench and D.E. Griffin. Immunocytochemical identification and quantitation of mononuclear cells in cerebrospinal fluid, meninges and brain during acute viral encephalitis. J. Exp. Med. 159:77-88 (1984).
10. D.E. Griffin (in press). Alphavirus Pathogenesis and Immunity. In: Comprehensive Virology: Togaviruses and Flaviviruses. (M. Schlesinger and S. Schlesinger, eds.). Plenum Publishing Corp.,N.Y.
11. D.E. Griffin. The Inflammatory Response to Acute Viral Infections. In: Concepts in Viral Pathogenesis. (A.L. Notkins and M.B.A. Oldstone, eds.). Springer-Verlag, New York. pp. 46-52 (1984).
12. J.J. Oppenheim. Lymphokines. In: Cellular Functions in Immunity and Inflammation (J.J. Oppenheim, D.L. Rosenstreich and M. Potter, eds). Elsevier, NY. pp. 259-282 (1981).
13. F. Mokhtarian, D.E. Griffin and R.L. Hirsch. Production of mononuclear chemotactic factors during Sindbis virus infection of mice. Infect. Immun. 35:965-973 (1982).

14. J.L. Platt, B.W. Grant, A.A. Eddy and A.F. Michael. Immune cell populations in cutaneous delayed-type hypersensitivity. J. Exp. Med. 158:1227-1242 (1983).
15. D.E. Griffin. Immunoglobulins in the cerebrospinal fluid: Changes during acute viral encephalitis in mice. J. Immunol. 126:27-31 (1981).
16. R.M. Zinkernagel and R.M. Welsh. H-2 compatibility requirement for virus-specific T cell-mediated effector functions in vivo. I. Specificity of T cells conferring antiviral protection against lymphocytic choriomeningitis virus is associated with H-2k and H-2D. J. Immunol. 117:1495-1502 (1976).
17. R.M. Zinkernagel. H-2 restriction of virus-specific T cell mediated effector function in vivo. II. Adoptive transfer of delayed-type hypersensitivity to murine lymphocytic choriomeningitis virus is restricted by the K and D region of H-2. J. Exp. Med. 144:766-787 (1976).
18. P.C. Doherty, M.B.C. Dunlop, C.R. Parish and R. Zinkernagel. Inflammatory process in murine lymphocytic choriomeningitis is maximal in H-2K or H-2D compatible interactions. J. Immunol. 117:187-189 (1976).
19. R.M. Zinkernagel and P.C. Doherty. MHC-restricted cytotoxic T cells: Studies on the biological role of polymorphic major transplantation antigens determining T-cell restriction-specific function, and responsiveness. Adv. Immunol. 27:51-171 (1979).
20. M.L. Berger. The role of the major histocompatibility complex in the adoptive transfer of ectromelia virus meningitis. J. Neuropathol. Exp. Neurol. 41:34-44 (1982).
21. D.E. Griffin and J.L. Hess. Cells with natural killer activity in the CSF of normal and athymic nude mice with acute Sindbis virus encephalitis. J. Immunol. 136:1841-1845 (1986).
22. R.T. Johnson, D.S. Burke, M. Elwell, C.J. Leake, A. Nisalak, C.H. Hoke and W. Lorsomrudee. Japanese encephalitis: Immunocytochemical studies of viral antigen and inflammatory cells in fatal cases. Ann. Neurol. 18:567-573 (1985).
23. R.T. Johnson, P. Intralawan and S. Puapanwatton (in press). Japanese encephalitis: Identification of inflammatory cells in cerebrospinal fluid. Ann. Neurol.

NEOPTERIN IN CEREBRO-SPINAL FLUID AS A PARAMETER OF LOCAL CELLULAR IMMUNE REACTIONS IN THE CENTRAL NERVOUS SYSTEM

W. Fierz[1], D. Dommasch[2] and A. Niederwieser[3]

[1] Section of Clinical Immunology, University Hospital Zürich, Switzerland
[2] Clinical Research Unit for Multiple Sclerosis, Max-Planck Society, Würzburg, FRG
[3] Division of Clinical Chemistry, Department of Pediatrics University of Zürich, Switzerland

SUMMARY

The clinical monitoring of cellular immune reactions still poses a problem that is partly based on the difficulty of sampling local cellular infiltrations. Diffusable factors which correlate with cellular immune responses could give at least some immune-nonspecific indication about cellular processes. A cellular interaction that is crucial for the development of immune responses in the central nervous system (CNS) is the induction of Ia (HLA-D) antigens in the primarily Ia-negative CNS by activated T lymphocytes. Since local Ia expression cannot be monitored clinically, we studied the cerebro-spinal fluid (CSF) levels of a small diffusable molecule, i.e. neopterin, that is produced by activated macrophages, similar to Ia antigen expression, as a response to low levels of immune interferon. Increased urinary excretion of neopterin has been previously reported in patients with malignancies, viral infections, rheumatoid arthritis, systemic lupus erythematosus, allograft rejections and graft versus host disease. We studied neopterin and biopterin levels in the CSF of patients with multiple sclerosis (MS) and other neurological diseases (OND) with high performance liquid chromatography (HPLC) and a radioimmunoassay (RIA). Increased levels of neopterin, but not biopterin, were found in two thirds of patients with inflammatory OND of the CNS compared to non-inflammatory OND and in half of the MS patients with relapses, in contrast to patients with inactive chronic progressive MS or MS patients in remission. Neopterin, but not biopterin, levels correlated with leucocyte counts but not with erythrocyte counts. Neopterin levels also correlated with IgG levels in the CSF, but much less so with albumin levels. The measurement of neopterin levels in CSF provides an additional parameter for the diagnosis and monitoring of inflammatory conditions of the CNS, but does not help to distinguish MS from OND.

INTRODUCTION

D-erythro 7,8-dihydroneopterin triphosphate (neopterin), a derivate of guanosine triphosphate (GTP), is a precursor molecule of biopterin which is an essential cofactor for hydroxylation of phenylalanine, tyrosine and tryptophan in the synthesis of the neurotransmitters dopamine and serotonin. Unexpectedly, it has recently been found that neopterin levels are increased during cellular immune responses (Huber et al., 1983) due to an induction of neopterin synthesis and release by macrophages upon a stimulus from T lymphocytes mediated by immune interferon (IFN-y) (Huber et al., 1984). The increased neopterin synthesis is accompanied by an increased intracellular activity of GTP cyclohydrolase I (GTP-CHI) that catalyzes the synthesis of neopterin from GTP (Blau et al., 1985). GTP levels are also increased in stimulated macrophages, in contrast to biopterin levels which remain low (Schoedon et al., 1985).

Activation of immune accessory cells such as macrophages is a pivotal step during the development of cellular immune responses, since the antigen-specific stimulation of T helper lymphocytes is dependent on the activity of antigen-presenting cells (APC) like macrophages. A particularly important mechanism is the induction of increased expression of class II major histocompatibility (MHC) antigens (Ia antigens, HLA-D antigens) through stimulation by T cell-produced IFN-y. Class II antigens are mandatory for the recognition of antigens by T helper cells, because of the MHC restriction of the T cell receptor. The role of APC is especially interesting to study in the CNS, since it has been found that in the normal CNS no class II MHC antigens are expressed (Williams et al., 1980, Momburg et al., 1986). However, in the course of cellular immune reactions in the CNS, class II antigens are found on various cell types within and around cellular infiltrates (Traugott et al., 1983, 1985; ter Laak and Hommes, 1986). The mechanism of class II antigen induction by IFN-y and consequent antigen presentation by cells of the CNS has recently been analysed in vitro with astrocytes (Fierz et al., 1985).

Since both class II antigen expression and neopterin release are induced by IFN-y, the measurement of neopterin levels in the CSF could give an indication about the activation of APC in the CNS, and indirectly about the expression of class II antigens which are otherwise not accessible for clinical examination. We found increased levels of neopterin, but not biopterin, in the CSF of patients with inflammatory CNS conditions and acute relapses of multiple sclerosis. Partial correlations to other inflammatory parameters in the CSF were observed.

MATERIALS AND METHODS

Patients

95 patients were recruited from the outpatient clinic at the Institute for Neurology of the University Hospital of Würzburg (FRG). They were not under immunosuppressive therapy or steroid treatment at the time of the CSF collection. MS patients were grouped into patients with acute relapses or active progression (n=20) and patients in remission or with inactive chronic progressive disease (n=19). Patients with OND were grouped into patients with inflammatory conditions of the CNS (n=19) and patients with noninflammatory conditions of the CNS or affections outside the CNS (n=37).

CSF

Fresh CSF samples were taken from the patients and after removal of the cells by centrifugation for other purposes, the supernatant CSF was alliquoted and immediately analyzed for immunoglobulin G (IgG) and albumin or stored at minus 70°C for pterin analysis. IgG and albumin levels were determined by using a laser nephelometric system (Behring).

Pterin analysis by radioimmunoassay (RIA) and high-performance liquid chromatography (HPLC)

Neopterin levels were determined with a commercial RIA kit (Neopterin-RIAcid, Henning Berlin GmbH) specially adapted to CSF, that measures the oxidized form of neopterin (Rokos et al., 1985a). Neopterin and biopterin were measured with HPLC as described (Niederwieser et al., 1984). Both reduced and oxidized pterins are detected with this technique. Twelve CSF samples were analysed for neopterin with both RIA and HPLC techniques. Comparison of the results gave a good correlation between the two detection methods ($r^2 = 0.98$) applying a linear regression to the logarithms of the neopterin levels. HPLC analysis, however, gave higher levels of neopterin than RIA analysis since neopterins are partially in reduced form in the CSF and therefore not detectable by RIA.

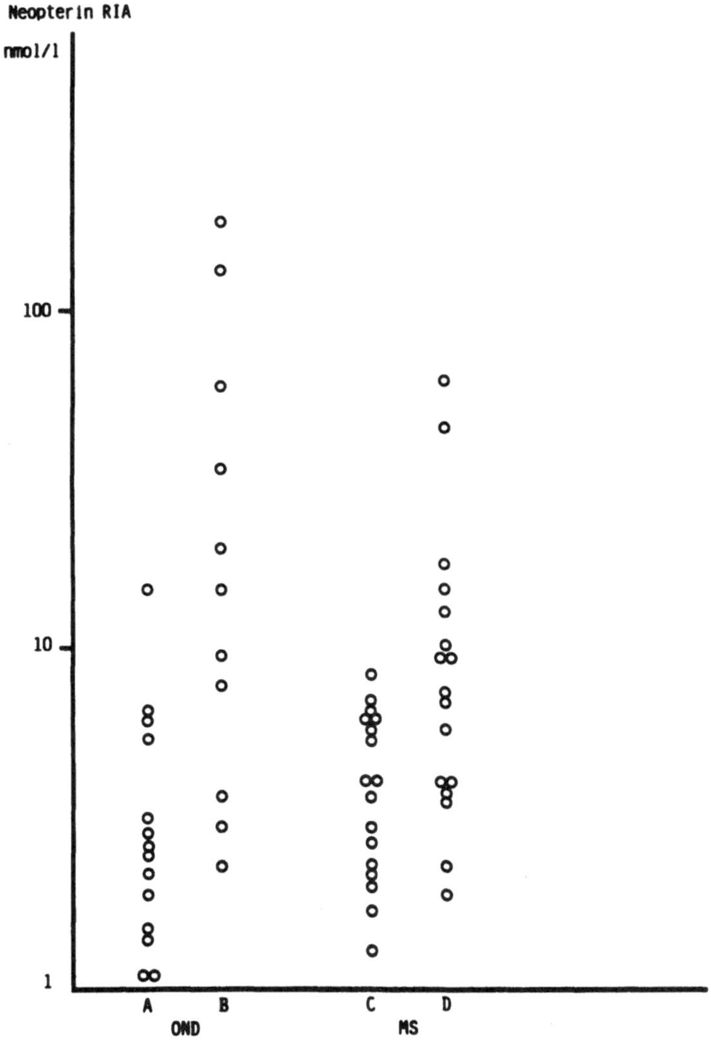

Fig.1. Neopterin levels determined with RIA in CSF from patients with extra-CNS OND or noninflammatory (A) or inflammatory (B) OND of the CNS patient with MS in remission or inactive chronic progression (C) or with acute relapse or active progression (D).

Evaluation of results

Linear regression analysis was performed using the logarithms of cell counts and of levels of neopterin, biopterin, IgG and albumin. Correlation coefficients (r) were tested for their significant departure from zero. Significant differences in pterin levels between groups of patients were calculated by using the Wilcoxon ranking test.

RESULTS

Neopterin and biopterin levels in the CSF of patients with MS and OND

Fig.1. shows levels of neopterin measured with RIA in CSF from patients with noninflammatory CNS diseases or affections outside the CNS (A), patients with inflammatory CNS diseases without MS (B), patients with

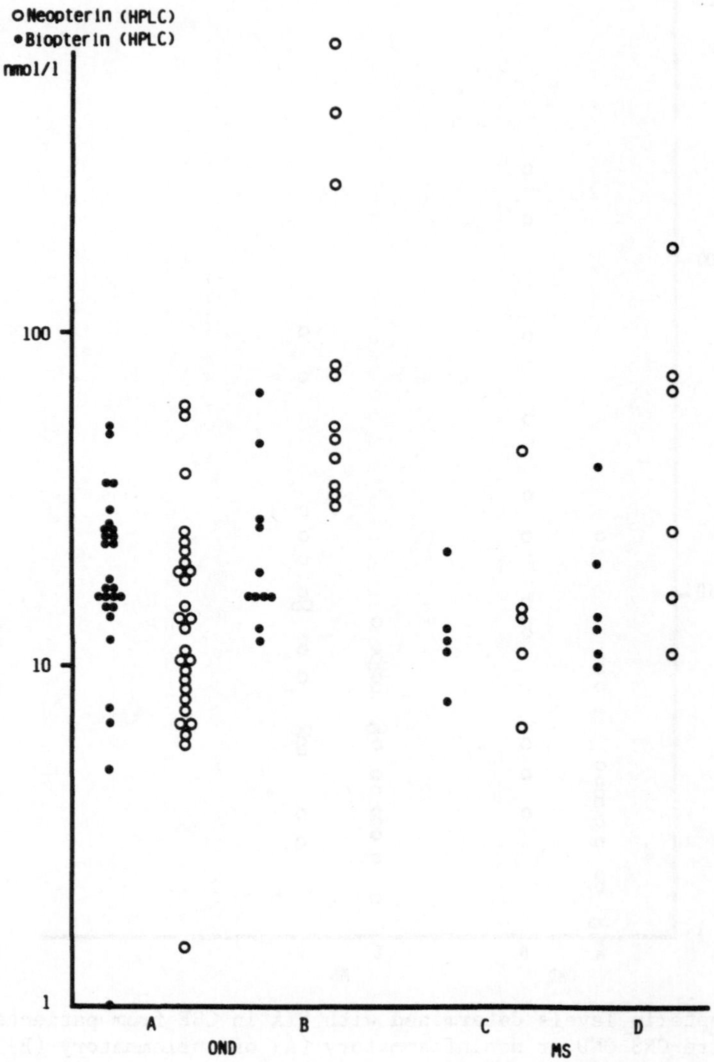

Fig.2. Neopterin (O) and Biopterin (●) levels determined with HPLC in CSF from patients as described in figure 1.

MS in remission or with inactive chronic progressive MS (C) and patients with acute relapses or active progression of MS (D). Neopterin levels are significantly higher in group B compared to group A ($p < 0.005$) and in group D compared to group C ($p < 0.01$). Similar results were reached by using HPLC for measuring neopterin (see Fig.2). Again group B values were significantly higher ($p < 0.001$) than group A values for neopterin. No significant difference, however, is observed for biopterin levels ($p > 0.1$). Group C and D show corresponding tendencies, but no significance is reached because of low numbers.

<u>Comparison of neopterin and biopterin levels with cell counts, IgG and albumin levels</u>

Neopterin levels measured with RIA are compared in Fig.3 with leucocyte and erythrocyte counts in the CSF by applying a linear regression analysis to the logarithms of the values. Neopterin levels correlate significantly ($r^2 = 0.41$) with leucocyte counts, not, however, with erythrocyte counts ($r^2 = 0.02$). A similar degree of correlation results when neopterin levels are compared with IgG levels ($r^2 = 0.44$), but only a minimal correlation is seen with albumin levels ($r^2 = 0.10$) (see Fig.4). These correlations were confirmed when the HPLC technique was used to measure neopterin (Fig. 5,6 and 7) with values of $r^2 = 0.47$ for the correlation with leucocytes, $r^2 = 0.36$ with IgG and $r^2 = 0.14$ with albumin. Biopterin levels, in contrast, did not correlate significantly with leucocyte counts ($r^2 = 0.00$) or albumin levels ($r^2 = 0.03$) and only marginally with IgG levels ($r^2 = 0.17$).

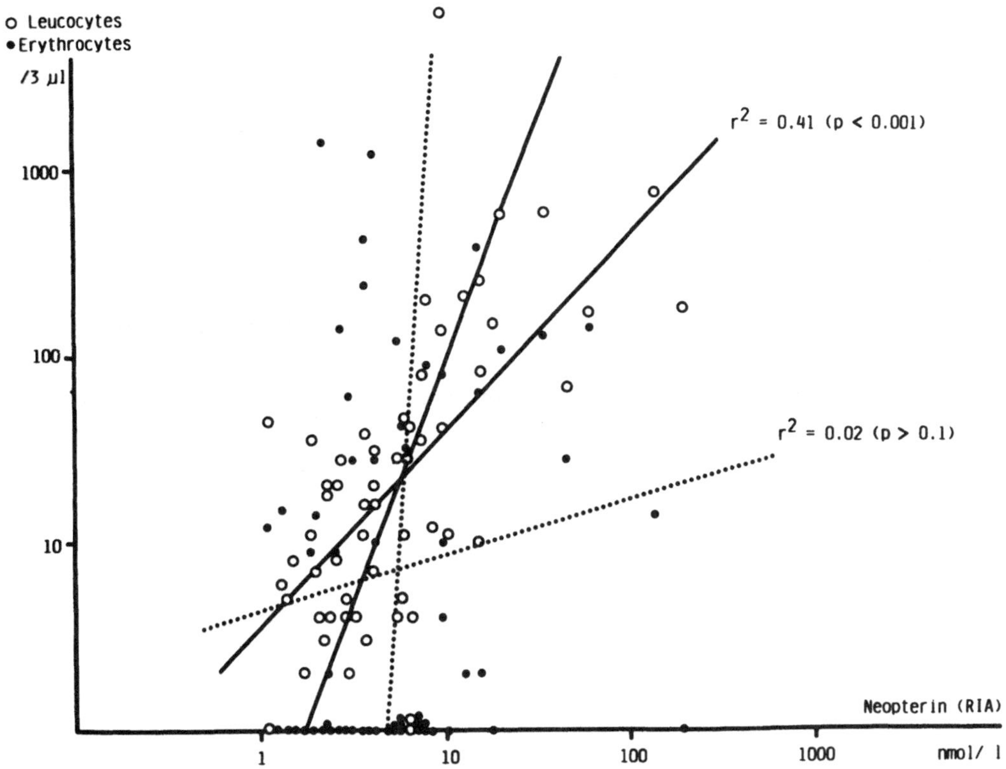

Fig.3. Correlations between neopterin levels (RIA) and leucocyte (O) or erythrocyte (●) counts in CSF.

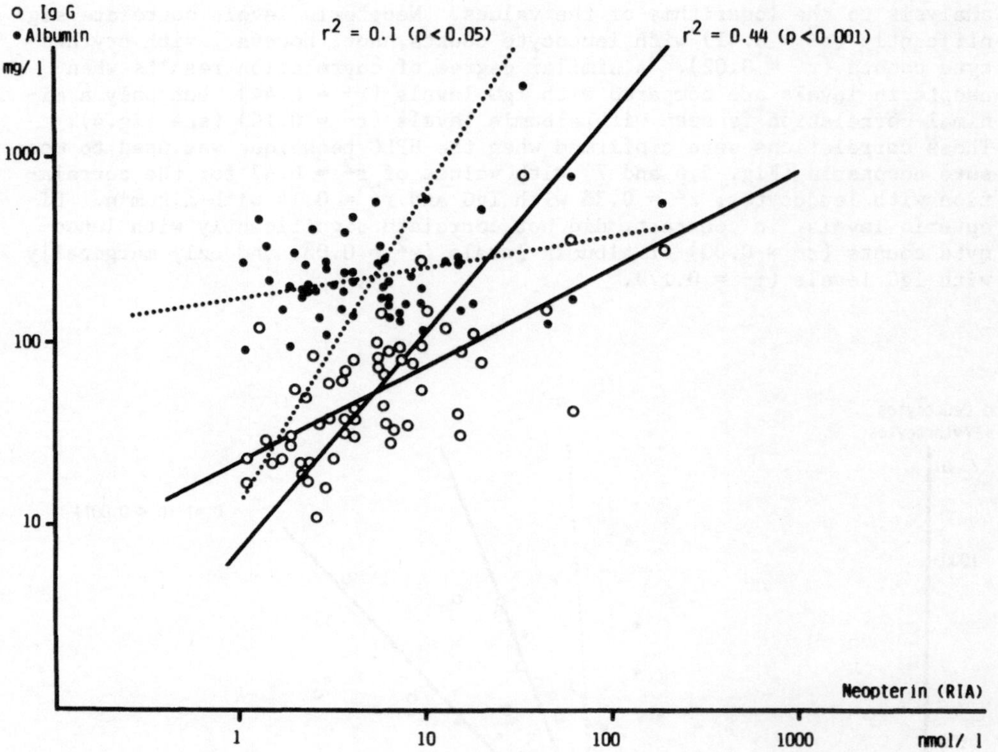

Fig.4. Correlations between neopterin levels (RIA) and IgG (○) or albumin (●) levels in CSF.

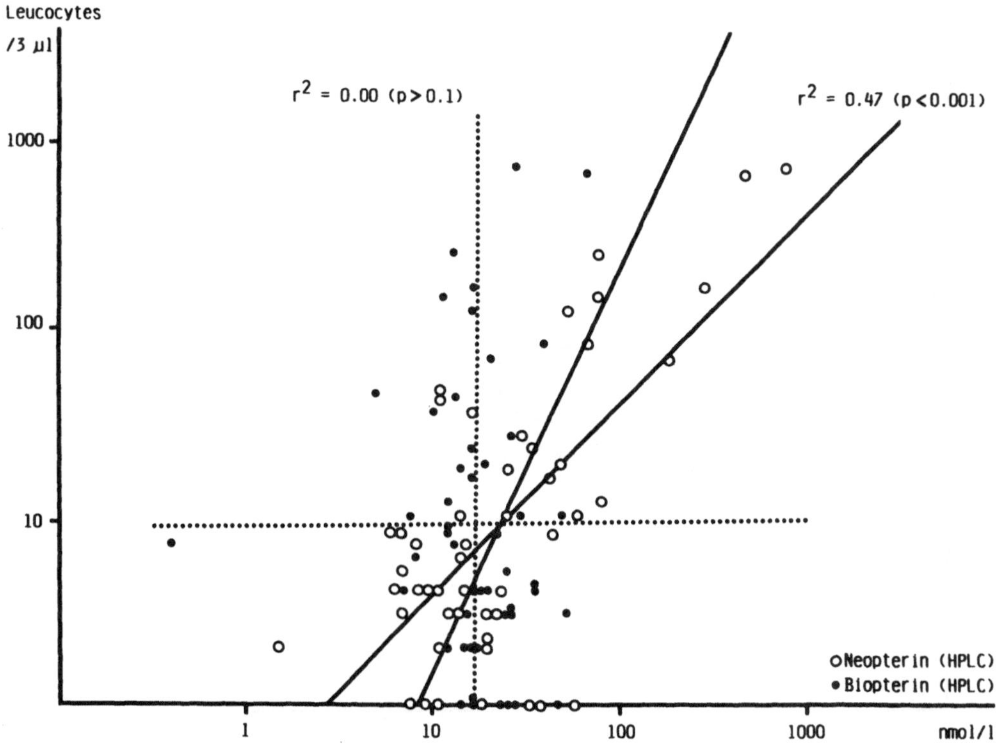

Fig.5. Correlations between neopterin (O) or biopterin (●) levels (HPLC) and leucocyte counts in CSF.

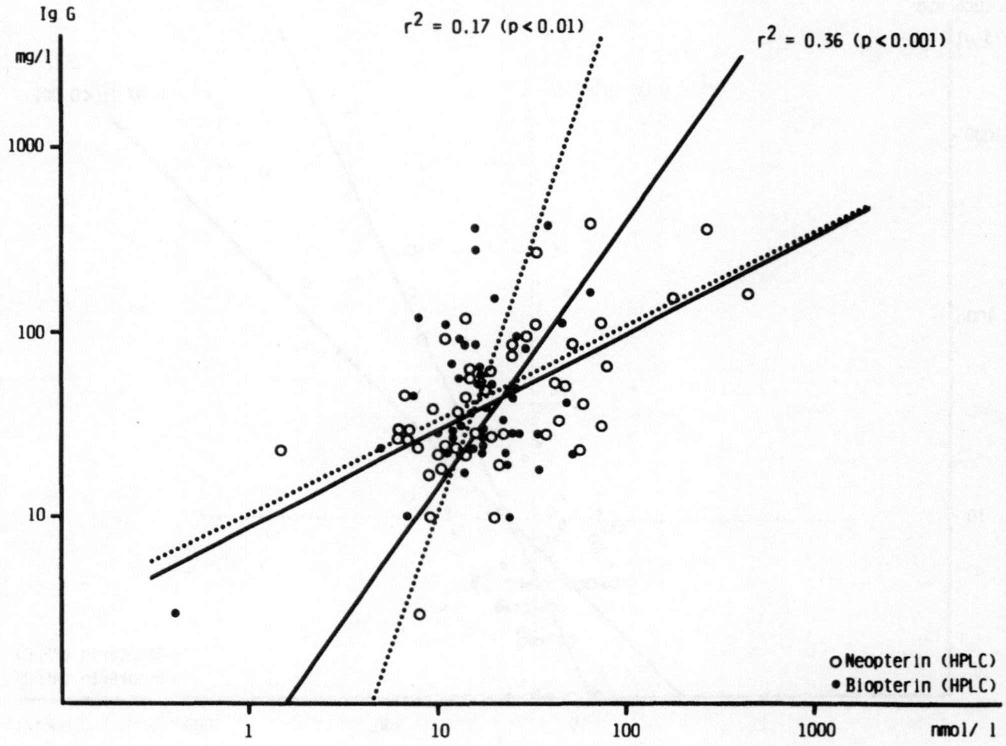

Fig.6. Correlations between neopterin (○) or biopterin (●) levels (HPLC) and IgG in CSF.

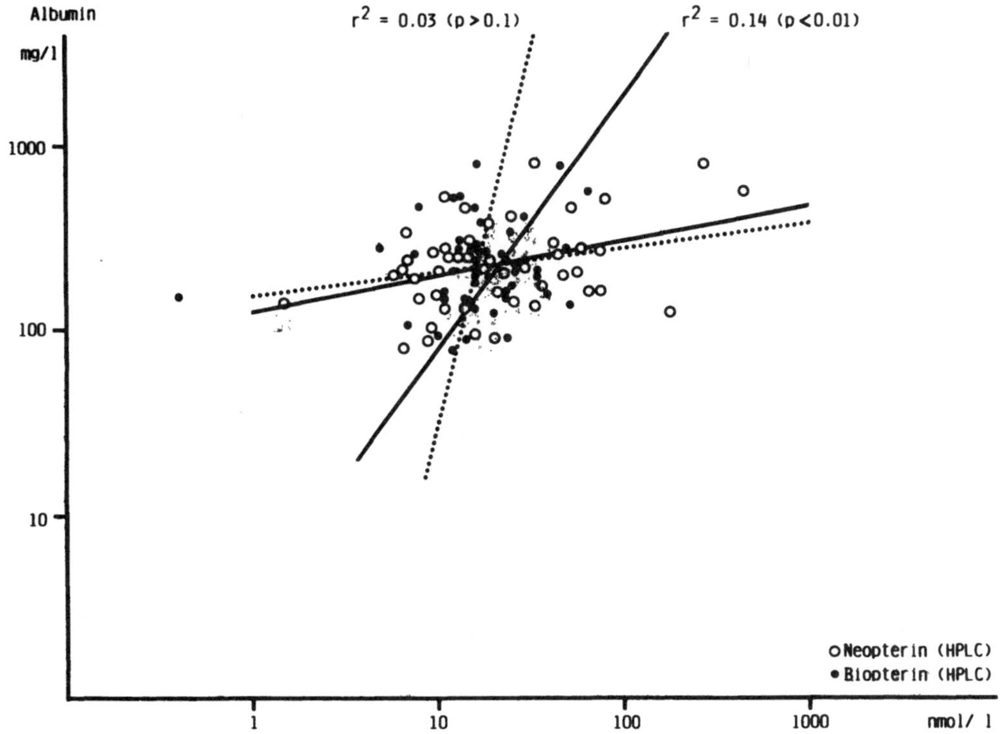

Fig.7. Correlations between neopterin (○) or biopterin (●) levels (HPLC) and albumin in CSF.

DISCUSSION

We studied neopterin and biopterin levels in CSF from patients with MS and OND. Elevated levels of neopterin were found in patients with acute relapses or active progression of MS or other inflammatory diseases of the CNS like viral meningitis/encephalitis, Lyme's disease or malignancies, as compared to patients with MS in remission or inactive chronic progressive MS and patients with noninflammatory CNS diseases or neurological affections outside the CNS like discus prolapse, cervical syndrome, stroke, headache, myasthenia gravis, and others. In contrast to neopterin levels, biopterin levels were not elevated in these inflammatory conditions of the CNS. Neopterin levels, but not biopterin levels, correlated with other parameters of CNS inflammation, i.e. leucocyte counts and IgG levels. In fact, these correlations were as high or higher as the correlation between leucocyte counts and IgG levels which gave a r^2 value of 0.37.

By using leucocyte, IgG and neopterin values of patients with noninflammatory OND (group A) to define upper limits of "normality" in such a way that 90% of group A values lie below these limits, the number of patients in group A,B,C and D was counted that showed elevated levels of leucocytes, IgG or neopterin. As demonstrated in Table 1, the 4 groups of patients are best discriminated with the leucocyte counts. This probably reflects the influence that this parameter had on the clinical diagnosis of inflammatory CNS disease. However, neopterin seems to be as good a parameter as IgG for discrimination between inflammatory and noninflammatory CNS disease. Further analysis showed that none out of 37 patients with noninflammatory OND (A) and only 1 out of 19 patients with MS in remission (C) were positive for all three parameters, i.e. false positive. Similarly, only 1 out of 19 patients with inflammatory CNS disease (B) and 1 out of 19 MS patients with acute relapse (D) were negative for all three parameters, i.e. false negative.

Table 1. Number of patients with elevated values for leucocytes, IgG, or neopterin in the CSF

		OND		MS	
		A	B	C	D
Leucocytes	+	3	16	8	18
> 10/3 µl	-	34	2	11	1
IgG	+	3	11	6	14
> 65mg/l	-	34	7	13	5
Neopterin	+	2	12	2	9
> 7nmol/l*	-	35	6	17	10

* RIA value, corresponds to 40 nmol/l for HPLC values.

In conclusion, measurement of neopterin levels in CSF seems to provide an additional parameter for the diagnosis of inflammatory CNS disease. As with other parameters, however, no specificity for MS was found. Further studies are under way to compare neopterin levels in the CSF with serum levels, and with levels of IFN-y, the inducer of neopterin in macrophages. At the same time, it will be studied whether the use of magnetic resonance imaging that gives a better definition of the degree of CNS inflammation, particularly in MS, will provide a better correlation between clinical course and neopterin levels.

The selective increase of neopterin as compared to biopterin is in accord with the hypothesis that the macrophages are the source of the excess neopterin, since stimulation of macrophages with IFN-y leads only to increased neopterin production but not to biopterin synthesis. In contrast, stimulated T lymphocytes produce only about 10% of neopterin, compared with macrophages, and T cells produce in addition biopterin (Schoedon et al., 1985). Since in parallel with increased neopterin production, macrophages respond to IFN-y also with Ia antigen expression, it would be interesting to know, whether other cells of the CNS also produce neopterin, like astrocytes which can also express Ia antigens when stimulated with IFN-y (Fierz et al., 1985). However, in vitro experiments to study this question are hampered by the fact that neopterin release is restricted to humans, and pterin metabolism in rodents, from which astrocytes are more readily accessible , is different from humans (Rokos et al., 1985b).

ACKNOWLEDGEMENTS

The neopterin RIA kit was kindly provided by Dr. H. Rokos, Henning Berlin GmbH. The Clinical Research Unit for Multiple Sclerosis of the Max-Planck Society is supported by funds from the Hermann and Lilly Schilling Foundation.

REFERENCES

1. N. Blau, P. Joller, M. Altares, J. Cardesa-Garcia and A. Niederwieser. Increase of GTP cyclohydrolase I activity in mononuclear blood cells by stimulation: detection of heterozygotes of GTP cyclohydrolase I deficiency. Clin. Chim. Acta. 148:47-52 (1985).
2. W. Fierz, B. Endler, K. Reske, H. Wekerle and A. Fontana. Astrocytes as antigen-presenting cells. I. Induction of Ia antigen expression on astrocytes by T cells via immune interferon and its effect on antigen presentation. J. Immunol. 134:3785-3793 (1985).
3. Ch. Huber, D. Fuchs, A. Hausen, R. Margreiter, G. Reibnegger, M. Spielberger and H. Wachter. Pteridines as a new marker to detect human T cells activated by allogeneic or modified self major histocompatibility complex (MHC) determinants. J. Immunol. 130:1047-1050 (1983).
4. Ch. Huber, J.R. Batchelor, D. Fuchs, A. Hausen, A. Lang, D. Niederwieser, G. Reibnegger, P. Swetly, J. Troppmair and H. Wachter. Immune response-associated production of neopterin. Release from macrophages primarily under control of interferon-gamma. J. Exp. Med. 160:310-316 (1984).
5. F. Momburg, N. Koch, P. Möller, G. Moldenhauer, G.W. Butcher and G.J. Hämmerling. Differential expression of Ia and Ia-associated invariant chain in mouse tissues after in vivo treatment with IFN-y. J. Immunol. 136:940-948 (1986).
6. A. Niederwieser, W. Staudenmann and E. Wetzel. High-performance liquid chromatography with column swithching for the analysis of biogenic amine metabolites and pterins. J. Chromatogr. 290:237-246 (1984).
7. H. Rokos, G. Bienhaus, A. Gadow and K. Rokos. Determination of neopterin and reduced neopterins by radioimmunoassay. In: "Biochemical and Clinical Aspects of Pteridines", Vol.4, H. Wachter, H.Ch. Curtius, W. Pfleiderer, eds. Walter de Gruyter & Co., Berlin, New York (1985a).
8. H. Rokos, G. Bienhaus and R. Kunze. Neopterin in serum of mammals? In: "Biochemical and Clinical Aspects of Pteridines", Vol.4, H. Wachter, H.Ch. Curtius, W. Ffleiderer, eds. Walter de Gruyter & Co., Berlin, New York (1985b).
9. G. Schoedon, A. Niederwieser, J. Troppmair and Ch. Huber. Metabolism of pterins in human peripheral blood mononuclear cells. In: "Biochemical and Clinical Aspects of Pteridines", Vol.4, H. Wachter, H.Ch. Curtius, W. Pfleiderer, eds. Walter de Gruyter & Co., Berlin, New York (1985).
10. H.J. Ter Laak and O.R. Hommes. Ia-presenting cells in early multiple sclerosis lesions and adjacent normal looking white matter; a morphological study. In: "Multiple Sclerosis Research in Europe, Report of a CEC Conference Nijmegen, 1985", O.R. Hommes, ed. MTP Press Lancaster, U.K. (1986).
11. U. Traugott, E.L. Reinherz and C.S. Raine. Multiple sclerosis: distribution of T cells, T cell subsets and Ia-positive macrophages in lesions of different ages. J. Neuroimmunol. 4:201 (1983).
12. U. Traugott, L.B. Scheinberg and C.S. Raine. On the presence of Ia-positive endothelial cells and astrocytes in multiple sclerosis lesions and its relevance to antigen presentation. J. Neuroimmunol. 8:1-14 (1985).
13. K.A. Williams, D.N.J. Hart, J.W. Fabre and P.J. Morris. Distribution and quantitation of HLA-ABC and DR (Ia) antigens on human kindly kidney and other tissue. Transplant. 29:274-279 (1980).

REGULATORY MOLECULES IN THE CSF AND CNS

Jean E. Merrill[1] and Florence M. Hofman[2]

[1]Department of Neurology, UCLA School of Medicine
Los Angeles, California
[2]Department of Pathology, USC School of Medicine
Los Angeles, California

INTRODUCTION

Recent evidence has shown activated leukocytes, macrophages (MO), and lymphocytes in cerebrospinal fluid (CSF) of multiple sclerosis (MS) patients. The activation of these cells in demonstrated by altered phenotype and the expression of membrane antigens or receptors characteristic of activation as well as by the increased capacity of these cells to produce and release immunoregulatory molecules not normally secreted by resting, inactive cells. Examination of cells and their secreted products in the CSF provides clues about the nature of the cells in the peripheral blood, from which the CSF cells are derived, as well as expectations of the types of cells and their state of activation to be found in situ in the CNS, the putative target organ for CSF cells. To fully assess the CSF cells, we have studied the production of alpha interferon (IFN-alpha), interleukin 2 (IL-2), IL-2 receptors, interleukin 1 (Il-1), glial growth promoting factor (GGPF), and prostaglandin E (PGE) by cells of CSF and peripheral blood. In addition, we have examined, using frozen sections, the production and expression of these cytokines in the CNS of patients with MS and other neurological diseases compared to healthy controls.

CYTOKINE PRODUCTION IN CSF AND CNS

IFN-alpha

Because of the debate over the nature of the exogenous infections agent(s) triggering the disease onset and/or perpetuating the pathologic condition, much attention has been paid to IFN production and response in MS patients. In MS where a viral etiology has been suggested though no virus specific to MS has been isolated, natural killer (NK) cells, and IFN produced by NK and other cells are of relevance and perhaps importance in the primary etiology and secondary immune imbalances in these patients.

In vitro production of IFN-alpha by blood cells in response to a variety of viral stimuli has been shown by some investigators (1-3) to be normal in MS patients. Other investigators have shown depressed IFN-alpha in vitro in response to tumor target cells, poly 1:C, viruses such as measles, Newcastles disease, mumps, rubella, Herpes simplex, and influenza (4-14). Even though 0.5 IU/ml of IFN produced in vivo might have been detected in CSF or serum of MS patients, using sensitive techniques, none was ever seen in 2 separate studies (15,16). In yet another study it was found to be elevated compared with controls (17). Recently, Kamin-Lewis examined in vitro IFN responsiveness of IFN-alpha-treated patients to Newcastle disease virus (NDV) or measles virus and poly I:C as well as proliferation in response to ConA. IFN treated patients exhibited normal proliferative responses but a decreased IFN production to all in vitro inducers (18).

In a study conducted in this laboratory, IFN-alpha production by NK cells was shown to be depressed both in peripheral blood and cerebrospinal fluid (CSF) cells of MS patients compared to controls (6). Production of IFN-alpha in response to antibody coated targets was not depressed.

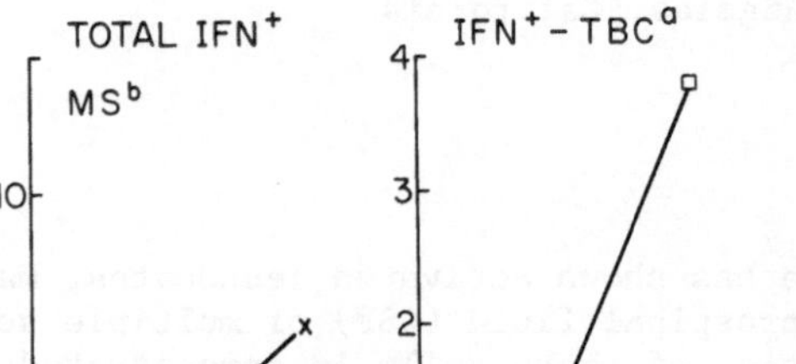

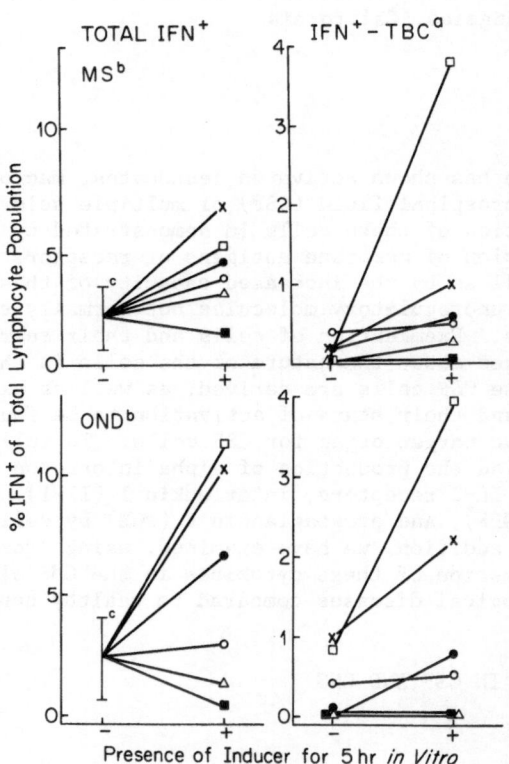

Fig.1. Comparison of direct IFN-alpha inducers on MS and OND NWP PBL. [a] NWP PBL incubated for 5 hr with (+) or without (-) target cell (E:T = 1:1) or soluble inducers indicated. At end of incubation fresh (identical to inducers) targets were added. MOLT 4 target was added to cells induced by poly IC and OKT3 and conjugated at E:T 1:1 for scoring IFN+-TBC. [b] Eleven MS patients (2 patients in relapse, experiencing an attack and 9 progressive patients) and five OND patients (all Friedreich's Ataxia) were studied concomitantly with their age- and sex-matched controls. [c] Total IFN+ cells at 5 hr without inducer is expressed as a mean ± SD. IFN inducers: X, MOLT 4; □, Chang + Ab; ●, K562; O, OKT3; △, poly IC; ■, Chang.

The production of IFN-alpha in relationship to NK and ADCC activity of peripheral blood and cerebrospinal lymphocytes was examined at the single cell level in patients with MS and other neurological diseases (OND) compared with age- and sex-matched controls. IFN-producing cells were assessed by indirect immunofluorescent scoring of cytoplasmic IFN+ cells. Peak production of cytoplasmic IFN-alpha in nylon wool-passed (NWP) cells occurred between 5 and 17 hr in vitro under the inductive stimulus of MOLT 4, K562, or antibody-coated Chang liver cells. The proportion of K562- and MOLT 4-induced IFN-alpha-positive cells in the total lymphocyte and target binding cell (TBC) population was significantly lower in MS NWP-peripheral blood lymphocytes (PBL) than in OND and normal controls (Fig.1). This was in direct relationship to a decreased percentage of NK cells in MS PBL (6). In contrast, MS cells responded the same as controls (total IFN+ cells) or higher than controls (IFN + - TBC) after IFN-alpha induction by antibody-coated Chang, the ADCC target, in parallel with elevated ADCC activity by MS PBL. MS CSF contained a higher proportion of total IFN+ cells but a similar proportion of IFN+-TBC as their homologous NWP PBL population. In OND CSF, both the percentage of total IFN+ and the percentage of IFN+-TBC were higher than in OND blood and higher than their respective MS CSF populations (Fig.2).

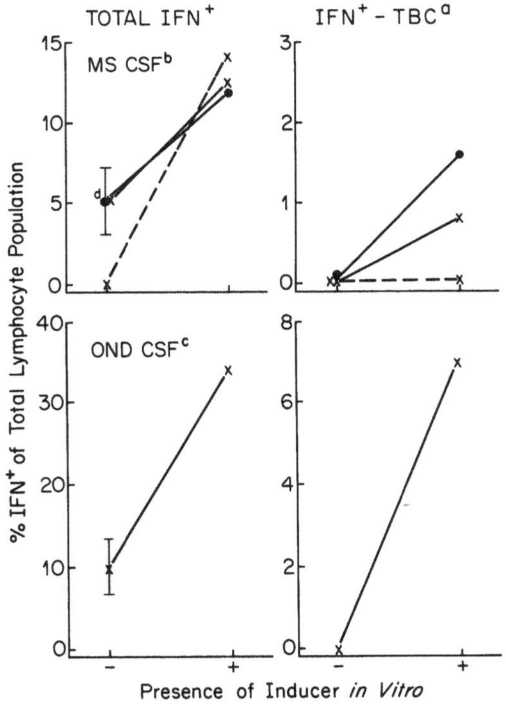

Fig.2. IFN-alpha induction in MS and OND CSF cells. [a] CSF lymphocytes incubated number of hours indicated with (+) or without (-) inducer target cells shown, E:T 1:1. At end of incubation, fresh target cells (identical to inducers) were added and conjugated at E:T = 1:1 for IFN +- TBC. [b] Ten CSF of MS in progression assayed. [c] Five OND CSF samples assayed. OND included three Friedreich's ataxia, one neurosyphylis, and one pseudotumor. X_, MOLT 4 incubated for 5 hr. X---, MOLT 4 incubated for 17 hr. ● , K562 incubated for 5 hr. [d] Total IFN+ cells without inducer expressed as mean ± SD.

Since there were high proportions of IFN+ cells in the CSF of MS and OND patients compared to the homologous PBL and no significant difference in IFN+ cells in the uninduced populations of CSF or PBL lymphocytes, IFN+ cells were induced to a greater extent in CSF than PBL. These data point out the CNS as the site of cells potentially already activated in vivo and the source of cells more easily activated in vitro compared to peripheral blood cells.

IL-2 and IL-2 receptors

In an effort to furhter characterize the defective proliferative response of T lymphocytes to mitogens in MS patients, we examined the response to and production of IL-2 by both PBL and CSF mononuclear cells. We also examined the proportion of cells bearing receptors for IL-2 and transferrin. The importance of IL-2 in induction of IFN (19) and subsequent enhancement of proliferation and differentiation of NK cells is well established (4,20). Thus, in addition to its effect on T cell proliferation, low IL-2 production or response could result in depressed IFN production (19,20) and NK activity (20,21). We showed in this study that PBL from chronic progressive MS patients gave an abnormally low response to exogenous IL-2 as compared to controls. Whereas acute relapse patients' PBL demonstrated a normal IL-2 response during an exacerbation, they showed reduced responsiveness during remission. These abnormalities could not be explained by different dose or kinetic response optima to PHA or IL-2 nor could they be explained by depressed numbers of IL-2 or transferrin receptor-bearing lymphocytes. Cerebrospinal fluid lymphocytes from MS patients had normal proportions of IL-2 receptor-bearing cells, but were deficient in their IL-2 response and production as compared to autochthonous or controls PBL (22).

Production of IL-2 by PBL was also normal in MS patients. Chronic progressive patients produced elevated levels of IL-2 whereas acute relapse patients undergoing an exacerbation produced diminished levels of IL-2. During remission, these levels returned to that of controls'. The effect of 1200 rad x-irradiation or nylon wool removal of adherent cells was a significantly greater augmentation of IL-2 produced in MS patients than in other neurologic disease or normal controls, suggesting suppression by a T suppressor cell, perhaps induced by macrophages (22). Production of IL-2 by CSF of MS or OND patients was less than half that produced by PBL (Table 1).

Using monoclonal antibodies to IL-2 (the generous gift of Dr. Steven Gillis) and the IL-2 receptor (anti-TAC, the generous gift of Dr. Thomas Waldmann), we examined cells in frozen sections of brain from 14 MS patients, 17 ONDs, and 6 normal individuals. OND patients included 1 progressive rubella panencephalitis (PRP), 1 progressive multifocal leukoencephalopathy (PML), 5 subacute sclerosing panencephalitis (SSPE), 1 chronic encephalitis of unknown etiology, 3 gliomas, 1 Alzheimer's disease, 1 Parkinson's disease, and 4 epilepsy patients. Twelve of 14 MS patients showed staining for IL-2 in the plaque region (center and edge). Eleven out of 19 MS patients showed TAC^+ cells predominantly within the plaque (23) (Table 1). None of the normal brain tissue exhibited IL-2 staining or TAC^+ cells. Only 3/17 ONDs showed IL-2 and 3/20 ONDs showed TAC^+ cells. For both markers these were the same 3 patients: the Parkinson's disease and 2/5 of the SSPE patients (Table 1). Only double staining with these antibodies and cell-specific markers will identify the source or cell association of the IL-2 and IL-2R. This need is due to the recent discovery that in addition to T cells, B cells (24-26), MO (27) and even oligodendrocytes (28) have receptors for and/or respond to IL-2. The role of IL-2 in the CNS will be very interesting in light of additional data from Fontana et al. that glioblastomas cells (and perhaps activated as-

Table 1. Immunoregulatory molecules in the CNS

	cell source		MS			OND			Normal control		
	CSF	CNS	blood	CSF	CNS	blood	CSF	CNS	blood	CSF	CNS
__cytokines__											
IL2 units/ ml	T cell	T cell or bound to glial cell B cell, or MØ	200 relapse 400 progression	<50	12/14⁺	300	<50	3/17⁺	300	N.D.	0/6⁺
IL1	MØ B cell	MØ, B cell, astroglia microglia	N.D.	N.D.	11/12⁺	N.D.	N.D.	1/13⁺	N.D.	N.D.	0/2⁺
IFN-alpha $\%^{+}$ cells	MØ, B cell NK cells	MØ, B cell NK cell	10 relapse 6 progression	14	N.D.	10	35	N.D.	10	N.D.	N.D.
GGPF	T cell	T cell	++	4/10⁺ or ±	N.D.	+++	+	N.D.	+++	N.D.	N.D.
PGE ng/ml	MØ	MØ, astroglia microglia	1.4	0.4	8/9⁺	0.7	0.1	0/8⁺	0.7	0.07	0/2⁺
__receptors__											
IL2 $\%TAC^{+}$ cells	T cell, B cell MØ	T cell, B cell MØ oligodendroglia	67	83 one relapse 64 progression	11/19⁺	70	49	3/20⁺	68	N.D.	0/7⁺

A6.mjtcytoc

trocytes?) release factors inhibiting interleukin 2-mediated effects (29).

IL-1

Interleukin 1 was examined in frozen sections of brains from 12 MS patients, 2 normal controls, and 13 ONDs including 1 Parkinson's disease, PRP, PML, 1 Alzheimer's disease, 1 chronic encephalitis, 3 epilepsy, and 5 SSPE patients. Only the PRP brain showed staining for IL-1 while 11/12 MS brains showed cells staining with IL-1, predominantly at the plaque edge (23). Because B cells (30) and astrocytes (31) make IL 1-like factors, it cannot be presumed that the IL-1 detected in our study is necessarily MØ-derived. Double-staining will have to be performed. Astrocytes behave, upon activation, much like macrophages in their ability to express Ia antigen *in vivo* (23) and *in vitro* after stimulation by T cell-derived gamma interferon (IFN-gamma) (32) and to function as accessory cells and present antigen to T cells (33,34). The transformation of cells of astrocyte lineage into MØ-like cells in organtypic cultures (35) may provide a putative source for the MØs and IL-1 found in the staining of MS plaques (23) (Table 1) as well as for IL 1-like material purified from injured brain tissue (36).

GGPF

We have reported that astrocyts and oligodendroglial cells proliferate in response to factors produced by the human T lymphocyte line Mo, human T cell leukemia-lymphoma virus (HTLV)-transformed peripheral blood T cells from healthy individuals, and phytohemagglutinin (PHA)-activated T cell from peripheral blood and cerebrospinal fluid of MS patients, normal, and other neurological disease controls (37). Two thirds of the MS patients examined, showed normal levels of GGPF produced by peripheral blood T cells. One third produced less GGPF. T cells from 40% of MS CSF samples tested produced GGPF though in lesser amounts than that produced by homologous PBL T cells (Table 1).

Our results showed that cerebrospinal fluid and peripheral blood T cells, when stimulated by PHA, make factors as stimulatory as those produced by the Mo line and HTLV-I and -II transformants. Characterization of factors produced by activated T cells may help to elucidate the pathogenesis of glial hyperplasia in MS as well as in other diseases involving chronic inflammation in the presence of infiltrating lymphocytes.

PGE

Depressed proliferative expansion and IFN production of MS peripheral lymphocytes in response to mitogens and antigens as well as depressed NK activity could be explained by the inability of MS lymphocytes to respond to IL-2 (22).

Both the MØ and T suppressor cell play a role in the suppression of Il-2 production. MØ make PGE (38) which will directly inhibit IL-2 production (39) or which induce T cells (40) that suppress IL-2 production (41). Increased IL-2 production after MØ depletion as we have shown (22) has also been demonstrated by other investigators: Rappaport and Dodge (39) showed a two- to 20-fold increase in IL-2 production, whereas Linker-Israeli et al. (42) showed a threefold increase when MØ were removed. If, like their NK cells (9), MS patients' T cells are more sensitive to the effects of PGE than control T cells, removal of adherent cells would be expected to boost IL-2 production to a greater extent in MS patients as compared to controls. We in fact demonstrated this (22) and in addition were able to show that MS patients' peripheral blood MNC spontaneously produced more prostaglandin $E_{1,2}$ *in vitro* than did OND or normal control

MNC. There were no differences between OND and normal controls (8). Higher levels of PGE correlated with lower levels of NK activity and endogenous interferon production in the peripheral blood. MS nylon wool adherent (NW Ad) cells also produced significantly more PGE than normals and ONDs. MS neat CSF contained significantly higher levels of measurable PGE with concomitantly lower NK activity and % IFN-positive cells than was seen in OND CSF (8) (Table 1). As with the lymphokines IL-2 and GGPF, levels of PGE in CSF are lower compared to peripheral blood cell-derived PGE. This may be due to a lower proportion of MØ in CSF compared to blood (8) or the metabolic processing of CSF PGE.

Using a rabbit anti-PGE antibody, we stained frozen sections of brain for PGE producing cells. None of the controls (normal, SSPE, chronic encephalitis, or epilepsy) showed any PGE staining. Eight out of 9 MS brains showed positive cells. PGE-positive cells were detected inside the plaque, at the lesion edge, and to some degree in adjacent white matter. Some of this staining was perinuclear while other staining identified cellular processes seen on cells like microglia and astrocytes (23). As with IL-1, sources of PGE other than blood MØ exist within the CNS. Astrocytes (31) and probably microglia may be contributing to the PGE production in MS brain. It is interesting that in spite of astrogliosis and presumed astrocyte activation in the other neurological diseases studied (SSPE, glioma, PRP, chronic encephalitis, etc) there is not an induction of IL-1 and PGE, whereas in MS gliosis, astrocytes may be activated to produce these cytokines and thus promote inflammation and a chronic feedback loop with cells of the immune response *in vivo.*

In summary, the presence of PGE, IFN-alpha, IL-1, IL-2 and GGPF, all immunoregulatory molecules secreted by activated cells and each a parameter of a turned on immune response, suggests an active immune mechanism in the pathogenesis of MS, possibly through the interaction of the lymphoid and nervous systems.

REFERENCES

1. D.R.Tovell, I. McRobbie, K.G. Warren and D.L. Tyrrell. Interferon production by lymphocytes from multiple sclerosis and non MS patients. *Neurol.* 33:640 (1983).
2. G. Vervliet, H. Claeys, H. Van Haver, H. Carton, C. Vermylen, E. Meulepas and A. Billiau. Interferon production and natural killer (NK) activity in leucocyte cultures from multiple sclerosis patients. *J. Neurol. Sci.* 60:137 (1983).
3. Santoli, W. Hall, L. Kastrokoff, R.P. Lisak, B. Perussia, G. Trinchieri and H. Koprowski. Cytotoxic activity and interferon production by lymphocytes from patients with multiple sclerosis. *J. Immunol.* 126:1274 (1981).
4. M. Benczur, G.Gy. Petranyi, Gy Palffy, M. Varga, M. Talas, B. Kotsy, I. Foldes and S.R. Hollan. Dysfunction of natural killer cells in multiple sclerosis: A possible pathogenic mechanism. *Clin. Exp. Immunol.* 39:657 (1980).
5. P.A. Neighbour. Studies of interferon production and natural killing by lymphocytes from multiple sclerosis patients. *Ann. N.Y. Acad. Sci.* 436:181 (1984).
6. J.E. Merrill, G.W. Ellison and L.W. Myers. Cytotoxic activity of peripheral blood and cerebrospinal fluid lymphocytes from patients with multiple sclerosis and other neurological diseases: Analysis at the single cell level of the relationship of cytotoxic effectors and interferon producing cells. *Clin. Immunol. Beta Immunopathol.* 31: 390 (1984).

7. P.A. Neighbour, A.I. Grayzel and A.E. Miller. Endogenous and interferon-augmented natural killer cell activity of human peripheral blood mononuclear cells in vitro. Studies of patients with multiple sclerosis, systemic lupus erythematosus, or rheumatoid arthritis. Clin. Exp. Immunol. 49:11 (1982).
8. J.E. Merrill, R.H. Gerner, L.W. Myers and G.W. Ellison. Regulation of natural killer cell cytotoxicity by prostaglandin E in the peripheral blood and cerebrospinal fluid of patients with multiple sclerosis and other neurological diseases. Part I: Association between amount of prostaglandin produced, natural killer, and endogenous interferon. J. Neuroimmunol. 4:223 (1983).
9. J.E. Merrill, L.W. Myers and G.W. Ellison. Regulation of natural killer cell cytotoxicity by prostaglandin E in the peripheral blood and cerebrospinal fluid of patients with multiple sclerosis and other neurological diseases. Part 2: Effect of exogenous PGE_1 on spontaneous and interferon induced natural killer. J. Neuroimmunol. 4:239 (1983).
10. E. Gyodi, M. Benczur, G. Gy. Palffy, M. Talas, Gy. Petranyi, I. Foldes and S.R. Hollan. Association between HLA B7, DR2 and dysfunction of natural and antibody-mediated cytotoxicity without connection with the deficient interferon production in multiple sclerosis. Human Immunol. 4:209 (1982).
11. R. Salonen, J. Ilonen, M. Reunanen and A. Salmi. Defective production of interferon associated with HLA DW2 antigen in stable multiple sclerosis. J. Neurol. Sci. 55:197 (1982).
12. P. Kaudewitz, H. Zander, J. Abb, H.W. Ziegler-Heitbrock and G. Riethmuller. Genetic influence on natural cytotoxicity and interferon production in multiple sclerosis studies in monozygotic discordant twins. Human Immunol. 7:51 (1983).
13. S. Haahr, A. Moller-Larson and E. Pedersen. Immunological parameters in multiple sclerosis patients with special reference to the herpes virus group. Clin. Exp. Immunol. 51:197 (1983).
14. G. Vervliet, H. Carton, E. Meulepas and A. Billiau. Interferon production by cultured peripheral leukocytes of MS patients. Clin. Exp. Immunol. 58:116 (1984).
15. S.L. Hauser, K.A. Ault, M.J. Levin, M.R. Garavoy and H.L. Weiner. Natural killer cell activity in multiple sclerosis. J. Immunol. 127:1114 (1981).
16. R. Salonen. CSF and serum interferon in multiple sclerosis: A longitudinal study. Neurol. 33:1604 (1983).
17. M. Degré, H. Dahl and B. Vandvik. Interferon in the serum and cerebrospinal fluid of patients with multiple sclerosis and other neurological disorders. Acta Neurol. Scand. 53:152 (1976).
18. R.M. Kamin-Lewis, H.S. Danitch, T.C. Merigan and K.P. Johnson. Decreased interferon synthesis and responsiveness to interferon by leukocytes from multiple sclerosis patients given natural alpha interferon. J. Interferon Res. 4:423 (1984).
19. T.J. Kasahara, J.J. Hooks, S.F. Dougherty and J.J. Oppenheim. Interleukin 2-mediated immune interferon (IFN-gamma) production by human T cells and T cell subsets. J. Immunol. 130:1784 (1983).
20. D.A. Weigert, G.J. Stanton and M.A. Johnson. Interleukin 2 enhances natural killer cell activity through induction of gamma interferon. Fed. Proc. 42:1072 (1983).
21. R.A. Dempsey, C.A. Dinarello, J.W. Mier, L.J. Rosenwasser, M. Allegretta, T.E. Brown and D.R. Parkinson. The differential effects of human leucocyte pyrogen/lymphocyte-activating factor, T cell growth factor, and interferon on human natural killer activity. J. Immunol. 129:2504 (1982).

22. J.E. Merrill, C. Mohlstrom, C. Uittenbogaart, V. Kermani-Arab, G.W. Ellison and L.W. Myers. Response to and production of interleukin 2 by peripheral blood and cerebrospinal fluid lymphocytes of patients with multiple sclerosis. J. Immunol. 133:1931 (1984).
23. F.M. Hofman, R.I. von Hanwehr, C.A. Dinarello, S.B. Mizel, D. Hinton and J.E. Merrill. Immunoregulatory molecules and IL-2 receptors identified in multiple sclerosis brain. J. Immunol. 136: in press (1986).
24. A.W. Bowd, D.C. Fischer, D.A. Fox, S.F. Schlossman and L.M. Nadler. Structural and functional characterization of IL-2 receptors on activated human B cells. J. Immunol. 134:2587 (1985).
25. R. Mittler, P. Rao, G. Olini, E. Westberg, W. Newman, M. Hoffmann and G. Goldstein. Activated human B cells display a functional IL-2 receptor. J. Immunol. 134:2393 (1985).
26. H. Kishi, S. Inui, A. Muraguchi, T. Hirano, Y. Yamamura and T. Kishimoto. Induction of IgG secretion in a human B cell clone with recombinant IL-2. J. Immunol. 134:3104 (1985).
27. W. Holter, R. Grunow, H. Stockinger and W. Knapp. Recombinant interferon-gamma induces interleukin 2 receptors on human peripheral blood monocytes. J. Immunol. 136:2171 (1986).
28. E.N. Benveniste and J.E. Merrill. Interleukin 2 stimulation of oligodendroglial proliferation and maturation. Nature. In press.
29. A. Fontana, H. Hengartner, N. de Tribolet and E. Weber. Glioblastoma cells release interleukin 1 and factors inhibiting interleukin 2-mediated effects. J. Immunol. 132:1837 (1984).
30. G. Scala, Y.L. Kuang, R.E. Hall, A.V. Muchmore and J.J. Oppenheim. Accessory cell function and human B cells, I. Production of both interleukin 1-like activity and interleukin 1 inhibitory factors by an EBV transformed human B cell line. J. Exp. Med. 159:1637 (1984).
31. A. Fontana, F. Kristensen, R. Dubs, D. Gemsa and E. Weber. Production of prostaglandin E and an interleukin 1-like factor by cultured astrocytes and C6 glioma cells. J. Immunol. 129:2413 (1982).
32. W. Fierz, B. Endler, K. Reske, H. Wekerle and A. Fontana. Astrocytes as antigen-presenting cells, I. Induction of Ia antigen expression on astrocytes by T cells via immune interferon and its effect on antigen presentation. J. Immunol. 134:3784 (1985).
33. A. Fontana, W. Fierz and H. Wekerle. Astrocytes present myelin basic protein to encephalitogenic T cell lines. Nature. 307:273 (1984).
34. B. Schnyder, E. Weber, W. Fierz and A. Fontana. On the role of astrocytes in polyclonal T cell activation. J. Neuroimmunol. 10:209 (1986).
35. H. Kusaka, A. Hirano, M.B. Bornstein, G.R.W. Moore and C.S. Raine. Transformation of cells of astrocyte lineage into macrophage-like cells in organotypic cultures of mouse spinal cord tissue. J. of the Neurol. Sci. 72:77 (1986).
36. D. Giulian and L.B. Lachman. Interleukin 1 stimulation of astroglial proliferation after brain injury. Science. 228:497 (1985).
37. J.E. Merrill, S. Kutsunai, C. Hohlstrom, F. Hofman, J. Groopman and D.W. Golde. Proliferation of astroglia and oligodendroglia in response to human T cell-derived factors. Science. 224:1428 (1984).
38. J.S. Goodwin, A.D. Bankhurst and R.P. Messner. Suppression of human T cell mitogenesis by prostaglandin. Existence of a prostaglandin producing suppressor cell. J. Exp. Med. 146:1719 (1977).
39. R.S. Rappaport and G.R. Dodge. Prostaglandin E inhibits the production of human interleukin 2. J. Exp. Med. 155:943 (1982).
40. H.V. Raff, K.C. Cochrum and J.D. Stobo. Macrophage-T cell interactions in the Con A induction of human suppressive T cells. J. Immunol. 121:2311 (1978).

41. M. Bullberg, F. Ivars, A. Coutinho and E.L. Larsson. Regulation of T cell growth factor production: Arrest of TCGF production after 18 hours in normal lectin-stimulated mouse spleen cell cultures. J. Immunol. 127:407 (1981).
42. M. Linker-Israeli, A.C. Bakke, R.C. Kitridou, S. Gendler, S. Gillis and D.A. Horwitz. Defective production of interleukin 1 and interleukin 2 in patients with systemic lupus erythematosis (SLE). J. Immunol. 30:2651 (1983).

INTERLEUKIN-1 IN THE CEREBROSPINAL FLUID IN CHRONIC RELAPSING EXPERIMENTAL ALLERGIC ENCEPHALOMYELITIS

J.A. Symons, R.V. Bundick*, A.J. Suckling and M.G. Rumsby

Department of Biology, University of York, YO1 5DD, U.K.
*Department of Pharmacology, Fison plc, Pharmaceutical Division, Loughborough, LE11, ORH, U.K.

SUMMARY

Paired cerebrospinal fluid (CSF) and plasma samples were taken from guinea pigs at various stages of chronic relapsing experimental allergic encephalomyelitis. The samples were assayed for interleukin-1 (IL-1) activity using a C3H/HeJ mouse thymocyte assay. IL-1 was detectable in low amounts (< 10U/ml) in plasma throughout the course of the disease and in control animals but raised in acute phase plasma. IL-1 in CSF was also present at < 10U/ml during the acute phase of the disease and in controls but elevated three-fold during the post-acute, relapse and remission phases of CR-EAE.

INTRODUCTION

Chronic relapsing experimental allergic encephalomyelitis (CR-EAE) in guinea pigs provides an animal model in which the pathogenesis of autoimmune demyelination may be investigated. Although there are vast differences in etiology and disease duration between CR-EAE and multiple sclerosis (MS), the animal model serves as a useful model for the human condition. It shares the relapsing and remitting course of MS and demonstrates a close similarity in respect of pathological changes in spite of differences in lesion size (1). The use of the guinea pig allows investigation of changes which occur in the cerebrospinal fluid (CSF) during the developing disease. Since CSF acts as a sink for molecules produced by the central nervous system such changes may give clues to key events, especially at the time of relapse, which occur during the pathogenesis of CR-EAE.

Few studies are available which document the presence or changes in activity of soluble mediators of immunity present in CSF either in MS or in CR-EAE. One of the first reports, from our laboratory, described the presence of a factor which promoted monocyte migration (2). The factor had a molecular weight of between 50 and 300Kd and was three times as active in the CSF from relapse animals compared with animals in remission. It is possible that this molecule is a lymphokine produced by cells residing within the parenchyma which have become activated before or during the onset of relapse. Its presence might induce monocytes to cross meningeal blood vessel walls and accumulate within the sub-arachnoid space (3).

Macrophages undoubtedly play an important, if not completely understood, role in lesion formation in CR-EAE and their presence led us to enquire about the presence of macrophage products in the CSF. In particular, was interleukin-1 (IL-1) detectable in the CSF? IL-1 is well known for being produced primarily by many types of phagocytic cells (4) but also from brain astrocytes and microglia (5). The following report describes the assessment of CSF samples from guinea pigs in various stages of CR-EAE for the presence of IL-1-like activity.

EXPERIMENTAL

Animals

CR-EAE was induced in juvenile strain 13 guinea pigs (University of York) by the inoculation into each hind foot dorsum of 0.1 ml of an emulsion consisting of equal parts of 50% whole spinal cord homogenate and Freund's adjuvant (Difco) containing 10 mg/ml *Mycobacterium tuberculosis* H37Ra. Other animals were inoculated with adjuvant alone or were left uninoculated. At various times post-inoculation (p.i.) anaesthetised animals were sampled for blood by cardiac puncture and for CSF by puncture of the cisterna magna. This method of CSF sampling occasionally incurred some degree of blood contamination, the degree of contamination was assessed by measuring the number of red blood cells (rbc)/µl CSF. Both red and white cell content of the CSF were determined in an improved Neubauer chamber using a 1:1 (v/v) dilution of CSF in 1% crystal violet, CSF samples containing > 5000 rbc/µl were discarded. Cell free CSF was obtained by centrifugation of samples at 10,000 g for 5 minutes and the CSF was then stored at -20°C. Disease onset was at 12-16 days p.i. (termed acute disease) followed by recovery between 25-42 days p.i. (post-acute). Animals then spontaneously developed the first relapse (relapse group in table) at about 70 days p.i. before showing a remission of clinical signs (remission group).

IL-1 assays

In order to assay plasma IL-1 it was necessary to remove previously described inhibitors of lymphocyte proliferation (6). Plasma was filtered through a PM30 Diaflo membrane supported in an MPS-1 micropartition system (Amicon). The filtrates were then stored at -20°C. Additionally, during the acute stages of the disease it was necessary to remove a low molecular weight (< 1000) inhibitor and this was achieved by extensive dialysis against RPMI 1640 medium at 4°C. Neither the filtration or dialysis techniques caused any loss of IL-1 activity as determined by the use of an IL-1 standard. CSF was used unfractionated.

For the IL-1 assay 4-8 week old C3H/Hej mouse thymocytes were cultured in serum-free RPMI 1640 containing 2mM L-glutamine, 100 IU/ml penicillin, 100 µg/ml streptomycin and 2 g/L sodium bicarbonate (Flow Laboratories), together with a suboptimal (0.05 µg/ml) concentration of PHA (Difco) and doubling dilutions of CSF or plasma. Thymocytes were incubated at 37°C in 5% CO_2/95% air for 48h and tritiated thymidine (0.5 µCi/well) was added 24h before the end of incubation and incorporated thymidine assayed by liquid scintillation counting. All IL-1 activities were quantitated by probit analysis (7) using ultrapure IL-1 (100 U/ml; Genzyme) as a standard.

IL-2 assays

CSF and plasma samples were assayed for IL-2 activity using both the IL-2 dependent cell line, CTLL (7) and a modification of the IL-2 assay described by De Vos and Libert (8) using dexamethasone-treated, PHA stimulated guinea pig splenocytes as the responsive cells.

RESULTS

The mean blood contamination of CSF was 995 rbc/μl, and 80% of the samples contained less than 2,500 rbc/μl, equivalent to 0.05% (v/v) blood contamination. A 0.05% (v/v) mixture of heparinised plasma in RPMI 1640, used at appropriate dilutions was inactive in the IL-1 assay.

IL-1 activity values are given in Table 1 and show that the activity of acute group plasma samples were significantly raised over adjuvant controls. All post-acute group activities were significantly lower than the acute group activity. In CSF, however, the acute group activity was not elevated over adjuvant controls but all post-acute groups were. Using the Mann-Whitney U test acute group plasma activity was significantly increased over paired acute CSF sample activity ($p = 0.01$) but CSF activity was significantly higher than plasma ($p = 0.01$) in the post-acute relapse and remission groups.

Table 1. IL-1 activity in paired plasma and CSF samples from guinea pigs in various stages of CR-EAE

animal group	IL-1 plasma	(U/ml) CSF
uninoculated (n = 6)	3.1 ± 1.5	1.1 ± 1.1
adjuvant controls (n = 6)	4.7 ± 2.9	3.2 ± 3.1
acute (n = 5)	13.9 ± 4.9*	6.1 ± 3.3
post-acute (n = 6)	5.5 ± 2.5°	18.5 ± 7.8°#
relapse (n = 6)	6.3 ± 3.4°	16.0 ± 6.9°#
remission (n = 8)	6.0 ± 3.2	18.8 ± 9.3°#

values are means ± s.d.
* differs from adjuvant controls ($p < 0.001$; t test)
° groups differ from acute group ($p < 0.05$; t test)
\# groups differ from adjuvant controls ($p < 0.01$; t test)

IL-2 in CSF/plasma

Using the two different assay systems referred to in the methods section we were unable to detect IL-2 activity in either CSF or plasma.

DISCUSSION

From the results presented above there is evidence of increased CSF IL-1 activity in all post-acute stages of CR-EAE. The increase in IL-1 activity is not due to increased plasma activity or leakage of blood during puncture. We suggest that the IL-1 detected in the CSF must therefore originate from within the central nervous system. Likely sources are the macrophages which populate in large numbers the meninges and parenchyma of the brain and spinal cord or astrocytes as suggested by the work of Fontana (9). Little IL-1 activity is found in normal human plasma but there do appear to be elevated levels in febrile or septic patients (10). We have also noted an elevated level of IL-1 in the plasma of animals in the acute stage of CR-EAE and this may account for the pyrexia seen during this stage of the disease.

What do higher levels of IL-1 activity indicate? Higher IL-1 levels might predispose affected animals to ongoing autoagressive changes, by its action on vascular endothelium. IL-1 can cause endothelial cells to become selectively adhesive for leucocytes (11). This effect may contribute to the processes involved in the formation of the dense foci of inflammation seen during the chronic stages of CR-EAE (3). IL-1 also has a major function in potentiating T-cell activation, B-cell proliferation and antibody formation all of which events are consistent with immunopathological findings in CR-EAE.

We do not think that the presence of increased IL-1-like activity in the CSF of CR-EAE animals is due either to IL-2 or peripherally derived IL-1. Its importance in the development of relapsing autoimmune disease and the definition of the source of IL-1 activity are under investigation at present.

ACKNOWLEDGEMENTS

This work was performed during the tenure of a SERC-CASE studentship (JAS) and was supported by funds from Fisons Pharmaceuticals Ltd. and the Multiple Sclerosis Society of Great Britain and Northern Ireland.

REFERENCES

1. H. Lassmann. Comparative Neuropathology of Chronic Experimental Allergic Encephalomyelitis and Multiple Sclerosis. Springer-Verlag, Berlin (1983).
2. J.A. Kirby, A.J. Suckling and M.G. Rumsby. Chronic relapsing experimental allergic encephalomyelitis: The presence in the cerebrospinal fluid of factors chemotactic for monocytes. J. Neuroimmunol. 5:271-281 (1983).
3. A.J. Suckling, N.R. Wilson, J.A. Kirby and M.G. Rumsby. Chronic relapsing experimental allergic encephalomyelitis: Cerebrospinal fluid cytology and a comparison with meningeal and spinal cord pathology. Neuropathol. Appl. Neurobiol. 9:237-249 (1983).
4. C.A. Dinarello. An update on human interleukin-1: From molecular biology to clinical relevance. J. Clin. Immunol. 5:287-297 (1985).
5. A. Fontana and P.J. Grob. Lymphokines and the brain. Springer Semin. Immunopathol. 7:375-386 (1984).
6. J.A. Symons, A.J. Suckling, R.V. Bundick and M.G. Rumsby. Chronic relapsing experimental allergic encephalomyelitis: Inhibition of lymphocyte mitogenesis by disease related serum factors. J. Neuroimmunol. In press (1986).
7. S. Gillis, M.M. Ferm, W. Ou and K.A. Smith. T cell growth factor: Parameters of production and a quantitative microassay for activity. J. Immunol. 120:2027-2032 (1978).
8. C. De Vos and W. Libert. A simple rapid method for detection of IL-2 in a physiological medium. J. Immunol. Methods. 74:375-384 (1984).
9. A. Fontana, F. Kristenson, R. Dubs, D. Gemsa and E. Weber. Production of prostaglandin E and an interleukin-1-like factor by cultured astrocytes and C_6 glioma cells. J. Immunol. 129:2413-2419 (1982).

10. C.A. Dinarello, G.H.A. Clowes, A.H. Gordon, C.A. Saravis and S.M. Wolff. Cleavage of human interleukin-1: isolation of a fragment isolated from the plasma of febrile humans and monocytes. J. Immunol. 133:1322-1338 (1984).
11. M.P. Bevclacqua, J.S. Pober, M.E. Wheeler, R.S. Cotran and M.A. Gimbrone. Interleukin-1 acts on cultured human vascular endothelium to increase the adhesion of polymorphonuclear leucocytes, monocytes and related leucocyte cell lines. J. Clin. Invest. 76:2003-2011 (1985).

DETERMINATION OF THE NEURAL CELL ADHESION MOLECULE (N-CAM) IN CEREBROSPINAL FLUID FROM PATIENTS WITH MULTIPLE SCLEROSIS

Angelo R. Massaro[1], Merete Albrechtsen[2] and Elisabeth Bock[2]

[1] Department of Neurology, Università Cattolica S. Cuore 00168 Roma, Italy
[2] The Protein Laboratory, University of Copenhagen, 34 Sigurdsade, DK-2200 Copenhagen, Denmark

SUMMARY

We studied longitudinally the cerebrospinal fluid (CSF) neural cell adhesion molecule (N-CAM) content of 20 multiple sclerosis (MS) patients in the acute phase, and 10 in the non-acute phase. Both groups were compared with a control group of 23 subjects without neurological diseases. All MS patients were subjected to two or three lumbar punctures for collection of CSF samples, one a week. N-CAM analysis was performed by an enzyme-linked immunosorbent assay (ELISA) method. Comparison of N-CAM concentrations of the first CSF drawings of each MS group with the control group values, showed statistically different (lower) levels in the non-acute MS patients. Furthermore, a statistically significant increase of CSF N-CAM was shown comparing the values of first, second and third drawings of the acute phase MS patients group. This increase paralleled the patient's clinical improvement.

INTRODUCTION

As a part of our effort to clarify the cellular and molecular basis for multiple sclerosis (MS) we have recently performed quantitative analyses of several cerebrospinal fluid (CSF) proteins in patients progressing through various phases of the disease. Variations in CSF concentrations of myelin basic protein and S-100 protein have been demonstrated and correlated with the clinical course of the disease (Massaro et al., 1982; Massaro et al., 1985). We here extend these studies to the neuronal cell adhesion molecule (N-CAM). The glycoprotein N-CAM, under the name of D2, was originally described as a neuronal membrane protein (Jörgensen and Bock, 1974). Antibodies against N-CAM/D2 were found to inhibit fasciculation of neurites from cultured sympathetic ganglia (Rutishauser et al., 1978; Jörgensen et al., 1980a), and a number of other studies likewise indicated that the protein is involved in inter-neuronal adhesion phenomena (Brackenbury et al., 1984; Fraser et al., 1984). In addition, a glial form of N-CAM has recently been demonstrated (Noble et al., 1985). A purification procedure for human N-CAM has been published (Rasmussen et al., 1983). Furthermore, a simple and sensitive enzyme-linked immunosorbent assay (ELISA) for human N-CAM has been developed, suited for routine analysis of CSF, amniotic fluid and serum (Ibsen et al., 1983).

Subnormal CSF concentrations of N-CAM have been found in patients with normal pressure hydrocephalus (NPH) (Soelberg Sörensen et al., 1983). Conversely, CSF N-CAM content increased during the recovery period in patients with delirium tremens and related clinical states (Jörgensen et al., 1980b), as well as in endogenously depressed patients during recovery (Jörgensen et al., 1977). Thus, abnormal N-CAM concentrations occur in patients with increased degradation or turnover of synapses, or with altered CSF flow.

PATIENTS AND METHODS

MS patients

30 patients with diagnosis of definite MS were selected on the grounds of clinical and laboratory criteria widely accepted (Brown et al., 1979). 20 patients were in the acute phase of the disease, and were admitted to our study 5-31 (median 13) days after onset of exacerbation, and followed-up until 16-76 (median 26) days after onset of exacerbation. 10 patients were in the non-acute phase of the disease (i.e. no acute exacerbation had been observed for at least six months when they were admitted to this study). The group of acute phase patients consisted of 16 females and 4 males with an age range of 10-56 years (median 31). The group of non-acute phase patients were 6 females and 4 males, 26-63 years old (median 41). All patients had 2-3 lumbar punctures performed at about one week interval for intrathecal steroid treatment with triamcinolone retard, 40 mg. Of the acute phase patients, 7 received two and 13 received three lumbar punctures; among the non-acute phase patients, 4 received two and 6 three punctures. The intrathecal steroid treatment was the same for both groups. Even if intrathecal triamcinolone retard in our hands, and according to our experience of many years (Massaro, 1978), was demonstrated to be an absolutely safe treatment (Neu et al., 1984), a prior informed consent was obtained from every MS patient studied by us.

Control group

The control group was made up of 23 subjects without signs of any neurological disease. They received the lumbar puncture while subjected to spinal anesthesia for surgical reasons (such as inguinal hernia, hemorroids, prostatic hypertrophy, ets.), or for diagnostic purposes in patients afterwards diagnosed as neurotic and free from any neurological disease. The group consisted of 13 males and 10 females, 30-70 years old (median 50).

Analytical methods

CSF N-CAM concentrations were determined by an inhibition ELISA previously set up and described (Ibsen et al., 1983). Briefly, solubilized human brain membranes were adsorbed to polystyrene microtest plates (Nunk, Denmark). The test solution to be measured was mixed with specific reference anti-N-CAM antibodies and this mixture incubated with the sensitized solid phase. After suitable washing, peroxidase-conjugated secondary antibodies were added. Finally, excess unbound reagent was removed by washing and the chromogenic enzyme substrate was applied. Statistical evaluations were made using analysis of variance and Student's t-test for unpaired data. CSF samples were stored at or below -20°C until analysis.

RESULTS

After the aforementioned therapy was administered, all the acute MS patients showed a more or less consistent clinical improvement, while the non-acute MS patients showed only minor signs of improvement, or no change at all. None of the patients presented signs of steroid overdosage, nor complications related to the lumbar puncture or to side effects of the drug vehicle.

Results are shown graphically in Fig.1 and 2. Fig.1 shows N-CAM concentrations in the first CSF sample taken from each MS patient and from the control subjects. At the time of this first sampling the MS patients had not yet received any treatment and therefore the three groups can be compared without regard to any possible influence of steroid treatment on CSF N-CAM levels. Mean values were 589 ± 321 ng/ml (median 510) for the acute phase patients; 497 ± 284 ng/ml (median 432) for the non-acute phase patients; and 765 ± 299 ng/ml (median 657) for the controls. Only the difference between patients in non-acute phase and the control group is statistically significant ($p < 0.025$). Subsequently, within each group of MS patients, mean values obtained from the first (I), second (II) and third (III) lumbar punctures were compared (Fig.2). No statistically significant differences were found in the group of non-acute phase patients. Conversely, mean N-CAM concentrations of first (583 ng/ml), second (1006 ng/ml) and third (1265 ng/ml) lumbar puncture samples from the acute phase patients did differ significantly from each other: $p < 0.02$ comparing I and II; $p < 0.005$ comparing I and III; and $p < 0.01$ when II and III are compared.

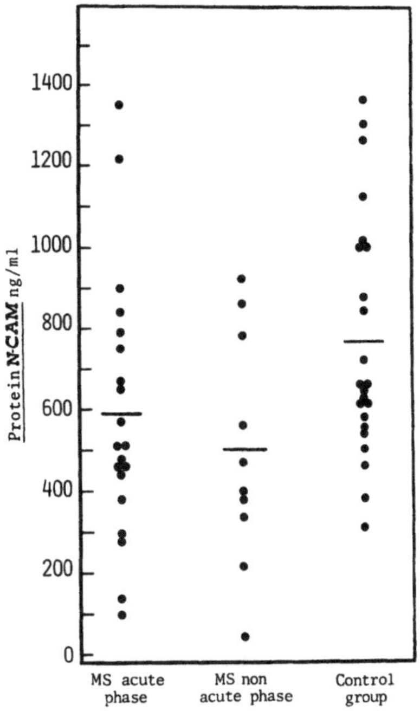

Fig.1. CSF concentrations of N-CAM in 20 MS patients in the acute phase, 10 MS patients in non-acute phase, and 23 control subjects without neurological disease. Only the first lumbar puncture sample from each MS patient is included. The bars represent mean values.

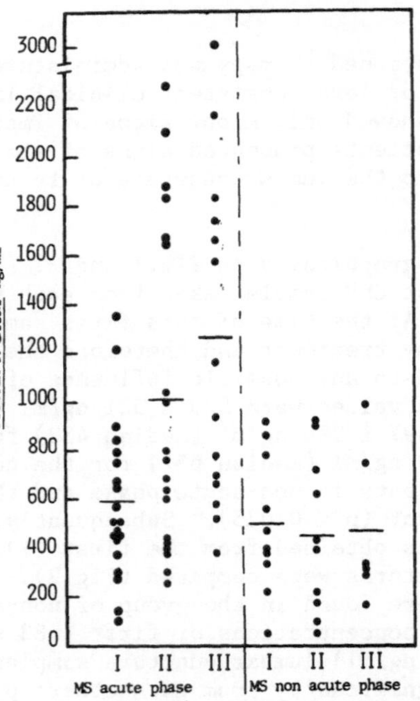

Fig.2. CSF concentrations of N-CAM in acute phase and non-acute phase MS patients. For each group, values obtained from first (I), second (II) and third (III) lumbar punctures are shown. The bars represent mean values.

DISCUSSION

N-CAM levels in CSF taken from two groups of MS patients (acute phase and non-acute phase) prior to steroid treatment, and from a control group of non-neurological patients were compared. The only statistical significant difference observed, was that of the non-acute phase patients having a lower mean CSF N-CAM content than the control group. The acute phase patients too showed on the average lower N-CAM levels than the control group, but this difference was not statistically significant. As a first hypothesis, the subnormal N-CAM levels in CSF could be caused by a lower than normal turnover of N-CAM in the brain. Alternatively, or at the same time, low N-CAM levels might be related to an altered CSF flow pattern, as suggested by the low N-CAM concentrations observed in CSF from NPH patients (Soelberg Sörensen et al., 1983). The fact that only the non-acute phase patients showed significantly decreased N-CAM levels might be related to differences in the state of progression of the disease in the two MS patients group. It is known that a relapsing course is more usual in the early stages of the disease, while a slowly worsening course is more common in the subsequent stages. In fact, the median age of acute phase patients in the present study is 31, while that of non-acute phase patients is 41. Further studies are needed to test this hypothesis.

The N-CAM content of CSF was found to increase significantly during the weeks following an acute exacerbation, reaching a mean value well above that of the control group. This development paralleled a pronounced clinical amelioration of the patients, who showed good or excellent recovery within one month after onset of exacerbation. A similar rise in CSF levels of N-CAM was observed during periods of recovery of manic-melancholic patients (Jörgensen et al., 1977) and of patients with delirium tremens and related clinical states (Jörgensen et al., 1980b). The biological basis for these findings can only be speculated upon at present. However, it seems reasonable to suppose, along with the latter authors, that the changes are related to synaptic remodelling and possibly neo-synaptogenesis. Alternatively, the rise in N-CAM levels may reflect the cleaning-up process with break-down and removal of damaged neurons and neuritic processes. The effect of the intrathecal steroid treatment cannot be assessed in the present study, because no control group of non-treated MS patients was available.

ACKNOWLEDGEMENTS

This research was supported in part by a grant from the Italian "Ministero della Publica Istruzione"; Warwara Larsens and Grosserer Sigurd Abrahamson og hustru Addie Abraham Abrahamson Mindelegat are thankfully acknowledged for their support.

REFERENCES

1. J.R. Brown, G.W. Beebe and J.F. Kurtzke. The design of clinical studies to assess therapeutic efficacy in multiple sclerosis. Neurology. 29:3 (1979).
2. R. Brackenbury, U. Rutishauser and G.M. Edelman. Distinct calcium-independent and calcium-dependent adhesion systems of chicken embryo cells. Proc. Natl. Acad. Sci. USA. 78:387 (1984).
3. S.E. Fraser, B.A. Murray, C.-M. Chuong and G.M. Edelman. Alteration of the retinothecal map in Xenopus by antibodies to neural cell adhesion molecules. Proc. Natl. Acad. Sci. USA. 81:4222 (1984).
4. S. Ibsen, V. Berezin, B. Nörgaard Pedersen and E. Bock. Enzyme-linked immunosorbent assay of the D2 glycoprotein. J. Neurochem. 41:356 (1983).
5. O.S. Jörgensen and E. Bock. Brain specific synaptosomal membrane antigens demonstrated by crossed immunoelectrophoresis. J. Neurochem. 23:879 (1974).
6. O.S. Jörgensen, E. Bock, P. Beck and O.J. Rafaelsen. Synaptic membrane protein D2 in the cerebrospinal fluid of manic-melancolic patients. Acta Psychiat. Scand. 56:50 (1977).
7. O.S. Jörgensen, A. Delouvée, J.-P. Thiery and J.M. Edelman. The nervous system specific protein D2 is involved in adhesion among the neurites from cultured rat ganglia. FEBS Lett. 111:39 (1980).
8. O.S. Jörgensen, R. Hemmingsen, P. Kramp and O.J. Rafaelsen. Blood-brain barrier selectivity and synaptic turnover during delirium tremens and related clinical states. Acta Psychiat. Scand. 61:356 (1980).
9. A.R. Massaro. Modifications of the cerebrospinal fluid IgG concentrations in patients with multiple sclerosis treated with intrathecal steroids. J. Neurol. 219:221 (1978).
10. A.R. Massaro, F. Michetti and G.L. Gigli. Marker liquorali di danno del sistema nervoso centrale. In:"L'analisi diagnostica del liquor", B. Tavolato and P. Livrea, eds., Piccin, Padova, pp.147-158 (1982).
11. A.R. Massaro, F. Michetti, A. Laudisio and P. Bergonzi. Myelin basic protein and S-100 antigen in CSF of patients with multiple sclerosis in the acute phase. Ital. J. Neurol. Sci. 6:53 (1975).
12. I.S. Neu, N.H. Koenig and W. Günther. Management of acute multiple sclerosis by a long acting intrathecally administered corticosteroid. In:"Immunological and clinical aspects of multiple sclerosis", R.E. Gonsette and P. Delmotte, eds. MTP Press Ltd., Lancaster pp.253-256 (1984).

13. M. Noble, M. Albrechtsen, C. Möller, J. Lyles, E. Bock, M. Watanabe, C. Goridis and U. Rutishauser. Glial cells express N-CAM/D2-CAM-like polypeptides in vitro. Nature. 316:725 (1985).
14. S. Rasmussen, V. Berezin, B. Nörgaard Pedersen and E. Bock. Purification of the glycoprotein D2 from fetal and adult human brain. In: "Protides of the biological fluids", H. Peeters, ed. Pergamon Press,Oxford. pp.83-86 (1983).
15. U. Rutishauser, W.E. Gall and G.M. Edelman. Adhesion among neural cells of the chick embryo. IV. Role of the cell surface molecule CAM in the formation of neurite bundles in cultures of spinal ganglia. J. Cell. Biol. 79:382 (1978).
16. P. Soelberg Sörensen, F. Gjerris, S. Ibsen and E. Bock. Low concentration of brain-specific protein D2 in patients with normal pressure hydrocephalus. J. Neurol. Sci. 62:59 (1983).

DETECTION OF Fc 'GAMMA' R-LIKE MATERIAL IN CEREBROSPINAL FLUID: A FACTOR MODIFYING THE IMMUNE REACTION?

D. Karcher, W. De Smet, F. Frank and A.Lowenthal

Laboratory of Neurochemistry, Born-Bunge Stichting, University of Antwerp (UIA), 2610 Antwerp, Belgium

INTRODUCTION

Fc-gamma receptors (Fc-gamma-R) are among the most important surface structures of a number of immunocompetent cells. They are present on most B lymphocytes, a subpopulation of T lymphocytes, macrophages, natural killer cells, killer cells and neutrophils. They have been implicated in several immune reactions such as phagocytosis, release of mediators of inflammation, antibody-dependent cell-mediated cytotoxicity, and antigen presentation (1,2). A regulatory role (for example suppressive activity on the antibody level) has also been ascribed to them (3). By means of monoclonal antibody (mAb) 2.4G2 (directed against the Fc-gamma-$_{2b/gamma-1}$R of mouse macrophages and B cells) the presence of circulating Fc-gamma-R in normal serum has recently been reported (4,5). It is of importance to note that an enhanced concentration of this soluble Fc-gamma-R was observed in serum of mice with certain autoimmune disorders (4,5). As multiple sclerosis (MS) can be considered as an autoimmune disease, we thought it worthwhile to examine the possible role these Fc-gamma-R might play in the immunoregulatory process in such patients.

MATERIAL AND METHODS

Preparation of cells and cell lysates

Mononuclear cells were prepared from venous peripheral blood (anticoagulated with heparin) on Ficoll-Paque (Pharmacia Fine Chemicals, Uppsala, Sweden). The sediments of these gradients were mixed with dextran and, after sedimentation of erythrocytes, granulocytes were recovered through lysis of the contaminating erythrocytes by hypotonic shock in distilled water. Both lymphocytes and granulocytes were washed extensively before solubilization in lysis buffer (phosphate buffered saline (PBS) containing NP-40, EDTA, aprotinin, pepstatin, iodoacetamide and phenylmethyl sulfonylfluoride) (1 ml lysis buffer/10^8 cells, 1 min at 4°C). The lysed cells were then centrifuged at 30,000 g (1 h,4°C). The supernatant was dialyzed overnight against PBS and kept frozen at -20°C.

Sepharose 4B immunosorbent

Human IgG were precipitated with Na_2SO_4 (18%) and purified on a DEAE

Sephadex A50 column (Pharmacia). Aggregated human IgG were prepared by heating human IgG (10 mg/ml PBS) at 63°C during 30'. $F(ab')_2$ fragments of human IgG were prepared by digestion with pepsin. Non digested IgG and contaminating Fc fragments were removed by affinity chromatography on a Sepharose-Protein A column (Pharmacia) and gel filtration on a Sephadex G200 column (Pharmacia). Ovalbumin was purchased from Sigma (A5503). The antigens were coupled to cyanogen bromide activated Sepharose 4B (Pharmacia) according to instructions. 10-15 mg of ovalbumin, human IgG, aggregated human IgG and $F(ab')_2$ fragments were bound to each ml of gel.

Free Fc-gamma receptor isolated from pooled human serum

400 ml pooled human plasma were run on a column (50 cm, Ø 1 cm) of aggregated human IgG coupled to cyanogen bromide activated Sepharose 4B. The column was washed with PBS/0.1 % NP-40 and eluted with 0.5 N acetic acid/ 0.1 % NP-40. The fractions eluted around pH 3.5 were found to contain the free Fc-gamma-R.

Binding activity of serum Fc-gamma receptor

The free Fc-gamma-R from pooled human serum was adsorbed on IgG, $F(ab')_2$ and ovalbumin immunosorbent. 1.5 ml Sepharose 4B immunosorbent was mixed for 2 h at 4°C with 250 µl sample. The unadsorbed and non-adherent fractions were tested in a solid phase radioimmunoassay (RIA) for the presence of residual Fc-gamma-R.

Cerebrospinal fluid samples

The cerebrospinal fluid (CSF) samples were collected after lumbar puncture from different sources but mainly from the Algemeen Ziekenhuis Middelheim, where the clinical data was readily made available. 118 CSF samples from patients affected with neurological diseases were studied. They run as follows: MS: 36; SSPE: 20; spongiform encephalopathy: 1; meningo encephalitis: 7; degenerative diseases: 4; peripheral nerve diseases: 11; vascular diseases: 10; metastases: 5; epilepsy: 5; intoxications: 6; cephalgia: 6; and miscellaneous: 7.

CSF IgG evaluation

Immunodiffusion plates (Behring Werke, Marburg, Germany) for qualitative determination of human IgG at low concentrations in CSF were used to test our samples.

CSF total proteins

The CSF total proteins were determined using Coomassie Page Blue (Electran Page Blue G90 BDH 44248).

Monoclonal antibodies

The mAb used are B73.1 (kindly provided by B. Perussia and G. Trinchieri, The Wistar Institute, Philadelphia, PA), and VEP13 (BMA 070, purchased from Behring Diagnostic Brussels). B73.1 is highly reactive with a subset of lymphocytes with natural killer and killer cell activity and in about half of the donors with neutrophils (6). VEP13 also reacts with an antigen present on virtually all natural killer cells and neutrophils from all donors (7). These two mAb are directed against and inhibit the functional properties of the Fc-gamma-R of these cells but recognize different epitopes (8). Both mAb were labelled with ^{125}I according to the method of Greenwood (9).

Solid phase radioimmunoassay

The solid phase radioimmunoassay (RIA) was carried out as described by Ran et al., (10). 50 µl of cell lysate or CSF samples were pipetted in flexible Falcon microtiter plates and air dried. 75 µl 80% acetone was then added to each well for 5'. The wells were emptied and a second portion of 80% acetone was added and left to incubate at room temperature for 15'. The wells were emptied, washed and saturated with 250 µl PBS/1% bovine serum albumin (BSA) for 60'. The wells were emptied and 50 µl labelled mAb diluted in PBS/1% BSA, the radioactivity measuring 50,000 cpm, were added to each well and incubated overnight at 4°C. After washing, the wells were cut out and the bound radioactivity counted in a gamma counter.

RESULTS

We have adapted to the human system a previously described solid phase RIA method (10, measuring soluble Fc-gamma-R in mouse serum, using two mAb directed against different epitopes of one type of Fc-gamma-R (present on natural killer cells, killer cells and neutrophils). To test the specificity of the assay, or in other words to check whether we were indeed measuring Fc-gamma-R-like material, a number of controls were carried out. From Fig.1 it is evident that ^{125}I-VEP13 reacts strongly with cell lysates of Fc-gamma-R$^+$ neutrophils and lymphocytes, while binding weakly to lysates prepared from Fc-gamma-R$^-$ cells. Similar data were obtained with ^{125}I-B73.1, except that this mAb gave higher counts with lysates of lymphocytes than of neutrophils. The latter phenomenon correla-

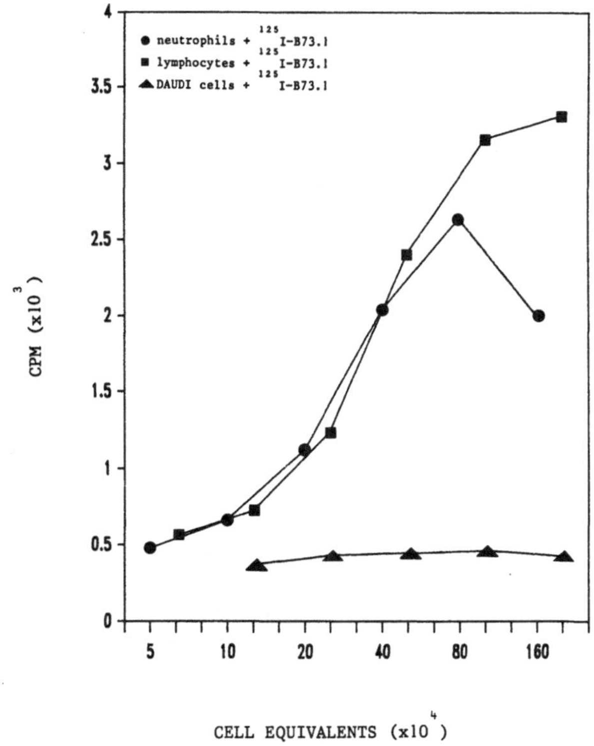

Fig.1. Binding of ^{125}I-VEP13 (closed symbols) and ^{125}I-BSA (open symbols) to cell lysates of Fc-gamma-R$^+$ lymphocytes (■) and neutrophils (●) and Fc-gamma-R$^-$ lyphocytes (▲) using solid phase RIA.

tes well with observations in flow microfluormetry, that indicate that the epitope recognized by mAb B73.1 is expressed only weakly on polymorphonuclear leukocytes (8). In addition, the results of the incubation of cell-lysates with ^{125}I-BSA can be considered as non specific binding. It is of importance to say that Daudi cells (which, in our hands, are Fc-gamma-R^{+} by rosetting, but which possess a Fc-gamma-R type that cannot be detected with the mAb used in this study) gave low values when incubated with ^{125}I-B73.1. This indicates that the observed binding to lymphocytes and neutrophils is not due to "aspecific" interaction of the Fc fragment of the labelled mAb with Fc-gamma-R which could eventually have retained their functional activity (Fig.2). In a second series of experiments, we compared the binding of the reactive material on immunosorbents consisting of Sepharose linked either to human IgG molecules, F(ab')$_2$ fragments or ovalbumin. As can be seen in Table 1, nearly all the reactive material was retained on a Sepharose-IgG column while some remained linked to ovalbumin. Immunosorbent-F(ab')$_2$ columns gave intermediary results.

Table 1. Binding of monoclonal ^{125}I-alpha-FcR (VEP13) to free Fc-gamma receptor isolated from pooled human serum (cpm)

	Exp 1	Exp 2
unadsorbed	3308	3091
human agg-IgG sepharose	966	896
human agg-F(ab')$_2$ sepharose	1445	1298
ovalbumin sepharose	2485	2137

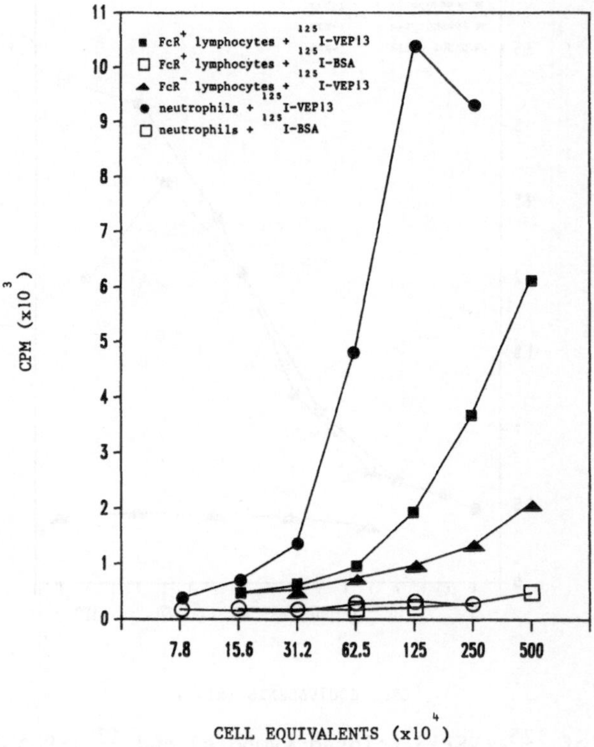

Fig.2. Binding of ^{125}I-B73.1 to Fc-gammaR^{+} lysates of lyphocytes (■), neutrophils (●) and Daudi cells (▲) using solid phase RIA.

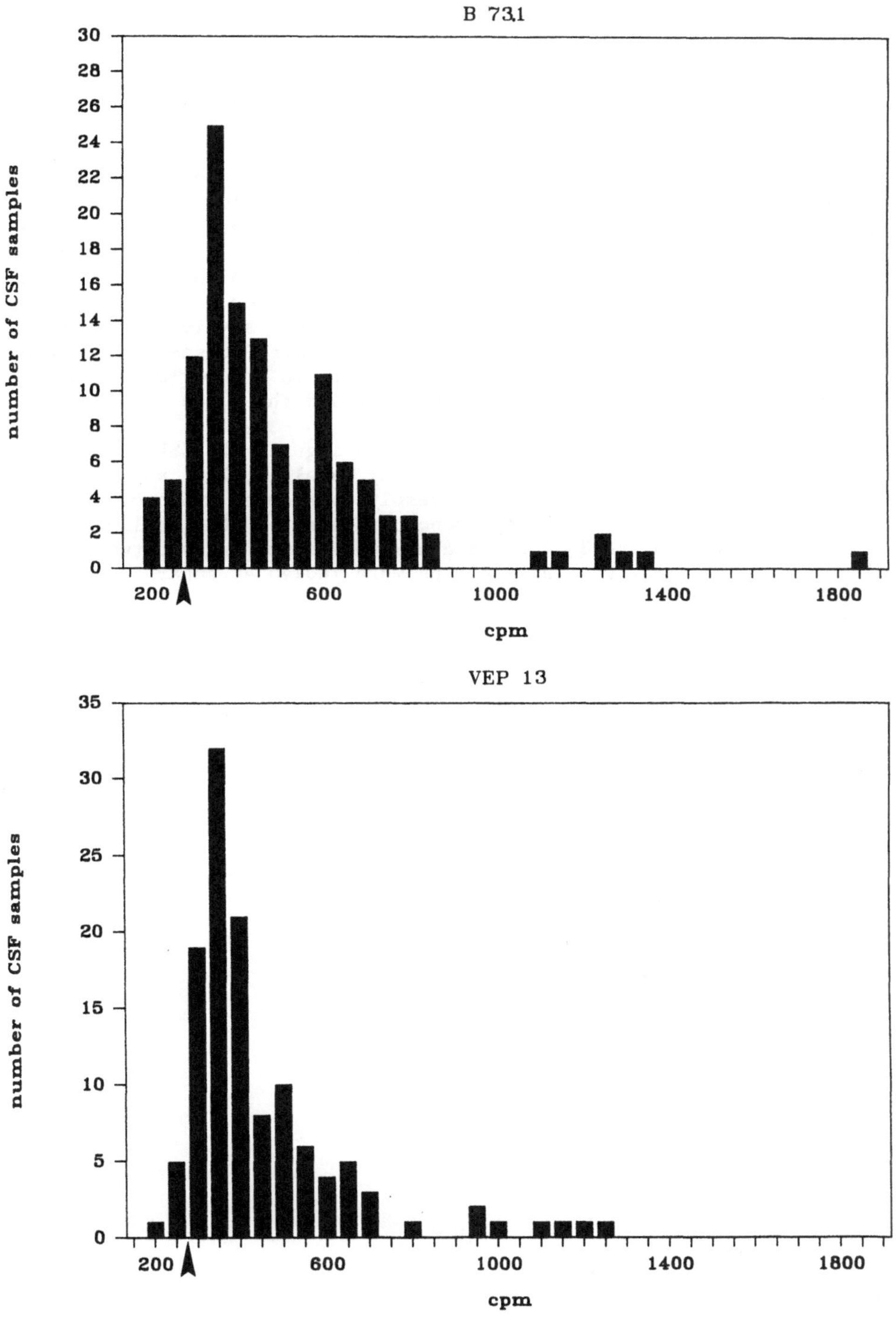

Fig.3. Histograms summarizing the results obtained for 118 CSF samples: binding of ^{125}I-B73.1 and ^{125}I-VEP13 to Fc-gamma R-like material.

We measured receptors for the Fc portion of the IgG in the CSF. The histograms show the distribution of free Fc-gamma-R in the CSF of 118 neurological patients, working with two different labelled mAb B73.1 and VEP13 (Fig.3).

All counts above 250 cpm were considered positive and this is a sufficient margin to account for nonspecific binding. Referring to the distribution pattern, all counts above 600 were taken as pathological.

The CSF samples from patients affected with neurological diseases were classified in three groups consisting of 36 MS patients, 20 SSPE patients, and 69 other neurological diseases (OND). For each group a correlation was looked for between the results obtained using both antibodies. The correlation coefficients (r) are judged to be very high when lying between .90- 1.00; high .78-.89; intermediate .64-.77; low .46-.63 and very low .00-.45. For MS the r was .69, only 3 cases were atypical, possibly corresponding with a clinical exacerbation. For SSPE, 15 cases registered high cpm using both mAb, and the r here was .88. In the series of OND, 8 cases out of 63 gave high values with both mAb and the r was .73 (Fig.4).

In addition we looked for a correlation using all the CSF samples studied and their total protein content using labelled B73.1 and VEP13. The r were respectively .61 and .65, a result considered average. The same approach was made using CSF IgG concentrations. With labelled B73.1 the r was .87 and with VEP13 .42. To check this discrepancy between the results for the two mAb, the three groups were looked at separately. When using VEP13, in MS CSF an r of .81 was calculated, in SSPE CSF an r of .72, and in the OND an r of .48.

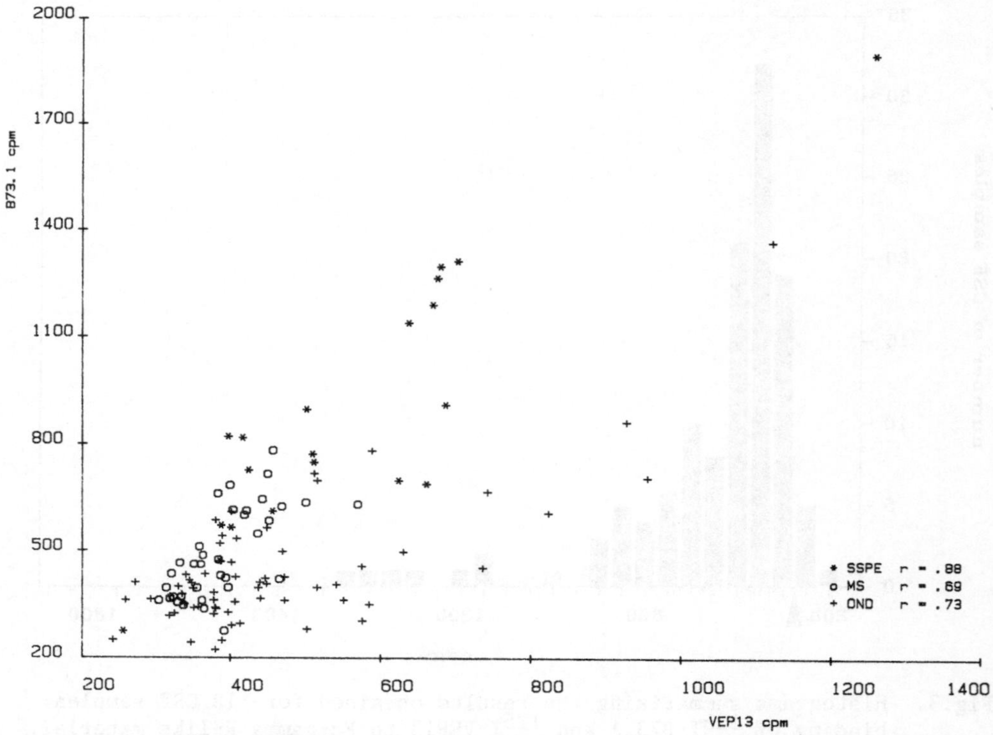

Fig.4. Correlation between B73.1 and VEP13 in cpm for Fc-gamma-R-like material present in the CSF of 20 SSPE (✱), 36 MS (□) and 69 OND (+).

DISCUSSION

The object of this study was to find another approach to the immune dysregulation observed in slow viral diseases, such as visna in sheep, SSPE in man, and MS, because of the oligoclonal reaction observed in the CSF. We have been looking for an inhibiting factor which might play a role in SSPE and eventually in MS.

The human immune reaction in SSPE is not impaired, and the antibodies in the CSF and in the serum of these patients do react with all the measles polypeptides. Therefore there is every reason to believe that there must, somewhere along the line, be a failure in the immune regulation.

To investigate the possible involvement of Fc-gamma-R in the immunoregulation of MS and SSPE, we measured (i) soluble Fc-gamma-R-like material in CSf by means of a solid-phase RIA, and (ii) percentage of Fc-gamma-R^+ cells (and their staining intensity) in peripheral blood by means of flow microfluorometry.

Specificity of the solid phase RIA was underlined by the following observations: (i) binding of ^{125}I-VEP13 or ^{125}I-B73.1 on cell extracts of Fc R^+ lymphocytes and neutrophils but not on extracts of Fc-gamma-R^- cells; (ii) no binding of an irrelevant ^{125}I-BSA probe; (iii) preferential adsorption of the reactive material on Sepharose-IgG as compared to Sepharose-ovalbumin columns.

SSPE patients (15 cases of a total of 20) showed a significantly enhanced concentration of Fc-gamma-R-like material in their CSF. A number of reports have indicated the existence of an inhibiting factor of the immune response in serum and CSF of SSPE patients, influencing, among others, the immune reactivity against measles virus (11,12). Soluble Fc-gamma-R could well be responsible for some of the observed facts. It would therefore be of interest to see whether a similar enhancement of soluble Fc-gamma-R is present in SSPE serum, and in case this material can be purified, to investigate its possible involvement in a number of "in vitro" tests. The CSF of MS patients measured for their Fc-gamma-R content with both mAb gave a normal number of cpm except 3 out of a total of 36 registered high counts.

By flow microfluormetry, 4 MS and 1 SSPE patient were studied. No marked differences in number of Fc-gamma-R^+ cells (in both lymphocyte and neutrophil preparations) or their staining intensity was observed (results not shown).

The high values found in the CSF of SSPE for Fc-gamma-R could be due to mthe following: 1) the measles virus in SSPE could induce disturbances of the normal cell membrane structure, thus causing an impairment of specialized membrane function; 2) comparing the CSF Fc-gamma-R level in MS, SSPE and OND with their IgG concentration, there appears to be a better correlation for those with high IgG content. In the course of immunological stimulation, it was demonstrated in vitro that different classes or subclasses of immunoglobulins could induce T cells to express specific receptors (13). These experiments refer to membrane linked Fc-gamma-R demonstrated with fluorescence-activated cell sorter analysis or by rosetting. The increases of free Fc-gamma-R cannot be ascribed to the cells present in the CSF. All CSF were handled in the same manner and in SSPE there is no increase of the CSF cell count. The release of Fc-gamma-R could be ascribed to the central nervous system. These observations suggest that FcR expression and release might act on the immunoregulatory system in SSPE and perhaps MS.

ACKNOWLEDGEMENT

The work was supported by grants awarded by the University of Antwerp (UIA); the Nationaal Fonds voor Wetenschappelijk Onderzoek (3.0004.81), the Nationale Loterij (9.0017.83), the Ministerie voor Nationale Opvoeding and the Programma voor Wetenschapsbeleid (84/89-68).

REFERENCES

1. J.C. Unkeless, H. Fleit and I.S. Mellman. Structural aspects and heterogeneity of immunoglobulin Fc receptors. Adv. Immunol. 31:247 (1981).
2. L. Fornusek and V. Vetvicka. Fc receptor - More answers, more questions. Folia Microbiol. 29:476 (1984).
3. W.H. Fridman, C. Rabourdin-Combe, C. Neauport-Sautes and R.J. Gisler. Characterization and function of T cell Fc receptor. Immunol. Rev. 56:51 (1981).
4. E. Pure, C.J. Durie, C.K. Summerill and J.C. Unkeless. Identification of soluble Fc receptors in mouse serum and the conditioned medium of stimulated B cells. J. Exp. Med. 160:1836 (1984).
5. D. Khayat, Z. Dux, R. Anavi, F. Shlomo, I.P. Witz and M. Ran. Circulating cell-free Fc $_{2b/1}$R in normal mouse serum; its detection and specificity. J. Immunol. 132:2496 (1984).
6. B. Perussia, S. Starr, S. Abraham, V. Fanning and G. Trinchieri. Human natural killer cells analysed by B73.1, a monoclonal antibody blocking Fc receptor functions. I. Characterization of the lymphocyte subset reactive with B73.1. J. Immunol. 130:2133 (1983).
7. H. Rumpold, D. Kraft, G. Obexer, G. Bock and G. Gebhart. A monoclonal antibody against a surface antigen shared by human large granular lymphocytes and granulocytes. J. Immunol. 129:1458 (1982).
8. B. Perussia, G. Trinchieri, A. Jackson, N.L. Warner, J. Faust, H. Rumpold, D. Kraft and L.L. Lanier. The Fc receptor for IgG on human natural killer cells: phenotypic, functional and comparative studies with monoclonal antibodies. J. Immunol. 133:180 (1984).
9. F.C. Greenwood, W.M. Hunter, J.S. Glover. The preparation of I^{131} labelled human growth hormone of high specific radioactivity. Biochem. J. 89:114-123 (1963).
10. M. Ran, Z. Dux, R. Anavi, N.I. Smorodinsky and I.P. Witz. A radioimmunoassay with monoclonal antibodies for the detection of antigenic cell-free Fc receptors. J. Immunol. Meth. 68:275 (1984).
11. A. Ahmed, D.M. Strong, K.W. Sell, G.B. Thurman, R.C. Knudsen, R. Wistar and W.R. Grace. Demonstration of a blocking factor in the plasma and spinal fluid of patients with subacute sclerosing panencephalitis. I. Partial characterization. J. Exp. Med. 139:902 (1974).
12. D. Karcher. Inhibiting factor: general review. In: "Humoral Immunity in Neurological Diseases", D. Karcher, A. Lowenthal, A.D. Strosberg, ed... Nato Advanced Study Institutes Series. Life Sciences, Plenum Press, New York, vol. 24:541-551 (1979).
13. M. Daeron and W.H. Fridman. Towards an isotypic network. 7e Forum d'Immunologie. Fc receptors as regulatory molecules. Ann. Inst. Pasteur Immunol. 136C:383-387 (1985).

IMMUNOSUPPRESSIVE ACIDIC PROTEIN (IAP) IN CEREBROSPINAL FLUID AND SERUM OF PATIENTS WITH MULTIPLE SCLEROSIS AND OTHER INFLAMMATORY NEUROLOGICAL DISEASES

Tetsuro Tsukamoto, Hisatomo Seki, Hisashi Aso*, Keiji Tamura*, Sadao Takase and Nakao Ishida*

*Department of Neurology, Institute of Brain Diseases and Department of Microbiology, Tohoku University School of Medicine, 1-1 Seiryo-machi, Sendai 980, Japan

SUMMARY

IAP has a molecular weight of 50,000 daltons, an isoelectric point of 3.0 and contains 31.5% carbohydrate. It is mainly produced by macrophages when stimulate in the presence of circulating immune complexes or some inflammatory substances. IAP acts immunosuppressively by inducing suppressor macrophages. We assayed the IAP levels in cerebrospinal fluid (CSF) and serum at the same time in patients with multiple sclerosis (MS), neuro-Behcet's disease (NBD), Guillain-Barré syndrome (GBS), amyotrophic lateral sclerosis (ALS) and control patients without intracranial organic lesion. In MS patients,, the CSF IAP increased during both the active and inactive stage, whereas serum IAP decreased significantly during the inactive stage. IAP% (CSF IAP/CSF protein) increased markedly during the active stage. These results suggest that intracranial production of IAP occurs and the efflux of IAP into blood might further induce suppressor macrophages and elevate the serum levels of IAP. In NBD patients, during the active stage, IAP levels, IAP% and IAP rate (CSF IAP/serum IAP) were all elevated, while during the inactive stage, CSF IAP significantly decreased. In GBS patients, CSF IAP increased greatly, being associated with an increase in protein levels in CSF, but an elevation of IAP% was only a little. IAP assay in CSF and serum at the same time could provide us many important informations about immunopathogenesis of MS and other inflammatory neurological disorders.

INTRODUCTION

We have recently assayed the serum levels of immunosuppressive acidic protein (IAP) in various neurological patients by a single radial immuno-usion method and found that IAP increased significantly in multiple sclerosis (MS) patients, especially during the active stage (1,2). The inflamflammatory and demyelinating processes, however, occur in the central nervous system (CNS) which is uniquely protected with blood brain barrier (BBB). We developed therefore a passive hemagglutination (PHA) - inhibition test (4) for the detection of scarce quantity of IAP in CSF to answer the question of where the production of IAP takes place, locally in the CNS or systemically elsewhere, by comparing with the serum levels of IAP. We also assayed the IAP levels in CSF of patients with neuro-

Behcet's disease (NBD), Guillain-Barré syndrome (GBS) and amyotrophic lateral sclerosis (ALS) to see whether the IAP in CSF can reflect the immunopathological process in these neurological diseases.

Briefly, we summarize here the physicochemical properties, the mechanism of the production of IAP and its function on the basis of several lines of evidence which were already reported (3,4,5,6); IAP has a molecular weight of 50,000 daltons, an isoelectric point of 3.0 and contains 31.5% carbohydrate. IAP is mainly produced by macrophages when stimulated in the presence of circulating immune complexes or some inflammatory substances and acts immunosuppressively by inducing suppressor macrophages (Fig.1).

MATERIALS AND METHODS

Serum and CSF samples were collected at the same time from the following neurological patients and control patients who were suffering from headache, epilepsy or hysteria without evidence of having any organic lesion in the nervous system, and stored at -20°C until use.

1. Control patients

Twenty-two samples were obtained from twenty-two patients between 16 and 58 years old, consisting of 5 patients with headache, four with epilepsy and thirteen with hysteria.

2. MS

Sixty-one samples were obtained from 32 patients between 8 and 69 years old. Among the samples, 24 were taken during the clinically active stage and 37 during the stable stage.

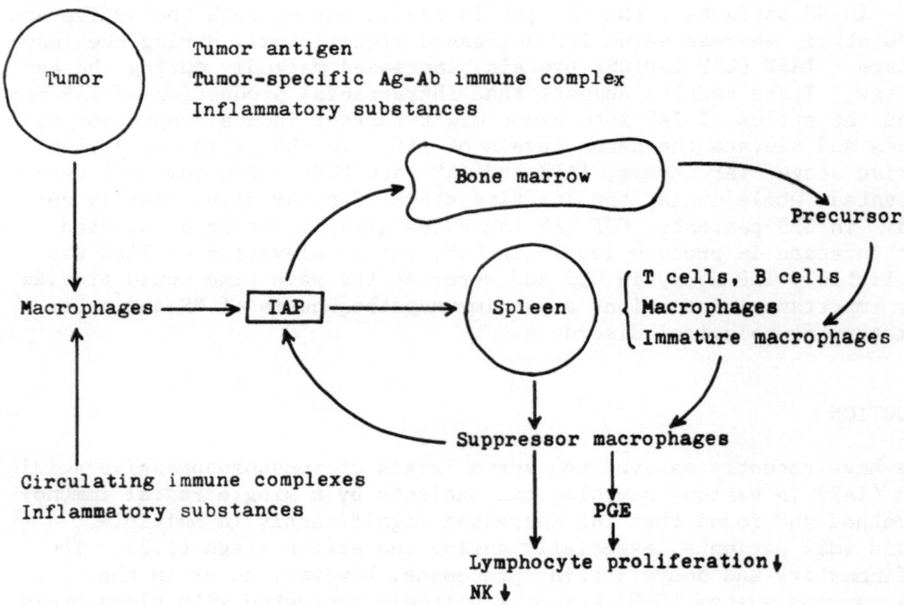

Fig.1. The mechanism of the production of IAP and its effect on inducing suppressor macrophages are summarized in a schema from several publications (3,4,5,6).

3. NBD

Twenty-nine samples were obtained from 13 patients between 21 and 46 years old. Among the samples, 18 were taken during the clinically active stage and 11 during the stable stage.

4. GBS

Forty samples were obtained during the illness from 11 patients between 10 and 67 years old.

5. ALS

Sixteen samples were obtained from 16 patients between 33 and 74 years old.

To assay the serum level of IAP we used a single radial immunodiffusion method (1,2,3,7). Five ul of serum was applied to an IAP agarose plate containing 5% nonspecific anti-IAP goat serum. After 48 hours' incubation in a moist chamber at 37°C, the diameter of the precipitating ring was measured and the concentration of IAP (μg/ml) was determined in a calibration curve between 50 and 1500-μg/ml concentration of purified IAP.

The IAP levels in CSF were assayed as follows by using a PHA-inhibition test (6). CSF was serially diluted with PBS containing 2% fetal calf serum (PBS-FCS) in a microtiter plate (Cooke Engineering, Alexandria, Va.), followed by the addition of an equal volume (25 μl) of rabbit anti-IAP serum dilution ($x10^{-5}$). After incubation at room temperature for 30 minutes, 50 μl of 0.4% IAP-coated SRBC suspension in PBS-FCS was added to each well and mixed. The plate was then incubated at room temperature for 2 hours and the inhibiting point of hemagglutination in the serially diluted CSF was determined. As a standard, IAP solution containing 2500 ng/ml was always assayed at the same time. By this method, the minimum amount of IAP detectable in CSF was as low as 10 ng/ml.

CSF-IAP% was calculated by [IAP(μg/ml) in CSF] x 100/ [protein(μg/ml) in CSF] and IAP rate by [IAP(μg/ml) in CSF] x 100/ [IAP(μg/ml) in serum].

The statistical significance was calculated by the Student's t-test or Cochran-Cox test.

RESULTS

The results of the present study are summarized in Table 1. Control patients had 1.66 ± 0.84 μg/ml (mean ± S.D.) of IAP in CSF. IAP% and IAP rate were 0.64 ± 0.27 and 0.35 ± 0.19 respectively.

In MS patients, IAP in CSF increased significantly both during the active stage (3.91 ± 2.85) and during the inactive stage (3.48 ± 2.68), but no difference was seen between the two stages. Although both IAP% and IAP rate were elevated, IAP% during the active stage increased more markedly than IAP rate. During the inactive stage, IAP% decreased, but was still much higher than that of control patients.

On the other hand, in patients with NBD, the difference of IAP amount in CSF between the active and inactive stage was very large. The value during the active stage was 6.21 ± 5.17 μg/ml and significantly higher

Table 1. CSF IAP values, serum IAP values, IAP% (CSF IAP/CSF protein) and IAP rate (CSF/IAP/serum IAP)in controls, and patients with multiple sclerosis (MS) during the active stage and inactive stage, neuro-Behcet's disease (NBD) during the active stage and inactive stage, Guillain-Barré syndrome (GBS) during the acute phase and recovery phase and amyotrophic lateral sclerosis (ALS). *The previous data (6.7) are shown to compare with this study.

Subjects	CSF IAP (μg/ml)	Serum IAP (μg/ml)	Serum IAP* (μg/ml)	IA%	IAP rate
control	1.66 ± 0.84	388.8 ± 142.8	385.0 ± 73.3	0.64 ± 0.72	0.35 ± 0.19
MS, active	3.91 ± 2.85	612.6 ± 217.6	630.4 ± 190.0	1.89 ± 1.93	0.78 ± 0.49
inactive	3.48 ± 2.68	441.9 ± 187.7	432.9 ± 169.9	1.14 ± 0.83	0.72 ± 0.55
NBD, active	6.21 ± 5.17	NT	678.3 ± 202.6	1.45 ± 0.75	
inactive	2.31 ± 1.67	NT	549.8 ± 109.1	0.46 ± 0.30	
GBS, active	9.85 ± 4.42	465.7 ± 120.4	NT	0.78 ± 0.19	2.02 ± 1.54
recovery	4.66 ± 3.28	452.0 ± 178.8	NT	0.72 ± 0.46	0.78 ± 0.45
ALS	1.75 ± 1.25	344.6 ± 114.8	449.4 ± 159.5	0.46 ± 0.19	0.46 ± 0.30

means ± S.D.

than the value during the inactive stage (2.31 ± 1.67). Although both IAP% and IAP rate were elevated during the active stage, IAP was more elevated than IAP%. During the inactive stage, however, both of the rates returned lower almost to the rates of control patients.

In GBS patients, the value of IAP in CSF was 7.29 ± 5.35 μg/ml. When the acute phase was arbitrarily regarded to be within 30 days after onset of the disease and the recovery phase to be after 50 days, the IAP value during the acute phase was 9.85 ± 4.42 μg/ml and the one during the recovery phase was 4.66 ± 3.28 μg/ml. Although the IAP levels in CSF during the recovery phase decreased markedly, it remained significantly higher for a long time than that of control patients. IAP rate was greatly elevated during the acute phase (2.02 ± 1.54), but IAP% (0.78 ± 0.19) was almost the same as that of control patients.

The IAP levels in CSF of patients with ALS was not different from those of control patients. IAP% abd IAP rate were also nearly the same.

DISCUSSION

IAP was found in 1977 in the serum and ascitic fluid of cancer hosts during a search for immunosuppressive mechanism in cancer patients (3). In fact, most of the IAP research until now have been done experimentally (3,5,6) or clinically (7) from this point of view, and many results have been accumulated. We tried to draw a schema in Fig.1 from those results to understand the mechanism of IAP production and its immunosuppressive role by inducing suppressor macrophages. Fig.1 shows that macrophages might be significantly stimulated not only by tumor, but also in the presence of circulating immune complexes or inflammatory substances to increase the production of IAP in serum. This increased IAP might then induce and activate suppressor macrophages. IAP itself has indeed immunosuppressive function, for example, in the inhibition of phytohemagglutinin -stimulated lymphocyte proliferation in vitro, but it is considered to be the induced suppressor macrophages that play the leading part in immunosuppression in these circumstances. Clinically, however, the elevated levels of IAP might indicate the presence of some ungoing inflammatory or immunopathological process and production of immune complexes in the patients (1,2).

Now, we assayed the IAP quantitiy in CSF and compared it with the serum level. The rise of IAP% in CSF could reflect the IAP production locally in the CNS, although it is not strictly proven, as in the case of IgG%. IAP rate might indicate two possibilities - a local production of IAP in the CNS and/or an increase in total protein level in CSF.

In MS patients, IAP in CSF increased significantly during both the active and inactive stages, whereas serum IAP decreased significantly during the inactive stage (1,2) (Table 1). IAP% was elevated markedly during the active stage and also moderately in the inactive stage. These results suggest that IAP might be produced locally in the CNS by infiltrating monocytes or macrophages, and even during the clinically inactive stage, there must be active plaques. The neuropathological evidence that in a MS brain there are always active demyelinating plaques with perivascular cuffing by mononuclear inflammatory cells mixed with inactive old plaques support this. During the active stage, locally produced IAP might flow out through the impaired BBB into blood and induce suppressor macrophages in the spleen., which further elevates the serum level of IAP. During the inactive stage, IAP efflux into blood might be inhibited probably because of partly repaired BBB, and serum IAP decreased. Another possibility is that some inflammatory substances produced in the CNS play a role in elevating the serum IAP, but in this case, the efflux of these substances into blood might also be inhibited during the inactive stage.

On the other hand, in NBD that is a systemic disease, IAP% as well as IAP amount in CSF decreased markedly during the inactive stage, whereas serum levels of IAP remained relatively high (1,2). This suggests that during the neurologically inactive stage, the inflammatory and immunopathological processes in the brain might also become inactive, but out of the brain, some inflammatory lesions are still progressing. During the active stage, IAP amount, IAP% and IAP rate in CSF were all elevated. These might reflect both a local production of IAP in the CNS and an increase in total protein level in CSF.

In GBS, although IAP amount and IAP rate in CSF were greatly elevated, especially during the acute phase, the elevation of IAP% was only small. Increases in IAP amount and IAP rate with almost normal IAP% might reflect the elevated total protein level in CSF, probably due to increased permeability of BBB. As serum levels of IAP increased also only a little (1,2), the production of IAP seems not to be significant, locally or systematically.

In conclusion, measuring IAP in CSF could give us many suggestive results. We pointed out the possibility that IAP is produced locally in the CNS and efflux of IAP into blood can induce suppressor macrophages and influence the serum level of IAP. As IAP is not only one of substances produced by immune competent cells, but also has a definite function, we believe that IAP assay in CSF and serum at the same time could provide us further important informations about immunopathogenesis of MS and other inflammatory neurological disorders.

ACKNOWLEDGEMENT

This study was supported by a Grant-in-Aid for Scientific Research from the Ministry of Education, Science and Culture of Japan.

REFERENCES

1. T. Tsukamoto, H. Seki, T. Sekizawa and S. Takase. Serum levels of immunosuppressive acidic protein (IAP) in patients with multiple sclerosis and other inflammatory disorders. The 13th World Congress on Neurology (Hamburg), (1985).
2. T. Tsukamoto, H. Seki, S. Takase, T. Sekizawa and S. Nakamura. Significant increase in immunosuppressive acidic protein (IAP) in serum of patients with multiple sclerosis and other inflammatory neurological disorders, submitted for publication.
3. K. Tamura, Y. Shibata, Y. Matsuno and N. Ishida. Isolation and characterization of an immunosuppressive acidic protein from ascitic fluids of cancer patients. Cancer Res. 41:3244-3252 (1981).
4. N. Ishida, Y. Shibata and K. Tamura. Serum protein factors against self-defence which are activated in cancer patients. In: D. Mizuno, Z.A. Cohn, K. Takeya and N. Ishida (Eds.). Self-defence mechanism, role of macrophages. University of Tokyo Press, Tokyo, pp.239-250 (1982).

5. Y. Shibata, K. Tamura and N. Ishida. In vivo analysis of the suppressive effects of immunosuppressive acidic protein, a type of alpha-acid glycoprotein, in connection with its high level in tumor-bearing mice. Cancer Res. 43:2889-2896 (1983).
6. Y. Shibata, K. Tamura and N. Ishida. Cultured human monocytes, granulocytes and a monoblastoid cell line (TPH-1) synthesize and secrete immunosuppressive acidic protein (a type of alpha-acid glycoprotein) Microbiol. Immunol. 28:99-111 (1984).
7. S. Matsuno, M. Kobari, Y. Matsuda and T. Sato. Diagnosis of carcinoma of the pancreas by assay of immunosuppressive acidic protein. Tohoku J. Exp. Med. 136:1-10 (1982).

A ROLE FOR THE INTERFERON SYSTEM IN MULTIPLE SCLEROSIS

A. Billiau, H. Carton, H. Heremans and K. Heirwegh

Rega Institute for Medical Microbiology, University of Leuven, B-3000 Leuven, Belgium

Interferons are defined by their ability to exert a direct antiviral effect on cells. However, they also possess other biological activities, in particular the ability to affect the function of and interactions between cells of the immune system. There exist 3 "types" of interferon: alpha, beta and gamma. An older classification, which is currently revived calls for only 2 types: I and II. Type I encompasses alpha and beta, which are in many ways similar to each other; type II or gamma is profoundly different from type I.

The possible role of interferons as immuno-regulators has generated speculations as to their involvement in pathology of the immune system, in particular in the pathogenesis of inflammation, allergic reactions and auto-immune diseases. Multiple sclerosis (MS) being a disease which bears some of the hallmarks of an auto-immune disorder, several research groups (including our own) have entertained the idea that interferon production might somehow be disturbed in MS patients. On the other hand, MS being a disease for which a viral etiology has often been postulated, some have also speculated that interferon therapy might exert a beneficial effect on disease course.

PRODUCTION OF INTERFERON IN MS

Production of interferon(s) can be elicited by viral as well as non-viral stimuli. Virtually any type of cells, in particular fibroblasts as well as lymphoid cells, produce both IFN-alpha and -beta after infection with viruses. At least two different mechanisms seem to exist: one which is based on replication of the virus in the cells, the other based on interaction of the outer cell membrane with viral antigen (1-4). Double-stranded RNAs are potent inducers of IFN-beta in fibroblasts. This and other types of evidence have led to the concept that the intracellular event which leads to IFN-alpha and -beta synthesis is the formation of double-stranded replicative forms of viral RNA. Induction of IFN-alpha as a result of interaction of viruses or virus-infected cells with the outer cell membrane occurs only in fresh spleen cells or peripheral blood mononuclear cells (1-4). It thus seems to be a specialized function of some as yet undefined population of lymphocytes. It should be mentioned that similar induction of IFN-alpha occurs when splenocytes or blood mononuclear cells are interacting with foreign or tumor cells (5-7).

In contrast to IFN-alpha and -beta, which can be produced by any type of cell, IFN-gamma is an exclusive product of T-cells (and possibly NK-cells). Typical inducers are mitogenic lectins (conA, PHA, PWM), antigens to which the T-cells have been sensitized (e.g. PPD, viruses) or foreign cells (e.g. mixed lymphocyte reactions). The successful induction of IFN-gamma in T-lymphocytes requires the help from monocytes, whose function seems to consist in providing interleukin-1 (8, 9). Another important or perhaps even necessary factor for IFN-gamma production is interleukin-2 (8, 10, 11) produced by T-helper cells.

In acute virus infections, interferon titers in the body coincide in time and space with virus replication. The type of interferon formed during the first few days of an acute virus infection in mice has not been analysed other than by showing that it is acid-resistant and neutralized by antisera with dual (alpha + beta) specificity. Most probably, therefore, it is a mixture of alpha and beta. One would expect IFN-gamma to be formed as soon as a cell-mediated immune response against the virus is mounted and in as far as viral antigens or virus-producing cells are still present in the body. Especially in persistent virus infections one would expect an IFN-gamma response to occur around the end of the acute phase. So far evidence for this is lacking.

There are some naturally occurring situations other than virus infections where we expect interferon-alpha and -beta to be produced. Injection of lipopolysaccharides of Gramnegative bacteria in experimental animals induces appearance of interferon in organs (e.g. spleen) and circulation. One may thus presume that naturally occurring infections with Gramnegative organisms are accompanied by production of interferon. Very little information is available about the molecular nature and cellular origin of this interferon. Circumstantial evidence (12) suggests that both alpha and beta types may be present and that B-lymphocytes as well as phagocytic cells are involved in the production. Phagocytes may be important, either because they are themselves the producers of the interferon or because they produce interleukin-1, which in turn induces interferon-beta by ordinary fibroblasts (13, 14).

Interferon-alpha, on the other hand, can be produced by an as yet unidentified mononuclear leukocyte (probably a B-cell) in response to foreign cells, tumor cells or cells carrying viral antigens (5-7). We may therefore presume interferon-alpha to be produced in the body whenever the immune system is confronted with cells carrying foreign antigens, e.g. in rejection reactions towards antigenic tumors, artificial transplants, or toward altered self antigens or virus-carrying cells.

If we think of MS as a persistent virus infection, it may be especially rewarding to ask the question what happens to the interferon system in experimental persistent virus infections. In approaching this question we should keep in mind that interferons exert toxic effects on various organs (15, 16) and that sustained high-level production of interferon may be incompatible with survival. Successful persistence of virus activity, meaning persistence compatible with long-term survival of the host, may therefore imply that interferon production is down-regulated. It has been known for a long time that a burst of interferon production, induced e.g. by massive virus challenge, is followed by a refractory period of several days. During this period responsiveness versus the same or other types of interferon stimuli is severely suppressed. Concordant with these considerations, high-level interferon production has not been found to occur in any known case of virus persistence, in man or animals. Evidence as to whether continuous low-level stimulation of the interferon system may occur during virus persistence is at best fragmentary.

Some states of virus persistence in humans have been examined from the point of view of interferon production: chronic HBV-infection, SSPE, and current infection with several herpesvirus infections. The investigators have mostly limited themselves to a search for low-level production of interferon. In SSPE interferon has been looked for in the CSF but not found (17). Serum and urine obtained from infants with congenital persistent rubella virus infection were found not to contain detectable interferon, although vaccination of such infants with live measles virus resulted in an interferon response similar to that of normal children (18). Reports on searches for systemic interferon production in such infections as chronic HBV or CMV-disease are not available.

From the discussion it clearly appears that we possess only fragments of information about the involvement of the interferon system in known persistent infections. However, two salient points have been raised. First, it is clear that continuous high-level activation of the interferon system would soon lead to irreversible tissue damage and, therefore, virus persistence might not only require the ability of the virus to avoid immune destruction of virus and virus-infected cells, but also to somehow suppress the interferon system. Hence, the level of activation of the interferon system might simply be so low as to escape our current detection procedures. Secondly, it is also clear that alternative means to look at possible involvement of the interferon system, e.g. by looking at altered reactivity towards restimulation in vitro or in vivo, have only sporadically been exploited. Ironically this is precisely what has been done with relative success in the case of MS.

The earliest investigation of the interferon system in MS dates from 1971 when Haahr et al. (19) found an interferon-like antiviral factor in CSF from 2 out of about 250 MS patients. In 1976 Degré et al. (20) found a similar antiviral factor in 13 out of 36 CSF samples and in 22 out of 36 serum samples from MS patients, against 8 out of 50 samples from normal blood donors. Titers in serum and CSF samples were correlated with each other. In our laboratory we have undertaken to confirm this finding but never could find antiviral activity that met the criteria for being an interferon in either sera or CSF samples of MS patients. Recently, Salonen (21) et al. (22) also reported failure to find interferon in body fluids of 31 MS patients. An explanation for the earlier findings could be that the assay system used picked up some non-interferon antiviral activity. Detection of low concentrations of interferon in crude biological fluids is indeed fraught with the difficulty that in trying to increase the sensitivity of the assay, one easily looses its specificity.

In a very recent study Hirsch et al. (23) employed a radio-immunoassay for detecting human interferon-gamma and found sizable quantities in the CSF of MS-patients, while control CSF samples were negative. While immunosorbent assays for interferons have several advantages over bioassays, they may not distinguish between active and inactive interferons. It will be interesting to see whether the finding of Hirsch et al. will be confirmed in other laboratories and whether the interferon has biological activity.

In 1979, while testing the possibility that MS patients might display signs of persistent measles virus infection, Neighbour and Bloom (24) found that blood leucocytes of MS patients produced less interferon when exposed to inactivated measles virus than did leucocytes of healthy individuals. The interferon was identified as alpha-type. In a subsequent study the same research group (25) confirmed and expanded this finding to include 3 additional inducers: inactivated Newcastle disease virus (NDV), the double-standed RNA poly-I:C and ConA. Reduced response rates as well as lower interferon titers were reported. These studies by Neighbour and

Bloom were followed by a series of publications, reporting failure to find MS-associated decreases in interferon production. Thus, Santoli et al. (26) used live rather than inactivated viruses (measles, SSPE and influenza virus). Not unexpectedly the interferon was found to have characteristics of alpha or beta (acid-resistant) rather than gamma. However, no differences were found in interferon-producing capacity of leucocytes between controls and MS patients. Salonen et al. (27) compared 29 MS patients with age- and sex-matched controls, testing interferon production by lymphocytes after in vitro stimulation with so-called "antigen preparations" of measles, rubella, herpes and mumps viruses. The authors did not specify whether these preparations contained live or inactivated viruses. However, the interferon produced was neutralizable by anti-IFN-alpha globulin, suggesting that virus infection rather than antigenic stimulation was responsible for the induction. Again, in contrast to the findings of Neighbour and Bloom (24), no difference in interferon-producing activity was found between MS patients and controls. Similarly, Tovell et al. (28) failed to find differences in amounts of interferon produced by MS patients and control lymphocytes stimulated by Sendai virus, herpes simplex virus or measles virus. Kaudewiz (29) studied interferon production in lymphocytes of MS patients, comparing them with their healthy monozygotic twins. He used phytohemagglutinin (inducer of IFN-gamma), influenza virus (inducer of interferon-alpha and/or -beta) and allogeneic T-cells (Molt-4; presumably inducing IFN-alpha). No differences in production between diseased and healthy siblings were seen.

While studying a possible association of NK-cell activity and HLA-phenotype in MS patients, Gyödi et al. (30) determined interferon production by lymphocytes after in vitro infection with vesicular stomatitis virus (VSV). It is not clear why the authors chose this virus for their study: VSV is not known as a particularly good or reliable interferon inducer in lymphocytes, nor does it have established or presumed relationships with MS or any other human disease. Remarkably, however, the interferon titers were on average 4-fold lower in cultures from MS patients than in those from healthy controls. Since an HLA-associated decrease in NK-cell activity was found in the MS group, the authors vaguely speculated that MS patients might have a generally aberrant immune response to viruses.

A problem in interpreting these data resides in the fact that many of the interferon induction systems that were used in these studies are poorly documented in the interferon literature and are not well characterized in the studies themselves.

Data obtained from induction of blood mononuclear cells with mitogens pose less of a problem because it is well-known that the interferon produced in these systems is of the gamma-type. We already mentioned the study of Neighbour et al. (25) who found that MS patients' leucocytes had a reduced responsiveness to ConA.

Salonen et al. (31) compared 39 MS patients with matched controls, testing interferon-inducing potential of their lymphocytes after stimulation with three mitogens: purified protein derivative, phytohemagglutinin (PHA) and pokeweed mitogen (PWM). With all three inducers, a lower response rate (2/39) was found among MS patients than among controls (11/39). Although characterization results were not reported, we may reasonably assume that the interferon studied here was of the gamma-type. In the MS patients the HLA-DR2^{+} phenotype tended to be associated with lower interferon titers in induced lymphocyte cultures. The authors could not find a correlation between interferon responsiveness and clinical parameters of disease.

In our own studies in this field, we tried to reconcile some of the apparent discordancies in published reports by using well characterized induction systems. We also tried to provide information concerning the mechanism, the specificity and the clinical correlates of the MS-associated aberrations in the interferon response.

In a first study (32) white blood cells were induced with either Sendai virus (a classical inducer of interferon-alpha) and ConA, a classical inducer of interferon-gamma. The formation of interferon-alpha was found to be normal in MS patients. In contrast, the leucocytes from a large number of MS patients (± 50%) appeared not to be able to mount an interferon response to stimulation with ConA, while leucocytes from virtually all normal volunteers did respond. However, while the response rate was different between MS patients and volunteers, the height of the response (titer of interferon-gamma) was not different between responding MS patients and responding normal volunteers. Furthermore, the response rate was lower in those subgroups of MS patients with clinically more advanced stages of the disease. Although the response rate was not correlated with the past duration of the disease, a good correlation was found with past progression rate (i.e. clinical score divided by number of years disease). Finally, the difference in response rate between MS patients and normal volunteers was more pronounced if only those individuals were considered who were DR2-positive.

In a second study (33), we evaluated the specificity of the defective interferon-gamma response with regard to the inducers used. In particular, we used other mitogens, PHA and PWM, in comparison with ConA. We confirmed that a high percentage of MS patients are non-responders when ConA is used as the inducer. These same patients were also non-responders towards phytohemagglutinin. In contrast, all patients did respond to PWM. This clearly demonstrated that, from the point of view of the underlying mechanism, all MS patients possess lymphocytes which are able to produce interferon-gamma, but that in some of the patients the reaction to only certain mitogens is disturbed. We also confirmed our earlier finding that formation of interferon-alpha is not aberrant in MS patients when Sendai virus is used as the inducer. The same was true with Newcastle disease virus, but with vesicular stomatitis virus a certain percentage of MS patients appeared to be low-responder, if not non-responder.

In a third study (34) we examined the specificity of the defect in interferon-gamma response with respect to disease. For this we determined ConA-induced interferon-gamma induction in leucocyte cultures from three population samples: MS patients, patients with other neurological diseases and normal volunteers. As it appeared, various neurological diseases are associated with a defect in interferon-gamma response to ConA: cerebrovascular accidents, meningo-encephalitis, Alzheimer's dementia, Huntington's chorea, myasthenia gravis, brain operations. In contrast, the response rates were normal in groups of patients with Parkinson's disease and with brain tumors. These observations indicate that organic lesions in the central nervous system can have a profound and lesion-specific influence on the immune system.

The production of IFN-gamma by T-lymphocytes is part of a general reaction involving production of several other lymphokines. It depends on antecedent production of IL-2 by the same or other T-lymphocytes, which in turn depends on production of IL-1 by monocytic cells. Hence, the MS-associated defect in IFN-gamma response could be due to defects in IL-1 or IL-2 responses. In examining this question Vervliet and Schandené (35) could correlated decreased IFN-gamma production with decreased IL-2 production but found IL-1 production to be normal in MS patients.

Prostaglandins (PG) are known to affect aspecific immune responses in various ways. Since PG metabolism may be altered in MS patients, the possibility also exists that MS-associated alterations in IFN-gamma responsiveness may be due to decreased or increased levels of PG-production. Vervliet et al. (36) examined this possibility by studying endogenous PGE_2 levels in stimulated lymphocytes as well as the effects of PGE_2 addition or blockage of PG synthesis on IFN-gamma production. Addition of PGE_2 to the induced lymphocytes caused depression of the IFN-gamma response, while indomethacin, a blocker of PG synthesis, caused increased production of IFN-gamma and could convert some of the nonresponding lymphocyte cultures into responders. Differences were observed between cultures from control donors and MS patients, in that the latter required lower doses of PG and higher doses of indomethacin to obtain maximal effects on interferon production. Although this suggested that nonresponsiveness of MS-patients' lymphocytes might be due to their increased PG-sensitivity or to higher levels of endogenous prostaglandins, a more detailed analysis led the authors (36) to conclude that the PG system was not the major cause of the defective interferon-gamma response in MS.

Whereas decreased responsiveness of MS patients, in terms of interferon-gamma production, is a rather general finding in various laboratories. Hirsch et al. (23) recently reported increased responsiveness. It should be mentioned that these authors used and immunosorbent assay for determining interferon-gamma yields: possibly MS patients' leucocytes produce an inactive variant of interferon-gamma.

ACTION OF INTERFERON IN MS

Before trying to answer the question how IFNs may act in MS, a brief reminder of the possible role of interferon in the immune network may be in place. Aside from their strong direct antiviral effect on cells, interferons-alpha and -beta exert two salient immunomodulatory effects. As first shown by De Maeyer et al. (38) the natural mixture of interferon-alpha and -beta can suppress inflammatory responses occurring as a result of delayed type hypersensitivity reactions. Secondly, interferons-alpha and -beta also enhance cytotoxic activity of NK-cells, sensitized T-cells and antibody-dependent cytotoxic T-cells.

One of the hallmarks of macrophage activation by interferon-beta is the enhanced expression of Class II antigens on the cell membrane. Such expression, in turn, is of high importance in antigen presentation. In the central nervous system Class II antigens can be induced on astrocytes by contact with T-lymphocytes, probably via interferon-gamma (39). Regulated expression of these antigens may play an important role in the pathogenesis of MS lesions. The obvious implication of this would be that local production of interferon-gamma may be disadvantageous.

In our laboratory we have examined the role of interferons-alpha, -beta and -gamma in inflammatory processes by studying footpad swelling in mice given local injections of S.marcescens lipopolysaccharide (LPS). Systemic induction of interferons-alpha and -beta by virus infection or systemic administration of these interferons alpha and beta were found to inhibit the LPS-induced footpad reaction (see Fig.1 and Table 1). This is in accordance with observations by De Maeyer et al. (38) who studied footpad reactions elicited by sheep red blood cells in sensitized mice. Systemic administration of interferon-gamma (Table 1) also inhibited the footpad reaction.

Systemic administration of neutralizing antibodies directed against interferons alpha and beta did not enhance the footpad reaction, sugges-

Table 1. Inhibition of LPS-induced footpad swelling by interferons

Interferon type	Dose units/mouse	% Inhibition of footpad swelling on : day 2	day 3
alpha,beta (nat.)	300,000	38	48
	100,000	32	41
	30,000	35.5	52.5
	3,000	-4	0
$alpha_1$ (rec.)	100,000	43	55.5
	10,000	5	2
beta (rec.)	100,000	16	22
	10,000	-6	-22
gamma (rec.)	100,000	26	51
	10,000	12	23
	1,000	11	22

Interferon was given intraperitoneally each day from day 0 till day 3 post LPS challenge. Each value represents the mean of 4 mice.

$$\%\text{Inhibition} = 100 - \frac{\text{mean swelling in experimental group}}{\text{mean swelling in control group}} \times 100$$

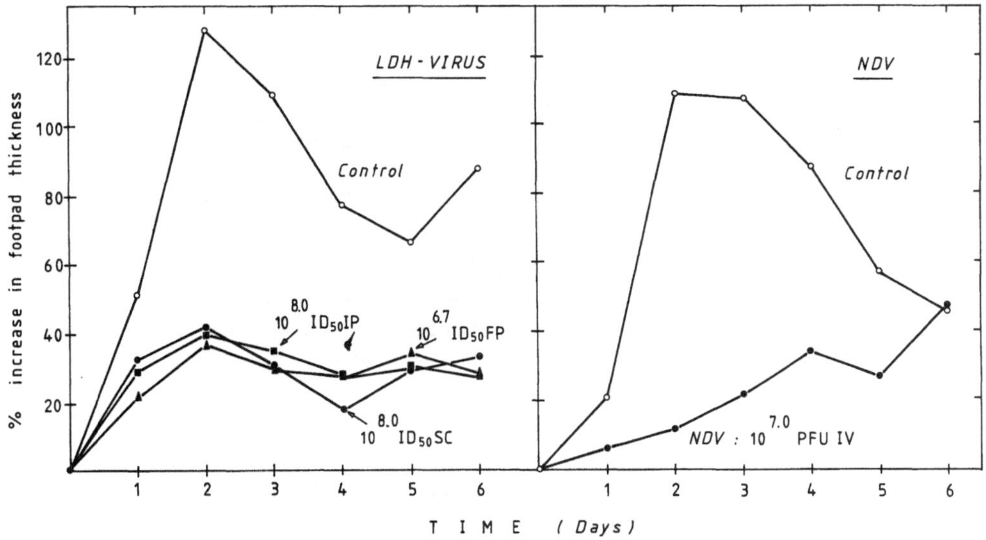

Fig.1. Effect of LDH-virus and NDV on the LPS-induced footpad swelling in NMRI mice.
Mice were injected into the right footpad with 5 µg (in 25 µl) of LPs of S. marcescens. PBS was injected as a control into the contralateral footpad. Open symbols (0): controls receiving only LPS challenge in the footpad. Closed symbols: virus inoculated mice. Left panel: mice inoculated with LDH-virus on day 0, 90 min. after LPS-challenge (●) subcutaneously; (■) intraperitoneally; (▲) locally in the footpad. Right panel: mice inoculated with NDV intravenously 5 hrs after LPS challenge.

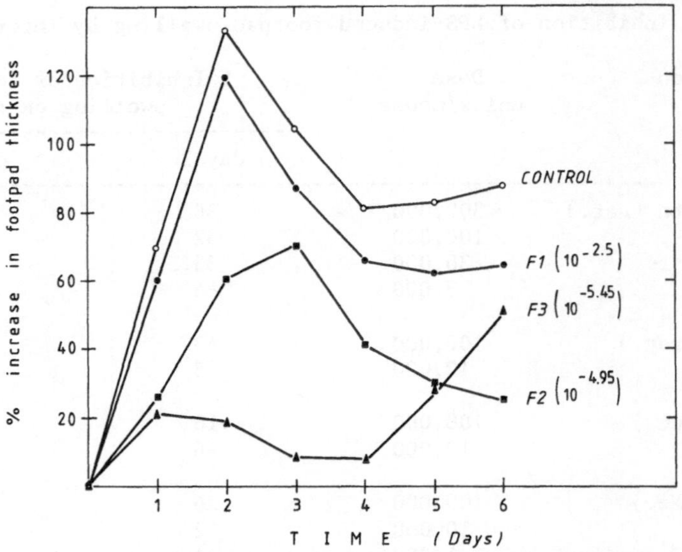

Fig.2. Effect of monoclonal antibodies against MuIFN-gamma on LPS-induced footpad swelling in NMRI mice.
Groups of 4 mice were injected intraperitoneally, 24 hr before LPS-challenge, with 0.1 ml of rat monoclonal antibodies to MuIFN-gamma. The control group received PBS. F_1, F_2 and F_3 are monoclonal antibodies derived from different rat x mouse hybridomas and possessing different neutralizing potential (titers in brackets) for the in vitro antiviral effect of MuIFN-gamma.

ting that endogenous production of these interferons was insufficient to regulate inflammation. Surprisingly, systemic administration of monoclonal antibodies to mouse interferon-beta caused a strong inhibition of the footpad reaction (Fig.2). Obviously, the effects of interferon-gamma on inflammatory responses are complex. One possibility may be that it enhances inflammation when acting locally, but inhibits it when acting systemically. Local production of interferon-gamma after injection of LPS in the footpad might be instrumental in bringing about the inflammation. Blockage of the action of this local interferon-gamma by monoclonal antibody would then inhibit the inflammatory response.

These observations raise a number of questions with regard to the role of interferons, - especially that of interferon-gamma -, in the pathogenesis of MS lesions. In particular, it is not clear, at this time, whether we are to expect benefit from a therapy with interferon or rather from one with agents that neutralize interferon.

REFERENCES

1. M.R. Capobianchi, J. Facchini, P. Di Marco, G. Antonelli and F. Dianzani. Induction of alpha interferon by membrane interaction between viral surface and peripheral blood mononuclear cells. Proc. Soc. Exp. Biol. Med. 178:551 (1985).
2. Y. Ito, Y. Nishiyama, K. Shimokata, I. Nagata, H. Takeyama and A. Kunii. The mechanism of interferon induction in mouse spleen cells stimulated with HVJ. Virology. 88:128 (1978).

3. P. Lebon, M.J. Commoy-Chevalier, B. Robert-Galliot and C. Chang. Different mechanisms for alpha and beta interferon induction. Virology. 119:504 (1982).
4. C.S. Reiss, L.C.M. Lin and S.L. Mowshowitz. Interferon production by cultured murine splenocytes in response to influenza-virus infected cells. J. Interferon Res. 1:81 (1984).
5. J.E. Blalock, M.P. Langford, J. Georgiades and G.J. Stanton. Nonsensitized lymphocytes produce leukocyte interferon when cultured with foreign cells. Cell. Immunol. 43:197 (1979).
6. I.K. Hughes, E.M. Smith and E.J. Blalock. Nonsensitized murine B lymphocytes produce mouse interferon alpha/beta in response to foreign cells. Cell. Immunol. 78:375 (1983).
7. G. Trinchieri, D. Santoli and B.B. Knowles. Tumor cell lines induce interferon in human leukocytes. Nature. 270:611 (1977).
8. W.L. Farrar, H.M. Johnson and J.J. Farrar. Regulation of the production of immune interferon and cytotoxic T lymphocytes by interleukin 2. J. Immunol. 126:1120 (1981).
9. J. Vilcek, D. Henriksen-De Stefano, D. Sieel and J. Le. IFN-gamma induction in peripheral blood leucocytes by interleukin-2: role of monocyte interleukin-1 and IFN-gamma. In: "The Interferon System", F. Dianzani and G.B. Rossi, eds. Serono Symposia. 24:43 (1985).
10. T. Kasahara, J.J. Hooks, S.F. Dougherty and J.J. Oppenheim. Interleukin-2-mediated interferon (IFN-gamma) production by human T-cells and T-cell subsets. J. Immunol. 130:1784 (1983).
11. G.H. Reem and N.H. Yeh. Interleukin-2 regulates expression of its receptor and synthesis of gamma interferon by human T lymphocytes. Science. 225:429 (1984).
12. N. Maehara and M. Ho. Cellular origin of interferon induced by bacterial lipopolysaccharide. Infect. Immun. 15:78 (1977).
13. J. Van Damme, M. De Ley, G. Opdenakker, A. Billiau, P. De Somer and J. Van Beeumen. Homogeneous interferon-inducing 22K factor is related to endogenous pyrogen and interleukin-1. Nature. 314:266 (1985).
14. J. Van Damme, G. Opdenakker, A. Billiau, P. De Somer, L. De Wit, P. Poupart and J. Content. Stimulation of fibroblast interferon production by a 22K protein from human leukocytes. J. Gen. Virol. 66:693 (1985).
15. I. Gresser, M. Aguet, L. Morel-Maroger, D. Woodrow, F. Puvien-Dutilleul, J.C. Guillon and C. Maury. Electrophoretically pure mouse interferon inhibits growth, induces liver and kidney lesions and kills suckling mice. Am. J. Pathol. 102:396 (1981).
16. I. Gresser, M.G. Tovey, C. Maury and I. Chouroulinkov. Lethality of interferon preparations for newborn mice. Nature. 258:76 (1975).
17. P.O. Behan. Interferon in treatment of subacute sclerosing panencephalitis. Lancet. i:1059 (1981).
18. J. Desmyter, W.E. Rawls, J.L. Melnick, M.D. Yaw and F.F. Barrett. Interferon in congenital rubella response to live attenuated measles vaccine. J. Immunol. 99:771 (1967).
19. S. Haahr. Virus inhibiting activity in the cerebrospinal fluid from patients with acute and chronic neurological disorders. Acta Path. Microbiol. Scand. Section B. 79:606 (1971).
20. M. Degré, H. Dahl and B. Vandvik. Interferon in the serum and cerebrospinal fluid in patients with multiple sclerosis and other neurological disorders. Acta Neurol. Scand. 53:152 (1976).
21. R. Salonen. CSF and serum interferon in multiple sclerosis: longitudinal study. Neurology. 33:1064 (1983).
22. R.J. Abbott, P.D. Giles and I. Bolderson. Absence of immunoreactive interferon-alpha in CSF from patients with multiple sclerosis. J. Neurol. Neurosurg. Psychiatry. 49:102 (1986).
23. R.L. Hirsch, H.S. Panitch and K.P. Johnson. Lymphocytes from multiple sclerosis patients produce elevated levels of gamma interferon in vitro. J. Clin. Immunol. 5:386 (1985).

24. P.A. Neighbour and B.R. Bloom. Absence of virus-induced lymphocyte suppression and interferon production in multiple sclerosis. Proc. Natl. Acad. Sci. USA. 76:476 (1979).
25. P.A. Neighbour, A.E. Miller and B.R. Bloom. Interferon responses of leukocytes in multiple sclerosis. Neurology. 31:561 (1981).
26. D. Santoli, W. Hall, L. Kastrukoff, R.P. Lisak, B. Perussia, G. Trinchieri and H. Koprowski. Cytotoxic activity and interferon production by lymphocytes from patients with multiple sclerosis. J. Immunol. 126:1274 (1981).
27. R. Salonen, J. Ilonen, M. Reunanen and A. Salmi. Defective production of interferon-alpha associated with HLA-DW2 antigen in stable multiple sclerosis. J. Neurol. Sci. 55:197 (1982).
28. D.R. Tovell, I.A. McRobbie, K.G. Warren and D.L.J. Tyrrell. Interferon production by lymphocytes for multiple sclerosis and non-MS patients. Neurology. 33:640 (1983).
29. P. Kaudewitz, H. Zander, J. Abb, H.W. Ziegler-Heitbrock and G. Riethmüller. Genetic influence on natural cytotoxicity and interferon production in multiple sclerosis studies in monozygotic discordant twins. Human Immunol. 7:51 (1983).
30. E. Gyödi, M. Benzcur, G. Pallfy, M. Talas, G. Petranyi, I. Földes and S.R. Hollan. Association between HLA B7, DR2 and dysfunction of natural- and antibody-mediated cytotoxicity without connection with the deficient interferon production in multiple sclerosis. Human Immunol. 4:209 (1982).
31. R. Salonen, J. Ilonen, M. Reunanen, J. Nikoskelainen and A. Salmi. PPD-, PWM-, and PHA-induced interferon in stable multiple sclerosis: association with HLA-DW2 antigen and clinical variables. Ann. Neurol. 11:279 (1982).
32. G. Vervliet, H. Claeys, H. Van Haver, H. Carton, C. Vermylen, E. Meulepas and A. Billiau. Interferon production and natural killer (NK) activity in leukocyte cultures from multiple sclerosis patients. J. Neurol. Sci. 60:137 (1983).
33. G. Vervliet, H. Carton, E. Meulepas and A. Billiau. Interferon production by cultured peripheral leucocytes of MS patients. Clin. Exp. Immunol. 58:116 (1984).
34. G. Vervliet, H. Carton and A. Billiau. Interferon-gamma production by peripheral blood leukocytes from patients with multiple sclerosis and other neurological diseases. Clin. Exp. Immunol. 59:391 (1985).
35. G. Vervliet and L. Schandené. In vitro correction of the interleukin-2 and interferon-gamma defect in multiple sclerosis. Clin. Exp. Immunol. 61:556 (1985).
36. G. Vervliet, H. Deckmyn, H. Carton and A. Billiau. Influence of prostaglandin E_2 and indomethacin on interferon-gamma production by cultured peripheral blood leucocytes of multiple sclerosis patients and healthy donors. J. Clin. Immunol. 5:102 (1985).
37. J. Le, W. Prensky, Y.K. Yip, Z. Chang, T. Hoffman, H.C. Stevenson, I. Balazs, J. Sadlik and J. Vilcek. Activation of human monocyte cytotoxicity by natural and recombinant immune interferon. J. Immunol. 131:2821 (1983).
38. E. De Maeyer, J. De Maeyer-Guignard and M. Vandeputte. Inhibition by interferon of delayed-type hypersensitivity in the mouse. Proc. Natl. Acad. Sci. USA. 72:1753 (1975).
39. W. Fierz, B. Endler, K. Reske, H. Wekerle and A. Fontana. Astrocytes as antigen-presenting cells. I. Induction of Ia antigen expression on astrocytes by T cells via immune interferon and its effect on antigen presentation. J. Immunol. 134:3785 (1985).

CSF ALPHA AND GAMMA INTERFERONS IN ACUTE AND SUBACUTE ENCEPHALITIS AND MULTIPLE SCLEROSIS: COMPARATIVE STUDY

Pierre Lebon[1], Edmond Schuller[2], Jean-Denis Degos[3], Olivier Lyon-Caen[4], Gérard Ponsot[5]

[1] Inserm U.43, Hôpital St. Vincent de Paul, 74 av. Denfert-Rochereau, Paris, France
[2] Laboratoire de Neuroimmunologie, Hôpital de la Salpêtrière Paris, France
[3] Clinique de Neurologie, Hôpital Henri Mondor, Créteil France
[4] Clinique de Neurologie, Hôpital de la Salpêtrière, Paris France
[5] Clinique de Pédiatrie, Hôpital St. Vincent de Paul, Paris France

INTRODUCTION

During viral chronic infections associated with an immune deficiency such as AIDS (Eyster et al., 1983) or congenital rubella (Lebon et al., 1985), an alpha acid labile interferon was detected in patients' sera. A similar interferon is also present in patients during relapses of systemic lupus erythematosis (Preble et al., 1982), rheumatoïd arthritis (Hooks et al., 1979), and psoriasis (Waschke and Diezal, 1984). Gamma interferon has been detected in the sera of patients with chronic CMV infections (Rhodes-Feuillette et al., 1983). It was also reported that peripheral blood mononuclear cells (PBMC) of patients, after a recurrence of herpes labialis, spontaneously secreted gamma IFN in vitro (Cunningham and Merigan, 1983).

Among the different hypotheses concernings its pathogenesis, multiple sclerosis is considered as a late auto-immune sequella of a neurological viral disease. For these reasons, we investigated the endogenous secretion of alpha and gamma interferon in MS patients in comparison with patients suffering from acute or chronic viral infections of the central nervous system.

METHODS AND PATIENTS

1) The measurement of the endogenous alpha IFN level in CSF was performed for 61 cases of definite MS (including ten cases studied during a relapse period), 129 cases of viral encephalitis, 20 cases of SSPE, 29 cases of Guillain Barré syndrome, 3 cases of amyotrophic lateral sclerosis (ALS), 13 cases of congenital rubella and 3 cases of systemic lupus erythematosis (SLE) with a neurological relapse. Partial results and the biological assay of IFN were previously reported (Lebon et al., 1979;

Dussaix et al., 1985). The sensitivity of the test is equal to 1 IU/ml. Ten MS cases were also investigated with a solid phase radioimmunoassay (RIA) (Abott) of 10 unit/ml sensitivity threshold.

2) The measurement of the endogenous gamma IFN level was performed for 24 cases of MS, including 10 cases studied during a relapse period, 20 cases of acute viral encephalitis and 8 cases of SSPE. Gamma IFN was measured by a commercial solid phase radioimmunoassay (Centocor Corporation). This test, described by Chang et al., (1984), could detect as little as 0.5 IU/ml. For limit values of 0.5 µ/ml, the specificity of the test was controlled by the addition of a polyclonal serum anti-recombinant gamma IFN to block the binding of the I^{125} labelled monoclonal IFN antibody.

3) The induction of alpha IFN in peripheral blood mononuclear cells (PBMC) was studied in 48 MS patients, 15 MS patients steroid-treated between two months and the day before the blood sampling, 20 other neurological diseases (Guillain Barré, myasthenic, Parkinson, medullar tumor, vascular malformation), 6 SSPE and 28 healthy controls. One ml of 10^6 PBMC was suspended in RPMI medium supplemented 10% fetal calf serum after separation by Ficoll paque density gradient centrifugation and incubated with 50 µl of viral suspension during 18 h at 37°C. The culture supernatants were then assayed for IFN titration after elimination of PBMC by centrifugation and the viruses by a 24-hour Ph2 treatment. IFN assays were performed in bovine cells (Madin-Darby bovine kidney cells, MDBK) with vesicular stomatitis virus as the challenge virus, as previously described by Lebon et al., 1985_2).

4) Different virus strains were used for alpha IFN induction. The Edmonton strain of measles virus and the herpes simplex virus type I (Shealey strain) were propagated in vero cells. The E 72 Sendaï virus strain was grown in embryonated chicken eggs. Viruses were titrated and stored in aliquots at minus 80°. Multiplicities of infection of infection of 0.1 for measles and HSV_1 viruses and 10 for Sendaï viruses were used in IFN induction tests.

5) The diagnosis of herpes encephalitis and SSPE was based on the increase of the intrathecal synthesis of specific antibodies. The diagnosis of post infectious encephalitis and congenital rubella was based on the presence of specific IgM antibodies in the patient serum.

6) Antibodies against alpha IFN were investigated for ten MS patients sera and CSF. Diluted sera at 1/10 and undiluted CSF were incubated with 4 IU of alpha IFN standard for 1h at 37°C and the IFN activity of the mixtures were titrated in parallel with controls.

7) A blocking activity of alpha IFN induction was investigated in CSF of ten MS patients. Two hundred µl of CSF were added at 0.5 ml of PBMC (10^6/ml) and incubated à 37°C for 1 h. Then 50 µl of diluted Sendaï virus (Moi.0.1) or herpes virus (Moi.0.5) were added. Supernatants were collected after an incubation of 18 h at 37°C and IFN yields were titrated as above.

RESULTS

Occurrence of alpha interferon production in CSF from patients with acute viral encephalitis

All CSF were collected before the 8th day of the neurological disease; endogenous alpha interferon was detected mainly in the CSF of 41 out of 43 (95%) patients with herpes encephalitis, 3/48 (6.2%) patients with post eruptive measles encephalitis and 2/8 (25%) patients with mumps meningo encephalitis, and in one case of influenza A infection (Table 1). All the levels of IFN CSF were higher than those of the sera (data not shown).

Table 1. Acute viral encephalitis: alpha IFN in CSF collected before the 8th day of the neurological disease

viral agents	N° of patients	N° of patients with CSF alpha IFN titre 8⩾IU	
measles	48	3++	6.2%
rubella	8	0	
mumps	8	2+	
adenoviruses	2	0	
influenza A	1	1+	
influenza B	1	0	
varicella-zoster	8	0	
Epstein-Barr	8	0	
herpes simplex	45	43+	95%

+ alpha IFN Ph2 resistant

++ alpha IFN Ph2 labile

<u>Incidence of intrathecal synthesis of alpha interferon in subacute or chronic viral infections of the CNS</u>

No IFN was detected in the CSF of 31 cases of herpes encephalitis investigated after the 12th day of the onset, nor in the CSF of 20 cases of SSPE. In active congenital rubella, an alpha interferon was present in 9 out of 13 CSF collected between 5 days to 4 months after birth (Table 2).

Table 2. Subacute and chronic viral infections of the CNS: intrathecal synthesis of alpha-IFN

	N° of patients	N° of patients with CSF alpha IFN titre ⩾ 2 IU
<u>herpes encephalitis</u>		
CSF collected after the 12th day of the neurological symptoms	31*	0
SSPE	20*	0
<u>congenital rubella</u>		
CSF collected between 5 days to 4 months after birth	13	9*

* Associated with intrathecal specific antibodies synthesis.

Patients with auto-immune neurological diseases

Alpha interferon was never detected in 29 cases of Guillain Barré syndrome, nor in 3 ALS cases, nor in 61 MS patients using biological assay (Table 3). Only in 1 out of 36 MS patients was the IFN serum level at 4 IU ml. The results were also negative using the RIA for ten sera and CSF of MS patients. Three cases of neurological complications of SLE were associated to an intrathecal synthesis of alpha IFN.

Alpha interferon production from PBMC of MS patients

No significant difference was noted for the mean IFN production between MS patients and controls. However, in MS patients treated with steroids, the capacity of alpha IFN production was strongly decreased compared to the controls when PBMC were induced with herpes or measles viruses, but the synthesis of Sendaï virus-induced interferon was not significantly affected (Table 4). Six cases of SSPE were also studied: the production of alpha IFN induced by measles virus was normal in two cases, 75% decreased in two other cases, and 90% decreased for the latter (data not shown). No alpha interferon antibodies were demonstrated in sera and CSF from 10 MS patients, nor any factor blocking its synthesis after induction with herpes and Sendaï viruses.

Incidence of gamma interferon titres in CSF from patients with acute, subacute encephalitis and MS

Gamma interferon was early synthetized in the central nervous system of herpes encephalitis (titres from 1 to 40 IU/ml), but not in measles or rubella encephalitis (Table 5); gamma IFN disappeared from CSF after about 10 days of illness. Three patients were studied 4 months after the onset of the encephalitis, and their IFN CSF levels were less than 0.5 IU/ml. One patient out of 9 with measles encephalitis had 0.5 IU/ml in the CSF collected 15 days after the onset of neurological symptoms.

Gamma interferon was detected neither in the sera and CSF in 8 cases of SSPE, nor in the 27 cases of MS (Table 6). For five CSF of MS patients, IFN levels seemed to be at about 0.3 IU/ml, but the specificity of the test could not be proved in a blocking test with a polyclonal anti-gamma interferon serum.

DISCUSSION

The intrathecal synthesis of alpha interferon during herpes encephalitis has already been largely discussed (Hamano et al., 1983; Hilfenhaus et al., 1981; Legaspi et al., 1980; Lebon et al., 1979; Vezinet et al., 1981). Alpha IFN was no longer detected in CSF collected between the 12th day and 4 months after the onset of encephalitis. In this report, gamma IFN was demonstrated for the first time to be present in the CSF early in the course of herpes encephalitis. It dissappeared at the same time as alpha IFN with the increase of specific antibodies in the CNS.

We confirm the absence of alpha IFN spontaneously produced in CSF of MS patients as has previously been reported (Salonem, 1983). No alpha IFN antibodies, nor blocking factors in sera and CSF of IFN induction, nor deficiency in alpha IFN production in untreated MS patients could be demonstrated. These last results agree with those of Santoli et al., (1981) and Vervliet et al., (1983), but not with those of Neighbour and Bloom (1979). Here the defect in alpha IFN production is significant only for the MS population treated with steroids. The absence of endogenous alpha IFN could be due simply to the absence of an inducer in the CNS of MS pa-

Table 3. Alpha interferon in CSF and sera from patients with "autoimmune" neurological diseases

	N° of patients:	with CSF IFN titre > 2 IU	N° of patients:	with sera IFN titre ⩾ 4 IU
Guillain Barré syndrome	29	0	27	0
amyotrophic lateral sclerosis	3	0	3	0
multiple sclerosis	61	0	36	1
neurological complications of SLE	3	3*	3	2

* Alpha IFN Ph2 labile, locally synthesized.

Table 4. Alpha interferon production from PBMC after induction with HSV, measles, Sendai virus

PBMC from	N° of cases	Herpes HSV_1	Sendai	N° of cases	measles
MS	48	300*	1200	40	180
MS steroid treated	15	40	800	13	30
other neurological diseases	20	200	ND		ND
healthy controls	28	360	1200	16	160

* Mean of IFN titers expressed in IU.

Table 5. Acute viral encephalitis: gamma interferon in CSF collected

	before the tenth day of the neurological disease		after the tenth day of the neurological disease	
viral agents	N° of cases	N° of cases with IFN titre ⩾ 0.5 IU	N° of cases	N° of cases with IFN titre ⩾ 0.5 IU
measles	6	0	9	1
rubella	2	0	2	0
herpes HSV_1	10	8**	15*	0

* Including 3 CSF collected 4 months after the onset of encephalitis.

** IFN intrathecally synthesized (titre from 1 to 40 IU).

Table 6. Gamma IFN in sera and CSF of SSPE and MS

	N° of cases	N° of sera	N° of CSF
SSPE	8	7	8
multiple sclerosis	27	24	29*

All the specimens are < 0.5 IU using a radioimmunoassay

* Including 10 CSF collected before 5th day of the relapse

tients or to the masking of an eventual inducer by specific antibodies present in the CNS as it probably occurs in SSPE or in patients with sequellae of herpes encephalitis. Indeed, it was reported that specific antibodies could neutralize the IFN-inducing activity of viruses (Lebon, 1985).

The presence of high amounts of an acid labile alpha interferon in the CSF during neurological relapses of SLE reported by Lebon et al., (1983) and Dussaix et al., (1985), and its absence in MS relapses suggest that the auto-immune processes of these diseases are different.

In this study, gamma IFN was not detected in the sera and CSF of MS patients using a sensitive method. We have observed that all the CSF from MS and non MS patients had a background in the RIA higher than that of the sera. We cannot demonstrate the specificity of low levels of about 0.3 IU/ml in five CSF from MS patients. These results are different from those reported by Hirsch et al., (1985). However, these negative results in multiple sclerosis do not exclude the possibility of small amounts of IFN in the CNS: indeed, it has recently been shown by Linnane et al., (1985) with immunofluorescent techniques that IFN was present in mononuclear cells of hepatitis B virus-infected livers, although no IFN was detected in the blood of the patients. Other techniques, such as molecular hybridation _in situ_ and immunochemistry applied on histologic material, are required to evaluate the real implication of the interferon system in MS.

ACKNOWLEDGEMENTS

This research was supported by a grant from ARSEP. P. Lebon is grateful to Mrs. G. Schlienger for her technical assistance.

REFERENCES

1. T.W. Chang, S. McKinney, V. Liu, P.C. Kung, J. Vilcek and J. Le. Use of monoclonal antibodies as sensitive and specific probes for biologically active human gamma interferon. _Proc. Natl. Acad. Sci._ 81: 5219-5222 (1984).
2. A.L. Cunningham and T.C. Merigan. Interferon production appears to predict time of recurrence of herpes labialis. _The J. of Immun._ 130:2397-2399 (1983).
3. E. Dussaix, P. Lebon, G. Ponsot, G. Huault and M. Tardieu. Intrathecal synthesis of different alpha interferons in patients with various neurological diseases. _Acta Neurol. Scand._ 75:504-509 (1985).

4. M.E. Eyster, J.J. Goedert, M.C. Poon and O.T. Preble. Acid-labile alpha interferon. A possible preclinical marker for the acquired immunedeficiency syndrome in hemophila. N. Engl. J. Med. 309:583-586 (1983).
5. K. Hamano, G. Ponsot, L. Gerbaut, P. Ploin and M. Arthuis. Encéphalites herpétiques du nourrisson et de l'enfant. Méthodes de diagnostic. Arch. Fr. Pédiatr. 40:709-714 (1983).
6. J. Hilfenhaus and R. Ackerman. Endogenous interferon in the cerebrospinal fluid of herpes encephalitis patients. Proc. Soc. Exp. Biol. 166:205-209 (1981).
7. R.L. Hirsch, H.S. Panitch and K.P. Johnson. Lymphocytes from multiple sclerosis patients produce elevated levels of gamma interferon in vitro. J. of Clin. Immunol. 5:6 386-389 (1985).
8. J.J. Hooks, H.M. Moutsoupoulos, S.A. Geis, N.I. Stahl, J.L. Decker and A.L. Notkins. Immune interferon in the circulation of patients with autoimmune disease. N. Engl. J. Med. 301:5-8 (1979).
9. O.T. Preble, R.J. Black, R.M. Friedman, J.H. Klippel and J. Vilcek. Systemic lupus erythematosus: presence in human serum of an unusual acid-labile leukocyte interferon. Science. 216:429-431 (1982).
10. P. Lebon, G. Ponsot, J. Aicardi, F. Goutieres and M. Arthuis. Early intrathecal synthesis of interferon in herpes encephalitis. Biomedicine. 31:267-271 (1979).
11. P. Lebon, G.R. Lenoir, A. Fischer and A. Lagrue. Synthesis of intrathecal interferon in systemic lupus erythematosus with neurological complications. Br. Med. J. 287:1165-1167 (1983).
12. P. Lebon, F. Daffos, A. Checoury, L. Grangeot-Keros, F. Forestier and J.E. Toublanc. Presence of an acid-labile alpha-interferon in sera from fetuses and children with congenital rubella. J. of Clin. Microb. 21:5, 775-778 (1985[1]).
13. P. Lebon. Inhibition of herpes simplex virus type 1-induced interferon synthesis by monoclonal antibodies against viral glycoprotein D and by lysosomotropic drugs. J. Gen. Virol. 66:2781-2786 (1985[2]).
14. R.C. Legaspi, B. Gatmaitan, E.J. Bailey and A.M. Lerner. Interferon in biopsy and autopsy specimens of brain: its presence in herpes simplex virus encephalitis. Arch. Neurol. 37:76-79 (1980).
15. A.W. Linnane, P.J. Hertzog, A.R. Jilbert, C.J. Burrel, E.J. Gowans and B.P. Marmion. Immunofluorescence demonstration of interferon-producing cells in hepatitis B infected livers. TNO ISIR, Meeting on the Interferon System (1985).
16. P.A. Neighbour and B.R. Bloom. Absence of virus-induced lymphocytes suppression and interferon production in multiple sclerosis. Proc. Natl. Acad. Sci. USA. 76:1, 476-480.
17. A. Rhodes-Feuillette, M. Canivet, H. Champsaur, E. Gluckman, M.C. Mazeron and J. Peries. Circulating interferon in cytomegalovirus infected bone-marrow-transplant recipients and in infants with congenital cytomegalovirus disease. J. of. Interferon Res. 3:1, 45-52 (1983).
18. R. Salonen. CSF and serum interferon in multiple sclerosis: longitudinal study. Neurol. 33:1604-1606 (1983).
19. D. Santoli, W. Hall, L. Kastrukoff, R.P. Lisak, B. Perussia, G. Trinchieri and H. Koprowski. Cytotoxic activity and interferon production by lymphocytes from patients with multiple sclerosis. J. of Immunol. 126:4, 1274-1278 (1981).
20. G. Vervliet, H. Claeys, H. Van Haver. Interferon production and natural killer cell activity in leukocyte cultures from multiple sclerosis patients. J. Neurol. Sci. 60:137-150 (1983).
21. F. Vezinet, P. Lebon, C. Amoury and C. Gibert. Synthèse d'interferon au cours des encéphalites herpétiques de l'adulte. Nouv. Press. Med. 10:1135-1138 (1981).
22. S.R. Waschke and W. Diezel. Interferon in patients with psoriasis. Contr. Oncol. 20:298-303 (1984).

MULTIPLE SCLEROSIS: ON SOMATOSTATIN IN CEREBROSPINAL FLUID AND ITS CORRELATION WITH DISEASE ACTIVITY

Kurt Virring Sörensen

Neurological Department, Central Hospital, DK - 8800 Viborg, Denmark; University Department of Neurology, Kommunehospitalet, DK - 8800 Aarhus C, Denmark; Institute of Experimental Clinical Research, University of Ärhus, DK - 8000 Ärhus C, Denmark

INTRODUCTION

The content of somatostatin in cerebrospinal fluid is reduced during relapses in multiple sclerosis (1). However, this is a reversible phenomenon and the somatostatin increases towards normal when the patients are in remission (2). Somatostatin in brain and cerebrospinal fluid is reported low in other diseases of the central nervous system, but in these cases low levels seem to be irreversible. For review see (3). The detection of peptides e.g. somatostatin within the central nervous system rises many questions regarding their source, distribution, mechanism of action, function and possible significance in central nervous system disorders. It was therefore tempting to look for abnormalities in the somatostatin release and occurrence in the brain and cerebrospinal fluid in patients with neurological diseases. An opening was achieved when Patel et al., and Kronheim et al., established that somatostatin was present in cerebrospinal fluid and reported on changes in various diseases of the central nervous system including one case of demyelinating disease (4,5).

A number of biochemical and physiological changes have previously been reported in patients with multiple sclerosis (6), but unfortunately nobody has succeeded in the search for the pathogenic mechanism behind the disease, and great efforts have been done to establish a dependable biochemical parameter, which could be of guidance in evaluation of the disease activity, which leads to the often erratic and unpredictable course of multiple sclerosis.

AN INDICATOR OF DISEASE ACTIVITY

A group of multiple sclerosis patients who all were clinically definite cases, were divided into one group in relapse and one in stable phase of the disease. It was demonstrated that the patients in relapse had low levels of somatostatin in the cerebrospinal fluid, whereas the patients in stable phase had a content of somatostatin in the cerebrospinal fluid similar to that found in normal controls (1). The idea that cerebrospinal fluid content of somatostatin was related to disease activity could therefore best be substantiated by examination of the individual patient in various phases of the disease.

16 of the multiple sclerosis patients were followed as out-patients and the content of somatostatin in the cerebrospinal fluid re-examined when a patient remitted from relapse and had been stable for at least six months, or when relapse followed a stable period (2). These repunctures, at different stages of disease activity in the same patient, showed that remission from a relapse was associated with increasing or normal values of cerebrospinal fluid somatostatin, and the opposite was found, when a patient after a stable period suffered from a new relapse, whereas a continuous progressive course of the disease was associated with permanent low or decreasing somatostatin content in the cerebrospinal fluid.

These changes in cerebrospinal fluid somatostatin necessitated experimental clinical trials and examinations to answer how and from where somatostatin arrives into the cerebrospinal fluid, the physiological and clinical importance of this parameter, and its usefullness in human pathophysiological research. It was also necessary to know if changes in the content of somatostatin in cerebrospinal fluid from lumbar punctures were representative only of local changes, or were representative of the concentration throughout the cerebrospinal fluid, which bathes the central nervous system.

RELATION TO GROWTH HORMONE SECRETION

If hypothalamic sources or blood borne somatostatin contribute to any significant extent to the cerebrospinal fluid content, it would be expected that cerebrospinal fluid somatostatin was indicative of the growth hormone release inhibiting activity of hypothalamic somatostatin, and an association might be expected with growth hormone concentrations. Intravenous arginine infusion revealed no difference in the plasma growth hormone concentrations before, during and after the infusion in 14 multiple sclerosis patients, 6 of whom were in stable phase of the disease and 8 in relapse, and 7 in controls. The levels of growth hormone in cerebrospinal fluid were also similar in the three groups (7). A similar result was demonstrated by Steardo et al., (8) in a study of the diurnal variation of plasma growth hormone in a group of Alzheimer-patients with low somatostatin in cerebrospinal fluid in single samples in the morning. In addition, identical diurnal profiles of plasma growth hormone were recently demonstrated in three groups of patients with significantly different diurnal patterns of cerebrospinal fluid somatostatin (9). This lack of association between cerebrospinal fluid somatostatin and plasma growth hormone during basal conditions, in the diurnal patterns and during arginine infusion, shows that cerebrospinal fluid somatostatin does not denote the activity or tone of hypothalamic somatostatin. It seems therefore unlikely that somatostatin in cerebrospinal fluid originates from hypothalamic or blood borne sources in any significant quantities. The results rather support that somatostatin originates within the extrahypothalamic central nervous system and that its action there is distinct from its action on the pituitary gland.

ROSTRAL-CAUDAL CONCENTRATION GRADIENT

There is a significant concentration gradient in protein concentrations from the cerebral ventricles to the lumbar part of the cerebrospinal fluid in accordance with the rostral excretion from the choroid plexus as shown by Rice (10). It is recently demonstrated that there is a considerable gradient in albumin and gamma-globulin concentration within the lumbar portion of the cerebrospinal fluid while the cerebrospinal fluid while there was no rostral-caudal concentration gradient in the somatostatin concentration (7). Gerner et al. (11) have demonstrated similar results for somatostatin, later also found for neurotensin and cholecystokinin (12). Recently, Thal et al. (13) reported identical somatostatin concentrations in ventricular and lumbar cerebrospinal fluid from patients with epilepsy and multiple sclerosis, and that somatostatin does not cross the blood-brain barrier.

The lack of a rostral-caudal concentration gradient in cerebrospinal fluid somatostatin, and of any association with hypothalamic growth hormone release inhibiting activity, provide further evidence for a disperse secretion of somatostatin from somatostatin containing cells within and all over the central nervous system directly into the cerebrospinal fluid through the extracellular space in both gray and white matter.

LOCALIZATION AND STABILITY

Radioimmunoassay and immunocytochemical examinations have revealed somatostatin in almost all areas of the central nervous system in various species (14, 15, 16). Examination of human brain obtained from neurosurgical biopsies demonstrated a widespread somatostatin cell system in all cortical layers and large somatostatin cells distributed throughout the white matter of the brain (17). Electron-microscopic examinations revealed somatostatin immunoreactivity within secretory vesicles, structures associated with exocytosis, (18, 19) and Foster and Johansson (20) have recently extended these examinations further in a study using colloidal gold technique. The morphology and the distribution of somatostatin cells within the central nervous system are indicative of neurophysiological functions throughout the brain.

In a study of the distribution of somatostatin in post-mortem human brain Geola et al. (21) demonstrated a time and temperature dependent stability of somatostatin. Cooper et al. (15) found that somatostatin was stable in brain tissue from 4 to 20 hours post-mortem. An immunocytochemical examination of somatostatin in post-mortem brains revealed a marked decomposition of the somatostatin cells and their processes within the first 6 hours post-mortem (22). There was not observed further significant decomposition in the period from 6 to 48 hours post-mortem. Lee et al. (23) found post-mortem decrease in somatostatin content in brains from rats and mice depending on extraction procedures. Others found a significant reduction in somatostatin content within the first hours post-mortem, however, at 6 to 24 hours post-mortem concentrations similar to those at zero time were found (24). These examinations demonstrate that storage conditions, preparation technique and methods must be considered in post-mortem examinations of peptides in the central nervous system.

DIURNAL OSCILLATION

Studies in subhuman primates revealed a diurnal variation of somatostatin content in the cerebrospinal fluid (25, 26). In vitro experiments demonstrated generation of somatostatin from hypothalamic and cortical tissues and secretion with diurnal variation (27). Measurement of the content of somatostatin and albumin in cerebrospinal fluid and plasma growth hormone hourly during a 24 hour period (9) showed that somatostatin in human cerebrospinal fluid exhibited a clearcut diurnal variation with basal levels during the day time, increasing values through the evening to a maximum around midnight, returning to basal levels about 5 a.m. and a small rise again about 8 a.m. A similar pattern was found in multiple sclerosis patients during stable phase of the disease, whereas no oscillation at all was found in patients in relapse. Their values remained consistently low throughout the 24 hour period on the same low level as reported in single samples obtained by lumbar puncture (1). The albumin content in the cerebrospinal fluid showed a rostral-caudal gradient without correlation to somatostatin. The diurnal patterns of plasma growth hormone were identical in the three groups, despite different concentration and lack of any oscillation in cerebrospinal fluid somatostatin in one of the groups.

DISCUSSION

The animal examinations (25,26,27) and the clinical findings in humans (9) provide evidence that somatostatin in cerebrospinal fluid originates from somatostatin containing cells within and all over the central nervous system including the spinal cord. It is most likely that the diurnal variation, and the localization of somatostatin within cell structures associated with exocytosis are indicative of secretory activity of neurophysiologically important somatostatin cells, whose mission is still mainly unknown. On the basis of the clinical examinations it seems sustained that the diurnal pattern of plasma growth hormone is without association with concentration or diurnal profile of somatostatin in the cerebrospinal fluid. The lack of a rostral-caudal gradient in somatostatin concentration indicates that the concentration measured in lumbar cerebrospinal fluid is representative of the mean concentration of somatostatin throughout the cerebrospinal fluid, which bathes the entire central nervous system. It seems therefore probable that cerebrospinal fluid somatostatin, generated in cells within the central nervous system and secreted directly into the cerebrospinal fluid, reflects the diurnal secretory activity of the somatostatin cells within the central nervous system. This does not exclude that alteration in somatostatin concentration takes place in localized areas in a magnitude insufficient to be reflected in levels detectable in the cerebrospinal fluid.

The low levels of somatostatin in cerebrospinal fluid during relapses in multiple sclerosis may represent reversible restrained secretory activity of somatostatin cells within the central nervous system, while the superimposed oscillating diurnal secretion in healthy subjects and during stable phases in multiple sclerosis expresses active secretory release governed by yet unidentified central nervous centers, which appear to be inactive during relapses in multiple sclerosis.

It is impossible on the basis of the present knowledge to suggest if the reduced levels and loss of oscillating activity of somatostatin in the cerebrospinal fluid in multiple sclerosis patients during relapses, are only secondary to the disease activity, or if abnormalities in somatostatin release may have pathogenic implications for some of the symptoms and disabilities in multiple sclerosis.

It seems evident, however, that the magnitude of and the variform nature of somatostatin release into the cerebrospinal fluid are dependable indicators of the disease activity in patients suffering from multiple sclerosis.

ACKNOWLEDGEMENTS

The Danish Medical Research Council, The Multiple Sclerosis Society, The Aarhus University Research Council, P. Carl Petersen Foundation, The

Fonden til Laegevidenskabens Fremme and The Institute of Experimental Research supported the study.

REFERENCES

1. K.V. Sörensen, S.E. Christensen, E. Dupont, Aa.P. Hansen, E. Pedersen and H. Örskov. Low somatostatin content in cerebrospinal fluid in multiple sclerosis. Acta Neurol. Scand. 61:186 (1980).
2. K.V. Sörensen, S.E. Christensen, Aa.P. Hansen, E. Pedersen and H. örskov. Cerebrospinal fluid somatostatin inversely correlated with disease activity in multiple sclerosis. The Lancet. I:988 (1983).
3. J. Epelbaum, Y. Agid, E. Enjalbert, M. Hamon, F. Javoy-Agid, C. Kordon, Y. Lamour and E. Mayse. Somatostatin alterations and brain disease. Adv. Exp. Med. & Biol. 188:261 (1985).
4. Y.C. Patel, K. Rao and M.D. Reichlin. Somatostatin in human cerebrospinal fluid. N. Engl. J. Med. 296:529 (1977).
5. S. Krohnheim, M. Berelowitz and B.L. Pimstone. The presence of immunoreactive growth hormone release-inhibiting hormone in normal cerebrospinal fluid. Clin. Endocrinol. (Oxf.) 6:411 (1977).
6. W.B. Matthews, E.D. Acheson, J.R. Batchelor and R.O. Weller. McAlpine's Multiple Sclerosis. Churchil Livingstone, London (1985).
7. K.V. Sörensen, S.E. Christensen, Aa.P. Hansen, E. Pedersen and H. Örskov. The origin of cerebrospinal fluid somatostatin: hypothalamic or disperse central nervous system secretion? Neuroendocrinology. 32:335 (1981).
8. L. Steardo, C.A. Taminga, P. Barone, N. Foster, R. Durso, S. Ruggeri and T.N. Chase. CSF somatostatin immunoreactivity and GH plasma levels in Alzheimers disease. Neuroendocrinol. Lett. 6:291 (1984).
9. K.V. Sörensen, T. Alslev, S.E. Christensen, N.B. Jensen and H. Örskov. Reversible loss of diurnal oscillation in cerebrospinal fluid somatostatin during relapses in multiple sclerosis. In press.
10. E.W. Rice. Total proteins in cerebrospinal fluid. In: Standard methods of clinical chemistry. S. Meiters, ed. Academic Press, New York (1965).
11. R.H. Gerner, D.P. Van Kammen and P.T. Ninan. Cerebrospinal fluid cholecystokinin, Bombesin and somatostatin in schizophrenia and normals. Prog. Neuro-Psychopharmacol. & Biol. Psychiat. 9:73 (1985).
12. C.A. Taminga, P.A. LeWitt and T.N. Chase. Cholecystokinin and Neurotensin gradients in human CSF. Arch. Neurol. 42:354 (1985).
13. L.J. Thal, N.S. Sharpless, D. Rosenbaum, D.P. Davis, I.M. Amin and J.M. Waltz. Ventricular fluid somatostatin concentrations decreases in childhood-onset dystonia. Neurology. 35:1742 (1985).
14. S.R. Vincent, C.H.S. McIntosh, A.M.J. Buchan and J.C. Brown. Central somatostatin systems revealed with monoclonal antibodies. The J. of Comp. Neurol. 238:169 (1985).
15. P.E. Cooper, M.H. Fernstrom, O.P. Rorstad, S.E. Leeman and J.B. Martin. The regional distribution of somatostatin, substance P and neurotensin in human brain. Brain Res. 218:219 (1981).
16. Ä. Ljungdahl, T. Hökfelt and G. Nilsson. Distribution of somatostatin immunoreactivity in the central nervous system of the rat. Neurosci. 3:945 (1978).
17. K.V. Sörensen. Somatostatin: Localization and distribution in the cortex and the subcortical white matter of human brain. Neurosci. 7:1227 (1982).
18. K.V. Sörensen, S.E. Christensen, E. Dupont, Aa.P. Hansen, J. Ingerslev, M.Kjaer, E. Pedersen, J. Törring and H. Örskov. Somatostatin in multiple sclerosis. In: Actual problems in multiple sclerosis research, E. Pedersen, J. Clausen and L. Oades, eds. FADL Copenhagen (1982).

19. G. Pelletier, D. Dubé and R. Puviani. Somatostatin: electron microscope immunohistochemical localization in secretory neurons of rat hypothalamus. Science. 196:1469 (1977).
20. G.A. Foster and O. Johansson. Ultrastructural morphometric analysis of somatostatin-like immunoreactive neurones in the rat central nervous system after labelling with colloidal gold. Brain Res. 342:117 (1985).
21. F.L. Geoloa, T. Yamada, R.J. Warwick, W.W. Tourtellotte and J.M. Hersman. Regional distribution of somatostatin-like immunoreactivity in the human brain. Brain Res. 229:35 (1981).
22. K.V. Sörensen. Rapid post-mortem decomposition of the somatostatin cells in human brain. An immunohistochemical examination. Biomed. & Pharmacotherapy. 38:458 (1984).
23. C.M. Lee, P.C. Emson and L.L. Iversen. Chromatographic behaviour and post-mortem stability of somatostatin in the rat and mouse brain. Brain Res. 220:159 (1981).
24. P. Davis and A. Thompson. Post-mortem stability of somatostatin-like immunoreactivity in mouse brain under conditions simulating handling of human autopsy material. Neurochem. Res. 6:787 (1981).
25. M. Berelowitz, M.J. Perlow, H.J. Hoffman and L.A. Frohman. The diurnal variation of immunoreactive thyrotropin-releasing hormone and somatostatin in the cerebrospinal of the Rhesus monkey. Endocrinol. 109:2102 (1981).
26. M.A. Arnold, S.M. Reppert, O.P. Rorstad, S.M. Sagar, H.T. Kentmann, M.J. Perlow and J.B. Martin. Temporal patterns of somatostatin immunoreactivity in the cerebrospinal fluid of the Rhesus monkey: effect of environmental lightning. The J. of Neurosci. 2:674 (1982).
27. M. Berelowitz, D. Dudlak and L.A. Frohman. Diurnal variation in release of somatostatin-like immunoreactivity from incubated rat hypothalamus and cerebral cortex. Endocrinol. 110:2195 (1982).

NEUROENDOCRINE PEPTIDE HORMONES AND THEIR RECEPTORS AS ENDOGENOUS COMPONENTS OF THE IMMUNE SYSTEM

J. Edwin Blalock

Department of Physiology and Biophysics, University of Alabama at Birmingham, Birmingham, Alabama 35294

INTRODUCTION

While the present paper may not appear to directly relate to our current knowledge of multiple sclerosis, it nonetheless may provide novel understandings of immune neuroendocrine interactions which could eventually be applied to this disease. Most simply, it seems that these two systems share a common set of hormones and their receptors which may be normally used for inter system communication as well as intra system regulation. The best studied system involves the proopiomelanocortin (POMC)-derived peptides, and these will be emphasized although others such as thyrotropin (TSH) will be discussed.

NEUROENDOCRINE PEPTIDE HORMONES IN THE IMMUNE SYSTEM

The first indication that cells of the immune system (immunocytes) might synthesize peptide hormones that are classically associated with the neuroendocrine system came as a result of the observation that during production of interferon-alpha in response to virus infection, human leucocytes coordinately expressed peptides which were antigenically related to corticotropin (ACTH) and endorphins (1). Since IFN-alpha was also synthesized by virus-infected immunocytes, one initial possibility was that the ACTH and endorphins were derived from a gene sequence within that family which codes for the IFNs. However, there were essentially no common nucleotide sequences shared by the cloned IFN and POMC cDNA (2,3). This data as well as other studies showed that these proteins often represent coordinately (and sometimes differentially) induced but differentially controlled products of separate genes (4,5). The immunocyte-derived ACTH was found to be similar, if not identical, to pituitary-derived ACTH with respect to its biological activity, molecular weight, antigenicity and retention time on a reverse phase high pressure liquid chromatography column (4-6). More recently, substantial evidence for the identity of the pituitary and immunocyte ACTH has come from the observation of the transcription of the POMC gene in virus-infected murine splenocytes as determined by dot and Northern blot analysis of total cellular and poly $(A)^+$ cytoplasmic RNA (7). Collectively, these data leave little doubt that cells of the immune system can produce at least one family of neuroendocrine peptide hormones.

While the production of the POMC-derived peptides was originally observed in response to virus infection, we now know that this is only one of a number of possible stimuli which include typhoid vaccination (unpublished observation), as well as bacterial endotoxin or lipopolysaccharide (8). Perhaps the most interesting new inducers are the classical hypothalamic signals for pituitary POMC production, corticotropin releasing factor (CRF) and arginine vasopressin (AVP). These peptides were shown to synergistically cause the de novo synthesis of ACTH and beta endorphin by human periphal leukocytes. As in the pituitary gland, such induction was suppressed by dexamethasone (9). These data strongly suggest that the POMC gene in pituitary cells and leukocytes is similarly controlled in both a positive and negative fashion. Interestingly, there can be alternate processing of POMC depending on the stimuli. In response to CRF or Newcastle disease virus, immunocytes seem to process POMC in a fashion that is analogous to a composition of the anterior and posterior lobes of the pituitary gland and this results in the release of ACTH (1-39) and beta endorphin. In contrast, LPS seems to cause a completely novel processing pattern which results in peptides with the molecular weights of ACTH (1-24 or 26) and alpha- or gamma-endorphin (8). As will be discussed below, this alternate processing may be quite important with respect to immunoregulation by these hormones.

The production of neuroendocrine peptide hormones by the immune system is now known to be limited to POMC-derived peptides. Depending on the leukocyte cell type and stimuli, we now know that they can make a number of molecules that are similar if not identical to known hormones. This includes TSH (10), chorionic gonadotropin (11), vasoactive intestinal peptide (12-14), somatostatin (14), follicle-stimulating hormone, luteinizing hormone, and growth hormone (J.E. Blalock, E.M. Smith, D. Harbour-McMenamin, K.L. Bost and D.A. Weigent, unpublished observations). Thus in many respects, the immune system looks like a circulating neuroendocrine organ.

NEUROENDOCRINE PEPTIDE HORMONE RECEPTORS IN THE IMMUNE SYSTEM

While there are numerous reports of specific binding sites for peptide hormones on immunocytes (for review see 15), until recently, there was no evidence that these sites are biochemically related to receptors on a particular hormone's classical target tissue. Such information, of course, is crucial to an understanding of the biochemistry of immune neuroendocrine interactions. Recently, we have developed a new approach for the purification of receptors and used it for the isolation and characterization of the adrenal ACTH receptor (16,17). This receptor was shown to have a total molecular weight of 225,000 and to be composed of 4 polypeptide chains of 83,000, 64,000, 52,000 and 22,000 Da. The ACTH binding site was located on the 83,000 Da polypeptide chain. Similar experiments were then done with mouse spleen and human peripheral blood mononuclear cells and a similar, if not identical receptor, was observed (K.L. Bost and J.E. Blalock, unpublished observation). Binding studies on mouse spleen cells show high affinity (K_d 0.1 nM) and low affinity (K_d 4.8 nM) binding sites (18). We believe these represent two confirmations of a single receptor (17) with K_ds that roughly correspond to those on rat adrenal cells (K_ds 0.25 and 10 nM, respectively) (19). A comparison of the average number of binding sites per cell shows approximately 3,000 high and 50,000 low affinity sites on splenocytes compared to 3,000 high and 30,000 low affinity sites on adrenal cells.

Binding sites on leukocytes for endogenous opiates have also been described. These include, but are not necessarily limited to, the following. Apparently, the first indirect evidence for opiate receptors resulted from the finding that morphine and methionine-enkephalin inhibited and enhanced, respectively T cell rosetting of sheep red blood cells (SRBC) (20). Both the inhibition and enhancement of rosetting could be reversed by the opiate antagonist naloxone, but not by an inactive enantimer, levomoramide.

By competitive binding experiments with a radiolabelled ligand, it was directly shown that methionine-enkephalin binding sites reside on mouse splenocytes (K_d = 0.6 nM) (18). Others measured stereospecific dihydromorphine binding to human phagocytic leukocytes. Both granulocytes and monocytes had specific receptors with apparent K_ds of 10 nM ns 8 nM, respectively (21). Hazum et al. (22) reported a high affinity beta-endorphin binding site on transformed human lymphocytes with an apparent K_d of 3 nM plus a lower affinity site. These, however, were not classic opiate receptors since the binding was not affected by opiate agonists and antagonists. Since binding to opiate receptors classically is through the amino terminal end of the peptide, this nonopiate receptor binding seems to be through the carboxyl end of beta-endorphin (22). This leads to the interesting possibility that a molecule such as beta-endorphin could bridge two different types of lymphocytes by binding through its amino terminus to an opiate receptor on one cell and through its carboxyl terminus to a nonopiate receptor on another lymphocyte.

NEUROENDOCRINE FUNCTIONS OF PEPTIDE HORMONES OF THE IMMUNE SYSTEM

The finding of neuroendocrine peptide hormones and their receptors in the immune system raises obvious questions about their function. In the case of ACTH, one immediate conclusion would be that the pituitary gland should not be required for an ACTH-mediated stress response if the immune system could be stimulated for hormone production <u>in vivo.</u> This appears to be the case since Newcastle disease virus (an inducer of leukocyte ACTH <u>in vitro</u>) infection of hypophysectomized mice caused a time dependent increase in corticosterone production which was inhibited by dexamethasone. Unless the mice were pretreated with dexamethasone, their spleens were positive for ACTH (5). Based on these observations, we have suggested a lymphoid-adrenal axis exists which may account for the increases in corticosteroid levels which are generally observed during infections. Further, such an axis might also explain the earlier observation of bacterial polysaccharide (Piromen) induced cortisol responses in 7 out of 8 patients who underwent pituitary stalk sectioning (23). More recently, a patient presented with the clinical ad laboratory features of the ectopic ACTH syndrome. While the absence of a gradient in ACTH concentration between the inferior petrosal sinuses and the periphery argued against pituitary overproduction, no ACTH producing tumor was found and bilateral adrenalectomy was performed to correct the hypercortisolism. Six months later, a pseudotumor containing only normal fat and inflammatory tissue was observed in the patient. Upon removal of this inflammatory tissue, basal plasma ACTH levels immediately returned to normal and leukocytes within the inflammatory tissue stained positively for ACTH by an immunoperoxidase procedure (24). Collectively, these studies seem to leave little doubt that cells of the immune system are able to directly influence adrenal function via ACTH production and consequently may also indirectly affect hypothalamic and pituitary function.

Gram-negative sepsis and endotoxin-induced shock may represent another situation in which leukocyte production of proopiomelanocortin-derived peptides play pivotal roles. For instance, endorphins have been implicated in the pathophysiology associated with these trauma since the opiate antagonist naloxone improved survival rates and blocked a number of cardiopulmonary changes associated with these conditions (25). Further, two separate pools of endorphins have been observed following endotoxin administration, and it was suggested that one might originate in the immune system (26). Considering the potent immunologic effects of endotoxin, as well as its ability to induce leukocyte production of endorphins in vitro (8), cells of the immune system seem the most likely source of endogenous opiates that are observed during Gram-negative sepsis and endotoxin shock. Consistent with this idea is the observation that lymphocyte depletion, like naloxone treatment, blocked a number of endotoxin-induced cardiopulmonary changes (27). Our interpretation of this results is that lymphocyte depletion removes the source of the endorphins while naloxone blocks their effector function. This may represent a situation where immune system-derived endorphins are involved in the manifestations of disease states. While possible immunocyte production of other peptide hormones in vivo has not yet been studied, we anticipate that they, like the POMC products, will be produced in physiologically meaningful amounts.

IMMUNOREGULATION BY NEUROENDOCRINE PEPTIDE HORMONES

Many neuroendocrine hormones have been shown to influence various parameters of immunity (for review see 28). Among them, perhaps the best studied are ACTH and the endorphins. While the in vivo immunosuppressive properties of ACTH were previously thought to be mediated through glucocorticoids, ACTH is now known to be directly suppressive for antibody production (18). In a plaque forming cell (PFC) assay in vitro which measures antibody secreting cells, $ACTH_{1-39}$ suppressed the response to both a T lymphocyte dependent antigen, sheep red blood cells (SRBC) and T independent antigen, dinitrophenol-Ficoll. Inhibition of antibody to SRBC required only one fourth of the amount of ACTH necessary for equal inhibition of the DNP-Ficoll response. This suggests that T cell function may be more sensitive to ACTH than B lymphocyte function. Interestingly, while highly purified and synthetic $ACTH_{1-39}$ is suppressive, $ACTH_{1-24}$ is not inhibitory (18). This is in contrast to ACTH's steroidogenic activity in which $ACTH_{1-39}$ or $ACTH_{1-24}$ are equally active (19). It was necessary for ACTH to be present at the time of addition of antigen for maximum inhibition and thiol-reducing agents blocked ACTH suppression of the antibody response. Since these characteristics are also associated with suppression of antibody by interferon (IFN), it seems that the mechanisms through which ACTH inhibits the antibody response may be quite similar to that of a lymphokine, IFN (18). Considering that $ACTH_{1-39}$ was immunosuppressive while $ACTH_{1-24}$ was without effect is particularly interesting in light of the aforementioned finding that CRF induced immunocytes to produce $ACTH_{1-39}$ while LPS caused $ACTH_{1-24}$ production. This leads to the interesting possibility that differential immunoregulation may result from alternate processing of the same hormone precursor. This idea is further supported by the recent observation that both $ACTH_{1-24}$ and $ACTH_{1-39}$ in conjunction with a B cell growth factor or recombinant IL-2 can enhance the growth and differentiation of human B cells (29).

Since ACTH and endorphins are products of the same polyprotein precursor and are both elevated during stress, endorphins were evaluated for immunomodulatory activity. Related peptides, the enkephalins, also were tested for modulation of antibody synthesis. Alpha-endorphin, the shortest of the three endorphin species, was the only one to affect PFC formation, and it was suppressive (18,30). Both leucine and methionine-enkephalin suppressed the antibody response in vitro to SRBC though to a lesser degree than alpha-endorphin. Since the endorphins and enkephalins share common amino terminal sequences and all bind to opiate receptors, the extra amino acid(s) on the carboxyl terminus of gamma- and beta-endorphin may be responsible for their inactivity in this system. Although beta-endorphin had no effect of its own, it, as well as naloxone, would compete with and block alpha-endorphin's suppressive effect. Thus it seems that binding of certain endogenous opioid peptides to an opiate-like receptor on lymphocytes will suppress antibody production. Interestingly, TSH caused an effect that was opposite to that of ACTH and alpha-endorphin. TSH enhanced the antibody response in vitro to SRBC and this effect required the addition of the hormone during the early phase of the response (1-2 days) (31). This effect is now known to occur through an effect of TSH on T cells which in turn enhance the B cell response (32). It is particularly intriguing that two different stimuli can elicit the leukocyte production of two different hormones (TSH and ACTH), and these in turn have opposite actions on the immune system.

Like B lymphocyte function, T cell function is also modulated by peptide hormones. Beta-endorphin enhanced the proliferative response of rat splenic lymphocytes to the T cell mitogens, concanavalin A (Con A) and phytohemagglutinin (PHA) (33). The enhancement was dose dependent but was not blocked by the opiate antagonist naloxone. The inability of naloxone to block the enhancement suggests that beta-indorphin does not act through a classic opiate receptor in this system. In contrast, others found that human T cell mitogenesis was effectively suppressed by beta-endorphin (34). While these results seem conflicting, they might be explained as being due to different species and relative concentrations. The latter study utilized higher beta-endorphin concentrations. Opiates frequently display opposite activities between high and low concentrations (35) which could account for these discrepancies. The enkephalins were subsequently found to enhance PHA-induced human lymphocyte mitogenesis (36).

Endogenous opiates have also been implicated in the regulation of natural killer (NK) cell activity. Beta-endorphin in a dose dependent fashion enhanced NK activity 20-55% (37,38). Again, the enhancement was observed with very low doses (1×10^{-14} M) and increased up to 1×10^{-6} M. Interestingly, gamma-endorphin also enhanced NK activity but was less potent and alpha-endorphin had very little effect at all (38). Thus, the endorphin enhancement of NK activity was opposite of that seen with antibody synthesis where the shorter alpha-endorphin was more suppressive than gamma- and beta-endorphin. NK enhancement seemed to be mediated through opiate receptor(s) since it was blocked by naloxone in both cases. Mononuclear cell chemotaxis is also stimulated by both beta-endorphin and methionine-enkephalin (39). The response to both neuropeptides was bimodal and active at very low concentrations (1×10^{-14} M). This effect also seems to be mediated through opiate receptors as evidenced by naloxone blockage of migration. Besides the endorphins and enkephalins, ACTH also modulates the cell-mediated immune response. ACTH was found to suppress lymphokine, IFN-gamma, production in vitro (40). Once again, $ACTH_{1-39}$ suppressed the induction of IFN-gamma while shorter fragments of ACTH, $ACTH_{1-24}$ and alpha-MSH ($ACTH_{1-13}$) did not. Also, CLIP (corticotropin-like intermediate lobe peptide) which corresponds to $ACTH_{18-39}$, did not affect IFN-gamma production. Thus, in two cases (IFN-gamma and antibody production), there seems to be no correlation between ACTH's steroidogenic and immunomodulatory activities since $ACTH_{1-24}$ has full steroidogenic capability and is not immunomodulatory.

A MOLECULAR BASIS FOR INTERACTIONS BETWEEN THE NEUROENDOCRINE AND IMMUNOLOGIC SENSORY SYSTEMS

Based on the above findings, it seems that a plausible and molecular explanation for bidirectional communication between the immune and neuroendocrine systems may in fact be quite simple. Both systems share a common set of peptide signals or hormones as well as their receptors. These combinations then are used for both inter- and intrasystem communications and regulation. This concept leads to the notion that the immune system may serve a sensory role (41).

Instead of classic sensory stimuli (physical, chemical, visual, etc.), the immune system recognizes immune type stimuli such as viruses, bacteria and tumors. Production of neuroendocrine hormones by the stimulated leukocytes could then alter homeostasis in a fashion similar to the pituitary gland during classic sensory stimuli recognition. Presumably, the hormones will also modulate host defense mechanisms. In the case of ACTH and endorphins, negative feedback through other endocrine hormones such as corticosteroids will shut off lymphocyte ACTH and endorphin synthesis. The ability of CRF to induce lymphocyte ACTH suggests that classic sensory stimuli can also induce the lymphocyte arm of the circuit. The possibilities for this system are numerous. One is the possibility for differential regulation. Since various immune inducers stimulate different hormones from leukocytes, there would be a variety of alterations in homeostasis. The particular responses elicited will correspond to the lymphocyte population, being induced or hormone being produced. Also, differential processing of the same hormone such as ACTH could cause alternate immunoregulation since the effects of ACTH on the immune system vary with the length of the molecule. An understanding of these interactions may help explain the pathophysiology of diseases which have both immune and neuroendocrine components. Furthermore, it may provide a rationale for new clinical therapies. As an example, it may be possible to partially reconstitute pituitary hormone deficiencies with the appropriate immune stimulus or hypothalamic releasing factor which in turn would act on the immune system. Indications that this may be possible come from the data showing the induction of corticosterone in hypophysectomized mice by a viral antigen (5).

POSSIBLE IMPLICATIONS FOR MULTIPLE SCLEROSIS

To this author's knowledge, no direct applications of the above findings to MS have yet been determined. However, one could envision any number of situations where the immunologic production and action of neuroendocrine peptide hormones may impinge on the disease. Among these are the possible alteration of leukocyte migration in response to neuropeptides as well as the immunologic enhancing and suppressing effects of TSH and ACTH, respectively. In this regard, it may be less than a chance occurrence that ACTH can ameliorate some aspects of MS in a fashion which may not be entirely via glucocorticoids (42). If this is in fact the case, then the induction of immunocyte ACTH by CRF might be one possible therapeutic measure.

ACKNOWLEDGEMENTS

This work was supported in part by Office of Naval Research Grant N0014-84-K-0486, NIH Grant R01 AM338-39-01 A1, the McLaughlin Foundation, and Triton Biosciences, Inc. The author thanks Drs. E.M. Smith, K.L. Bost and W.J. Meyer for many helpful scientific discussions, and Diane Weigent for her skillful typing of this manuscript.

REFERENCES

1. J.E. Blalock and E.M. Smith. Human leucocyte interferon: structural and biological relatedness to andrenocorticotropic hormone and endorphins. Proc. Natl. Acad. Sci. USA. 77:5972 (1984).

2. M. Uhler and E. Herbert. Complete amino acid sequence of mouse pro-opiomelanocortin derived from the nucleotide sequence of pro-opiomelanocortin cDNA. J. Biol. Chem. 258:257 (1983).
3. G.D. Shaw, W. Boll, H. Taira, N. Mantci, P. Lengyel and C. Weissman. Structure and expression of cloned murine IFN-alpha genes. Nucleic Acids Res. 11:555 (1983).
4. E.M. Smith and J.E. Blalock. Human lymphocyte production of ACTH and endorphin-like substances: Association with leukocyte interferon. Proc. Natl. Acad. Sci. USA. 78:7530 (1981).
5. E.M. Smith, W.J. Meyer and J.E. Blalock. Virus-induced increases in corticosterone in hypophysectomized mice: A possible lymphoid-adrenal axis. Science. 218:1311 (1982).
6. J.E. Blalock and E.M. Smith. A complete regulatory loop between the immune and neuroendocrine systems. Fed. Proc. 44:108 (1985).
7. H.J. Westley, A.J. Kleiss, K.W. Kelley, P.K.Y. Wong and P.-H. Yuen. Newcastle disease virus-infected splenocytes express the pro-opiomelanocortin gene. J. Exp. Med. In press (1986).
8. D.V. Harbour-McMenamin, E.M. Smith and J.E. Blalock. Bacterial lipopolysaccharide induction of leukocyte derived ACTH and endorphins. Infect. Immun. 48:813 (1985).
9. E.M. Smith, A.C. Morrill, W.J. Meyer and J.E. Blalock. Corticotropin releasing factor induction of leukocyte derived immunoreactive ACTH and endorphins. Nature (London). In press (1986).
10. E.M. Smith, M. Phan, D. Coppenhaver, T.E. Kruger and J.E. Blalock. Human lymphocyte production of immunoreactive thyrotropin. Proc. Natl. Acad. Sci. USA. 80:6010 (1983).
11. D. Harbour-McMenamin, E.M. Smith and J.E. Blalock. Production of immunoreactive chorionic gonadotropin during mixed lymphocyte reactions: a possible selective mechanism for genetic diversity. Proc. Natl. Acad. Sci. USA. Submitted (1986).
12. A. Giachetti, A. Goth and S.I. Said. Vasoactive intestinal polypeptide (VIP) in rabbit platelets, and rat mast cells. Fed. Proc. 37:657 (1978).
13. M.S. O'Dorisio, T.M. O'Dorisio, S. Cataland and S.P. Balcerzak. Vasoactive intestinal peptide as a biochemical marker for polymorphonuclear leukocytes. J. Lab. Clin. Med. 96:666 (1980).
14. I. Lygren, A. Revhaug, P.G. Burhol, K.E. Giercksky and T.G. Jenssen. Vasoactive intestinal peptide and somatostatin in leukocytes. Scand. J. Clin. Lab. Invest. 44:347 (1984).
15. J.E. Blalock, K.L. Bost and E.M. Smith. Neuroendocrine peptide hormones and their receptors in the immune system-production, processing and action. J. Neuroimmunol. 10:31 (1985).
16. K.L. Bost, E.M. Smith and J.E. Blalock. Similarity between the corticotropin (ACTH) receptor and a peptide encoded by an RNA that is complementary to ACTH mRNA. Proc. Natl. Acad. Sci. USA. 82:1372 (1985).
17. K.L. Bost and J.E. Blalock. Molecular characterization of a corticotropin (ACTH) receptor. Molec. Cell. Endocrinol. 44:1 (1986).
18. H.M. Johnson, E.M. Smith, B.A. Torres and J.E. Blalock. Neuroendocrine hormone regulation of in vitro antibody production. Proc. Natl. Acad. Sci. USA. 79:4171 (1982).
19. R.A.J. McIlhinney and D. Schulster. Studies on the binding of ^{125}I-labelled corticotropin to isolated rat adrenocortical cells. J. Endocrinol. 64:175 (1975).
20. J. Wybran, T. Appelbroom, J.-P. Famaey and A. Govaerts. Suggestive evidence for receptors for morphine and methionine-enkephalin on normal blood T lymphocytes. J. Immunol. 123:1068 (1979).
21. A. Lopker, L.G. Abood, W. Hoss and F.J. Lionetti. Stereoselective muscarinic acetylcholine and opiate receptors in human phagocytic leukocytes. Biochem. Pharmacol. 29:1361 (1980).

22. E.K. Hazum, K. Chang and P. Cuatrecasas. Specific non opiate receptors for beta-endorphin. Science. 205:1033 (1979).
23. J.J. Van Wyk, G.S. Dugger, J.F. Newsome and P.Z. Thomas. The effect of pituitary stalk section in the adrenal function of women with cancer of the breast. J. Clin. Endocrinol. Metab. 20:157 (1960).
24. A.G. Dupont, G. Somers, A.C. Van Steirteghem, F. Warson and L. Vanhaelst. Ectopic andrenocorticotropin production: disappearance after removal of inflammatory tissue. J. Clin. Endocrinol. Metab. 58:654 (1984).
25. D.G. Reynolds, N.V. Guill, T. Vargish, R.B. Hechner, A.I. Fader and J.W. Holaday. Blockade of opiate receptors for naloxone improves survival and cardiac performance in canine endotoxic shock. Circ. Shock. 7:39 (1980).
26. D.B. Carr, R. Bergland, A. Hamilton, H. Blume, N. Kasting, M. Arnold, M.B. Martin and M. Rosenblatt. Endotoxin stimulated opioid peptide secretion: two secretory pools and feedback control in vivo. Science. 217:845 (1982).
27. C.T. Bohs, J.C. Fish, T.H. Miller and D.L. Traber. Pulmonary vascular response to endotoxin in normal and lymphocyte depleted sheep. Circ. Shock. 6:13 (1979).
28. J.E. Blalock. Relationships between neuroendocrine hormones and lymphokines. Lymphokines. 9:1 (1984).
29. M. Mon-Alvarez, J.H. Kehrl and A.S. Fauci. A potential role for adrenocorticotropin in regulating B lymphocyte functions. J. Immunol. 135:3823 (1985).
30. C.J. Heijnen, C. Bevers, A. Kavelaars and R.E. Ballieux. Effect of alpha-endorphin on the antigen induced primary antibody response of human B cells in vitro. J. Immunol. 136:213 (1986).
31. J.E. Blalock, H.M. Johnson, E.M. Smith and B.A. Torres. Enhancement of the in vitro antibody response by thyrotropin. Biochem. Biophys. Res. Commun. 125:30 (1985).
32. T.E. Kruger and J.E. Blalock. Cellular requirements for thyrotropin enhancement of in vitro antibody production. J. Immunol. In press (1986).
33. S.C. Gilman, J.M. Schwarz, R.J. Milner, F.E. Bloom and J.D. Feldman. Beta-endorphin enhances lymphocyte proliferative responses. Proc. Natl. Acad. Sci. USA. 79:4226-4230.
34. H.W. McCain, I.B. Lamster, J.M. Bozzone and J.T. Grbic. Beta-endorphin modulates human immune activity via non-opiate receptor mechanisms. Life Sci. 31:1619 (1982).
35. R.E. Faith, N.P. Plotnikoff and A.J. Murgo. Effects of opiates and enkephalins-endorphins on immune functions. In: "Proc. Natl. Inst. Drug Abuse Techn. Meet. on Mechanisms of Tolerance and Dependence" (1983).
36. N. Plotnikoff and G.C. Miller. Enkephalins as immunomodulators. Int. J. Immunopharmacol. 5:437 (1983).
37. P.M. Mathews, C.J. Froelich, W.L. Sibbitt, Jr. and A.D. Bankhurs. Enhancement of natural cytotoxicity by beta-endorphin. J. Immunol. 130:1658 (1983).
38. N. Kay, J. Allen and J.E. Morley. Endorphins stimulate normal human peripheral blood lymphocyte natural killer activity. Life Sci. 35:53 (1984).
39. D. Van Epps and L. Saland. Beta-endorphin and met-enkephalin stimulate human peripheral blood mononuclear cell chemotaxis. J. Immunol. 132:3046 (1984).
40. H.M. Johnson, B.A. Torres, E.M. Smith, L.D. Dion and J.E. Blalock. Regulation of lymphokine (gamma-interferon) production by corticotropin. J. Immunol. 132:246 (1984).

41. J.E. Blalock. The immune system as a sensory organ. J. Immunol. 132:1067 (1984).
42. W.W. Tourtellotte, R.W. Baumhefner, A.R. Potvin, B.I. Ma, J.H. Potvin, M. Mendez and K. Syndulko. Neurology. 30:1155 (1980).

CEREBROSPINAL FLUID PROSTAGLANDINS IN MULTIPLE SCLEROSIS

Paula Dore-Duffy

Multiple Sclerosis Center, Department of Neurology
University of Connecticut School of Medicine Farmington,
Connecticut 06032

INTRODUCTION

One of the most exciting developments in physiology and biochemistry over the last two decades is the emerging knowledge of the prostaglandins (PGs). PGs are synthesized by most tissues in the body, and in brain tissue, have been implicated in cerebrospinal hemodynamics (1), neurotransmission (1), temperature regulation (2), behaviour (3), regulation of food intake (1,4) and motor functions (1). Following a few brief general comments, this paper will be limited to a discussion of PGs in the cerebrospinal fluid (5) and in multiple sclerosis (MS).

The PGs are unsaturated twenty carbon cyclopentane carboxylic acids (6). The type designation for the primary PGs (E,F,D,B etc.) is based on structural differences in the cyclopentane ring. They are further subclassified according to the number of carbon-carbon doubled bonds. PGs are not stored in cells but are synthesized and released on stimulation. A wide range of stimuli activate mobilization of fatty acid precursors such as arachidonic acid from plasma membrane phospholipids by the action of phospholipase A_2 (7). The action of phospholipase C (8) and diglyceride lipase (9) may also be operative. Fatty acid precursors then serve as substrate for oxygenation by both the cyclooxygenase (PGs) and 5-lipoxygenase (leukotriene) pathways. Nonsteroidal anti-inflammatory drugs such as aspirin and feldene inhibit the cycloxygenase enzyme. Steroids act by inhibiting phospholipase activity. Upon release PGs may be converted to less active metabolites if appropriate enzymes are present.

CENTRAL NERVOUS SYSTEM

Cerebrospinal fluid

The existence of PG material in cerebrospinal fluid (CSF) was first reported by Ramwell (10) in 1964. Since that time there have been numerous reports of CSF PGs both in animals and humans. Although the exact origin of the CSF prostaglandins is not clear, it is thought that both cisternal and lumbar concentrations reflect a steady state equilibrium between CNS synthesis and transport into the general circulation. Further, the brain, in contrast with other tissues, has low catabolic enzyme activity for the conversion of PGE_2 and PGF_{2alpha} into the less active 15-Keto-13,14, dihydrometabolites (11).

Reports of CSF prostaglandin levels vary considerably. Interpretation of these studies to a large extent depends of the species examined; the sampling technique; the technique used to measure the PGs (radioimmunoassay, high pressure liquid chromatography (HPLC), mass spectometry etc.) and the particular PG looked for. The lack of availability of large amounts of normal CSF samples has made it difficult to calculate basal levels. It is clear however that, in general, the basal level of unesterfied arachidonic acid and PGs in normal brain tissue (12,13) and CSF is very low (11,4,15,16).

The concentration of CSF PGF_{2alpha} in human subjects without neurological disease has been reported to range from about 30-140 pg/ml (11,17). PGF_{2alpha} is either undetectable (11,16) or at low levels ranging from 15-30 pg/ml (11-17). The concentration of 6-Keto PGF_{1alpha} (stable metabolite of prostacyclin) and thromboxane B_2 were very low (5-30 pg/ml) (16). PGD_2 is undetectable in normal human lumbar CSF (17), although it is a major constituent of rat brain (18). Measurements of stable metabolites have not yielded additional new information because of lack of catabolic enzymes in the CNS.

Marked increases in PGF and PGE are seen during the disease state. CSF PG or arachidonate concentrations have been reported to be increased in patients with trauma (19,20), schizophrenia (21), febrile illness (22,23,24), Stroke (25) and subarachnoid hemorrhage (26,27). These increases probably reflect actual changes in synthesis by brain tissue. Elevations in CSF PGE_2 have also been reported in patients with epilepsy (1) and migraine headache!

Prostaglandins in MS

Although the evidence is equivocal, PG-mediated control of immune function may be altered in patients with MS. In early studies, Kirby and Morely and co-workers (28) reported a decreased leukocyte response to PGE-mediated inhibition of leukocyte migration inhibition (LIF) activity. These studies were not confirmed by Willoughby et al. (29) or by Goodwin and Messner (30). Neither group used aspirin or indomethacin to inhibit endogenously PGs. Different concentrations of PHA were used, and small numbers of patients with significantly different clinical pictures were studied.

Lymphocytes from patients with MS adhere to most virus-infected cells to a significantly greater degree than control lymphocytes (31,32,33). The lymphocyte adherence determination (LAD) is not virus specific (34), but is PGE sensitive (35). Treatment of control lymphocytes with PGE_1 or E_2 and cyclic AMP increased T-lymphocyte adherence to MS levels. PGF and cyclic GMP had no effect while PGI also increased adherence. The ability of PGE to increase LAD may be via its ability to increase cellular cyclic AMP.

Incubation of MS lymphocytes with PG inhibitors significantly decreased MS LAD to levels normally exhibited by control cells (36). Ingestion of aspirin in single dosages of 975 mg or 1.3g significantly reduced LAD. Values returned to pretreatment levels by 8 hours. Aspirin does not reduce MS LAD values to below control levels, and does not significantly reduce control LAD despite inhibition of PG synthesis. These observations might suggest that, although the attachment of normal lymphocytes is not entirely dependent on PGE synthesis, a PGE-mediated event may account for the increased LAD exhibited by MS lymphocytes.

Increased LAD in patients with MS may be due to the ability of MS monocytes to produce significantly greater amounts of PGE than control monocytes (37). Removal of monocytes reduced the LAD. Addition of PGE to either monocyte-depleted cells or to aspirin-treated mononuclear cells restores LAD to pretreatment levels. Furthermore, MS cells are more sensitive to low concentrations and less sensitive to high concentrations of PGE (37,38).

Together the data that increased expression of adherence in MS may be the result of increased synthesis and exposure of cells to PGE. Exposure to high levels of PGE in vivo may result in loss of PG receptors and down regulation. Cells may not be responsive to PGE signals until the high PGE is removed or cells are treated with a PG inhibitor. The reappearance of PG receptors would result in concomitant increase in PG sensitivity. Such a condition may explain why in the Kirby et al. (28) study the lymphocytes were responsive to PGE whereas in our studies (37) and those of Merrill et al. (39) lymphocytes treated with aspirin or monocyte-depleted lymphocytes were shown to be more sensitive to PGE.

PGE modulation of lymphocyte responses may in part explain much of the epiphenomena observed in MS. It has been suggested that increased PGE synthesis by MS monocytes may explain the decrease in natural killer cell activity observed by some investigators (40-42). In these studies Merrill and colleagues confirmed increased synthesis of PGE by MS monocytes both from the peripheral blood and cerebrospinal fluid and showed that this correlated with decreased NK cell activity and responsiveness to interferon (39,43).

PGE can suppress modulation of T cell surface antigens (44). Incubation of mononuclear cells from patients with MS at 37°C increases the number of OKT8 positive cells. PGE inhibits this increase. Our results suggest that exposure of MS leukocytes to high levels of endogenous PGE may be responsible for modulation of T suppressor cells. A similar mechanism of modulation may explain the observations of Booss et al. (45) In perivascular lymphocyte infiltrates, in contrast to CNS parenchyma, lymphocyte populations were in roughly equal proportions. That cytotoxic-suppressor cells are in preponderance in parenchyma suggest that some type of antigenic modulation may play a role. The role of PGs in MS has recently been reviewed (38).

CSF prostaglandins in MS

CSF mononuclear cells from patients with MS synthesize increased concentrations of PGE (43,46). We compared PGE synthesis by peripheral blood mononuclear cells and CSF mononuclear cells from patients currently experiencing an exacerbation. CSF mononuclear cells produced significantly more PGE over a 48 hour period than peripheral blood cells (Fig.1). In previous studies we have reported that PGE synthesis by peripheral blood monocytes dramatically decreases during the early stages of an exacerbation (47). These results suggest that the decreased synthesis of PGE during exacerbation may be the result of migration of PGE producing cells into the CNS.

Previous measurements of MS CSF PGs have shown that PGE and PGF_{2alpha} are elevated (48,49). Bolton and colleagues (48) showed that PGE and PGF levels decreased in clinically documented exacerbation although they continued to remain higher than controls. Merrill et al. (42) showed no change with clinical activity, although they confirm elevated CSF PGE.

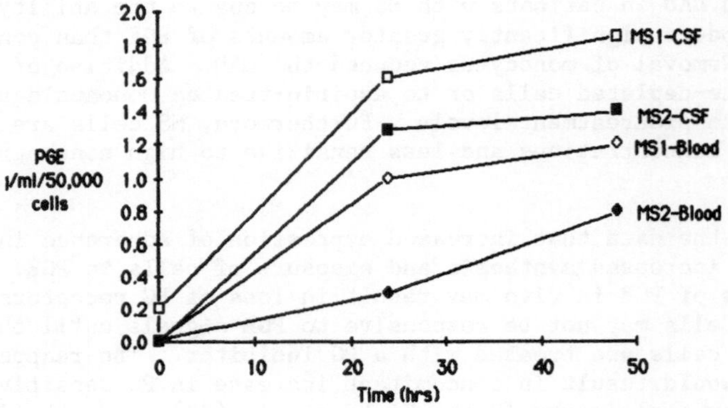

Fig.1. Mononuclear cells from patients in exacerbation (first few days) were placed in culture (50,000 cells in 0,5 ml RPMI 1640). Released PGE was measured by RIA at the times indicated.

We have measured CSF PGs HPLC in patients with MS and neurological and inflammatory disease controls (Table 1,2) (50). We have expanded on previous studies by examining a number of PGs by HPLC following extraction of CSF. All the major CNS PGs were found to be elevated in the diseased state. However, significantly different patterns were seen in different disease groups. CSF PGE and PGF_{2alpha} levels were found to be higher than normal in all MS and neurological and inflammatory disease controls. MS PGF_{2alpha} levels ranged from 2 to 37 ng/ml. PGE levels ranged from 300 pg/ml to 5 ng/ml. PGD_2 was consistently found in all patients with MS and in one patient with myasthenia gravis. PGA was not detectable in all samples examined.

Table 1. CSF prostaglandins in multiple sclerosis

PG ng/ml

patients	PGF_2	PGE	PGD_2	PGA
MS1	2.0	4.0	1.2	--
2	9.2	1.6	7.6	--
3 (ex)	36.9	0.3	4.5	--
4	3.2	3.2	5.2	--
5 (ex)	3.4	1.9	5.3	--
6	3.5	4.8	5.3	--
7	4.8	8.4	6.0	--
8	6.2	4.4	5.8	--
Control 1*	7.1	1.9	--	--
2	0.02	--	--	--
3	0.10	0.01	--	--
4	--	--	--	--

* chronic depression

Table 2. CSF prostaglandins in neurological controls

patients	PGF_2	PG ng/ml PGE	PGD_2	PGA
manic depression	3.1	3.2	--	--
myasthenia gravis	28	8.0	11	--
	11	5.6	--	--
Guillain Barré	20	4.9	--	--
CNS manisfestation of lyme arthritis	1.8	4.1	--	--
CNS lupus	2.0	5.6	--	--

While it is clear that these numbers must be increased, it is interesting that the ratios of PGF: PGE: PGD appear to be substantially different (Table 3). In all neurological diseases examined PGF_2 levels were higher than PGE levels. In CNS lupus and Lyme arthritis PGE was higher than PGF_{2alpha}. MS was the only disease with consistently measurable PGD_2.

Table 3. CSF prostaglandin ratios

	PGF_2: PGE: PGD_2
MS	3:1:2
MG	6:2:1
GB	4:1:0
depression	1:1:0
lyme arthritis	1:2:0
CNS lupus	1:3:0

DISCUSSION

That prostaglandins are formed by CNS tissue has been established clearly. The basic principles governing stimulation, synthesis and release of PGs in nonneural tissue also apply to synthesis in the CNS (1,5). Only PGF_{2alpha}, PGE and small amounts of PGI were detectable in human brain homogenates. Thromboxane was undetectable in normal human brain (50). However, measurements must be considered relative as exogenous precursor fatty acid does not appear to equilibrate with endogenous pools. Thus, there is a low conversion of tritiated arachidonate into PGs by brain homogenates (1,5).

The presence of large amounts of PGD_2 in all MS CSF examined may be potentially important. PGD_2 has been shown by a number of investigators to be the predominant PG in rodent brain (18,51). Synthesis of PGD_2 was found to be exceedingly low in human brain homogenates and absent in CSF

(17). It's presence in MS CSF may therefore be related to changes induced by the disease.

It is possible that PGD may be produced by MS specific inflammatory cells within the CNS. PGD has been reported to be synthesized by human platelets and mast cells (11). Preliminary evidence indicates PGD_2 may also be produced by human astrocytes (Dore-Duffy, unpublished data). Astrogliosis associated with demyelination may result in production of large quantities of PGD_2.

The potential effect of PGD_2 in the CNS of MS patients can be speculative at best. Both PGD_2 and D_3 have been shown to inhibit sympathetic nerve transmission at the nictitating membrane of the cat (52,53), apparently via presynaptic inhibition of norepinephorine release (52). In contrast PGE_2 has been shown to enhance the effects of nerve stimulation and exogenously added norepinephrine. Indomethacin, but not other nonsteroidal anti-inflammatory agents, antagonized the ability of PGE to enhance neurotransmission (52). Such opposing effects of PGE and PGD have not been seen at other synapses (54,55) at the majority of synapses tested PGE depressed transmitter release and PGD_2 had either no effect or caused enhancement (56).

In the CNS, rat studies indicated that PGE reduced the electrically stimulated release of noradrenalin and dopamine from cerebral cortex (57). Variable results have been seen in other sections of rat brain and in the cerebral cortex of other animals (11). Exogenously administered PGD_2, although the major prostaglandin produced by rodent CNS tissue had no effect. However, as with most prostaglandin studies, one must be careful to separate pharmacologic effects from the effects of endogenously synthesized PGs.

That PGD appears to be present in MS CSF, and that it has been shown to be involved in neurotransmission (11) temperature regulation (58,59) and inflammation (60-62) certainly justify further study.

REFERENCES

1. L.S. Wolf and F. Coceani. The role of prostaglandins in the central nervous system. Ann. Rev. Physiol. 41:669 (1979).
2. W.G..Clark and J.M. Lipton. Changes in body temperature after administration of acetylcholine histamine, morphine, prostaglandins and related agents. Neurosci. Biobehav. Rev. 9:479 (1985).
3. H.A. Gross, D.L. Dunner, D. Lafleur, H.L. Meltzer, H.L. Muhlbauer and R.R. Fieve. Prostaglandins. A review of neurophysiology and psychiatric implications. Arch. Gen. Psychiatry. 34:1189 (1977).
4. O.E. Scaramuzzi, C.A. Baile and J. Mayer. Prostaglandins and food intake of rats. Experientia. 27:256 (1971).
5. F. Coceani. Prostaglandins and the central nervous system. Arch. Int. Med. 133:119 (1974).
6. B. Samuelsson. Biosynthesis of prostaglandins. Fed. Proc. 31:1442 (1972).
7. H. Kunze and W. Vogat. Significance of phospholipase A_2 for prostaglandin formation. Ann. NY Acad. Sci. 180:122 (1971).
8. S. Rittenhouse-Simmons. Production of diglyceride from phosphatidylinositol in activated platelets. J. Clin. Invest. 63:580 (1979).
9. R.L. Bell, D.A. Kennerly, N. Stanford and P. Majerus. Diglyceride lipase: a pathway for arachidonic acid from human platelets. Proc. Nat. Acad. Sci. (USA). 76:3238 (1979).

10. P.W. Ramwell. The action of cerebrospinal fluid on the frog rectus abdominus muscle and other isolated tissue preparations. J. Physiol.(London). 170:21 (1964).
11. L.S.Wolfe. Eicosanoids: prostaglandins, thromboxanes, leukotrienes and other derivatives of carbon-20 unsaturated fatty acids. J. Neurochem. 38:1 (1982).
12. E. Bosisio, C. Galli, G. Galli, S. Nicosia, C. Spagnuolo and L. Tosi. Correlation between release of free arachidonic acid and prostaglandin formation in brain cortex and cerebellum. Prostaglandins. 11: 773 (1976).
13. J. Marion and L.S. Wolfe. Increase in vivo of unesterfied fatty acids, prostaglandin F_2 but not thromboxane in rat brain during drug induced convulsions. Prostaglandins. 16:99 (1978).
14. D. Egg, M. Herold, E. Rumpl and R. Gunther. Prostaglandin F_2 levels in human cerebrospinal fluid in normal and pathological conditions. J. Neurol. 222:239 (1980).
15. L.S. Wolfe and O. Mamer. Measurement of prostaglandin F_2 levels in human cerebrospinal fluid in normal and pathological conditions. Prostaglandins. 9:183 (1975).
16. S.D. Romero, D. Chyatte, D.E. Byer, J.C. Romero and T.L. Yaksh. Measurement of prostaglandins in the cerebrospinal fluid in cat, dog and man. J. Neurochem. 43:1642 (1984).
17. M.S. Abdel-Halim, J. Ekstedt and E. Anggard. Determination of prostaglandin F_2 in cerebrospinal fluid. Prostaglandin. 17:405 (1979).
18. M.S. Abdel-Halim, M. Hamburg, B. Sjoquist and E. Anggard. Identification of prostaglandin D_2 as a major prostaglandin in homogenates of rat brain. Prostaglandins. 14:633 (1977).
19. C.K. Ellis, R.K. Narayan and E.F. Ellis. GC/MS analysis of prostaglandins in ventricular cerebrospinal fluid from head injured humans. Prostaglandins and Medicine. 7:157 (1981).
20. C.Y. Hsu, P.V. Halushka, E.L. Hogan, N.L. Banik, W.A. Lee and P.L. Perot. Alteration of thromboxane and prostacyclin levels in experimental spinal cord injury. Neurol. 35:1003 (1985).
21. M. Linnoila, A.R. Whorton, D.R. Rubinow, R.W. Cowdry, P.T. Ninan and R.N. Waters. CSF prostaglandin levels in depressed and schizophrenic patients. Arch. Gen. Psychiatry. 40:405 (1983).
22. I. Tamai, T. Takei, K. Maekawa and H. Ohta. Prostaglandin F_2 concentrations in the cerebrospinal fluid of children with febrile convulsions, epilepsy and meningitis. Brain Develop. 5:357 (1983).
23. C.A. Harbey, A.S. Milton and D.W. Straughan. Prostaglandin E levels in cerebrospinal fluid of rabbits and the effects of bacterial pyrogen and antipyretic drugs. J. Physiol.(Lond.). 248:26 (1975).
24. F. Coceani, I. Bishai, C.A. Dinarello and F.A. Fitzpatrick. Prostaglandin E_2 and thromboxane B_2 in cerebrospinal fluid afebrile and febrile cat. Am. Physiol. Soc. 83:785 (1983).
25. V.S. Kostic, B.M. Djuricic and B.B. Mrsuljia. Cerebrospinal fluid prostaglandin F_2 in stroke patients: no relationship to the degree of neurological deficit. Eur. Neurol. 23:291 (1984).
26. R.R. Baena, P. Gaetani, G. Folco, V. Branzoli and P. Paoletti. Cisternal and lumbar CSF concentration of arachidonate metabolites in vasospasm following subarachnoid hemorrhage from ruptured aneurysm: biochemical and clinical considerations. Surg. Neurol. 24:428 (1985).
27. C. Patrano and E. LaTorre. Prostaglandin F_2 in cerebrospinal fluid in a patient with subarachnoid hemorrhage. Clin. Res. 23:346 (1974).
28. I. Kirby, J. Morley, J.R. Ponsford and W.I. McDonald. Defective PGE reactivity in leukocytes of multiple sclerosis patients. Prostaglandin. 11:621 (1976).
29. E.W. Willoughby, B. Dupont and R.A. Good. Prostaglandin effect on lymphokine production in multiple sclerosis. Ann. Neurol. 5:391 (1979).

30. J.S. Goodwin and R.P. Messner. Prostaglandin E inhibition of mitogen stimulation in patients with multiple sclerosis. Prostaglandins. 15:281 (1978).
31. B.P. Barna, H. Goren, B.S. Jacobs, L. Conomy and S.D. Doedhar. Analysis of leukocyte adherence to measles infected cells in multiple sclerosis. Ann. Neurol. 9:28 (1981).
32. P. Dore-Duffy, R.B. Zurier, J.O. Donaldson, S.S. Nystrom, M.V. Viola, B. Rothman and H.G. Thompson. Lymphocyte adherence in multiple sclerosis. Neurology. 29:232 (1979).
33. N.L. Levy, P.S. Aubach and E.C. Hayes. A blood test for multiple sclerosis based in the adherence of lymphocytes to measles infected cells. N. Engl. J. Med. 294:1423 (1976).
34. P. Dore-Duffy and R.B. Zurier. Lymphocyte adherence in multiple sclerosis: Lack of virus specificity. Cell. Immunol. 77:215 (1983).
35. R.B. Zurier, P. Dore-Duffy and M.V. Viola. Adherence of human peripheral blood lymphocytes to measles-infected cells. Enhancement by prostaglandin E. N. Engl. J. Med. 296:1443 (1977).
36. P. Dore-Duffy and R.B. Zurier. Lymphocyte adherence in multiple sclerosis. Effects of aspirin. J. Clin. Invest. 63:154 (1979).
37. P. Dore-Duffy and R.B. Zurier. Lymphocyte adherence in multiple sclerosis. Role of monocytes and increased sensitivity of MS lymphocytes to prostaglandin E. Clin. Immunol. Immunopathol. 19:303 (1981).
38. P. Dore-Duffy, S.-Y. Ho and M. Longo. The role of prostaglandins in altered leukocyte function in MS. Springer Seminar Immunopathol. 8: 305 (1985).
39. J.E. Merrill, L.W. Myers and G.W. Ellison. Regulation of natural killer cell cytotoxicity by prostaglandin E in the peripheral blood and cerebrospinal fluid of patients with multiple sclerosis and other neurological diseases. II. Effect of exogenous PGE on spontaneous and interferon induced NK. J. Neuroimmunol. 4:238 (1983).
40. S.J. Hauser, K.A. Ault, M.J. Levin, M.R. Garouay and H.L. Weiner. Natural killer cell activity in multiple sclerosis. J. Immunol. 127: 1114 (1981).
41. J.E. Merrill, M. Jondal, J. Seely, M. Ullberg and A. Siden. Decreased NK killing in patients with multiple sclerosis. An analysis on the level of the single effector cell from peripheral blood and cerebrospinal fluid in relation to the activity of the disease. Clin. Exp. Immunol. 47:419 (1982).
42. J.E. Merrill, A. Scott, L. Myers and G. Ellison. Cytotoxic activity of peripheral blood and cerebrospinal fluid lymphocytes from patients with multiple sclerosis and other neurological diseases. Analysis at the single cell level using morphological and surface marker phenotype criteria. J. Neuroimmunol. 3:123 (1982).
43. J.E. Merrill, R.H. Gerner, L.W. Myers and G.W. Ellison. Regulation of natural killer cell cytotoxicity by prostaglandin E in the peripheral blood and cerebrospinal fluid of patients with multiple sclerosis and other neurologcial diseases. I. Association between amount of prostaglandin produced, natural killer and endogenous interferon. J. Neuroimmunol. 4:223 (1983).
44. P. Dore-Duffy, H.-H. Huo and M.M. Dowling. Role of prostaglandin E in modulation of T-cell differentiation antigens: implication for multiple sclerosis. Neurology (NY). 33:142 (1983).
45. J. Booss, M.M. Esiri, W.W. Tourtellotte and D. Mason. Immunohistological analysis of T lymphocyte subsets in the central nervous system in chronic progressive multiple sclerosis. J. Neurol. Sci. 62:219 (1983).
46. P. Dore-Duffy, S.-Y. Ho and M. Longo. The role of prostaglandins in altered leukocyte function in MS. Springer Seminar Immunopathol. 8: 305 (1985).

47. P. Dore-Duffy, M. Longo, M. Leuze and J.O. Donaldson. Prostaglandin synthesis in multiple sclerosis. Correlation to disease activity. Neurol. (In press). (1986).
48. C. Bolton, A.M. Turner and J.L. Turk. Prostaglandin levels in cerebrospinal fluid from multiple sclerosis patients in remission and relapse. J. Neuroimmunol. 6:151 (1984).
49. D. Egg, M. Herald, E. Rumpl and R. Gunther. Prostaglandin F_2 levels in human cerebrospinal fluid in normal and pathological conditions. J. Neurol. 222:239 (1980).
50. M.S. Abdel-Halim, H. Von Holst, B. Myerson, C. Sachs and E. Anggard. Prostaglandin profiles in tissue and blood vessels from human brain. J. Neurochem. 34:1331 (1980).
51. F.F. Sun, J.P. Chapman and J.C. McGuire. Metabolism of prostaglandin endoperoxide in animal tissue. Prostaglandins. 14:1055 (1977).
52. D.P. Hemker and J.W. Aiken. Actions of indomethacin and prostaglandins E_2 and D_2 on nerve transmission in the nictitating membrane of the cat. Prostaglandins. 22:599.
53. D.P. Hemker and J.W. Aiken. Modulation of autonomic neurotransmission by PGD_2: comparison with effects of other prostaglandins in anesthetized cats. Prostaglandins. 20:321.
54. P. Hedquist, L. Stjarne and H. Wennmalm. Facilitation of sympathetic nerve transmission in the cat spleen after inhibition of prostaglandin synthesis. Acta. Physiol. Scand. 83:430 (1971).
55. D.V. Malik. Prostaglandin modulation of adrenergic nervous system. Fed. Proc. 37:203 (1978).
56. J.R. Bedwani and S.E. Hill. Facilitation of sympathetic neurotransmission in the rat anoccygeus muscle by prostaglandins D_2 and F_2. Br. J. Pharmacol. 69:609 (1980).
57. S. Bergstrom, L.O. Farnebo and K. Fuxe. Effect of prostaglandin E_2 in central and peripheral catecholamine neurons. Eur. J. Pharmacol. 21:362 (1973).
58. R. Ueno, S. Narumiya, T. Ogorochi, T. Nakayama, Y. Ishikawa and O. Hayaishi. Role of prostaglandin D_2 in the hypothermia of rats caused by bacterial lipopolysaccharide. Proc. Nat. Acad. Sci.(USA). 79:6093 (1982).
59. D.J. Heavey, P. Lumley, S.E. Barrow, M.B. Murphy, P.P.A. Humphrey and C.T. Dollery. Effects of intravenous infusions of PGD_2 in man. Prostaglandins. 28:755 (1984).
60. S.W. Burchiel and A.D. Bankhurst. PGI_2 and PGD_2 effects on cyclic AMP and human T-cell mitogenesis. Prostaglandins and Medicine. 3:315 (1979).
61. R.J. Flower, E.A. Harvey and W.P. Kingston. Inflammatory effects of prostaglandin D_2 in rat and human skin. Br. J. Pharmacol. 56:229 (1976).
62. R.A. Lewis, N.A. Soter, P.T. Diamond, K.F. Austen, J.A. Oates and L.J. Roberts. Prostaglandin D_2 generation after activation of rat and human mast cells with anti-IgE. J. Immunol. 129:1627 (1982).

MYELIN CONTAINING MACROPHAGES/MICROGLIA ARE PRESENT IN NORMAL APPEARING WHITE MATTER IN MULTIPLE SCLEROSIS

N. Groome*, G. Hayes, M.N. Woodroofe, P. Glynn and M.L. Cuzner

Multiple Sclerosis Society Laboratory, Department of Neurochemistry, Institute of Neurology, 33 John's Mews London WC1N
*Department of Biology, Oxford Polytechnic Oxford, U.K.

Demyelinating plaques in post mortem multiple sclerosis (MS) brain are characterized by a hypercellular zone at the advancing edge of myelin loss, which consists predominantly of macrophages (Prineas and Connell, 1978). Macrophages, the most likely primary agents of myelin phagocytosis and its subsequent degradation by proteases and phospholipases, also function as accessory cells in lymphocyte activation and could have a role in the induction stage of inflammatory demyelination. In an electron microscopic study of MS tissue myelin-containing macrophages were found in white matter beyond the lesion edge, in which the number and morphology of myelin sheaths appeared normal (Prineas et al., 1984). In the present study we have examined the immunocytochemical characteristics of macrophages/microglia in white matter, both near and far from established lesions, with a pan macrophage marker and two anti basic protein (BP) monoclonal antibodies, one reacting with the intact molecule and the other requiring cleavage of the phenylalanine-phenylalanine band at position 88 (Groome et al., 1985).

MATERIALS AND METHODS

CNS tissue

Brain and spinal cord from 4 MS cases with post-mortem times of less than 24 h were obtained at autopsy. In three cases of long-standing MS macroscopic plaques were distributed throughout the brain while in one acute case of only 2 years duration active demyelination was widespread. Control brain samples were obtained from 5 cases of coronary heart disease, with similar post mortem times.

Blocks of normal appearing white matter (NAWM) and macroscopic plaques were mounted in OCT embedding medium (R.A.Lamb, London) on a cork disc and snap-frozen in isopentane cooled on liquid nitrogen. Blocks were sectioned in a Slee cryostat (Slee, London) at -20°C and 10 µm sections collected on gelatin-coated slides. Sections were stained for routine histology by both haematoxylin and eosin (H & E) and Oil Red O neutral lipid stain, for estimation of cellular infiltration and demyelination respectively.

Immunocytochemistry

Sections were fixed in acetone at 4°C for 10 min prior to incubation with monoclonal antibodies and were immunostained, following the Vector Laboratories "ABC" avidin-biotin peroxidase method (Seralab Ltd., Crawley, U.K.). Sections were counterstained with haematoxylin, dehydrated and mounted in DPX (R.A. Lamb, London). Slides were examined on a Leitz dialux microscope fitted with interference contrast optics. The relative distribution of positively stained cells in plaque border and normal appearing white matter was examined qualitatively.

Three monoclonal antibodies were used in this study - EBM/11 (Dakopatts), a pan macrophage marker, reacts with a cytoplasmic determinant in infiltrating macrophages and in microglia from both normal and pathological brain tissue (Esiri and McGee, 1986). Clone 2 reacts with intact myelin basic protein and peptides containing the amino acid sequence 116-128 and clone 10 recognizes an epitope 79-88 of BP only in the context of its conformation at the C-terminal end of the peptide (Groome et al., 1985). The epitopes specificities of clones 2 and 10 were confirmed by immunoblotting; clone 10 reacted uniquely with MBP 1-88 (Fig.1).

RESULTS

In serial sections of active lesions in which numerous Oil Red O lipid macrophages were present, staining with EBM/11, clone 2 and clone 10 was localized in the hypercellular areas in the centre of small plaques or at the border of chronic progressive ones. The morphology of the EBM/11+ cells at the plaque edge was predominantly macrophage-like, with foamy cytoplasm and a patchy staining pattern. Intact myelin beyond the plaque edge was positively stained with clone 2 (Fig.2a) but clone 10 (Fig.3a) reactivity was largely restricted to cells containing myelin fragments in

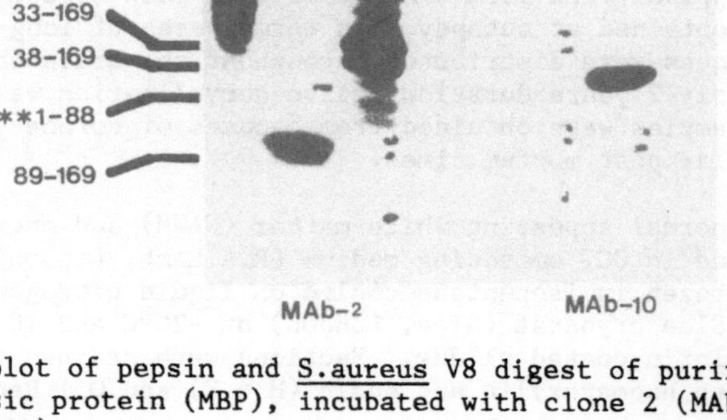

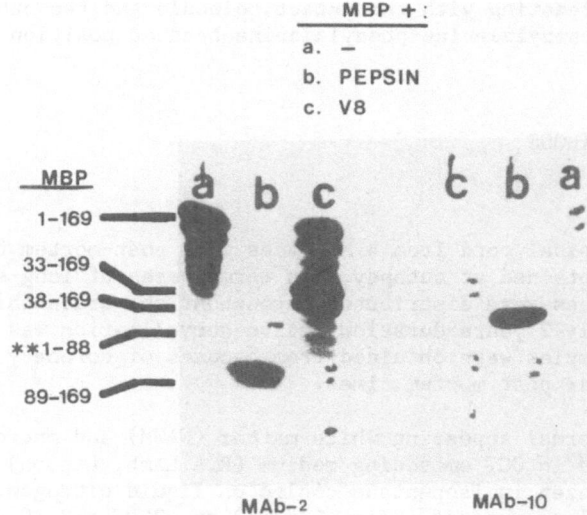

Fig.1. Immunoblot of pepsin and S.aureus V8 digest of purified human myelin basic protein (MBP), incubated with clone 2 (MAb2) and clone 10 (MAb10).

the centre and at the edge of plaques. The clone 2 staining in macrophage-like cells was granular while that seen with clone 10 was more diffuse, which may suggest that in the latter case the myelin is more degraded. Proteolysis of basic protein by cathepsin D, the major acid proteinase of macrophages, results in the appearance of peptide fragments, including ones with Phe-88 as their C-terminal residue, required for clone 10 reactivity.

A systematic examination of white matter blocks taken both near and far from the rim of plaques revealed the presence of clone 2^+ cells, predominantly in the vicinity of blood vessels, but also scattered throughout the parenchyma (Fig.2b). Clone 10 staining was restricted to white matter bordering hypercellular zones of plaque (Fig.3b). Appropriate controls white matter sections contained no positively stained cells in the parenchyma or around blood vessels.

EBM/11^+ cells, readily visualized in MS white matter at a 1:25 dilution of the antibody, were macrophage-like around vessels while cells in the parenchyma distant from lesions appeared to be microglia, with branching processes radiating from the cell antibody (Fig.4a). Microglia in control white matter demonstrated a similar staining pattern at a lower dilution (1:2) of the same antibody (Fig.4b). This difference may reflect microglia/macrophage activation in MS white matter, a complex phenomenon requiring a "blend" of lymphokines and inflammatory stimuli.

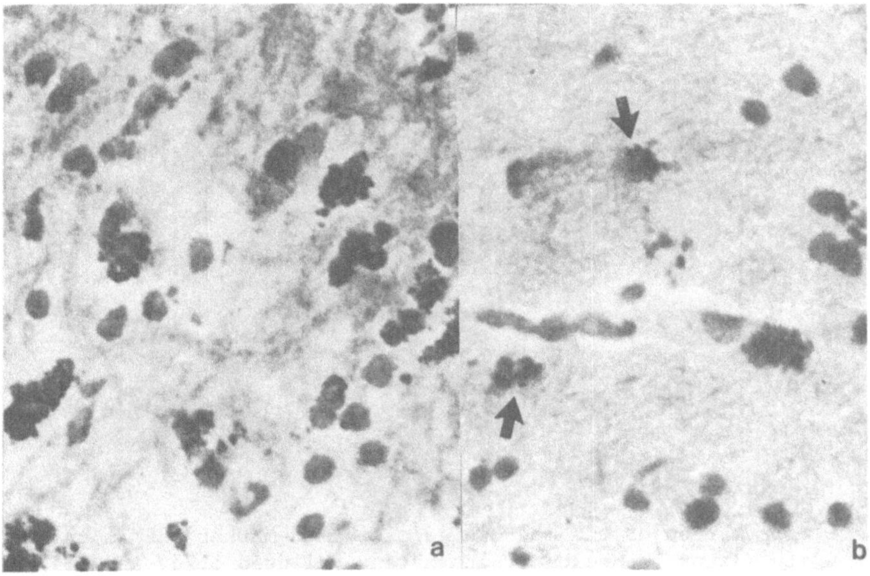

Fig.2. Immunoperoxidase staining of (a) MS plaque edge and (b) normal-appearing white matter with clone 2 (x750). Against a background of intact myelin, granular staining of myelin is seen within cells (arrows). The monoclonal ascites was diluted 1:100.

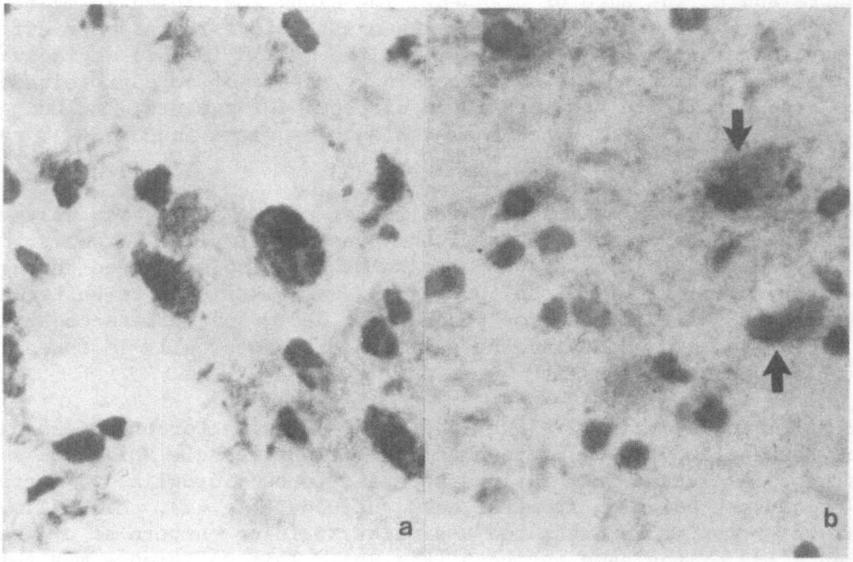

Fig.3. Immunoperoxidase staining of (a) MS plaque and (b) bordering white matter with clone 10 (x750). Positive staining is largely confined to myelin within macrophage-like cells (arrows). The monoclonal ascites was diluted 1:100.

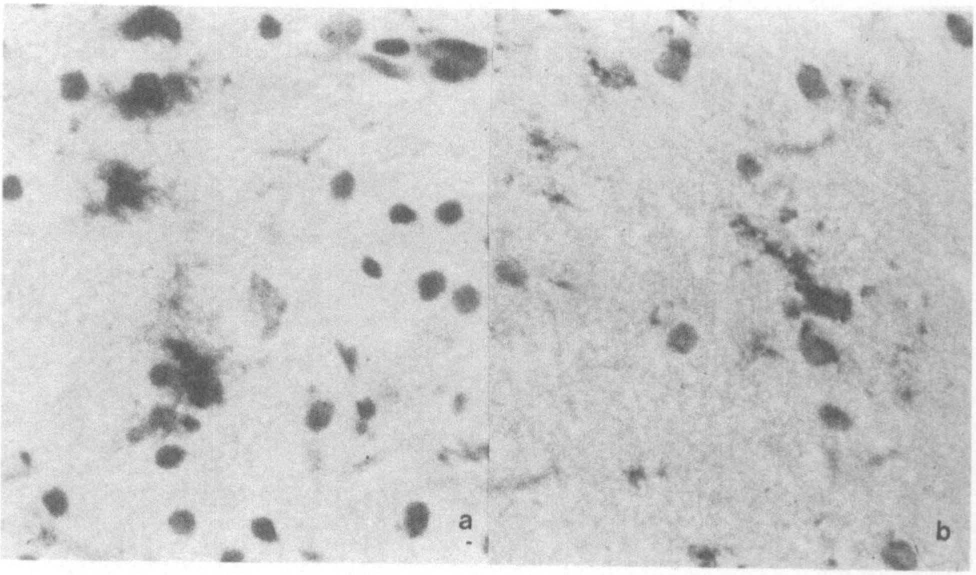

Fig.4. Demonstration of the macrophage/microglia marker, EBM11 in (a) MS white matter (monoclonal supernatant, diluted 1:25) and (b) control white matter (diluted 1:2).

DISCUSSION

The presence of peptides of basic protein within phagocytic cells in MS plaques reinforces the evidence implicating infiltrating macrophages as the agent primarily responsible for myelin destruction at the edge of progressive lesions (Prineas et al., 1984). Our results also confirm previous observations of Prineas and Graham (1981) who found, in an acute case of MS, that extensive infiltration of white matter bordering active plaques by microglia (macrophages) preceded any detectable reduction in staining for myelin basic protein. Although undetectable pathological changes cannot be ruled out, the present evidence that myelin-containing, macrophage-like cells are found in apparently unaffected white matter suggests a primary role for them in the demyelinating process.

Macrophages and their products are important in the induction phases of inflammation as well as performing their effector function (Roitt et al., 1985). Cultured resident rat brain macrophages can be stimulated by lymphokine-containing supernatant to express MHC class II antigen (Ia) on their surface (DuBois et al., 1985) and, using a monoclonal antibody against the cytoplasmic invariant chain of class II MHC, macrophages and microglia in MS plaques and normal-appearing white matter have been demonstrated as potential antigen-presenting cells (Woodroofe et al., 1986).

Thus the macrophage-like cells in the white matter in MS tissue, which have internalised myelin, are suitable candidates for the processing and presentation of autoantigen to sensitized T cells sequestered in the CNS, resulting in plaque formation or extension. As this is a post sensitization event, recruitment of these cells in the white matter may be facilitated by diffusion of lymphokines through the white matter or by T cells sparsely scattered throughout the white matter.

REFERENCES

1. J. Dubois, G.D. Hammond-Tooke and M.L. Cuzner. Expression of MHC antigens in neonate rat primary mixed glial cultures. J. Neuroimmunol. 9:363-377 (1985).
2. M.M. Esiri and J. O'DMcGee. EBM11 is a marker for microglia in brain tissue. J. Clin. Pathol. In press (1986).
3. N. Groome, J. Harland and A. Dawkes. Preparation and properties of monoclonal antibodies to myelin basic protein and its peptides. Neurochem. Int. 7:309-317 (1985).
4. J.W. Prineas and F. Connell. The fine structure of chronically active multiple sclerosis plaques. Neurology. 28 (9, Part 2):68-75 (1978).
5. J.W. Prineas and J.S. Graham. Multiple sclerosis: capping of surface immunoglobulin G on macrophages engaged in myelin breakdown. Ann. Neurol. 10:149-158 (1981).
6. J.W. Prineas, E.E. Kwon, E.-S. Cho and L.R. Sharer. Continual breakdown and regeneration of myelin in progressive multiple sclerosis. Ann. N.Y. Acad. Sci. 436:11-32 (1984).
7. I. Roitt, J. Brostoff and D. Male. Immunology. Churchill Livingstone and Gower Medical Publishing London. pp. 11.7-11.11. (1985).
8. M.N. Woodroofe, A.S. Bellamy, M. Feldman, A.N. Davison and M.L. Cuzner. Immunocytochemical characterization of the immune reaction in the central nervous system in multiple sclerosis. J. Neurol. Sci. In press (1986).

ANALYSIS OF FACTORS INVOLVED IN CELL-MEDIATED DEMYELINATION

Celia F. Brosnan[1,3], Wendy Cammer[2,3], Ellen A. Goldmuntz[3], Harry J. Sacks[1] and William T. Norton[2,3]

Departments of [1]Pathology, [2]Neurology and [3]Neuroscience
Albert Einstein College of Medicine, Bronx, N.Y. 10461

The pathological lesion of multiple sclerosis is characterized by perivascular inflammation, demyelination, sclerosis and edema. The formation of the lesion, which contains T-lymphocytes and macrophages, is generally acknowledged to be related to a cell-mediated immune response. We have used the animal model, experimental autoimmune encephalomyelitis (EAE), to investigate mechanisms by which such an immune response might initiate inflammation, edema and demyelination. We summarize here our recent studies on the degradation of myelin by macrophages and the role of complement in the process, and the involvment of catecholamines in the induction of edema and inflammation.

POSSIBLE ROLE OF PROTEINASES SECRETED BY ACTIVATED MACROPHAGES

A rather large body of evidence has accumulated over the years that implicates both macrophages and elevated proteinase activity in the process of inflammatory demyelination. Macrophages are consistently found in perivascular cuffs in both MS and EAR (1-8), and, in the latter condition, can sometimes be seen penetrating between myelin lamellae (4,6). Additional observations suggest that the macrophages can damage nearby myelin sheaths without actually contacting them. The supporting evidence in EAE is the occurrence of splits between the myelin lamellae and extensive vesicular disruption of myelin sheaths in the proximity of macrophages (6). Rather similar observations in MS are the net-like disruptions of the myelin sheaths in acute MS, the apparent melting away of myelin in contact with macrophages in an active plaque, and the presence of myelin debris in the extracellular space as well as in macrophages (8). In MS there is some evidence for neutral proteinases, including macrophage proteinase, in brain and of basic protein fragments in the CSF (11-13). In EAE, elevated neutral proteinase activities are found within lesions (14-15). Marion Smith and her colleagues have presented evidence that the increased proteinase activities in EAE can be traced to invading lymphocytes and macrophages (14) and that the proteinase activity in EAE spinal cords is most elevated at pH's close to neutrality (16).

These observations assumed more coherence with the demonstration some years ago that stimulated macrophages secreted several neutral proteinases, including plasminogen activator (17). This discovery led to our hypothesis that inflammatory demyelination could be initiated by macrophage secretion products (18). We proposed that infiltrating lymphocytes "called in" and activated macrophages which in turn secreted plasminogen activator. Since the blood-brain barrier is destroyed in the area of the inflammatory reaction, serum proteins, including plasminogen, are present in the CNS parenchyma. The plasminogen activator catalyses the formation of the neutral proteinase, plasmin, providing for amplification of proteolytic activity. Plasmin then degrades myelin proteins.

We showed that macrophage-secreted enzymes can degrade the basic protein of lyophilized myelin in vitro, and that the degradation is considerably enhanced by the addition of plasminogen (18), thus indicating our hypothesis is feasible. Cuzner et al. (19) have also shown that macrophage proteinases can degrade basic protein in myelin neutral pH. These results led to the further proposal that the specificity of the macrophage proteinases lay in the extreme sensitivity of basic protein to proteolytic degradation (20,21). Some support for this is the evidence that basic protein is selectively depleted at the margins of MS plaques (22).

POSSIBLE ROLE OF COMPLEMENT IN THE POTENTIATION OF PROTEINASE ACTIVITY

Although macrophage secretion products alone, or together with plasminogen, could degrade myelin proteins in lyophilized myelin, the were ineffective when either freshly isolated myelin or fresh white matter was used as a substrate. We reasoned that some additional factor was needed to disrupt the myelin structure making it accessible to the proteinases. Two possible candidates for such factors were phospholipases and complement, both known to be secreted by macrophages under appropriate conditions (reviewed in 23). The addition of phospholipase or lysolecithin to plasmin, or to macrophage conditioned media plus plasminogen, potentiated the degradation of basic protein in fresh bovine myelin from none to 35-90% (23).

Perhaps more significant was the finding that pretreatment of fresh myelin with complement was also effective in potentiating the action of plasmin, or of macrophage conditioned media plus plasminogen. Complement depleted (heated) sera, C_3-deficient sera or C_4-deficient sera were ineffective (23). These data indicated that complement, activated by the classical pathway, could render the basic protein in fresh myelin vulnerable to proteolytic enzymes.

The properties and availability of complement strongly support its hypothetical role in demyelination. Once activation of complement has taken place, there is generation of the C5b-9 membrane-attack complex, which can form pores in membranes. Furthermore, myelin is known to be the only brain fraction that can activate complement in the absence of antibody or immune complexes (24,25), and this activation, by means of the classical pathway, results in the incorporation of the membrane-attack complex into the myelin (26,27).

There is some evidence for a role of complement in inflammatory demyelination in vivo. In guinea pigs decomplemented with cobra venom factor EAE is delayed and the symptoms attenuated (28,29). While this finding is commonly interpreted to show a role for antibody in EAE, an alternative explanation could involve a direct alteration of myelin by complement. The finding of a subnormal amount of complement component C_9 in the CSF of multiple sclerosis patients has suggested that the complement membrane attack complex might be involved in the damage to myelin that occurs in this disease (30). However, the hypothetical role for complement as a potentiator of the action of proteinases in vivo should be distinguished from its role in antibody-mediated complement-dependent demyelination in vitro (31,32) and from the presumably similar role of complement in augmenting antibody-mediated demyelination in vivo (33,34). The present hypotheses does not require a role for antibody. Since complement and plasminogen could enter the CNS through lesions in the blood brain-barrier, we believe that the combined effects of complement, plasminogen and macrophage-secreted plasminogen activator provide an attractive hypothetical mechanism for the initiation of demyelination in inflammatory lesions.

ROLE OF FACTORS INVOLVED IN THE BREAKDOWN OF THE BLOOD-BRAIN-BARRIER

It is clear that alteration in BBB permeability is an early and significant event in EAE. Several studies have shown that clinical signs of disease correlate more closely with the extent of edema in the spinal cord than with histological evidence of inflammation (35,37). The factors involved in this alteration of BBB function are not well understood, but in the mouse the histamine sensitizing factor of B. pertussis appears to play a major role (36). Furthermore, in the Lewis rat EAE can be reactivated by resensitizing the animal with MBP plus CFA plus B. pertussis (38). In both the mouse model and the reactivated rat model (but not in the primary clinical episode in the rat) antagonists of histamine can suppress clinical signs of disease, thus implicating this vasoactive amine in the disease process. In addition to a role in edema, a possible requirement for vasoactive amines in the development of a delayed-type hypersensitivity (DTH) reaction has been proposed (39). In DTH reactions the augmenting inflammatory response is known to play a major role in the initiation of tissue damage. This augmenting inflammatory response consists primarily of cells of the monocyte-macrophage lineage that do not normally leave the blood. Gershon et al. (39) have suggested that vasoactive amines cause constriction of the endothelial cells thus facilitating the egress of the bone marrow derived cells from the circulation.

If this hypothesis is correct than one would predict that only the specifically sensitized T-cell would elicit lymphokine production that results in vasoconstriction, edema, and a non-specific augmentation of the immune response. Linked together with this hypothesis is the concept that all activated T-cells cross the endothelium into the parenchyma, and there is preliminary evidence from work with the T-cell lines that this is indeed the case. Thus, there would be two levels at which the response could be blocked: the receptor that mediates perivascular transit of activated T-cells, and the action of lymphokines on the vascular endothelium. Much interest is currently focused on the role of Ia as the receptor that participates in perivascular transit of activated T-cells (40,41), and our work has come to focus on the vascular response.

ROLE OF CATECHOLAMINES IN THE INITIATION OF EDEMA AND INFLAMMATION

Evidence for the involvment of the alpha$_1$-adrenergic receptor

Preliminary studies indicated that antagonists of histamine and serotonin could not significantly suppress the development of clinical signs of EAE in the Lewis rat, and we focused our attention on the catecholamines.

In most of the vasculature norepinephrine and epinephrine mediate vasoconstriction via the alpha-receptor and vasodilation via the beta-receptor. We, therefore tested the ability of antagonists of alpha and beta adrenergic receptors to modulate the expression of EAE in the Lewis rat. The results indicated that significant suppression of EAE could be obtained by treatment with prazosin, a specific alpha$_1$-adrenoceptor antagonist (42). This effect is specific for the $alpha_1$-receptor since treatment with the antagonists yohimbine ($alpha_2$) or propranolol (beta) exacerbated the disease, whereas phenoxybenzamine (mixed $alpha_1$ and $alpha_2$) had some suppressive activity. Since the presynaptic $alpha_2$-adrenoceptor exerts a negative feedback control on the release of norepinephrine, antagonism of this receptor could lead to unrestrained release of NE, which could account for the exacerbation of the disease observed in animals treated with yohimbine.

Effect of antagonism of the $alpha_1$-receptor on edema and inflammation

Ongoing studies have shown that treatment with prazosin (2 mg twice a day) delays and reduces perivascular inflammation, reduces leakage of serum proteins into the CNS, and delays increased immunohistochemical staining of glial fibrillary acidic protein in astrocytes. Prazosin also suppresses clinical signs of EAE in animals passively sensitized with activated lymphocytes. Prazosin, therefore, is able to suppress the two most significant correlates of EAE in Lewis rats: cellular infiltration and edema (42-44). Since perivascular cellular infiltration and leakage of serum proteins into the CNS are features of the early lesion in acute MS, the results in rats suggest that prazosin may have potential benefit for patients with MS.

Catecholamines modulate a diverse array of cellular functions through interaction with cell surface receptors, and we have considered two, not necessarily exclusive, sites of action to account for the suppressive effect of prazosin: the immune response and the vasculature. In order to explore the mechanism of action of prazosin further we have now tested the effect of prazosin on the early, inductive phase and on the late, effector phase of the disease. Additional experiments have also explored the effect of lymphocyte responses to mitogen and antigen _in vitro_.

The results of these studies have shown that treatment with prazosin has no effect on the early, inductive phase of EAE but can still significantly suppress disease when treatment is begun at the time on onset of early clinical signs (day 10). Leakage of serum proteins and perivascular inflammation were also suppressed in these animals, particularly in the early stages of the acute response. Analyses of lymphocyte response from treated animals, and from sensitized animals incubated in the presence of prazosin _in vitro_ showed that prazosin had no effect on lymphocyte responses to antigen or mitogen. These results support the hypothesis that prazosin suppresses EAE through a direct vascular effect although they do not preclude an immunologic component to its mechanism of action.

This drug, therefore, provides us with a tool with which to explore the factors involved in the development of edema. The use of prazosin will allow us to dissect which factors correlate with clinical disease, and at which level they can be blocked.

Effect of antagonism of the alpha-1receptor on astrocyte activation

Since prazosin also delays astrocytic reactivity this drug allows us to explore the factors involved in enhanced immunohistochemical expression of glial fibrillary acid protein (GFAP) in EAE.

Reactive astrocytes are now frequently detected by their strong immunocytochemical staining for glial fibrillary acidic protein (GFAP). The terms fibrous gliosis or reactive astrocytosis are applied rather loosely to a spectrum of glial reactions that range from enhanced GFAP staining of enlarged fibrous astrocytes (hypertrophy) to the full-blown glial scar with a greatly increased number of fibrous astrocytes (hyperplasia).

Intense fibrous astrocytosis is prominent in multiple sclerosis, and reactive astrocytes can constitute the major cell type in MS plaques (8). Such glial scars stains intensely for GFAP, and biochemical studies have confirmed that there are large amounts of this protein in gliotic tissue (45,46). There is much speculation, but little evidence, that the mat of reactive astrocytes in glial scars inhibits the regeneration of axons in wounds and remyelination in plaques.

Reactive gliosis of this extreme nature is not seen in acute EAE but is present in chronic models in the guinea pig and mouse (47,48) in which plaque formation occurs. A few years ago, however, Smith et al. (49) showed that in Lewis rats sensitized to develop EAE, enhanced immunocytochemical staining for GFAP was evident early in the course of the disease (10-12 dpi). This glial reaction was widespread in both grey and white matter of the spinal cord, was morphologically unrelated to the inflammatory perivascular lesions, and continued to persist after the animals recovered from the clinical signs of disease. The onset of enhanced staining correlated with the initiation of inflammation and with the onset of disease. These investigators noted, however, that there was no apparent increase in GFAP content in the spinal cords of these animals.

We have confirmed and extended these results and shown that there was no increase in GFAP synthesis in spinal cord slices when there was a dramatic increase in immunostaining, nor was there an increase in GFAP content in cytoskeletal fractions of spinal cords from EAE animals. Prazosin treatment delayed this astrocyte reaction, but at 15 dpi the GFAP staining in the prazosin-treated animals was similar to that in the saline-treated animals. GFAP staining was also reduced in prazosin-treated animals with passively-transferred disease (43).

The prazosin treatment permits us to dissect the glial reaction more completely. We find that:

1. Enhanced GFAP staining does not correlate with clinical signs; the glial reaction is still intense at 20 dpi when the animals have recovered, and enhanced staining occurs in prazosin-treated animals in the absence of clinical signs.
2. Enhanced staining does not correlate with the amount of edema. At 15 dpi edema in prazosin-treated rats is about one-tenth that in saline-treated rats, yet GFAP staining is similar.
3. The enhanced staining does correlate with the onset of inflammation in either prazosin- or saline-treated animals and both pathological signs persist after animals have recovered clinically.

The mechanisms for induction of reactive astrocytes and proliferative gliosis are not known but many may exist. Astrocytes are known to swell and imbibe plasma proteins in areas of vasogenic edema, induced, for example, by freeze lesions or stab wounds that cause destruction of the BBB (50,51). Serum is known to induce GFAP expression *in vitro* (see ref. 52 for review) and serum factors might be assumed to have the same effect *in vivo*.

In EAE, however, the astrocyte reaction correlated more with the influx of inflammatory cells. A large number of factors have been found that stimulate astrocyte proliferation *in vitro* (for review see ref. 53). Of particular interest here are glial stimulating factor (54) and glial growth promoting factor (55,56), both released by activated lymphocytes, and interleukin-1, released by activated macrophages (57). These are all diffusible proteins and could act at a distance from the inflammatory lesion. These factors, however, have been identified only by their ability to induce proliferation. We have no evidence of astrocyte hyperplasia in

EAE, and, in fact the lack of an increase in GFAP content argues against hyperplasia.

In EAE, therefore, we have a condition where there is a unmistakable increase in immunocytochemical staining for GFAP without an apparent increase in chemically detectable GFAP. We believe the EAE model, together with prazosin suppression, gives us a means to test several hypotheses to explain this phenomenon, as well as other questions of the nature of reactive gliosis.

CONCLUSION

The studies discussed here concern several aspects of the induction and development of the cell-mediated immune lesion in EAE - from the opening of the BBB to the molecular mechanisms that may be responsible for demyelination. Although we recognize that EAE is an imperfect model of multiple sclerosis, the similarity in the pathology of the lesions in these two conditions justifies the use of this model disease to investigate what we believe may be universal mechanisms of inflammatory demyelination.

From our work and that of others, the following sequence of events can be proposed. Sensitized T-cells either invade the CNS and react with antigen (myelin basic protein in the case of EAE) or react with antigen presented by the endothelial cell. Lymphokines are released which amplify the response by "calling in " monocytes and other lymphocytes. Cellular products from one or more of these inflammatory cell types induce the release of vasoactive amines which cause vasospasm leading to an increase in vascular permeability. Our evidence indicates that in EAE vasospasm is maintained by agonists acting on $alpha_1$-adrenergic receptors. The resultant breakdown in the blood-brain barrier leads to vasogenic edema and increased perivascular transit of inflammatory cells. We have some evidence from our studies of passively-transferred disease that the increase of edema slightly precedes the increase in cellular infiltration.

The effector stage of disease, discussed above, leads subsequently to the augmented inflammatory response and a greatly increased infiltration of inflammatory cells. We believe that the activated macrophages are largely responsible for the tissue damage (demyelination) in the lesion, which is initiated by secretion products of these cells.

We have shown this sequence of events can be interferred with at several stages, leading to suppression of various manifestations of the disease. For example, blockade of the $alpha_1$-receptor by prazosin during the inductive phase has no effect, suggesting that it has no effect on the immune response. However, blockade during the effector stage suppresses edema and clinical signs, but only delays inflammation and the astrocyte response (42-44). We are thus able to show that clinical disease correlates better with edema than with inflammation, whereas the astrocyte response is related to inflammation. We have also shown previously that clinical signs can be suppressed by depletion of macrophages (58) and by treatment with proteinase inhibitors (59). In some cases the proteinase inhibitors also suppressed inflammation but in other cases clinical signs were suppressed but the development of inflammatory lesions was unaffected. Thus proteinases may be important not only for initiating demyelination but also for development of the inflammatory response.

It is our hope that detailed studies of the pathogenesis of the model disease, EAE, will lead to logical ways of interfering with the progression of multiple sclerosis.

REFERENCES

1. R.D. Adams. A comparison of the morphology of the human demyelination disease and experimental "allergic" encephalomyelitis. In: "Allergic encephalomyelitis". M.W. Kies, E.C. Alvord, eds. Charles C. Thomas, Springfield, Illinois (1959).
2. C.W.M. Adams. Pathology of multiple sclerosis: progress of the lesion. Br. Med. Bull. 33:15 (1977).
3. J.W. Prineas, E.E. Kwon, E.-S. Cho and L.R. Sharer. Continual breakdown and regeneration of myelin in progressive multiple sclerosis plaques. In: "Multiple sclerosis: Theory and Practice". L.C. Scheinberg, C.S. Raine, eds. N.Y. Acad. Sci. 436:11 (1984).
4. P.W. Lampert. Demyelination and remyelination in experimental allergic encephalomyelitis: further electron microscopic observations. J. Neuropathol. Exp. Neurol. 24:371 (1965).
5. C.S. Raine, D.H. Snyder, M.P. Valsamis and S.H. Stone. Chronic experimental allergic encephalomyelitis in inbred guinea pigs: an ultrastructural study. Lab. Invest. 31:369 (1974).
6. M.C. Dal Canto, H.M. Wisniewski, A.B. Johnson, S.W. Brostoff and C.S. Raine. Vesicular disruption of myelin in autoimmune demyelination. J. Neurol. Sci. 24:313 (1975).
7. H. Lassmann and H.M. Wisniewski. Chronic relapsing EAE. Time course of neurological symptoms and pathology. Acta Neuropath. 43:35 (1978).
8. C.S. Raine. Multiple sclerosis and chronic relapsing EAE: comparative ultrastructural neuropathology. In: "Multiple sclerosis, Pathology, Diagnosis and Management". J.F. Hallpike, C.W.M. Adams, W.W. Tourtellotte, eds. Chapman and Hall, London (1983).
9. D.M. Bowen and A.N. Davison. Macrophages and cathepsin. A activity in multiple sclerosis brain. J. Neurol. Sci. 21:227 (1974).
10. S. Sato, R.H. Quarles and R.O. Brady. Susceptibility of the myelin-associated glycoprotein and basic protein to a neutral protease in highly purified myelin from human and rat brain. J. Neurochem. 39: 97 (1982).
11. S.R. Cohen, R.M. Herndon and G.M. McKhann. Radioimmunoassay of myelin basic protein in spinal fluid: an index of active demyelination. New. Eng. J. Med. 295:1455 (1976).
12. J.N. Whitaker. Myelin encephalitogenic protein fragments in cerebrospinal fluid of persons with multiple sclerosis. Neurology. 27:911 (1977).
13. J.H. Carson, E. Barbarese, P.E. Braun and T.A. McPherson. Components in multiple sclerosis cerebrospinal fluid that are detected by radioimmunoassay for myelin basic protein. Proc. Natl. Acad. Sci. USA. 75:1976 (1978).
14. M.E. Smith, L.M. Sedgewick and J.S. Tagg. Proteolytic enzymes and experimental remyelination in the rat and monkey. J. Neurochem. 34: 965 (1974).
15. K.R. Govindavajan, H.C. Rauch, J. Clausen and E.R. Einstein. Changes in cathepsins B-1 and D, neutral proteinase and 2',3'-cyclic nucleotide-3'-phosphohydrolase activities in monkey brain with experimental allergic encephalomyelitis. J. Neurol. Sci. 23:295 (1974).
16. G.F. Buletza and M.E. Smith. Enzymatic hydrolysis of myelin basic protein and other proteins in central nervous system and lymphoid tissues from normal and demyelinating rats. Biochem. J. 156:627 (1976).
17. J.C. Unkeless, S. Gordon and E. Reich. Secretion of plasminogen activator by stimulated macrophages. J. Exp. Med. 139:834 (1974).
18. W. Cammer, B.R. Bloom, W.T. Norton and S. Gordon. Degradation of basic protein in myelin by neutral proteases secreted by stimulated macrophages: a possible mechanism of inflammatory demyelination. Proc. Natl. Acad. Sci. USA. 75:1554 (1978).

19. M.L. Cuzner, N.L. Banik and A.N. Davison. The metabolism of myelin proteins by macrophages and by lymphocytes. Abs. Int. Soc. Neurochem, Barcelona. (1975).
20. M.E. Smith. A lymph node neutral proteinase acting on myelin basic protein. J. Neurochem. 27:1077 (1976).
21. N.L. Banik. The degradation of myelin basic protein by serum proteinase in experimental allergic encephalomyelitis and control rats. Neurosci. Lett. 11:307 (1979).
22. Y. Itoyama, N.H. Sternberger, H.deF. Webster, R.H. Quarles, S.R. Cohen and E.P. Richardson. Immunocytochemical observations on the distribution of myelin-associated glycoprotein and myelin basic protein in multiple sclerosis lesions. Ann. Neurol. 7:167 (1980).
23. W. Cammer, C.F. Brosnan, C. Basile, B.R. Bloom and W.T. Norton. Complement potentiates the degradation of myelin proteins by plasmin: implications for a mechanism of inflammatory demyelination. Brain Res. 364:91 (1986).
24. C.-J. Cyong, S.S. Witkin, B. Rieger, E. Barbarese, R.A. Good and N.K. Day. Antibody-independent complement activation by myelin via the classical complement pathway. J. Exp. Med. 155:587 (1982).
25. P. Vanguri, C.L. Koski, B. Silverman and M.L. Shin. Complement activation by isolated myelin: activation of the classical pathway in the absence of myelin-specific antibodies. Proc. Natl. Acad. Sci. USA. 79:3290 (1982).
26. W.T. Liu, P. Vanguri and M.L. Shin. Studies on demyelination in vitro: the requirement of membrane attack components of the complement system. J. Immunol. 131:778 (1983).
27. B.A. Silverman, D.F. Carney, C.A. Johnston, P. Vanguri and M.L. Shin. Isolation of membrane attack complex of complement from myelin membranes treated with serum complement. J. Neurochem. 42:1024 (1984).
28. H. Pabst, N.K. Day, H. Gewurz and R.A. Good. Prevention of experimental allergic encephalomyelitis with cobra venom factor. Proc. Soc. Exp. Biol. Med. 136:555 (1971).
29. M.A. Morari and A.P. Dalmasso. Experimental allergic encephalomyelitis in cobra venom factor-treated and C4-deficient guinea pigs. Ann. Neurol. 4:427 (1978).
30. B.P. Morgan, A.K. Campbell and D.A.S. Compston. Terminal component of complement (C_9) in cerebrospinal fluid of patients with multiple sclerosis. Lancet. i:251 (1984).
31. S.H. Appel and M.B. Bornstein. The application of tissue culture to the study of experimental allergic encephalomyelitis. II. Serum factors responsible for demyelination. J. Exp. Med. 119:303 (1964).
32. M.B. Bornstein and C.S. Raine. Multiple sclerosis and EAE: specific demyelination of CNS in culture. Neuropathol. Appl. Neurobiol. 3: 359 (1977).
33. H. Lassman, H. Stemberger, K. Kitz and H.M. Wisniewski. In vivo demyelinating activity of sera from animals with chronic experimental allergic encephalomyelitis. J. Neurol. Sci. 59:123 (1983).
34. K. Saida, T. Saida, M.J. Brown, D.H. Silberberg and A.K. Asbury. Antiserum mediated demyelination in vivo. A sequential study using intraneural injection of experimental allergic neuritis serum. Lab. Invest. 39:449 (1978).
35. S. Leibowitz and L. Kennedy. Cerebral vascular permeability and cellular infiltration in experimental allergic encephalomyelitis. Neurology. 22:859 (1972).
36. D.S. Linthicum and J.A. Frelinger. Acute autoimmune encephalomyelitis in mice. II. Susceptibility is controlled by the combination of H-2 and histamine sensitization genes. J. Exp. Med. 155:31 (1982).

37. N.K. de Rosbo, C.C.A. Bernard, R.D. Simons and P.R. Carnegie. Concomitant detection of changes in myelin basic protein and permeability of blood-spinal cord barrier in acute experimental autoimmune encephalomyelitis by electroimmunoblotting. J. Neuroimmunol. 9:349 (1985).
38. F.J. Waxman, R.K. Bergman and J.J. Munoz. Abrogation of resistance to the reinduction of experimental allergic encephalomyelitis by pertussigen. Cell. Immunol. 72:375 (1982).
39. R.K. Gershon, P.W. Askenase and M.D. Gershon. Requirement for vasoactive amines for production of delayed-type hypersensitivity skin reactions. J. Exp. Med. 142:732 (1975).
40. L. Steinman, J.T. Rosenbaum, S. Friram and H.O. McDevitt. In vivo effects of antibodies to immune response genes products: prevention of experimental allergic encephalitis. Proc. Natl. Acad. Sci. 78:7111 (1981).
41. H. Werkerle. The lesion of acute EAE. Isolation of membrane phenotypes of perivascular infiltrates from encephalitogenic rat brain white matter. Lab. Invest. 51:199 (1984).
42. C.F. Brosnan, E.A. Goldmuntz, W. Cammer, S.M. Factor, B.R. Bloom and W.T. Norton. Prazosin, an $alpha_1$-adrenergic receptor antagonist, suppresses experimental autoimmune encephalomyelitis in the Lewis rat. Proc. Natl. Acad. Sci. USA. 82:5915 (1985).
43. E.A. Goldmuntz, C.F. Brosnan, F.-C. Chiu and W.T. Norton. Astrocytic reactivity and intermediate filament metabolism in EAE: the effect of suppression with prazosin. Brain Res. In press.
44. E.A. Goldmuntz, C.F. Brosnan and W.T. Norton. Prazosin treatment suppresses edema in both acute and passively-transferred EAE in the Lewis rat. Submitted.
45. L.F. Eng, J.J. Vanderhaegen, A. Bignami and B. Gerstl. An acidic protein isolated from fibrous astrocytes. Brain Res. 128:351 (1971).
46. J.E. Goldman, H.H. Schaumburg and W.T. Norton. Isolation and characterization of glial filaments from human brain. J. Cell. Biol. 78: 426 (1978).
47. M.E. Smith, F.P. Somera, K. Swanson and L.F. Eng. Glial fibrillary acidic protein in acute and chronic relapsing experimental allergic encephalomyelitis (EAE). In: "Experimental allergic encephalomyelitis. A useful model for multiple sclerosis". E.C. Alvord, M.W. Kies and A.J. Suckling, eds., Alan R. Liss. Inc., New York. (1984).
48. C. Linington, A.J. Suckling, M.D. Weir and M.L. Cuzner. Changes in the metabolism of glial fibrillary acid protein (GFAP) during chronic relapsing experimental allergic encephalomyelitis in the strain 13 guinea-pig. Neurochem. Int. 6:393 (1984).
49. M.E. Smith, F.P. Somera and L.F. Eng. Immunocytochemical straining for glial fibrillary acidic protein and the metabolism of cytoskeletal proteins in experimental allergic encephalomyelitis. Brain Res. 264:241 (1983).
50. L. Amaducci, K.I. Forno and L.F. Eng. GLial fibrillary acidic protein in cryogenic lesions of the rat brain. Neurosci. Lett. 21:27 (1981).
51. N. Latov, G. Nilaver, E.A. Zimmerman, W.G. Johnson, A.-J. Silverman, R. Defendini and L. Cote. Fibrillary astrocytes proliferate in response to brain injury. Devel. Biol. 72:381 (1979).
52. F.-C. Chiu and J.E. Goldman. Synthesis and turnover of cytoskeletal proteins in cultured astrocytes. J. Neurochem. 42:166 (1984).
53. B. Pettman, G. Labourdette, M. Weibel and M. Sensenbrenner. Glial growth factors. In: "Dynamic properties of glial cells: cellular and molecular aspects". T. Grisar, G. Franck, L. Hertz, W. Norton, M. Sensenbrenner and D. Woodburry, eds. Pergamon Press, Oxford. (1986).

54. A. Fontana, R. Dubs, R. Merchant, S. Balsiger and P.J. Grob. Glia cell stimulating factor (GSF): a new lymphokine. Part 1. Cellular sources and partial purification of murine GSF, role of cytoskeleton and protein synthesis in its production. J. Neuroimmunol. 2:55 (1981).
55. G.E. Lemke and J.P. Brockes. Identification and purification of glial growth factor. J. Neurosci. 4:75 (1984).
56. J.E. Merrill, S. Kutsunai, C. Mohlstrom, F. Hofman, J. Groopman and D.W. Golde. Proliferation of astroglia and oligodendroglia in response to human T cell-derived factors. Science. 223:1428 (1984).
57. D. Giulian and L.B. Lachman. Interleukin-1 stimulation of astroglial proliferation after brain injury. Science. 229:497 (1985).
58. C.F. Brosnan, M.B. Bornstein and B.R. Bloom. The effects of macrophage depletion on the clinical and pathologic expression of EAE. J. Immunol. 126:614 (1981).
59. C.F. Brosnan, W. Cammer, W.T. Norton and B.R. Bloom. Proteinase inhibitors suppress the development of experimental allergic encephalomyelitis. Nature. 285:235 (1980).

ENZYMES IN CEREBROSPINAL FLUID: EVIDENCE FOR A CALCIUM-ACTIVATED NEUTRAL PROTEINASE IN CSF

E.L. Hogan, N.L. Banik, J.M. Goust and D. Lobo

Departments of Neurology and Basic and Clinical Immunology and Microbiology, Medical University of South Carolina Charleston, S.C. 29425

INTRODUCTION

A substantial number of enzymes have been assayed in cerebrospinal fluid and the majority of them have been examined in neurological diseases. Although the CSF enzymes originate from cells indigenous to the CNS, the major source of CSF enzymes is serum because of the greater activities in serum. They probably enter CSF by traversing the blood-CSF barrier and/or blood-brain barrier. Activities of most enzymes in CSF are lower in health than disease leading to attempts to employ CSF enzyme activities as an index of disease. To date, a consistent and clinically significant correlation exists only for lactic dehydrogenase in pyogenic meningitis (Nelson et al., 1975), and beta-glucuronidase in meningeal carcinomatosis and globoid-cell leukodystrophy (Shuttleworth and Allen, 1968).

In the demyelinating diseases, including MS, fragments of cells with myelin morphology have been found in CSF (Herndon et al., 1970). This suggests than an increase in the CSF level of enzymes or other components may be used as a marker for white matter. Thus, increased levels of 2', 3'-cyclic nucleotide 3'-phosphohydrolase (CNPase) activity have been found in CSF of MS patients by some (Sprinkle and McKhann, 1978; Banik et al., 1979; Tsukada et al., 1983). Others did not find any difference in CNPase activity comparing CSF of normal and patients with MS (Raes et al., 1986; Clapshaw et al., 1984). Lymphocytic cells in MS CSF contain increased levels of hydrolases (Cuzner et al., 1979; Riekkenen et al., 1972). Since there is neutral proteinase in CSF (Cuzner et al., 1979) and a calcium-activated neutral proteinase (CANP) in CNS and circulating red cells we examined the CANP activity in normal CSF. CANP is associated with myelin (Sato et al., 1982a; Banik et al., 1985) and we are now studying its activity in the CSF of MS patients as a possible indicator of the disease process and its activity.

ENZYMES IN CSF

The enzymes which have been determined in CSF include energy-yielding enzymes (e.g. glycolytic and mitochondrial); neurotransmitter synthesis enzymes (e.g. acetylcholine esterase (AChE); lysosomal hydrolases (e.g. acid phosphatase, glucuronidase); lipid metabolizing enzymes (e.g. cholesterol ester hydrolase); peptidases and proteinases (e.g. acid and neutral proteinase) and miscellaneous enzymes (e.g. 2', 3'-cyclic nucleotide 3'-phosphohydrolase).

Of the energy yielding enzymes, creatine phosphokinase (CPK) and lactic dehydrogenase (LDH) have been the most widely studied in CSF. LDH has been used for assessing cellular damage in CNS disease with the idea that its release into CSF implicates involvement of the brain and its level in CSF would determine the extent of neurological damage (Viallard et al., 1978). LDH activity has been determined in CSF in many neurological diseases (see review Banik and Hogan, 1983) and found elevated in meningitis, epilepsy, dementia, Huntington's Chorea, Tay Sachs and Niemann-Pick disease. The increased activity was greater in bacterial than viral meningitis. The source of LDH activity may be due to alterations in the blood-CSF or the blood brain barriers or stem from cells in brain or CSF (Table 1).

Enzymes involved in the metabolism of neurotransmitters (e.g. AChE, CHAT) and lipids (e.g. Cholesterol ester hydrolase, cholesterol acyl transferase) have been determined in several different diseases (Johnson and Domino, 1971; Shah and Johnson, 1978) and the changes related to human disorders (see review Banik and Hogan, 1983).

Lysosomal enzymes (e.g. acid phosphatase, glucuronidase and others) in CSF have proved to be a useful indicator of disease in many neurological disorders especially inflammatory and demyelinating diseases. The increased activity found in patient CSF reflects increased permeability in such disease (Arstilla et al., 1973; Cuzner and Davison, 1973, see reviews Banik and Hogan, 1983; Wood, 1982; Table 2).

A number of other enzymes (e.g. 2', 3'-cyclic nucleotide-3'-phosphohydrolase (CNPase), adenosine deaminase, ribonuclease and others) have been examined (see review Banik and Hogan, 1983; Wood, 1982). Since the report of myelin fragments in CSF in MS (Herndon et al., 1970) the activity of CNPase, a myelin marker enzyme has been studied in several laboratories. The initial enthusiasm for CNPase activity as a measure of active demyelination has waned. The increases first reported in MS CSF (Sprinkle and McKhann, 1978; Banik et al., 1979; Tsukada et al., 1983) have not been confirmed by others (Raes et al., 1981; Clapshaw et al., 1984). Still, the demonstration of the CNPase protein in CSF by specific antisera may be useful in determining the release of CNPase into CSF due to insult to myelin or oligodendrocytes (see review by Banik and Hogan, 1983; Wood, 1982) and is now being pursued.

PROTEINASES IN CSF

Activities of proteolytic enzymes and peptidases in the CSF of healthy and neurologically disordered patients were found more than two decades ago (Chapman and Wolf, 1959; Green and Perry, 1963; Riekkinen and Rinne, 1968) and are known to be elevated in CSF of patients with MS and other neurological disorders (see review Banik and Hogan, 1983; Table 2).

Peptidases in CSF are well known. These include leucine aminopeptidase (LAP) gamma-glutamyl peptidase and gamma-glutamyl-transpeptidase (Green and Perry, 1963, Riekkinen and Rinne, 1968; Rinne and Riekkinen, 1968; Swinen, 1967). The substrate specificity of these enzymes is the same as those of brain. Upon fractionation of CSF by DEAE-Sephadex chromatography and starch-gel electrophoresis, Riekkinen and Rinne (1968) found several different peptidase activities. One was a leucine amino peptidase hydrolysing leucyl-beta-napthylamide and its activity was elevated in MS CSF (Rinne and Riekkinen, 1968). Since LAP is associated with

Table 1. Activity of energy-yielding enzymes in CSF[a]

Clinical state	CPK	(IU)	LDH	(IU)	Predominant LDH isoenzymes
control	0.40	(0-1)[b]	10.6	(3-17)	1,2,3
meningitis					
bacterial	40.4	(1.4-256)	316	(31-1498)	5,4,3
viral	6.6	(3-18)	22.9	(14-36)	1,2,3
epilepsy					
generalized	6	(2-14)	17-28		1,2,3
petit mal	5	-	-		-
febrile seizures	5.2	(2-7)	3-21		1,2,3
CNS neoplasia	-		19-55		1,2,3
primary CNS tumors	-		-		-
metastatic to CNS	-		-		-
multiple sclerosis					
acute	-		-		-
chronic	-		-		-
dementia	-		-		-
peripheral neuropathy	-		-		-
carcinomatous neuromyopathy	-		-		-
muscular dystrophy	3.4	(0-12.9)	-		-
cerebellar degeneration	-		-		-
hydrocephalus	-		17-53		1,2,3

[a] One IU equals 1 μmole/min per ml.

[b] Ranges of values recorded are in parenthesis.

Table 2. Proteolytic enzymes in CSF

clinical state	leucine aminopeptidase (µg beta-naphthylamine hydrolyzed/hr per ml)	acid proteinase (µg myelin basic protein hydrolized/hr per ml ± S.D.)	neutral proteinase (µg myelin basic protein hydrolized/hr per ml ± S.D.)
control	1.42 (0.42-2.38)[b]	18.5 ± 28.1	1.55 ± 3.93
cerebral infarction	2.55 (1.08-5.46)	-	-
CNS neoplasia	4.43 (3.06-6.36)	-	-
astrocytoma	3.93	-	-
oligodendroglioma	3.90	-	-
meningioma	6.36	-	-
lymphosarcoma	5.20	-	-
multiple sclerosis			
acute	-	60.2 ± 26.8	6.11 ± 3.34
progressive	-	36.8 ± 29.0	3.87 ± 4.17
other CNS disorders[a]	2.48 (1.23-5.95)	-	-

[a] Amyotrophic lateral sclerosis, Meniere's syndrome and others.

[b] Range of values recorded are in parenthesis.

myelin (Adams et al., 1963; Banik and Davison, 1969; Beck et al., 1968; Marks et al., 1976) this suggests that myelin destruction may be responsible for the increased LAP activity in CSF.

Activities of proteinases have been found in CNS tissues plasma and white cells, in normal as well as in patients with MS and other neurological diseases. The activities of both neutral and acid proteinase are increased in plaque lesions and in inflammatory cells taken from patients with MS (Cuzner et al., 1973, 1975; Hallpike et al., 1970; Hirsch et al., 1976) and it was suspected that CSF proteinases would be increased as well. Studies of MS CSF revealed greatly elevated neutral and acid proteinase activities in CSf of patients with MS while no changes were found in patients with epilepsy and myelopathy (Cuzner et al., 1979; Rinne and Riekkinen, 1968). Fractionation of CSF by DEAE-Sephadex chromatography revealed three distinct proteinases: an acid proteinase at pH 5.0, a neutral proteinase at pH 7.1 and an alkaline proteinase at pH 8.0 (Rinne and Riekkinen, 1968). The molecular weight of these proteinases are 74,000; 39,000 and 27,000 respectively. Both acid and neutral proteinases are sulfhydryl-containing enzymes while the alkaline proteinase is activated by calcium and resembles the calcium-activated neutral proteinase (CANP) of brain and muscle (Guroff, 1962, see review Nixon).

CALCIUM-ACTIVATED NEUTRAL PROTEINASE IN CSF

Although the source of proteinases in CSF is not clearly defined, it is noteworthy that neutral proteinase and calcium-activated neutral proteinase have been found associated with purified myelin (Sato et al., 1982, Banik et al., 1985). The presence of proteinase(s) in myelin may foster autodigestive disease with consequent enzyme release into CSF. This led us to examine the activity of calcium-activated neutral proteinase (CANP) in human CSF.

Assay of enzyme activity: the CANP activity in CSF was determined by two different methods: 1) Incubation of 0.1 ml of CSF in 50 mM Tris HCl buffer, pH 7.6, 2 mM DTT, with and without $CaCl_2$ (5 mM), 15 ug of purified proteolipid protein (PLP) as a substrate and sodium azide (NaN_3) (1 mM) at 37°C for different time intervals; controls included a) CSF incubated in buffer alone and b) CSF incubated in buffer plus EGTA (5 mM). After incubation, the samples were freeze-dried and the proteins separated by SDS-PAGE (sodium dodecyl sulphate polyacrylamide gel electrophoresis). 2) Incubation of CSF (0.24 ml) in 50 mM Tris acetate buffer, pH 7.4, 0.1% mercaptoethanol, 100 mM KCl, 50 ul azocasein (6.0%), NaN_3 (1 mM), with either $CaCl_2$ (5 mM) or EGTA (5 mM) at 37°C for 24 hours. The incubation was stopped with 20% TCA. Hydrolysis of azocasein in the supernatant was determined colorimetrically at 366 nm.

Enzyme activity was also determined in CSF after centrifugation. A few samples of MS CSF were examined. The results are expressed as percent of PLP degraded compared to EGTA control, for method 1 and increase in O.D. (caseinolytic activity) by calcium compared to EGTA control taken as unit of enzyme per ml of CSF for method 2.

SDS-PAGE analysis of CSF revealed progressive degradation of both PLP (which consists of a mixture of two proteins PLP (25 Kd) and DM-20 (20 Kd) Agrawal et al., 1972) by calcium compared to EGTA control. The DM-20 protein was more susceptible. There was a 14% loss of PLP at 2 hrs. following incubation and a greater decrease (39%) at 24 hours. Similarly the loss of DM-20 amounted to 37% at 2 hours and 58% at 24 hours. Mg^{2+} was ineffective in provoking degradation of both proteins. Some endogenous CSF proteins were also found susceptible to Ca^{2+}-mediated degradation.

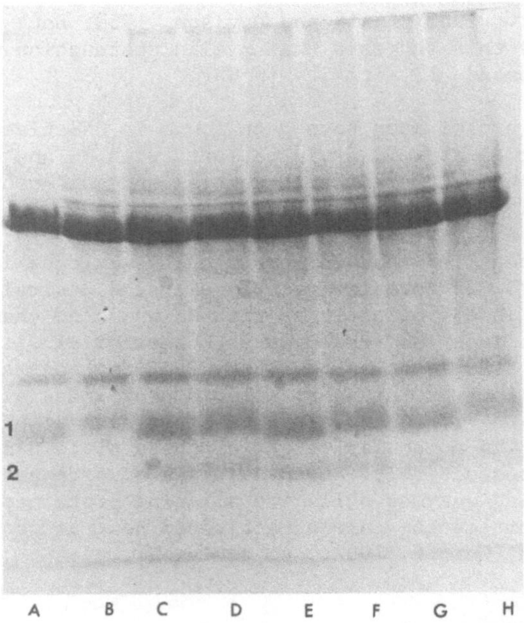

Fig.1. SDS-PAGE protein pattern of CSF after incubation. The method of incubation is described in the text. Lanes; A, CSF with PLP incubated in buffer for 24 hr.; B, CSF incubated in buffer alone for 24 hr; C, E, G, CSF incubated with PLP and EGTA for 2, 4 and 24 hrs.; D, F and H, CSF incubated with PLP and calcium for 2, 4 and 24 hrs. respectively. 1, PLP; 2, DM-20.

(Fig.1). The enzyme activity was inhibited by EGTA (5 mM) and leupeptin (1 mM).

Calcium-mediated caseinolytic activity in CSF was also demonstrated in a number of samples. This suggests that CSF contains a factor, a neutral proteinase which is activated by calcium. The level of activity (i.e. an increase in O.D. in the presence of calcium as caseinolytic activity) compared to control ranged from .004 - 1.377 up to 24 hours of incubation. The greatest increase was found in the CSF of a patient with intracerebral hemorrhage and may result from the increased number of white cells in the CSF. Neutral proteinase activity in CNS and leukocytes is well known (Marks and Lajtha, 1963; Riekkinen et al., 1977) and an increased neutral proteinase activity in circulating leukocytes as well as in MS CSF was reported by Cuzner et al. (1975, 1979).

Our finding of greater CANP activity in the precipitate (cells) than in the CSF supernatant confirms this report (Cuzner et al., 1979) that demonstrated an association of neutral proteinase (Ca^{2+}-independent) with macrophages and of acid proteinase with the soluble supernatant. These cells are found in MS CSF in acute MS disease. CANP degrades myelin (MBP and PLP) and cytoskeletal proteins (Banik et al., 1983, 1985; Nixon, 1984). Recently an increased activity of neutral proteinase (whether Ca^{2+}-dependent or not, was not determined) was found in myelin, isolated from MS CNS (Sato et al., 1984). The association of neutral proteinase and/or CANP with myelin (Sato et al., 1982a,b; Banik et al., 1985) and its possible localization in glial cels (and/or neurons) is potentially important in demyelinating disease (e.g. MS). The increased CANP in MS may derive from destroyed myelin, glial cells or from infiltrating macrophages.

It is noteworthy that CANP has been found in granulocytes although no difference in activity was found on comparing normal and MS (Konat et al., 1986). Preliminary studies indicate that there is CANP activity in CSF. A larger number must be studied before the significance of this is clear. The correlation of CANP activity and disease stage may be clinically valuable for assessing disease activity, affect of therapy etc.

ACKNOWLEDGEMENTS

This study was supported in part by NIH-NINCDS grants NS-11066, NS-12044 and NS-21353. We are grateful to Elaine Tidwell for secretarial assistance.

REFERENCES

1. C.W.M. Adams, A.N. Davison and N.A. Gregson. Enzyme inactivity of myelin: histochemical and biochemical evidence (1963).
2. H.C. Agrawal, R.M. Burton, M.A. Fishman, R.F. Mitchell and A.L. Prensky. Partial characterization of a new myelin protein component. J. Neurochem. 19:2083 (1972).
3. A.V. Arstilla, P. Riekkinen, U.K. Rinne and L. Laitinen. Studies on the pathogenesis of multiple sclerosis: participation of lysozymes in demyelination in the central nervous system white matter outside plaques. Eur. Neurol. 9:1-20 (1973).
4. N.L. Banik and A.N. Davison. Enzyme activity and composition of myelin and subcellular fraction in the developing rat brain. Biochem. J. 115:1051-1062 (1969).
5. N.L. Banik, L. Mauldin and E.L. Hogan. Activity of 2', 3'-cyclic nucleotide 3'-phosphohydrolase in human CSF. Ann. Neurol. 5:539-541 (1979).
6. N.L. Banik and E.L. Hogan. Cerebrospinal fluid enzymes in neurological disease, in Neurobiology of Cerebrospinal Fluid. Vol.2, J.H. Wood, ed. Plenum Press, New York. pp. 205-231 (1983).
7. N.L. Banik; E.L. Hogan, M.G. Jenkins, J.K. McDonald, W.W. McAlhaney and M. Sostek. Purification of a calcium-activated neutral proteinase from bovine brain. Neurochem. Res. 8:1389-1405 (1983).
8. N.L. Banik, E.L. Hogan and W.W. McAlhaney. Calcium-stimulated proteolysis in myelin: evidence for a Ca^{2+}-activated neutral proteinase associated with purified myelin of rats CNS. J. Neurochem. 45:581-588 (1985).
9. C.S. Beck, C.S. Hasinoff and M.E. Smith. L-Alanyl-beta-napthylamidase in rat spinal cord myelin. J. Neurochem. 15:1297-1301 (1968).
10. L.F. Chapman and H.G. Wolf. Studies of proteolytic enzymes in CSF. Arch. Intern. Med. 103:86-90 (1976).
11. P.A. Clapshaw, H.W. Miller, H. Wietholter and W. Seifert. Simultaneous measurement of 2', 3'-cyclic nucleotide 3'-phosphodiesterase and RNase activities in sera and spinal fluids of multiple sclerosis patients. J. Neurochem. 42:12-15 (1984).
12. M.L. Cuzner and A.N. Davison. Cerebral lysosomal enzyme activity and lipids in multiple sclerosis. J. Neurol. Sci. 19:29-36 (1973).
13. M.L. Cuzner, A.N. Davison and P. Rudge. Proteolytic enzyme activity of blood leukocytes and cerebrospinal fluid in multiple sclerosis. Ann. Neurol. 4:337-344 (1979).
14. M.L. Cuzner, W.I. McDonald, P. Rudge, A.N. Davison and N. Borshell. Leukocyte proteinase activity and acute multiple sclerosis. J. Neurol. Sci. 26:107-111 (1975).
15. J.P. Green and M. Perry. Leucine amino peptidase activity in cerebrospinal fluid. Neurology. 13:924-926 (1963).

16. G. Guroff. A neutral, calcium-activated proteinase from the soluble fraction of rat brain. J. Biol. Chem. 239:149-155 (1964).
17. J.B. Hallpike, C.W.M. Adams and O.B. Bayliss. Histochemistry of myelin: proteolytic activity around multiple sclerosis plaques. Histochem. J. 2:199-208 (1970).
18. R.M. Herndon and M.A. Johnson. A new method for the electron microscopic study of cerebrospinal fluid sediment. J. Neuropathol. Exp. Neurol. 29:320-329 (1970).
19. H.E. Hirsch. The role of acid hydrolases in demyelination. Neurology. 26:39-41 (1976).
20. S. Johnson and E.F. Domino. Cholinergic enzymatic activity of cerebrospinal fluid of patients with various neurological diseases. Clin. Chim. Acta. 35:421-428 (1971).
21. G. Konat, N.L. Banik, J.M. Goust and E.L. Hogan. Digestion of myelin proteins by granulocytic proteases. Trans. Am. Soc. Neurochem. 17 (1986).
22. N. Marks and A. Lajtha. Protein breakdown in the brain: subcellular distribution and properties of neutral and acid proteinases. Biochem. J. 89:438-447 (1963).
23. N. Marks, A. Grynbaum and A. Lajtha. The breakdown of myelin-bound proteins by intra and extracellular proteases. Neurochem. Res. 1:93-111 (1976).
24. P.V. Nelson, W.F. Carey and A.C. Pollard. Diagnostic significance and source of lactate dehydrogenase and its isoenzymes in CSF of children with a variety of neurological diseases. J. Clin. Pathol. 28:828-833 (1975).
25. R.A. Nixon. Proteolysis of neurofilaments, in neurofilaments. C.A. Marotta, ed. University of Minnesota Press, Minneapolis. pp. 117-154 (1983).
26. I. Raes, S. Weissbarth, H.S. Maker and G.M. Lehrer. 2', 3'-cyclic nucleotide 3'-phosphodiesterase in cerebrospinal fluid. Neurology. 31:1361-1363 (1981).
27. P.J. Riekkinen and U.K. Rinne. Proteinases in human cerebrospinal fluid. J. Neurol. Sci. 7:97-106 (1968).
28. P.J. Riekkinen, J. Palo and I. Askikainen. Lysosomal enzymes in the lymphocytes and granulocytes of patients with MS. Acta Neurol. Scand. 56:83-86 (1977).
29. U.K. Rinne and P.J. Riekkinen. Esterase, peptidase and proteinase activities of human cerebrospinal fluid in multiple sclerosis. Acta Neurol. Scand. 44:156-167 (1968).
30. S. Sato and T. Miyatake. Degradation of myelin basic protein by calcium-activated neutral protease (CANP)-like enzyme in myelin and inhibition by E-64 analogue. Biomed. Res. 3:461-464 (1982a).
31. S. Sato, R.H. Quarles and R.O. Brady. Susceptibility of the myelin associated glycoprotein and basic protein to a neutral protease in highly purified myelin of human and rat brain. J. Neurochem. 39:97-105 (1982b).
32. S. Sato, R.H. Quarles, R.O. Brady and W.W. Tourtellotte. Elevated neutral proteinase activity in myelin from multiple sclerosis brain. Ann. Neurol. 15:264-267 (1984).
33. S.N. Shah and R. Johnson. Cholesterol ester hydrolase activity in human cerebrospinal fluid. Exp. Neurol. 58:68-73 (1978).
34. E.C. Shuttleworth and N. Allen. Early differentiation of chronic meningitis by enzyme assay. Neurology. 18:534-542 (1968).
35. T.J. Sprinkle and G.M. McKhann. Activity of 2', 3'-cyclic nucleotide 3'-phosphohydrolase in CSF of patients with demyelinating disorders. Neurosci. Lett. 7:203-206 (1978).
36. J. Swinnen. Peptidase and transpeptidase activities in CSF. Methods for the calorometric determination of leucine aminopeptidase, gamma-glutamyl-peptidase and gamma-glutamyl transpeptidase activities. Clin. Chem. Acta. 17:255-263 (1967).

37. Y. Tsukada, H. Suda, T. Hosokawa, R. Ohno and K. Hamaguchi. 2', 3'-cyclic nucleotide 3'-phosphohydrolase in human cerebrospinal fluid with neurological diseases. J. Neurochem. 41 Suppl. 157B (1983).
38. J.L. Viallard, J. Gaulne, B. Dalens and B. Dastugue. Cerebrospinal fluid enzymology, creatine kinase, lactate dehydrogenase activity and isoenzyme pattern as a brain damage index. Clin. Chim. Acta. 89:405-409 (1978).
39. J.H. Wood. Physiological neurochemistry of cerebrospinal fluid, in Handbook of Neurochemistry Second Edition, Vol.1, A, Lajtha, ed. Plenum Press, New York. pp. 415-487 (1982).

DEGRADATION OF MYELIN BASIC PROTEIN IN MYELIN BY CEREBROSPINAL FLUID AND EFFECTS OF PROTEASE INHIBITORS

Takashi Inuzuka, Shuzo Sato, Hiroko Baba and Tadashi Miyatake

Department of Neurology, Brain Research Institute, Niigata University, Niigata 951, Japan

Neutral proteases have been reported to exist in cerebrospinal fluid (CSF), but the functional role of these proteases on myelin breakdown has not been elucidated. We examined the degradation of myelin basic protein (MBP) by the neutral proteases in CSF and the effect of protease inhibitors.

CSF was taken from patients with psychosomatic disease, multiple sclerosis, acute viral meningoencephalitis or amyotrophic lateral sclerosis. After centrifugation at 700g for 10 min, the CSF was stored at -70°C until use. Myelin was purified from white matter of patients without neurological disease.

Neutral protease is demonstrated to exist in cell free human CSF. Incubation of heated human myelin with CSF at 25°C resulted in marked reduction of MBP and the degradation products appeared at apparent mol. wt. 14 kDa and 12 kDa on polyacrylamide gel electrophoresis. Optimal pH of the protease was 7.0. This protease was activated by calcium ion. Degradation of MBP was inhibited by FOY305 (camostat mesilate), Trasylol, Leupeptin, but was not inhibited by a specific calcium activated neutral protease (CANP) inhibitor, E-64-a. FOY305 was the strongest inhibitor that is synthesized as a specific serine protease inhibitor. The protease activity was significantly elevated in CSF of patients with multiple sclerosis in exacerbation and acute phase of acute viral meningoencephalitis.

INTRODUCTION

Although a number of neutral proteases which degrade myelin basic protein (MBP) have been reported to exist in cerebrospinal fluid (CSF) (1, 2,3,4), the origin and functional role of these proteases in myelin breakdown has not yet been elucidated. Since digestion of MBP has been implicated as an initial step in degradation of myelin in demyelinating disease (5,6,7) and the periventricular zone is an area of prediction for the plaque in multiple sclerosis (8), it might be expected that the protease in CSF would reflect these changes.

In this paper we demonstrate that the neutral protease in CSF degrades MBP in purified myelin and is inhibited by protease inhibitors, including drugs such as FOY305 and Trasylol^{R}. Elevation of the protease activity in CSF in patients with multiple sclerosis (MS) in exacerbation and acute viral meningoencephalitis in acute phase is also demonstrated.

EXPERIMENTAL PROCEDURES

CSF was immediately centrifuged at 700 g for 10 min. at 4°C. CSF was stored at -70°C until use. For the characterization of this protease, we used CSF from a patient with psychosomatic disease (PSD). The laboratory examination of this CSF was within normal limits. We studied the neutral protease activity in CSF from 6 patients (10 relapses) with definite MS (9) in exacerbation (MS-E) and in remission (MS-R), 6 patients with acute viral meningoencephalitis in acute phase (MAE-A) and in recovery phase (AME-R), 7 patients with amyotrophic lateral sclerosis (ALS) and 4 patients with PSD. The periods of taking CSF between MS-E and MS-R range from 11 days to 4 months, and those between AME-A and AME-R range from 7 days to 52 days. Protein, IgG % of total protein, cell count of polymorphonuclear cell (PMN) or mononuclear cell (MNC), sugar and chloride ion of all these CSFs were examined. Correlation between neutral protease activity and each of these was studied.

Myelin was purified from human white matter without neurological disease by the procedure of Norton and Poduslo (10). The endogenous proteases were inactivated by pretreatment of the myelin with heat, by placing the suspension of myelin in an 80°C water bath for 5 min. Unheated fresh myelin suspension was used as control. Fifty microliters of CSF were preincubated with or without an inhibitor in 100 µl of 20 mM Tris-HCl buffer pH 7.5 for one hour at 25°C. Incubation began with addition of 40 µl of heated myelin suspension (200 µg protein), 5 µl of 10% Triton and 5 µl of 200 mM $CaCl_2$ to the preincubated material. Control was prepared by the same procedure with the exception that CSF was from PSD and the material was immediately frozen without incubation.

To study the influence of calcium ion, 5 µl of 200 mM $MnCl_2$ or 200 mM $MgCl_2$, was added to the incubation mixture instead of 200 mM $CaCl_2$. Incubations were done at 25°C for 15 hr for characterization of the protease and 4 hr for study on protease among diseases, except where indicated in the legend to the figures, and terminated by freezing. In one experiment, as a control, CSF was heated at 80°C for 5 min to inactivate protease in CSF. Assessment of proteolytic activity at various pHs was done by adjusting the pH of Tris with HCl. The following protease inhibitors were used: FOY305 (Ono Pharmaceutical Co., Japan), E-64-a (Taisho pharmaceutical Co., Japan), Leupeptin (kindly provided by Dr. T. Aoyagi of the Institute of Microbial Chemistry, Japan), Phenylmethylsulfonyfluoride (PMSF) (Sigma Chem. Co., MO, USA), Di-isopropyl fluorophosphate (DIFP) (Sigma Chem. Co., MO, USA), Tranexamic acid (Di-ichi Pharmacent Co., Japan), Trasylol^R (aprotinin) (Boehringer-Mannheim Co., FRG).

Concentration of inhibitors was adjusted to 1 mM except where indicated in the table. 100 µM FOY305 was studied to see whether it inhibited protease in CSF from patients with MS-E. The effect of the calcium chelator, 1 mM EGTA, was investigated when $CaCl_2$ was omitted from incubation.

Incubated mixtures were lyophilized and electrophoresed on 11% of polyacrylamide slab gel after partial delipidation with 3:2 (vol/vol) ethyl ether-ethanol. Coomassie blue stained gels were densitometrically scanned with a spectrodensitometer (Shimadzu, CS-910, Japan) operating at 540 nm for quantitation of MBP. Each gel has a control lane to avoid differences of staining intensity among gels. The percentage of remaining MBP compared with that in control indicates protease activity. A higher percentage of remaining MBP means lower protease activity. The myelin proteins on other gels were transferred to nitrocellulose sheets by the procedure of Towbin et al. (11) and immunostained with anti-human MBP antibody (DAKO Co., CA, USA).

RESULTS

Incubation of purified myelin with CSF at pH 7.5 resulted in degradation of only MBP with time but not other myelin proteins such as Wolfgram's protein and proteolipid protein. The percentage of remaining MBP was 80% after 4 hr and 12% after 15 hr of incubation. Degradation products appeared at apparent mol wt 14 KDa and 12 KDa on polyacrylamide gel electrophoresis (Fig.1). They were determined as degradation products of MBP by immunoblot analysis with anti-human MBP antibody. No degradation of MBP was observed when myelin was incubated with heated CSF.

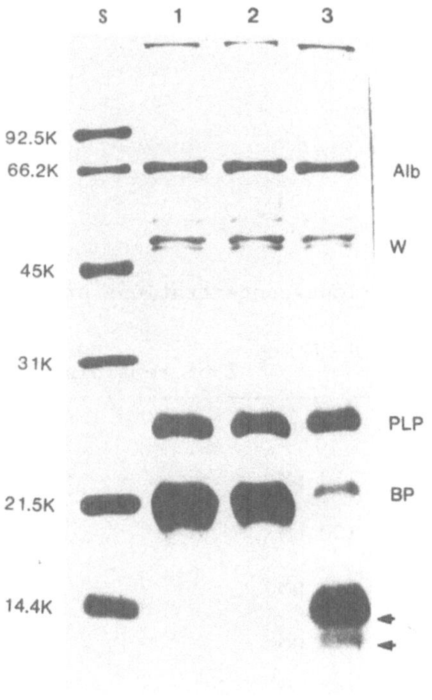

Fig.1. Degradation of MBP in human myelin as a function of incubation time. The sample in lane 1 was from myelin suspension frozen without incubation, whereas the incubation times for the samples in other lanes were 2, 4h;3, 15h;4. Each lane was loaded with 10 µg myelin protein. Molecular weight standards indicated are in the left lane. Alb, Albumin: W. Wolfgram protein: PLP, Proteolipid protein: BP, Basic protein. Arrows indicate degradation products.

The optimal pH for degradation of MBP in myelin by the protease in CSF was 7.0. Inhibition of degradation of MBP was shown by 1 mM of FOY305, Leupeptin, or 100 μM of Trasylol[R]. However, 1 mM of the other inhibitors, including a specific CANP inhibitor E-64-a, PMSF, DIFP and Tranexamic acid, failed to inhibit the degradation of MBP (Table 1). The inhibitory effects at various concentrations of the three inhibitors are shown in Table 2. FOY305 had the strongest effect on inhibition of protease activity on MBP at neutral pH in CSF. At 10 μM of FOY305 or Trasylol[R] intact MBP remained 74%, 29% respectively, whereas 10 μM Leupeptin almost failed to inhibit.

Table 1. Effect of various protease inhibitors on degradation of MBP

	% of remaining intact MBP
control (immediately frozen)	100
no protease inhibitor	12
1 mM FOY305	100
1 mM E-64-a	12
1 mM Leupeptin	100
1 mM PMSF	11
1 mM DIFP	16
1 mM Tranexamic acid	14
100 μM Trasylol	100

Table 2. Effect of various concentrations of FOY305, Trasylol and Leupeptin

		% of remaining intact MBP
FOY305	1 μM	12
	10 μM	74
	100 μM	100
Trasylol	1 μM	15
	10 μM	29
	100 μM	100
Leupeptin	1 μM	9
	10 μM	17
	100 μM	58

As shown in Table 3, the protease was activated by calcium ion but not by magnesium ion. Manganese ion slightly inhibited. Protease was inhibited by 1 mM EGTA, if $CaCl_2$ was omitted from the incubation.

Table 3. Effect of various metal ions and EGTA on degradation on MBP

	% of remaining intact MBP
control (immediately frozen)	100
no exogenous metal ion	77
$CaCl_2$	12
$MgCl_2$	77
$MnCl_2$	93
1 mM EGTA without exogenous metal ion	94

The average of neutral protease activity in CSF from patients with MS-E was significantly higher than that of the same patients in remission by paired t-test [$P(t) < 0.005$], and was also significantly higher than that of PSD or ALS by Student t-test. [$P(t) < 0.05$] (Table 4). In each relapse, protease activity was higher in exacerbation than in remission.

Table 4. Comparison of the protease activity among diseases

	% of remaining intact MBP
MS-E	50.6 ± 21.6 (n=10)
MS-R	83.0 ± 8.4 (n=10)
AME-A	43.2 ± 25.7 (n=6)
AME-R	68.3 ± 20.7 (n=6)
ALS	80.6 ± 10.1 (n=7)
PSD	80.3 ± 4.6 (n=4)

Longitudinal analysis of the MS patient showed a relationship between protease activity and disease activity (Table 5). The average of protease activity in CSF from patients with AME-A was significantly higher than that of the same patients with AME-R by paired t-test [$P(t) < 0.005$], and was also significantly higher than that of PSD or ALS. The coefficients of correlations between the percentage of remaining intact MBP and protein of CSF, and the percentage of remaining intact MBP and IgG % of protein of CSF were -0.658 and -0.416 respectively. No significant correlation was found between the percentage of remaining intact MBP and cell count of MNC or PMN.

Table 5. Longitudinal analysis of the MS patient

relapse	date	stage	% of the remaining intact BP
1	Jan. 14 '82	E	55
	Jan. 25 '82	R	79
2	May 18 '82	E	60
	Jun. 4 '82	R	83
3	Sept.17 '84	E	49
	Oct. 12 '84	R	95
4	Sept.13 '85	E	24
	Oct. 4 '85	R	76

E: exacerbation
R: remission

As shown in Table 6, increased activity of the patient with MS-E was totally inhibited by 100 μM FOY305.

Table 6. Effect of FOY305 on protease in CSF from a patient with MS-E

	% of remaining intact BP
control	100
CSF (MS-E)	55
CSF (MS-E) + 100 μM FOY305	100

DISCUSSION

The presence in human purified myelin of endogenous neutral protease which is inactivated by heating at 70°C for 5 min, has been reported (12). Heated CSF failed to degrade MBP, which clearly demonstrates that the neutral protease is present in cell free CSF, as was predictable from some of the earlier investigations (13, 14). Our study also revealed that FOY305 strongly inhibited the protease even at 10 μM level.

The formation of two degradation products on gel at apparent mol wt 14 KDa and 12 KDa may suggest that this protease has a specific cleaving site on MBP. It is interesting that increased levels of low-molecular-weight proteins around 10 KDa to 13 KDa which have an antigenicity to MBP, have been reported in CSF of multiple sclerosis (4).

Although this protease is activated by calcium ion and inhibited by EGTA, CANP specific inhibitor E-64-a cannot inhibit it. Furthermore, this protease is inhibited by FOY305 and Trasylol^R, which are serine protease inhibitors, also by Leupeptin, which is a serine-thiol protease inhibitor. FOY305 has been developed as a drug for pancreatitis and disseminated intravascular coagulation, and strongly inhibits trypsin, plasmin, thrombin and plasma kallikrein. These enzymes affect the bond of the carboxyl end of L-Arginine or L-Lysine in peptides or esters (13). Riekkinen et al. (14) reported that neutral protease in CSF was an SH-sensitive enzyme. However, our finding of a strong inhibition by FOY305 of the protease suggests that it has the character of a serine protease. Although Alvord et al. (3) reported neutral protease in CSF which resembled thrombin, plasmin and kallikrein, our investigation showed that common serine protease inhibitors such as PMSF, DIFP and plasmin inhibitor tranexamic acid did not inhibit the degradation of MBP. Therefore, neutral protease in CSF may not be thrombin, plasmin or kallikrein despite its similarity in character. Thus, the protease has a part of the character of CANP on a point of activation by calcium, but failure of inhibition by E-64-a suggests it is different from CANP. On the other hand, inhibition of serine protease by FOY305 or Trasylol suggests it has some characteristics of serine protease, but failure of inhibition by PMSF or DIFP suggests it is not a common serine protease. After all, this peculiar protease in CSF may be an uncommon serine protease which is activated by calcium or a complex of some kinds of protease. Purification of this protease will make possible further characterization.

Statistically elevated neutral protease activity, using denatured hemoglobin as substrate, in cell free CSF was reported in the acute stage of MS compared with the chronic stage of MS and normal control (15). But Alvord et al. (3) could not find any correlation between the type of disease and neutral protease activity using bovine purified MBP as substrate. Our data clearly show the increased protease activity in cell free CSF from a patient with MS-E and AME-A using human central nervous system (CNS) MBP in myelin as substrate. Increased neutral protease in MS-E and that in AME-A are considered to be the same protease because of the same pattern of degradation products (Fig.2). Longitudinal analysis shows good correlation between neutral protease activity and disease activity of MS. Thus the elevation of this protease is not unique to MS, however, it may be one good marker of disease activity of MS.

Possible origins of this protease are peripheral blood, cells in the central nervous system or cells in CSF. Leucocytes especially PMN and macrophage in peripheral blood are known to have neutral protease activity as well as acid protease and these proteases have been reported to be increased in acute MS or central nervous system infection. (2,16,17,18,19) This protease is not considered to be derived from plasma, because proteolytic enzymes in plasma are immediately bound to various enzyme inhibitors (20), which would inhibit their transport across the blood-CSF barrier. These cells may gather to inflammatory lesion or demyelinating lesion, where PMN is seen rarely, in CNS throughout the vessel wall and may release proteases. Indeed elevation of various kinds of proteolytic activities, which are thought to be from infiltrating cells or astrocytes, has been reported in the lesions of MS and experimental allergic encephalomyelitis (7).

Although neutral protease in CSF seems to correlate to total protein in CSF, there are some cases which have discrepancy between protease activity and protein. Therefore, increased protease activity may not be simply due to increase of permeability of blood-CSF barrier.

Normal human brain tissue has also been reported to have neutral proteases (21). Riekkinen et al. (14) reported the similarity of SH-enzyme which they found in CSF and that in rat brain. This SH-enzyme was not activated by calcium and it was not known if it degraded MBP. Human brain neutral protease which degrades MBP has been reported (22,23,24) and this is inhibited by E-64-a. The existence of neutral protease in cellular

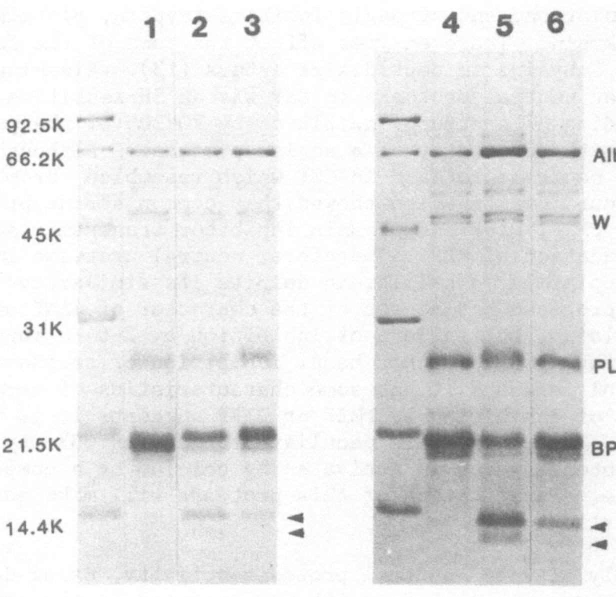

Fig.2. Degradation of MBP by CSF from MS-E (Lane 2), MS-R (Lane 3), AME-A (Lane 5) and AME-R (Lane 6). Incubation time of these samples is 4 hrs. Lane 1 or 4 is a control of each gel. Left side lanes of gels are molecular standards. Alb, Albumin: W. Wolfgram protein: PLP, Proteolipid protein: BP, Basic protein. Arrows indicate degradation products.

fraction of CSF was reported, however, this did not show any increase of neutral protease activity in cell free CSF in spite of an increase of it in cellular fraction of CSF in acute stage of MS. (1,2) Besides our data show no correlation between neutral protease activity and cell count of PMN or MNC. Thus the origin of the neutral protease in CSF in physiological condition is still obscure.

This neutral protease may be related to physiological turnover of MBP in CSF and is shown to be closely related to the activity of some neurological diseases such as MS. One hundred micro molar of FOY305 inhibited increased neutral protease activity in MS-E, which suggests the possibility of the clinical application of this protease inhibitor for MS.

ACKNOWLEDGEMENT

Supported by grants from the Neuroimmunological Disorder Research Committee and the New Drug Development (Ministry of Health and Welfare of Japan). The authors thank Dr. T. Aoyagi of the Institute of Microbial Chemistry for kindly providing Leupeptin, Ono Pharmaceutical Co. for providing FOY305 and Taisho Pharmaceutical Co. for providing E-64-a.

REFERENCES

1. P.T. Richards and M.L. Cuzner. Proteolytic activity in CSF. Adv. Exp. Med. Biol. 100:521 (1978).
2. M.L. Cuzner, A.N. Davison and P. Rudge. Proteolytic enzyme activity of blood leucocytes and cerebrospinal fluid in multiple sclerosis. Ann. Neurol. 4:337 (1978).

3. E.C. Alvord, S. Hruby and L.R. Sires. Degradation of myelin basic protein by cerebrospinal fluid: Preservation of antigenic determinants under physiological conditions. Ann. Neurol. 6:474 (1979).
4. B. Carlson and C. Alling. Molecular size of myelin basic protein immunoactivity in spinal fluid. J. Neuroimmunol. 6:141 (1984).
5. J.F. Hallpike and C.W.M. Adams. Proteolysis and myelin breakdown: a review of recent histochemical and biochemical studies. Histochem. J. 1:559 (1969).
6. E.R. Einstein, J. Csejtey, K.B. Dalal, C.W.M. Adams, O.B. Bayliss and J.F. Hallpike. Proteolytic activity and basic protein loss in and around multiple sclerosis plaques. Combined biochemical and histochemical observations. J. Neurochem. 19:653 (1972).
7. M.E. Smith. Proteinase inhibitors and the suspension of EAE. In: "The suppression of experimental allergic encephalomyelitis and multiple sclerosis". A.N. Davison and M.L. Cuzner, eds. Academic Press, London. (1980).
8. C.W.M. Adams. Pathology of multiple sclerosis: progression of the lesion. Br. Med. Bull. 33:15 (1977).
9. D. McAlpine, C.E. Lumsden and E.D. Acheson. "Multiple Sclerosis - A Reappraisal" 2nd ed. Churchill Livingston, Edingburgh (1972).
10. W.T. Norton and S.E. Poduslo. Myelination in rat brain: method of myelin isolation. J. Neurochem. 21:749 (1973).
11. H. Towbin, T. Staehelin and J. Gordon. Electrophoretic transfer of proteins from polyacrylamide gels to nitrocellulose sheets: procedure and some applications. Proc. Natl. Acad. Sci. USA. 76:4350 (1979).
12. S. Sato, R.H. Quarles and R.O. Brady. Susceptibility of the myelin-associated glycoprotein and basic protein to a neutral protease in highly purified myelin from human and rat brain. J. Neurochem. 39:97 (1982).
13. Y. Tamura, M. Hirado, K. Okamura and Y. Minato. Synthetic inhibitors of trypsin, plasmin, kallikrein, thrombin, C_1 r and C_1 esterase. Biochim. Biophys. Acta. 484:417 (1977).
14. P.J. Riekkinen and U.K. Rinne. Proteinases in human cerebrospinal fluid. J. Neurol. Sci. 7:97 (1968).
15. U.K. Rinne and P. Riekkinen. Esterase, peptidase and proteinase activities of human cerebrospinal fluid in multiple sclerosis. Acta Neurol. Scandinav. 44:156 (1968).
16. M.L. Cuzner, W.I. McDonald, P. Rudge, M. Smith, N. Borshell and A.N. Davison. Leucocyte proteinase activity and acute multiple sclerosis. J. Neurol. Sci. 26:107 (1975).
17. I. Goto, N. Shinno and Y. Kuroiwa. Proteolytic enzyme activities in mononuclear cells and granulocytes of patients with various neurological disorders. J. Neurol. Sci. 59:323-329 (1983).
18. Y. Aoki, T. Miyatake, N. Shimizu and M. Yoshida. Medullasin activity in granulocytes of patients with multiple sclerosis. Ann. Neurol. 15:245 (1984).
19. B. Guarnieri, F. Lolli and L. Amaducci. Polymorphonuclear neutral protease activity in multiple sclerosis and other disease. Ann. Neurol. 18:620-622 (1985).
20. A.J. Barrett and P.M. Starkey. The interaction of alpha2-macroglobulin with proteinases, characteristics and specificity of the reaction and a hypothesis concerning its molecular mechanism. Biochem. J. 133:709 (1973).
21. A. Pope and R.A. Nixon. Proteases of human brain. Neurochem. Res. 9:291 (1984).
22. S. Sato and T. Miyatake. Degradation of myelin basic protein by calcium-activated neutral protease (CANP)-like enzyme in myelin and inhibition by E-64 analogue. Biomed. Res. 3:461 (1982).

23. S. Sato, K. Yanagisawa and T. Miyatake. Conversion of myelin-associated glycoprotein (MAG) to a smaller derivative by calcium-activated neutral protease (CANP)-like enzyme in myelin and inhibition by E-64 analogue. Neurochem. Res. 9:629 (1984).
24. K. Yanagisawa, S. Sato, N. Amaya and T. Miyatake. Degradation of myelin basic protein by calcium-activated neutral protease (CANP) in human brain and inhibition by E-64 analogue. Neurochem. Res. 8:1285 (1983).

CSF RIBONUCLEASES IN MULTIPLE SCLEROSIS

B. Allinquant, C. Mussenger and E. Schuller

Laboratoire de Neuroimmunologie (INSERM U 134) Hôpital de la Salpêtrière - 75651 Paris Cédex 13 - France

Ribonucleic acid fragments and polynucleotides are known to be amplifiers of specific signals in immunity (Braun, 1973; Johnson, 1979). The capacity of certain synthetic polynucleotides to act as adjuvants for induction of experimental allergic encephalomyelitis in guinea-pigs when added to emulsions of spinal cord in incomplete Freund's adjuvant has already been reported (Gruenewald et al., 1977; Gumbiner et al., 1973; Paterson and Drobish, 1974; Paterson, 1976). Thus endogenous or exogenous nucleic acid fragments not (or insufficiently) catabolized, would be able to entertain an inflammatory process inside the central nervous system.

Ribonucleases (RNases) constitute the first step of RNA catabolism. The action of such enzymes in brain, is to produce fragments terminated by 2'3' cyclic phosphate (Fig.1) (Niedergang et al., 1974; Okazaki et al.,

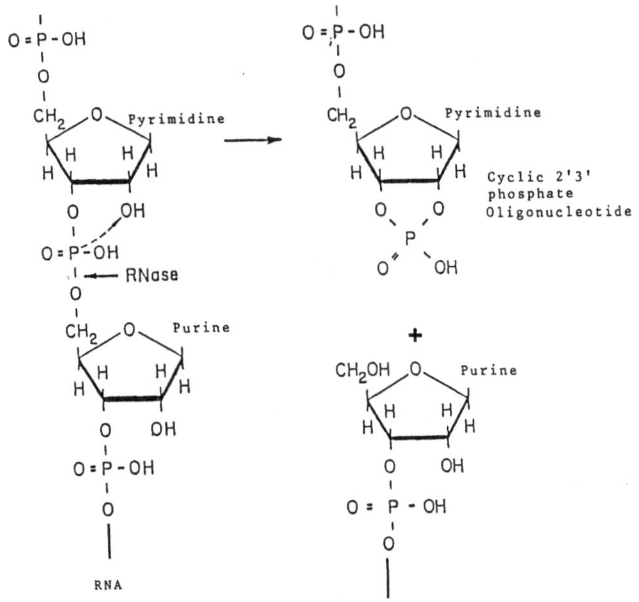

Fig.1. Action of ribonucleases in brain cells

1975) which could be potential targets for 2'3' cyclic phosphodiesterase. Such cyclic oligonucleotide 2'3' phosphates are only intermediate products for pancreatic RNases, giving at the end of the enzymic reaction oligonucleotide 3' phosphate only. Alkaline RNases are associated with an inhibitor in tissues (Takashi et al., 1967, 1970). The function of RNases in tissues remains unknown, but it is probable that they may be involved in RNA maturation and splicing (Abelson 1979; Levy 1975; Perry 1976) after depression of their interaction with the inhibitor. These enzymes are excreted in biological fluids. Thus, variations in CSF RNases might reflect their variations in brain cells.

Our first study of CSF RNase activity in neurological diseases (Allinquant et al., 1984) has shown in controls and in patient groups devoid of any transudation phenomena: 1) a very high ratio of CSF/Serum RNase activity. 2) an absence of correlation between serum and CSF RNase activity, two facts suggesting that the major part of CSF RNase activity originates in brain tissue.

The highest CSF RNase activity observed in CNS infectious processes was significantly different from CSF RNase activity in MS ($p < 0.01$).

Such variations could affect certain types of RNase isoenzymes or their totality. Five groups (1-5) of RNase isoenzymes have already been

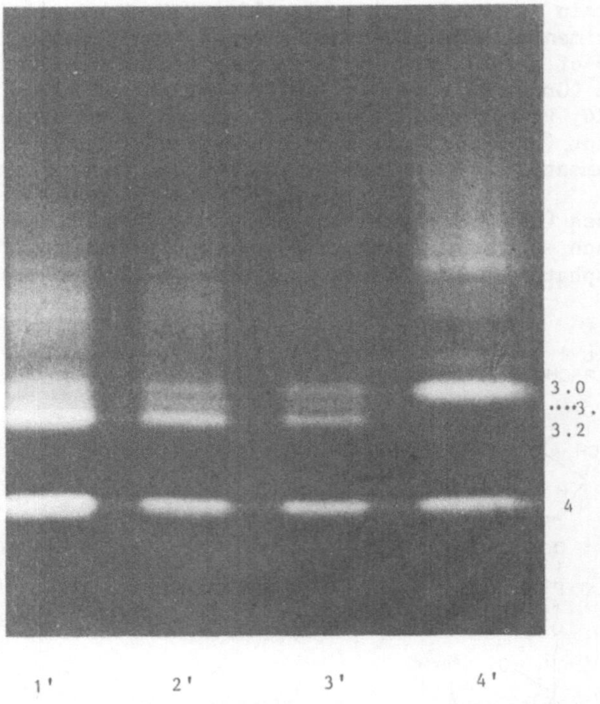

Fig.2. RNase isoenzymes separated by SDS-electrophoresis (15% polyacrylamide gels cast with Poly (C) and stained according to (Blank and Dekker, 1981).
Left to right:
* 0.01 unit of RNases from white matter (1')-grey matter (2')-crude fresh myelin (3')-peripheral nerve (4')
- 1 unit of RNase was defined as the amount of enzymes which produce in 1 minute 1.0 OD 278 nm of acid soluble material from Poly (C) used as substrate under the assay conditions (Allinquant et al., 1984).

reported by SDS-electrophoresis (Blank and Dekker, 1981), and two CSF RNase isoenzymes of group 3 (a major one, RNase 3.2 of MW 18700 and a minor one, RNase 3.1 of MW 19200) which are absent from serum and urine and have been demonstrated (Schieven et al., 1982).

RNase 3.1 and RNase 3.2 were found absent in peripheral nerves and present in brain tissue extracts (Fig.2) (grey, white matter, crude fresh myelins released from human oligodendrocyte purification) by using SDS-polyacrylamide gels (cast with substrate). Thus variations in these 2 RNase isoenzymes in CSF probably rather reflect their variations in brain tissue. CSF RNases of group 3 are the major CSF RNase isoenzymes (Fig.3). One of these RNases 3, RNase 3.0 is present in serum too (Blank and Dekker, 1981; Schieven et al., 1982). Using samples by SDS-electrophoresis with greater activity than 0.01 RNase unit, RNase 3.1 and RNase 3.2 could not be distinguished one from the other (Fig. 3).

A study of CSF RNase isoenzymes in multiple sclerosis (MS) comparatively to other CNS diseases was undertaken. The population included a)6 CNS infectious processes: 3 meningitis, 1 trypanosomiasis, 1 herpes zoster, 1 syphilis. b)12 MS. c)15 other neurological diseases (non infectious and non SEP). The 33 CSF were chosen for being devoided of any transudation phenomena to prevent contamination by serum RNase 3.0. The major variations of CSF RNase isoenzymes were observed in RNases of group 3, and sometimes in RNases of group 4. The variations of CSF RNases of group 3 were evaluated by the ratio of RNases $\frac{3.1 + 3.2}{3.0}$. Even though the population investigated is small, results presented in Table 1 showed a significant decrease of such ratio in CNS infectious processes and in MS, in absence of any significant increase of serum RNase. In 2 MS out of the 12 studied, this ratio was 0.3 and in 2 other, 0.4. In some cases, a decrease in this ratio was associated to a decrease in RNase 4. Such dis-

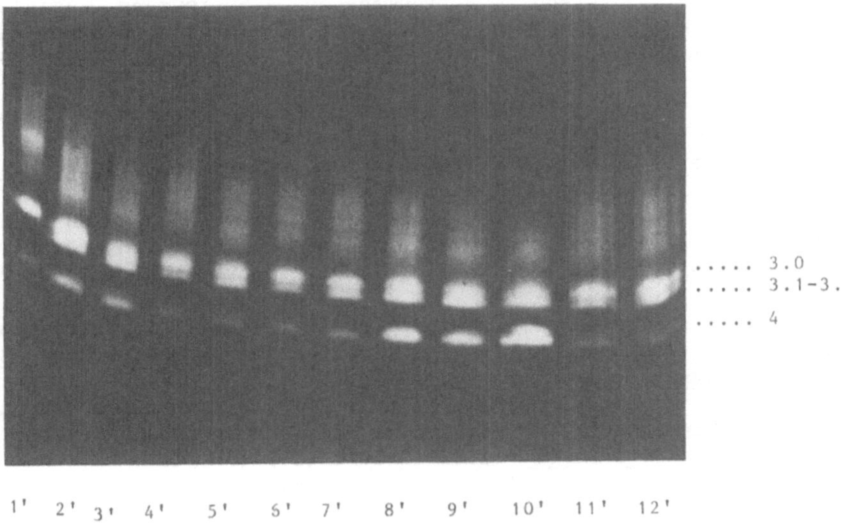

Fig.3. Serum and CSF RNase isoenzymes separated by SDS-electrophoresis (12.5% polyacrylamide gels cast with Poly (C) and stained according to Blank and Dekker, 1981.
Left to right:
0.7 to 1.0 unit of RNases from: normal serum (1')-OND CSFs (2'-3') -MS CSFs (4'-5'-6') Meningitis CSF (7')-grey matter (8')-white matter (9')-crude fresh myelin (10')-MS CSF (11'-12').

crepancy in RNases 3 seems more the result of a decrease in specific CNS RNases 3.1 and 3.2 than an increase in RNase 3.0 (Fig.3).

CONCLUSION

The variations of these CSF RNases 3 and the decrease in specific CNS RNases 3.1 and 3.2 could result of an absence of synthesis (or of a proteolysis) of such RNases 3.1 and 3.2 by infected cells (in infectious processes) and by cells around plaques (in MS). Their presence in brain tissue, in absence of excretion into CSF in such diseases, could be another possibility. The biological role of these CNS specific RNase isoenzymes and their variations in MS and infectious processes need to be further investigated.

REFERENCES

1. J. Abelson. RNA processing and the intervening sequence problem. Ann. Rev. Biochem. 48:1035-1069 (1979).
2. B. Allinquant, C. Musenger and E. Schuller. Intrathecal origin of CSF ribonuclease. Differences between infectious processes of the nervous system and multiple sclerosis. Acta Neurol. Scand. 70:12-19 (1984).
3. A. Blank and C.A. Dekker. Ribonucleases of human serum, urine, cerebrospinal fluid and leucocytes. Activity staining following electrophoresis in sodium dodecyl sulfate-polyacrylamide gels. Biochem. 20:2261-2267 (1981).
4. W. Braun. RNAs as amplifiers of specific signals in immunity. Annals of the N.Y. Acad. Sci. 207:17-28 (1973).
5. R. Grünewald, S. Levine and R. Sowinski. Experimental allergic encephalomyelitis in the rat: enhancement and suppression by synthetic polyribonucleotides. Proc. Soc. Exp. Biol. Med. 154:175-179 (1977).
6. C. Gumbiner, P.Y. Paterson, G.P. Youmans and A.S. Youmans. Adjuvanticity of mycobacterial RNA and Poly A:U for induction of experimental allergic encephalomyelitis in Guinea pigs. J. Immunol. 110:309-312 (1973).
7. A.G. Johnson. Modulation of the immune system by synthetic polynucleotides. Springer Semin. Immunopathol. 2:149-168 (1979).
8. C.C. Levy. Roles of RNases in cellular regulatory mechanisms. Life Sci. 17:311-315 (1975).
9. C. Niedergang, H. Okazaki, M.E. Ittel, D. Munoz, F. Petek and P. Mandel. Ribonucleases of beef brain nuclei. Purification and characterization of an alkaline RNase. Bioch. Biophy. Acta. 358:91-104 (1974).
10. H. Okazaki, M.E. Ittel, C. Niedergang and P. Mandel. Purification of an alkaline ribonuclease from soluble fraction of beef brain. Biochim. Biophys. Acta. 391:84-95 (1975).
11. P.Y. Paterson and D.G. Drobish. Adjuvanticity of synthetic polynucleotides for induction of experimental allergic encephalomyelitis in guinea pigs. J. Immunol. 113:1942-1946 (1974).
12. P.Y. Paterson. Experimental allergic encephalomyelitis-inducing activity of synthetic polyadenylic and polyuridylic homopolymers and complexes in guinea pigs. Cell. Immunol. 21:48-55 (1976).
13. R.P. Perry. Processing of RNA. Ann. Rev. Biochem. 45:605-624 (1976).
14. C.L. Schieven, A. Blank and C.A. Dekker. Ribonucleases of human cerebrospinal fluid: detection of altered glycosylation relative to their serum counterparts. Biochem. 21:5148-5155 (1982).

15. Y. Takahashi, K. Mase and Y. Suzuki. Purification of ribonuclease inhibitor from pig cerebral cortex. Experientia. 23:525-529 (1967).
16. Y. Takahashi, K. Mase and Y. Suzuki. Purification and characteristics of RNase inhibitor from pig cerebral cortex. J. Neurochem. 17:1433-1440 (1970).

CONCLUSIONS

It is a difficult task to draw conclusions a few months after the end of the symposium. We have listened attentively to all speakers and discussants. We have read the manuscripts and are convinced that still a lot remains to be learned from them. Nevertheless we shall draw the following conclusions:

1. the clinical defintion of multiple sclerosis remains an important starting point for research in this disease. The clinical examination should be completed with examination with evoked potentials, nuclear magnetic resonance imaging and the electrophoretic analysis of cerebrospinal fluid proteins. Scientifically only cases examined according to these 4 methods, can be accepted and discussed.

2. chronic relapsing experimental allergic encephalomyelitis remains the best model for multiple sclerosis. However total similarity with multiple sclerosis is not yet accepted.

3. classification of the different demyelinating diseases should be made with the utmost care. A loss of myelin, associated with an immune reaction or due to an immune reaction does not necessarily mean multiple sclerosis. Undoubtedly in this aspect confusion arises in human as well as in animal pathology.

4. neuropathology still plays a major role in the examination of samples from multiple sclerosis patients. Neuropathology should however be enriched with new techniques inspired from biochemistry and immunology.

5. the antigen responsible for multiple sclerosis is still unknown. It can be an antigen or antigens of viral origin, it can be autoantigens. The specificity of the immunoglobulins observed in multiple sclerosis is still unknown. Some research workers even suggest the existence of a nonsense immune reaction in the cerebrospinal fluid. It is a fact that an immune reaction can be detected in multiple sclerosis and is induced by one or more unknown antigen(s) with production of immunoglobulins which specificity is still unknown. The way this immune reaction is controlled or modulated remains to be questioned. Different factors influencing the immune regulation, were described.

6. the study of the cellular immunology in multiple sclerosis has made major progress due to the introduction of monoclonal antibodies, cell cultures and cell cloning. The role played by lymphocytes and monocytes can be very accurately investigated. It is not to be excluded that among these cellular reactions the astrocytes play a role. The specificity of the changes observed, remains unknown. Serum and cerebrospinal fluid do not run completely parallel. Does the immune reaction start within the central nervous system or extraneously to the nervous system? How and why do

the reacting cells reach the central nervous system, how do they leave one compartment to develop in another one and more precisely in the central nervous system? These are questions which momentarily cannot be answered.

7. it is generally accepted that demyelination induces or maintains the immune reaction, humoral as well as cellular. The question raised is whether this demyelination provokes the disease or whether this demyelination is secondary to another pathological factor which provoked the disease. This is a question which since long has preoccupied research workers studying multiple sclerosis.

Summarizing, we can say that the Hengelhoef symposium has shown new ways to follow. The symposium did not provide definite answers. A lot of work awaits future research workers.

Dr. J. Raus Dr. A. Lowenthal

CELLULAR AND HUMORAL COMPONENTS OF CEREBROSPINAL FLUID

IN

MULTIPLE SCLEROSIS

DIRECTORS:
A. Lowenthal (Antwerp, Belgium)
J. Raus (Diepenbeek, Belgium)

SCIENTIFIC COMMITTEE:
B.G.W. Arnason (University Chicago - USA)
A. Lowenthal (Born-Bunge-Stichting, Universitaire Instelling Antwerp - Belgium)
D.E. McFarlin (National Institutes of Health - USA)
J. Raus (Dr. L. Willems-Instituut - Belgium)
B.H. Waksman (National MS Society - USA)
H.L. Weiner (Center for Neurological Disease - USA)
H. Wekerle (Max-Planck-Gesellschaft - BRD)

PARTICIPANTS

O. ABRAMSKY	Hadassah Univ.Hosp., Kiryat Hadassah, P.O.B. 12000, IL-91120 Jerusalem - Israel
B. ALLIQUANT	Lab. de Neuroimmunologie, Hopital de la Salpetrière, 47 Boulevard de l'Hopital, 75651 Paris Cedex 13 - France
L. AMADUCCI	Dept.Neurol., Clinica Neurologica, Viale Morgagni 85 Careggi, 50134 Firenze - Italy
J. ANTEL	Dept.Neurology, Univ.Chicago, 5841 S.Maryland, Chicago Ill 60637 - USA
B.G.W. ARNASON	Dept.Neurology, Univ.Chicago, BH Box 425 5841 South Maryland Av., Chicago Ill 60637 - USA
M.-A. BACH	Pathol.de l'Immunité, Institut Pasteur, 28 Rue du Dr Roux, F-75724 Paris Cedex 15 - France
A. BILLIAU	Rega Instituut, Kath.Univ.Leuven, Minderbroeders-straat 10, B-3000 Leuven - Belgium
G. BIRNBAUM	Dept.Neurology, Univ.Minnesota, Box 241 Mayo Building, Minneapolis Mn 55455 - USA
J.E. BLALOCK	Dept.Microbiology, Univ.Texas, Medical Branch, Galveston Texas 77550 - USA
A. BLANCHER	Service de Neurologie, CHU Toulouse, Place Docteur Baylac, Toulouse 31059 - France
E. BOSMANS	Dept.Immunol., Dr Willems Instituut, Univ.Campus, B-3610 Diepenbeek - Belgium
C. BROSNAN	Dept.Pathology, Alb.Einstein Coll.Med., 1300 Morris Park Aven., Bronx NY 10461 - USA
W. BUURMAN	Afd.Heelkunde, Akademisch Ziekenhuis, Maastricht - The Netherlands

H. CARTON	MS Kliniek, 16 Vanheylenstraat, B-1910 Melsbroek - Belgium
I. CATZ	Dept.Lab.Med., Univ.of Alberta, 11282-84 Avenue, Edmonton Alberta, 76G 2G3 - Canada
M. CLANET	Service de Neurologie, CHU Toulouse, Place Docteur Baylac, Toulouse 31059 - France
D. COMPSTON	Dept.Neurol., Univ.Hospit.Wales, Heath Park, Cardiff CF4 4XW - United Kingdom
P. COYLE	Dept.Neurology, SUNY at Stony Brook, HSC T-12, Stony Brook NY 11794 - USA
M.L. CUZNER	MS Society Lab., Institute of Neurology, Queen Square, London WC1N3BG - England
A. CZLONKOWSKA	Dept.Neurol., Psych.Institute, Sobieskiego 1/9, 02-957 Warsaw - Poland
L. DE RIJCK	Dept WNF, Limburgs Univ.Centrum, Univ.Campus, B-3610 Diepenbeek - Belgium
E. DEFREITAS	Dept.Immunol., Wistar Institute, 36th Street at Spruce, Philadelphia PA 19104 - USA
J. DEGOS	108 Rue de la Tour, 75116 Paris - France
P. DELMOTTE	MS Kliniek, 16 Vanheylenstraat, B-1910 Melsbroek - Belgium
W. DE SMET	U.I.A., 2610 Wilrijk-Antwerpen - Belgium
P.C. DOHERTY	Dept.Exp.Pathology, John Curtin Sch.Med.Research, P.O.Box 334, Canberra City ACT 2601 - Australia
P. DORE-DUFFY	Dept.Neurology, Univ.Connecticut, Health Center, Farmington Ct 06032 - USA
R. DöRRIES	Inst.Virologie Immunbiol., Univ.Würzburg, Versbacher Str.7, 8700 Würzburg - W.Germany
G.C. EBERS	Dept.Neurology, Univ.Hospital, London Ontario, NGA 5A5 -Canada
W. FIERZ	Dept.Innere Medizin, Universitatsspital Zurich, Haldeliweg 4, CH-8044 Zurich - Switzerland
T. FREEMAN	Univ. Texas, Medical Branch, Galveston,Texas - USA
J. FRIEDMAN	The Rockefeller University, 1230 York Avenue, New-York, NY 10021 - USA
W. GERHARD	Dept.Neurology, The Wistar Institute, 36th street at Spruce, Philadelphia PA 19104 - USA
J. GHEUENS	Born Bunge Stichting, UIA, Universiteitsplein 1, B-2610 Wilrijk - Belgium
J.-M. GOUST	Dept.Immunol.Microbiol., Med.Univ.South Carolina, 171 Ashley Aven., Charleston SC 29425 - USA
D.E. GRIFFIN	Meyer 6-181, The Johns Hopkins Univ., Sch.Medecine, Baltimore MD 21205 - USA
A. GUSEO	Dept.Neurol., Székesfehérvar, Central Hosp.County Fejér, Seregélyesiu 3, 8001 - Hungary
D.A. HAFLER	Div.Neurology, Harvard Med.School, 75 Francis Street, Boston Ma 02115 - USA
E.L. HOGAN	Dept.Neurology, Med.Univ.South Carolina, Charleston, South Carolina 29425 - USA
O.R. HOMMES	Instituut voor Neurologie, Kath.Univ.Nijmegen, Reinier Postlaan 4 Postbus 9101, 6500 Nijmegen - The Netherlands
V. HUKKANEN	Dept.Virology, Univ.Turku, Kiinamyllynkatu 13, SF-20520 Turku - Finland
T. INUZUKA	Dept.Neurology, Brain Research Institute, Niigata University, Niigata, 951 - Japan
K. JOHNSON	Dept. Neurology, Univ.Maryland School of Medecine, 22 South Greene Street, Baltimore MD 21201 - USA
D. KARCHER	Born Bunge Stichting, UIA,Universiteitsplein 1, B-2610 Wilrijk - Belgium
R. KELLY	Chairman, Internat.Med.Adv.Board IFMSS, 60 Montagu Square, London W1 - England

P. KERZA-KWIATECKI	Health Sc.Administrator, NINCDS-NIH, Fed.Building Rm 710, Bethesda Maryland 20205 - USA
H. KOPROWSKI	The Wistar Institute, 36th and Spruce streets, Philadelphia Penn 19104 - USA
H.W. KRETH	Immunol.Labor., Universit.Kinderklinik,Josef Schneider Str.2, D-87 Wurzburg - W.Germany
LAMERS	Instituut voor Neurologie, Kath.Univ.Nijmegen, Reinier Postlaan 4 Postbus 9101, 6500 Nijmegen - The Netherlands
H. LASSMANN	Neurol.Institut, Univ.Wien,Schwarzspanierstr.17, 1090 Wien - Austria
K. LAUER	Neurol.Klinik, 379 Heidelberger Landstr., 6100 Darmstadt-Eberstadt - W.Germany
P. LEBON	Unité 43, Hopital St Vincent de Paul, 74 Aven.Denfert Rochereau, Paris 75014 - France
H. LINK	Dept.Neurol., Karolinska Institutet, S-14186 Huddinge, Stockholm - Sweden
A. LOWENTHAL	Born Bunge Stichting, UIA, Universiteitsplein 1, B-2610 Wilrijk - Belgium
C.J. LUCAS	Central Lab., Blood Transfusion Service, Plesmanlaan 125, 1066 CX Amsterdam - The Netherlands
R. MARTIN	MPG Klin Forschungsgruppe MS, Max-Planck Gesellschaft, Dr. Josef Schneiderstr.11 Postfach 6120, D-8700 Würzburg 1 - W.Germany
A.R. MASSARO	Facoltà di Medicina e Chirurgica, Università Cattolica Del Sacro Cuore, 8 Largo Agostino Gemelli, Roma - Italy
D.E. MCFARLIN	Neuroimmunol.Branch, National Inst.of Health, Building 10 Rm 5B16, Bethesda Maryland 20205 - USA
R. MEDAER	MS Kliniek, Boemerangstraat, B-3583 Overpelt - Belgium
P.D. MEHTA	Inst.Bas.Res.Dev.Disabilities, 1050 Forest Hill Road, Staten Island NY 10314 - USA
F. MELCHERS	Basel Institute for Immunology, Grenzacherstr 487, CH-4005 Basel - Switzerland
J.E. MERRILL	Dept.Neurology, Reed Neurol.Res.Center, 710 Westwood Blvd, Los Angeles CA 90024 - USA
T. MIYATAKE	Dept.Neurol.Brain Res.Instit., Niigata University, Asahimachi-1, Niigata 951 - Japan
E. MOENS	Middelheim Algemeen Ziekenhuis, Lindenstraat 1, 2020 Antwerpen - Belgium
R. MONTANINI	Prim.Neurol.Ospedale, Via Palestro 29, 21013 Gallarate - Italy
J. OGER	Dept Medecine, Health Sci Center Hospital, 2211 Wesbrook Mall, Vancouver BC V6T 1W5 - Canada
T. OLSSON	Dept.Neurology, Karolinska Institutet, Huddinge Hospital, S-14186 Huddinge - Sweden
T.A. OUT	Central Lab., Blood Transfusion Service, Postbus 9190, 1006 AD Amsterdam - The Netherlands
C. PAPAGEORGIOU	Dept.Neurol. Athens Nat.Univ., Eginition Hospital, 74 Vasilissis Sophias Av., Athens (611) - Greece
J. RAUS	Dr Willems Instituut, Universitaire Campus, B-3610 Diepenbeek - Belgium
F. ROTTEVEEL	Central Lab., Blood Transfusion Service, Plesmanlaan 125, 1066 CX Amsterdam - The Netherlands
R.A. RUDICK	Dept.Neurology, Strong Memorial Hospital, Box 605, Rochester NY 14642 - USA
M.G. RUMSBY	Dept Biology, University of York, York YO1 5DD - United Kingdom
B. RYBERG	Dept.Neurol., Univ.Hospital, Univ.Lund, S-22185 Lund - Sweden

J.-P. SALIER Un.Rech.Génét.Prot.Hum., Inst.Natl.Santé et Rech. Medic., 543 Chemin de la Bretèque, 76230 Bois-Guillaume - France

A. SALMI Dept.Med.Microbiol., Univ.Alberta, Med.Sc.Building Rm 168, Edmonton Alberta, T6G 2H7 - Canada

M. SANDBERG Dept.Neurol.Univ.Hospital, Univ.Lund, S-22185 Lund - Sweden

E. SCHULLER Lab. de Neuroimmunologie, Hopital de la Salpetrière, 47 Boulevard de l'Hopital, 75651 Paris Cedex 13 - France

T.A. SEARS Sobell Department of Neurophysiology, Institute of Neurology, Queen Square,London WC1N 3BG - England

C.J.M. SINDIC ICP, UCL-MEXP, 75 Avenue Hippocrate, B-1200 Bruxelles - Belgium

SLAVENKA Karolinska Institutet, S-14186 Huddinge, Stockholm - Sweden

E. SLUGA Dept.Neurology, Wilhelminenspital,Montleartstr., A-1160 Vienna - Austria

C. SMITH 889 Pacific Street, Monterey, California 93940 - USA

K.V. SORENSEN Dept.Neurol., Central Hospital Viborg, 8800 Viborg - Denmark

A. STECK Service de Neurologie, CHUV, 1011 Lausanne - Switzerland

A.J. SUCKLING Dept.Biology, University of York, York Y01 5DD - England

B. TAVOLATO Universita degli Studi Padova, Ist.Clin. Mal.Nervose, Via Giustiniani 5, 35128 Padova - Italy

V. TER MEULEN Inst.Virologie Immunbiol., Univ.Würzburg, Versbacher-str. 7, 8700 Würzburg - W.Germany

K. THIELEMANS Inst.Klin.Research, Vrije Univ.Brussel, Laarbeeklaan 103/E, B-1090 Brussel - Belgium

U. TRAUGOTT Dept.Pathol., Albert Einstein Coll.Med., 1300 Morris Park Av., Bronx NY 10461 - USA

T. TSUKAMOTO Dept.Neurology Institute of Brain Dis., Tohoku Univ. Sch.Medecine, Seiryo-machi 1-1, Sendai 980 - Japan

B. UITDEHAAG Instituut voor Neurologie, Kath.Univ.Nijmegen, Reinier Postlaan 4 Postbus 9101, 6500 Nijmegen - The Netherlands

A.A. VANDENBARK Immunol.Res.1515, Veterans Adm.Hospital, Medical Center, Portland Or 97207 - USA

M. VANDERMEEREN Dept.Immunol., Dr Willems Instituut, Universit.campus 3610 Diepenbeek - Belgium

B. VANDVIK Dept.Neurol., Rikshospitalet,Oslo 1 - Norway

D. VASSILOPOULOS Dept.Neurol. Athens Nat.Univ., Eginition Hospital, 74 Vasilissis Sophias Av., Athens (611) - Greece

B.H. WAKSMAN Dir.Research Progr., Natl.MS Society, 205 East 42nd street, New-York NY 10017 - USA

T-B. WANG Dept.Pathophysiology, Friendship Hospital, 95 Yong An Road, Beijing - China

K.G. WARREN Neurol.Unit, Univ.Alberta, 9-101 Clin.Sci.Building, Edmonton Alberta, T6G-2G3 Canada

W. WEBER Dept.Immunol., Dr Willems Instituut, Universit.campus 3610 Diepenbeek - Belgium

H.L. WEINER MS Clin.Res.Unit, Center for Neurol.Dis., Brigham and Women's Hospit., Boston Ma 02115 - USA

H. WEKERLE MPG Klin Forschungsgruppe MS, Max-Planck-Gesellschaft Josef Schneiderstr.11, Postfach 6120, D-8700 Würzburg 1 - W.Germany

J.N. WHITAKER Dept.Neurol., Univ.Alabama, University Station, Birmingham Alabama 35294 - USA

U. WURSTER	Labor der Neurologischen Klinik, Medizinische Hochschule Hannover, Postfach 610180, 3000 Hannover - W.Germany
J.B. ZABRISKIE	Dept.Immunol., The Rockefeller Univ., 1230 York Aven. New York NY 10021 - USA

INDEX

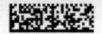